FIFTH EDITION

INTRODUCTION TO
HEALTH
CARE

LEE HAROUN
DAKOTA MITCHELL

CENGAGE

Australia • Brazil • Canada • Mexico • Singapore • United Kingdom • United States

Introduction to Health Care, **Fifth Edition**
Lee Haroun and Dakota Mitchell

SVP, GM Skills & Global Product Management: Erin Joyner

Product Director: Matthew Seeley

Product Manager: Laura Stewart

Product Assistant: Nicholas Scaglione

Executive Director, Content Creation: Mara Bellegarde

Learning Design, Senior Manager: Leigh Hefferon

Senior Learning Designer: Deb Myette-Flis

Vice President, Strategic Marketing Services: Jennifer Ann Baker

Marketing Manager: Jonathan Sheehan

Director, Content Creation: Juliet Steiner

Senior Content Manager: Kenneth McGrath

Digital Delivery Lead: Lisa Christopher

Manufacturing Planner: Beverly Breslin

Production Service/Composition: SPi Global

Senior Designer: Angela Sheehan

Cover image credit: iStockPhoto.com/andresr

For product information and technology assistance, contact us at
**Cengage Customer & Sales Support,
1-800-354-9706 or support.cengage.com.**

For permission to use material from this text or product,
submit all requests online at **www.cengage.com/permissions**.

Library of Congress Control Number: 2019912555

Student Edition:
ISBN: 978-0-357-12307-2

Loose-leaf Edition:
ISBN: 978-0-357-12316-4

Cengage
200 Pier 4 Boulevard
Boston, MA 02210
USA

Cengage is a leading provider of customized learning solutions with employees residing in nearly 40 different countries and sales in more than 125 countries around the world. Find your local representative at **www.cengage.com**.

To learn more about Cengage platforms and services, register or access your online learning solution, or purchase materials for your course, visit **www.cengage.com**.

Notice to the Reader

Printed in Mexico
Print Number: 5   Print Year: 2023

Contents

Preface   xi

Dedication   xviii

About the Authors   xviii

Acknowledgments   xviii

About this Book   xix

Unit 1 | Health Care Today

CHAPTER 1

Your Career in Health Care   1

Your Future in Health Care   2

Getting Off to a Good Start   3

    Essential Core Qualities of Health Care Professionals   3

    Learning for Mastery   4

    Volunteering   5

    Professional Organizations   5

    Returning Adult Students   5

Learning to Think Like a Health Care Professional   6

    Problem-Solving Process   6

Making a Career Decision   9

    Educational Requirements   9

    Standards for Health Care Professionals   10

Occupational Profiles   11

    Therapeutic and Treatment Occupations   12

    Diagnostic Occupations   24

    Sources of Additional Information   32

CHAPTER 2

Health Care Yesterday, Today, and Tomorrow   36

The History of Western Health Care   37

Trends and Issues in Health Care Today   42

    Specialization   42

    Aging Population   43

    Cost of Health Care   43

Variety of Approaches to Health Care   44

    Wellness   44

    Holistic Medicine   44

    Complementary, Alternative, and Integrative Medicine   45

The Future of Health Care   48

Challenges in Health Care Today   48

    Providing Affordable Health Care   48

    Providing Long-Term Care   49

    Improving Social Conditions   49

    Eliminating Racism in Health Care   50

    Maintaining the Quality of Care   50

    Treating Alzheimer's and Other Forms of Dementia   51

    Addressing Public Health Concerns   52

    Encouraging Medication Adherence   52

    Managing the Opioid Crisis   52

    Preventing Antibiotic Resistance   52

    Preventing Suicides   53

    Dealing with TV Prescription Drug Ads   53

Health Care Facilities and Services   53

    Hospitals   53

    Ambulatory Services   55

    Long-Term Care Facilities   55

    Home Health Care Providers   56

    Hospice   57

    Consolidation of Health Care Services   57

    New Types of Health Care Facilities   57

    Government Health Services   58

    State Health Departments   58

    Local Health Departments   58

CHAPTER 3

Ethical and Legal Responsibilities   64

The Purpose of Ethics   65

Ethics and the Law   65

Ethics and Health Care   66

    Professional Codes of Ethics   68

    Personal Values   69

    Professional Values   69

Guiding Principles of Health Care Ethics ... 69
   Preserve Life ... 69
   Do Good ... 73
   Respect Autonomy ... 73
   Uphold Justice ... 76
   Be Honest ... 77
   Be Discreet ... 78
   Keep Promises ... 80
   Do No Harm ... 81
Patient Rights ... 82
Handling Ethical Dilemmas ... 84
Who Decides? ... 84

Unit 2 | The Language of Health Care

CHAPTER 4

Medical Terminology ... 89
Importance of Medical Terminology ... 90
The Building Blocks of Medical Language ... 90
   Word Roots and Combining Forms ... 90
   Suffixes ... 93
   Prefixes ... 95
Deciphering Medical Terms ... 96
   Example # 1 cardiology ... 96
   Example # 2 polyarthritis ... 97
   Example # 3 echocardiogram ... 97
Eponyms ... 97
Words with Special Meanings in Medicine ... 97
Names of Drugs ... 97
Spelling and Pronunciation ... 97
Medical Abbreviations
   and Symbols ... 99
Medical Dictionary ... 101
Mastering Medical Terminology ... 101

CHAPTER 5

Medical Math ... 106
Importance of Math in Health Care ... 107
Math Anxiety ... 107
Basic Calculations ... 107
   Whole Numbers ... 109
   Decimals ... 109
   Fractions ... 110
   Percentages ... 111
   Ratios ... 112
   Converting Decimals, Fractions,
     Percentages, and Ratios ... 112
   Rounding Numbers ... 112
   Solving Problems with Proportions ... 114
Estimating ... 116
Statistics ... 116
Military Time ... 116
Roman Numerals ... 118
Angles ... 118
Systems of Measurement ... 119
   Household System ... 119
   Metric System ... 120
   Apothecary System ... 122
   Converting Systems of Measurement ... 122
Medication Safety ... 124
Temperature Conversion ... 124

Unit 3 | The Human Body

CHAPTER 6

Organization of the Human Body ... 129
The Basis of Life ... 130
   Cells ... 130
   Tissues ... 133
Describing the Body ... 133
   Body Planes ... 134
   Directional Terms ... 134
   The Body Cavities ... 134
   Abdominal Descriptions ... 136

CHAPTER 7

Structure and Function of the Human Body ... 140
The Importance of Anatomy and Physiology ... 141
Genetics ... 141
The Systems of the Body ... 142
Systems for Movement and Protection ... 142
   Skeletal ... 142
   Muscular ... 150
   Integumentary ... 152
Systems for Providing Energy and
   Removing Waste ... 154
   Circulatory ... 154
   Respiratory ... 161

Digestive 164
Urinary 166
Systems for Sensing, Coordinating, and Controlling 168
Eyes and Ears 168
Nervous 172
Endocrine 177
Systems for Producing New Life 180
Female Reproductive 180
Male Reproductive 182

CHAPTER 8

Growth and Development 187
Knowing Your Patient 188
Life Stages 188
Prenatal 189
Infancy 191
Toddler 191
Preschooler 192
School-Age Child 192
Adolescence 193
Young Adulthood 193
Middle Adulthood 194
Later Adulthood 194
Care Considerations 196
Other Developmental Theories 198
Jean Piaget 198
Lawrence Kohlberg 198
Carol Gilligan 199
Future Trends 199
Death and Dying 200

Unit 4 | Personal and Workplace Safety

CHAPTER 9

Body Mechanics 205
The Importance of Prevention 206
Repetitive Motion Injuries 206
Computer Use and Repetitive Motion Injuries 207
Preventing Repetitive Motion Injuries 207
Visual Problems 208
Exertion Injuries 210
Preventing Exertion Injuries 212
Treatment of Musculoskeletal and Nerve Injuries 213
Back Belts 214

CHAPTER 10

Infection Control 217
Importance of Infection Control in Health Care 218
Scope of the Problem 218
Regulatory Agencies 219
Microorganisms 219
Types of Microbes 220
Defense Mechanisms 224
How Infections Spread 224
Preventing Infection 224
Breaking the Chain of Infection 225
Handwashing 226
Personal Protective Equipment 229
Patient-Care Equipment 232
Antiseptics, Disinfectants, and Sterilization 232
Surgical Asepsis 236
Standard Precautions 236
Environmental Control 239
Blood-Borne Pathogens 239
Transmission Precautions 241
Disposal of Hazardous Waste 243
Neutropenic Precautions 244
The Challenges 245
Influenza 245
Workplace Risks 245
Other Infectious Diseases 251
Drug-Resistant Organisms 251
Reporting Accidental Exposure 253

CHAPTER 11

Environmental Safety 258
Importance of Environmental Safety in Health Care 259
General Safety Guidelines 259
Moving Safely 259
Dressing for Safety 259
Working Safely with Patients 260
Protecting Yourself and Others 261
Reporting for Safety 262
Workplace Violence 262
Fire and Electrical Hazards 263
Chemical Hazards 268

Radiation Hazards   268

Infectious Waste   268

Oxygen Hazards   269

Bioterrorism   269

Emergency Code System   270

Emergency Preparedness Plan   270

Triage   271

Unit 5 | Behaviors for Success

CHAPTER 12

Lifestyle Management   275

Importance of a Healthy Lifestyle   277

Habits and Health   277

Diet and Nutrition   277

Nutrients   277

Calories   279

Carbohydrates   279

Sugars   279

Fats   279

Salt (Sodium)   280

Processed Foods   280

Organic Foods   280

Healthy Eating   281

Maintaining a Healthy Weight   282

Body Mass Index   283

Weight-Loss Diets   283

Vegetarian Diets   283

Eating Disorders   284

Physical Activity   284

Sleep   285

Preventive Measures   285

Stress in Modern Life   286

External and Internal Stressors   286

Dealing with Stress   287

Minimizing Health Risks   290

Smoking   290

Substance Abuse   291

Occupational Hazards   291

Safe Sex   292

Burnout   292

Helping Patients Develop Healthy Lifestyles   293

CHAPTER 13

Professionalism   298

The Meaning of Professionalism   299

Professional Attitude   299

Professional Behaviors   300

Technical Skills   301

Professional Appearance   301

Professional Distance   302

Handling Difficult Situations Professionally   302

Professional Acceptance of Criticism   303

Professionalism Outside the Workplace   303

Professional Leadership   303

CHAPTER 14

Professional Development and Lifelong Learning   307

Professional Development   308

Professional Organizations   308

Importance of Lifelong Learning   309

Keeping Up with Changes in Health Care   309

Continuing Education Units   310

Ways to Earn CEUs   311

Self-Directed Learning   312

Learn from Role Models and Mentors   313

Career Ladders   314

Unit 6 | Communication in the Health Care Setting

CHAPTER 15

The Patient as an Individual   317

Patients as Individuals   318

Philosophy of Individual Worth   319

Understanding Patients   319

The Meaning of Culture   320

Dominant Culture   321

Individuals and Culture   321

Cultural Differences   322

Health Care Beliefs   324

Religious Beliefs and Health   324

Harmony and Health   324

Herbs and Plant Medicines   325

Human Needs   327

Implications for Health Care Professionals   327

Defense Mechanisms 330
Dealing with Loss 330
Treating Patients as Individuals 331

CHAPTER 16

The Communication Process 337
Importance of Communication in Health Care 338
Communication with Patients 338
The Communication Process 340
The Six Steps of the Communication Process 340
Communication through the Life Span 347
Overcoming Communication Barriers 348
Patients Who Are Terminally Ill 348
Patients Who Are in Pain, Medicated,
Confused, or Disoriented 349
Patients with Dementia 349
Patients Who Are Depressed 349
Patients Who Are Anxious 350
Patients Who Have Hearing Impairments 350
Patients Who Have Visual Impairments 351
Patients Who Have Speech Impairments 351
Patients Who Are Angry 352
Patients Who Do Not Speak English 352
Special Applications of Communication Skills 352
Telephone Communication 353
Patient Education 353
Presentations to Groups 354
Gossip and Patient Privacy 354

CHAPTER 17

Written Communication 359
Written Communication: A Vital Link in Health Care 360
The Components of Good Writing 361
Organizing Content 361
Preparing to Write 361
Starting to Write 362
Spell Your Way to Success 362
Spelling Tips 363
Grammar at a Glance 363
Capitalization Rules 363
Punctuation Rules 364
Writing Numbers Correctly 367
Writing Titles Correctly 367

Business Letters 367
Using Form Letters 368
Writing Effective Letters 368
Business Letter Formats 368
Preparing Letters for Mailing 372
Memos 372
Meeting Agendas 372
Minutes of Meetings 372
Patient Education Materials 373
Confidentiality of Written Materials 374
Proofreading Written Work 374

CHAPTER 18

Computers and Technology in Health Care 378
Computers in Health Care 379
Information Management 380
Creation of Documents 382
Spreadsheets 382
Diagnostics 384
Medical Lab Testing 385
Patient Monitoring 388
Research 388
Education 389
Communication 389
Virtual Communities 391
Telemedicine 391
Using Computers Effectively 392
Computer Security 393
Maintaining the Human Touch 394
Learning More about Computers 394

CHAPTER 19

Documentation and Medical Records 398
Medical Documentation and Recordkeeping 399
Purposes of Medical Documentation 399
Characteristics of Good Medical
Documentation 400
Making Corrections on Medical Documentation 401
Contents of the Medical Record 402
Progress Notes 404
Electronic Health Recordkeeping 405
Example of a Computerized System 406
Advantages of Computerized Systems 407

Challenges of Computerized Systems 407

Providers' Concerns 408

Personal Health Record 408

Safeguarding Health Records 408

HIPAA 409

Cybersecurity 409

Sending Protected Information 409

Unit 7 | Health Care Skills

CHAPTER 20

Physical Assessment 413

General Assessment 414

Noting Variances from Normal 415

General Survey 415

Psychosocial Observations 416

Physical Observations 416

Pain Evaluation 419

ADL Evaluation 419

Vital Signs 419

Temperature 420

Pulse 424

Respirations 428

Blood Pressure 429

Height and Weight 433

CHAPTER 21

Emergency Procedures 441

Emergency Situations 442

When an Emergency Occurs 443

Cardiopulmonary Resuscitation (CPR) 444

First Aid Procedures 444

Allergic Reactions 445

Bleeding and Wounds 447

Bone, Joint, and Muscle Injuries 447

Injuries to Facial Structures 452

Burns 452

Drug Abuse 461

Poisoning 461

Temperature-Related Illness 462

Other Conditions 466

Bandaging 466

Unit 8 | Business of Caring

CHAPTER 22

Paying for Health Care 481

The Rising Costs of Health Care 482

Impact of Costs on Individuals 483

Health Care Institutions 483

History of Health Care Reimbursement 484

Health Care Payment Methods 484

Government Programs 484

Veterans Health Care 485

Medicare and Medicaid Reimbursement 485

Managed Care 486

Types of Managed Care Plans 486

Prepaid Plans 486

Negotiated Fees 487

Primary Care Providers 487

Review of Services 487

Providing Affordable Health Care 488

Controlling Organizational Costs 489

Health Care Professionals' Impact on Costs 490

Personal Efficiency 491

Acting with Thought 492

CHAPTER 23

Quality Control and Customer Service 497

Quality of Care 498

Approaches to Measuring Quality of Care 498

Quality Improvement 499

Centers for Medicare and Medicaid Services 499

The Joint Commission 499

Agency for Healthcare Research and Quality 500

American Hospital Association 500

Internal Monitoring 500

Reducing Medical Errors 501

Medication Errors 502

Customer Service 502

Taking Responsibility for Quality 504

Customer Satisfaction 505

Internal Customers 505

Unit 9 | Securing and Maintaining Employment

CHAPTER 24

Job Leads and the Resume 512
Overview of the Job Search 513
  What Do You Have to Offer? 513
  What Are Your Expectations? 513
  Organizing Your Time 514
  Organizing Your Space and Supplies 514
  Projecting a Professional Image 514
Finding Job Leads 515
  School Career Service 515
  Community Career Centers 515
  Networking 515
  Internet 516
  Clinical Experience 518
  Cold Calls and Visits 518
  Job Fairs 518
The Resume 519
  Resume Contents 519
  Formatting the Resume 521
  Important Resume Guidelines 524
  Recent Resume Trends 524
Cover Letters 524
  Writing Good Cover Letters 528

CHAPTER 25

Interview, Portfolio, and Application 531
The Job Interview 532
  The Importance of Proper Preparation 532
  Learn About the Employer 532
  Prepare to Demonstrate Your Qualifications 532
  Prepare Your Questions 533
  Questions to Avoid 533
  Anticipating an Employer's Questions 533
  Creating a Professional Appearance 535
  Securing References 536
  Creating a Portfolio 537
  What to Take to an Interview 537
  Practice, Practice, Practice 538
  Starting Off on the Right Foot 538
  Recent Trends in Interviews 539
  After the Interview 539
  Additional Requirements 540

Accepting the Job 540
Declining the Job 542
Dealing with Rejection 542
Filling out Applications 542

CHAPTER 26

Successful Employment Strategies 549
Getting Off to a Good Start 550
  Learning about the Job 550
  Policies and Procedures 550
  Probationary Period 551
Guidelines for Workplace Success 552
  Act with Integrity 552
  Demonstrate Loyalty 552
  Follow the Chain of Command 552
  Give a Full Day's Work 553
  Become Part of the Team 554
  Go Beyond the Minimum 554
Employment Laws 555
  Grievances 555
  Sexual Harassment 557
Tracking Your Progress 557
Moving Up 558
Moving On 559
If You Are Fired 561

APPENDIX 1

Health Care Professional Organizations 565
Therapeutic and Treating Occupations 565
  Dental Occupations 565
  Emergency Medical Occupations 565
  Home-Care and Long-Term Care Occupations 565
  Massage Therapy Occupations 565
  Medical Office Occupations 565
  Mental Health Occupations 566
  Nursing Occupations 566
  Occupational Therapy Occupations 566
  Pharmacy Occupations 566
  Physical Therapy Occupations 566
  Respiratory Therapy Occupations 567
  Surgical Occupations 567
  Veterinary Occupations 567
  Vision Care Occupations 567

Diagnostic Occupations 567
   Diagnostic Imaging Occupations 567
   Medical Laboratory Occupations 568
Health Information Management
   Occupations 568
Environmental Occupations 568
   Biomedical Engineering Occupations ... 568
   Dietary Services Occupations 568

APPENDIX 2

Useful Spanish Expressions for
Health Care Professionals 569

Glossary 571

References 583

Index 589

Preface

Introduction to Health Care, Fifth Edition, is designed as an introductory text for students who are entering college-level health care programs or for those who believe they may be interested in pursuing a career in health care. The fundamentals common to all health care professions are presented in this full-color text to create a foundation on which students can build when they take their specific professional courses. The topics included are appropriate for professions that involve direct patient care, such as nursing and dental assisting, as well as those that provide support services, such as health information technology and pharmacy technician. The goal of the text is to present a broad base of health care essentials. Therefore, skills and procedures that apply only to specific professions are not included.

The text is written in easy-to-understand language. A variety of learning exercises are included in each chapter. These exercises are designed to appeal to the different ways that students comprehend and learn material. The text can be used by students as a reference book after completion of their introductory courses.

CONTENT FOR TODAY'S HEALTH CARE PROFESSIONAL

Introduction to Health Care, Fifth Edition, includes topics essential for today's student and tomorrow's health care professional. The basic concepts that create the foundation for health care education have been expanded beyond those usually included in an introductory text. The following topics have been included in response to the current needs of health care educators and employers:

- Thinking skills
- Study techniques
- Complementary and alternative medicine
- Prevention and wellness strategies
- Lifelong learning and continuing education
- Documentation
- Cost-control measures
- Performance improvement
- Personal efficiency
- Customer service

EMPHASIS ON THINKING SKILLS

The dramatic growth of the health care industry promises to provide increasing numbers of employment opportunities for graduates of health care programs. At the same time, today's graduates face new challenges. Changes in health care are rapid and continuous. Professionals at all levels are being given additional responsibilities. Efficiency and flexibility, combined with competency, are vital to workplace success. To be competent and successful in this ever-changing environment, health care professionals must be able to think for themselves and learn and adapt as necessary to meet current employment demands.

The authors recognize the need of health care educators for materials that can assist them in preparing students to assess new situations, determine appropriate action, and apply on the job what they learned in the classroom. This text is designed to help meet this need. Students are introduced to the concept of thinking like a health care professional (also called "critical thinking") in Chapter 1. The specific skills that make up applied thinking are explained in everyday language. A five-step problem-solving model is clearly described to help students systematically approach new situations. Every chapter includes exercises called "Thinking It Through" that require students to apply the concepts presented in the text to typical on-the-job situations. Each chapter then concludes with two application exercises and one problem-solving exercise that provide opportunities to summarize and apply the chapter content. For a detailed review of the features in this book, see *About This Book* on page xix.

ORGANIZATION OF THE TEXT

Introduction to Health Care, Fifth Edition, is divided into nine units that contain between two and five chapters of related topics. The following overview highlights many of the major concepts included in the text.

Unit 1 | Health Care Today

- Characteristics and trends of modern health care, including changing patient demographics, challenges in health care today, and complementary and alternative medicine
- Descriptions of many health occupations, organized by type of work performed
- Explanation of how to think like a health care professional
- Personal characteristics required of health care professionals
- Legal and ethical responsibilities of health care professionals

Unit 2 | The Language of Health Care

- Introduction to basic concepts of medical terminology
- Examples of common word elements
- Suggested ways to approach the study of terminology and to learn it systematically
- Review of math skills necessary for health care applications
- Measurement systems and methods of converting between systems
- Calculating drug dosages
- Tips for dealing with math anxiety

Unit 3 | The Human Body

- Brief overview of the basic organization, structure, and functions of the body systems, intended as an introduction rather than a complete anatomy and physiology course
- Examples of diseases and conditions related to each body system
- Preventive measures for each system, including lifestyle management tips
- Physical and mental milestones of growth and development over the life span and the implications when providing health care

Unit 4 | Personal and Workplace Safety

- Basic skills and habits needed to protect both health care professionals and patients
- Explanations of body mechanics and infection control
- Hands-on skills, such as using a fire extinguisher

Unit 5 | Behaviors for Success

- Self-care practices important for health care professionals, including dealing with stress
- Characteristics of professionalism essential for career success
- Lifelong learning and continuing education strategies

Unit 6 | Communication in the Health Care Setting

- Patients as individuals
- Basic human needs
- Acknowledging diversity while avoiding cultural stereotypes
- The six-step communication process
- Using questions and observations to assess specific patient needs
- Basic oral and written communication techniques
- Overview of computer applications in health care
- Basics of health care documentation and medical records

Unit 7 | Health Care Skills

- Basic assessment skills
- Hands-on skills, such as taking vital signs and measuring height and weight
- Normal ranges and significant changes
- Step-by-step instructions for performing basic emergency procedures (Cardiopulmonary resuscitation is not included because certification is often required of health care students and the course is taught by certified instructors who use annually updated, written materials instead of a textbook.)

Unit 8 | Business of Caring

- Health care as a business
- Improving care while controlling costs
- Working efficiently
- Customer service

Unit 9 | Securing and Maintaining Employment

- Application of job search skills to health care employment
- Tips for remaining successfully employed
- Behaviors for job success, including teamwork and leadership skills
- Employment legalities

MAJOR CHANGES TO THE FIFTH EDITION

Book Chapter	Description of Changes
Chapter 1	• Reordered material in chapter to be more logical: beginning chapter with "Getting Off to a Good Start" and ending with career profiles • Added more specific study tips and resources • Deleted references to learning styles, now considered inaccurate • Added information and suggestions about volunteering and joining a professional organization in preparation for a career in health care • Updated career information and added Occupational Outlook Handbook web addresses for each within the text • Added information about the levels of education needed for various health care careers
Chapter 2	• Reorganized chapter content for more logical presentation • Updated health care industry statistics • Expanded list of advancements in medicine and health care • Added section on future of health care, including discussion of precision/personalized medicine • Added topics: health disparities, racism in health care, managing the opioid crisis and increase in suicides, and concerns about TV drug ads • Added definition of western medicine • Deleted some events in table on history of health care to make more manageable for students
Chapter 3	• Added sections on professional values, patient rights, and legalization of medical marijuana • Updated information on physician-assisted suicide • Expanded information on the Patient Care Partnership
Chapter 4	• Added root words for colors, how drugs are named, eponyms, and acronyms
Chapter 5	• Revised section on solving problems with proportions to make more clear • Added the basic formula method for calculating medication dosages • Added section on statistics in health care
Chapter 7	• Added a few diseases and conditions related to the various body systems
Chapter 8	• Revised Erikson's stages of psychosocial development
Chapter 9	• Major reorganization of content for more logical flow • Added section specific to exertion injuries • Revised discussion about back belts, including opinions that they should not be used routinely. Replaced all figures showing health care professionals wearing back belts • Included ways to help prevent back injuries
Chapter 10	• Reorganized chapter content for better flow • Updated current disease threats • Added information about influenza
Chapter 11	• Added sample contents of an incident report • Updated safety data sheets, previously called material safety data sheets • Added information about violence in the health care workplace

(continued)

Book Chapter	Description of Changes

Chapter 12	• Reorganized section on nutrition for better flow
	• Updated information on effects of cholesterol in foods
	• Revised definitions of carbohydrates and fiber
	• Distinguished between different types of fats
	• Added information about sodium and its effects
	• Added discussion about sugar
	• Expanded section on causes of overweight and obesity
	• Updated statistics for:
	  ○ Leading causes of death in the United States
	  ○ Prevalence of overweight and obesity
	  ○ Deaths due to smoking and secondhand smoke
	  ○ Incidence and deaths from substance abuse
	  ○ Cases of HIV

Chapter 13	• Added discussion about empathy • Updated information about tattoos and piercings in the workplace • Added professionalism outside the workplace, including on social media
Chapter 14	Added new sections on professional development, learning from role models and mentors, and career ladders
Chapter 15	• Deleted table listing characteristics of various cultural and ethnic groups • Expanded information on bias, including strategies for recognizing bias Added explanation of implicit bias • Expanded view of culture to include factors such as socioeconomic status (poverty) • Revision of section on Abraham Maslow, including deletion of his hierarchy
Chapter 16	• Added discussion of health literacy • Explained "teach back" as a communication-check technique • Added discussion of communication through the life span • Expanded section on communicating with people who have dementia • Revised and updated the patient education section
Chapter 17	• Added material on writing emails and email etiquette
Chapter 18	• Added guidelines for writing and sending professional emails • Added section on computerized testing in medical labs • Moved information on electronic medical records to Chapter 19
Chapter 19	• Reorganized content for more logical flow • Added information on purposes of medical documentation • Added negative consequences of poor records • Moved electronic records to this chapter from Chapter 18 and expanded to include advantages, sample situation with a patient, challenges • Added section on cybersecurity • Expanded section on HIPAA, including sending protected information
Chapter 21	• Added RICE mnemonic for treating bone, joint, and muscle injuries and SAMPLE for getting information about an illness or injury • Updated information on properly removing ticks from the skin
Chapter 22	• Expanded information on Medicaid • Added section on Veterans' Health Administration • Added section on impact of health costs on individuals

(continued)

Book Chapter	Description of Changes

Chapter 23	• Added information about the following:
	  ° Partnership for Patients
	  ° The Joint Commission
	  ° Agency for Healthcare Quality and Research
	  ° American Hospital Association: Patient Care Partnership
	• Added sections on reducing medical errors, including medication errors

Chapter 24	• Updated job-search websites, deleting those no longer available • Added discussion about avoiding job-search scams on the Internet • Expanded information about using the Internet in the job search
Chapter 26	• Added section on advancing in one's career ("Moving Up")

STUDENT RESOURCES

Online Resources

Online resources are available to enhance the learning experience. Additional resources include:

- PowerPoint® presentations
- Anatomy and pathophysiology videos
- Health care–related videos
- Mathematics tutorials

Redeeming an Access Code:

1. Go to: http://www.cengage.com
2. Register as a new user or log in as an existing user if you already have an account with Cengage Learning or cengage.com
3. Select **Go to My Account**
4. Open the product from the My Account page

Animations and Videos Included on the Online Resources

Chapter	Animation Topic
4	Word Parts Work Together
4	Combining Word Roots
4	Dangerous Abbreviations
6	Anatomy of a Typical Cell
6	Body Planes
7	Shoulder Injuries
7	Skin
7	The Heart (Conduction System)
7	The Blood
7	Types of Fractures
7	Respiration

Chapter	Animation Topic
7	Digestion
7	Urine Formation
7	Vision
7	Hearing
7	Endocrine System
7	Female Reproductive System
7	Male Reproductive System
7	Types of Muscle Tissue
7	Anatomy of the Heart
7	Firing of Neurotransmitters

Chapter	Video Topic
9	Body Mechanics
10	Infection Control
10	Controlling Disease
10	Sterile Gloves and the Sterile Field
10	The Chain of Infection
10	Transmission-Based Precautions
10	Proper Handwashing
10	Removing Contaminated Gloves
10	Sterilizing Instruments in Autoclave
11	Fire Safety
11	Using a Fire Extinguisher
17	Business Correspondence

(continued)

(continued)

Chapter	Video Topic
20	Thermometers (Chemical-dot)
20	Digital/Electronic Thermometers
20	Measuring a Tympanic Temperature
20	Measuring a Temporal Artery Temperature
20	Measuring Apical and Radial Pulse
20	Counting Respirations
20	Measuring Height and Weight
20	Measuring Blood Pressure
21	Allergic Reaction Management
21	Burns
21	Obstructed Airway

Math Tutorials for Chapter 5
Convert between Celsius and Fahrenheit Temperatures
Weight and Volume Equivalents
The Metric System
The Apothecary System
An Introduction to Decimals
Adding and Subtracting Fractions
Fractions, Decimals, Ratios, and Percent
Dividing Fractions
Fractions and Decimals

INSTRUCTOR RESOURCES

Resources for instructors include:

- Cognero® Testbank makes generating tests and quizzes a snap. You can create customized assessments for your students with the click of a button. Add your own unique questions and print tests for easy class preparation.
- Customizable instructor slide presentations created in PowerPoint® focus on key concepts from each chapter.
- Electronic Instructor's Manual includes the following items to help instructors most effectively use the text in planning and teaching an introductory course:
  - Suggested answers to "Thinking It Through" and "Application Exercises" found in the text

  - Procedure check-off forms for evaluating skills
  - Suggestions for class activities
  - Teaching thinking skills
  - Answers to review questions found at the end of each chapter in the text
  - Websites and corresponding activities to support and expand on the information presented in the text and provide enrichment assignments for students.

MINDTAP: EMPOWER YOUR STUDENTS

MindTap is a platform that propels students from memorization to mastery. It gives you complete control of your course, so you can provide engaging content, challenge every learner, and build student confidence. Customize interactive syllabi to emphasize priority topics, then add your own material or notes to the eBook as desired. This outcomes-driven application gives you the tools needed to empower students and boost both understanding and performance.

Access Everything You Need in One Place

Cut down on prep with the preloaded and organized MindTap course materials. Teach more efficiently with interactive multimedia, assignments, quizzes, and more. Give your students the power to read, listen, and study on their phones, so they can learn on their terms.

Empower Students to Reach their Potential

Twelve distinct metrics give you actionable insights into student engagement. Identify topics troubling your entire class and instantly communicate with those struggling. Students can track their scores to stay motivated towards their goals. Together, you can be unstoppable.

Control Your Course –and Your Content

Get the flexibility to reorder textbook chapters, add your own notes, and embed a variety of content including Open Educational Resources (OER). Personalize course content to your students' needs. They can even read your notes, add their own, and highlight key text to aid their learning.

Get a Dedicated Team, Whenever You Need Them

MindTap isn't just a tool, it's backed by a personalized team eager to support you. We can help set up your course and tailor it to your specific objectives, so you'll be ready to make an impact from day one. Know we'll be standing by to help you and your students until the final day of the term.

To learn more, visit www.cengage.com/mindtap

INFECTION CONTROL AT A GLANCE

Topic	Content Summary	Page Number(s)
Infection Control	Scope of the problem, regulatory agencies	218–219
Microorganisms	Types of microorganisms	219–224
How Infections Spread and Preventing Infection	Breaking the chain of infection by using various methods, including standard and transmission precautions and asepsis	224–245
Procedures		
10–1 Handwashing	These procedures show step-by-step directions and rationales with accompanying figures to illustrate the steps.	227–228
10–2 Nonsterile Gloves		230–231
10–3 Applying and Removing PPE		232–235
10–4 Sterile Gloves		237–239
The Challenges	The most common contagions that health care professionals may encounter, including drug resistant organisms	245–253
Reporting Accidental Exposure	OSHA regulations that apply to all health care facilities	253

LIST OF VITAL SIGNS PROCEDURES

Procedure Number	Procedure	Purpose	Page Number(s)
20–1	Temperature	Measures how much heat is in the body. An elevation may indicate that an infection or other disease process is present	421–423
20–2	Radial Pulse	Measures how fast the heart is beating when felt at the wrist	424–425
20–3	Apical Pulse	Measures how fast the heart is beating by listening over the heart with a stethoscope	426–427
20–4	Respirations	Measures how fast the patient is breathing	428
20–5	Blood Pressure	Indicates how hard the heart is working to distribute blood to all parts of the body	431–432

LIST OF FIRST AID PROCEDURES

Procedure Number	First Aid Procedure	Page Number(s)
21–1	Allergic Reactions	445–447
21–2	Bleeding and Wounds	448–452
21–3	Bone, Joint, and Muscle Injuries	453–455
21–4	Facial Injuries	456–457
21–5	Burns	459–461
21–6	Drug-Related Problems	462
21–7	Poisonings	463
21–8	Temperature-Related Illnesses	464–465
21–9	Other Common Conditions	466–473
21–10	Applying a Triangular Sling	474–475
21–11	Applying a Spiral Wrap	475–476
21–12	Applying a Figure-Eight Wrap	476–477
21–13	Applying a Bandage to a Finger	478

Dedication

In memory of David, who continues to inspire.

—Lee Haroun

To the future health care professionals who will dedicate their time and energy to taking care of those in need of their services. May your career be as rewarding to you as mine is to me.

—Dakota Mitchell

About the Authors

Lee Haroun has a Master's of Art in Education from Portland State University (Oregon), a Master's in Business Administration from National University in San Diego, and a Doctorate of Education from the University of San Diego.

She has more than 35 years' experience in teaching and educational administration and has developed curricula for a variety of postsecondary programs, including occupational therapy assistant, health information professional, insurance coder, and patient care technician.

Lee is the author of *Career Development for Health Professionals* (Elsevier Science); co-author of *Teaching Ideas and Classroom Activities for Health Care* with Susan Royce (Cengage Learning); co-author of *Occupational Therapy Fieldwork Survival Guide* with Bonnie Napier-Tibere (F. A. Davis; out of print); and technical writer for *Essentials of Health and Wellness* by James Robinson and Deborah McCormick (Cengage Learning).

Dakota Mitchell has a Master's of Science degree in Nursing from the University of California, San Francisco, and a Master's in Business Administration degree from the University of Santa Clara. The combination of these two degrees provides a framework for understanding and functioning within the current and rapidly evolving world of health care today.

Dakota has 30-plus years of experience in health care, including education, management, and curriculum consultation. Besides many years in classroom and clinical teaching, she has developed and implemented unique and innovative health care programs at both the vocational and associate's degree levels.

Acknowledgments

The authors wish to acknowledge the help, support, and continual good humor of Laura Stewart, Managing Editor, Deb Myette-Flis, Senior Product Manager, and Ken McGrath, Senior Content Manager, at Cengage Learning who patiently shepherded us through the process of producing a fifth edition. A special thank you to all the reviewers who offered many wonderful suggestions.

Dr. Susan Grant
Assistant Professor
Harper College- Health Science Palatine, IL

Mischelle Monagle, MSN, MBA, RN
Dean of College of Nursing & Health Professions
Carl Sandburg College Galesburg, Illinois

Shirley J. Cherry, Ed.D., R.T. (R)
Associate Professor and Program Director
Radiologic Science East Tennessee State University
Johnson City, TN

S. Summers
Adjunct Professor
Johnson County Community College Overland Park, Kansas

Dedication

In memory of David, who continues to inspire.

—Lee Haroun

To the future health care professionals who will dedicate their time and energy to taking care of those in need of their services. May your career be as rewarding to you as mine is to me.

—Dakota Mitchell

About the Authors

Lee Haroun has a Master's of Art in Education from Portland State University (Oregon), a Master's in Business Administration from National University in San Diego, and a Doctorate of Education from the University of San Diego.

She has more than 35 years' experience in teaching and educational administration and has developed curricula for a variety of postsecondary programs, including occupational therapy assistant, health information professional, insurance coder, and patient care technician.

Lee is the author of *Career Development for Health Professionals* (Elsevier Science); co-author of *Teaching Ideas and Classroom Activities for Health Care* with Susan Royce (Cengage Learning); co-author of *Occupational Therapy Fieldwork Survival Guide* with Bonnie Napier-Tibere (F. A. Davis; out of print); and technical writer for *Essentials of Health and Wellness* by James Robinson and Deborah McCormick (Cengage Learning).

Dakota Mitchell has a Master's of Science degree in Nursing from the University of California, San Francisco, and a Master's in Business Administration degree from the University of Santa Clara. The combination of these two degrees provides a framework for understanding and functioning within the current and rapidly evolving world of health care today.

Dakota has 30-plus years of experience in health care, including education, management, and curriculum consultation. Besides many years in classroom and clinical teaching, she has developed and implemented unique and innovative health care programs at both the vocational and associate's degree levels.

Acknowledgments

The authors wish to acknowledge the help, support, and continual good humor of Laura Stewart, Managing Editor, Deb Myette-Flis, Senior Product Manager, and Ken McGrath, Senior Content Manager, at Cengage Learning who patiently shepherded us through the process of producing a fifth edition. A special thank you to all the reviewers who offered many wonderful suggestions.

Dr. Susan Grant
Assistant Professor
Harper College- Health Science Palatine, IL

Mischelle Monagle, MSN, MBA, RN
Dean of College of Nursing & Health Professions
Carl Sandburg College Galesburg, Illinois

Shirley J. Cherry, Ed.D., R.T. (R)
Associate Professor and Program Director
Radiologic Science East Tennessee State University
Johnson City, TN

S. Summers
Adjunct Professor
Johnson County Community College Overland Park, Kansas

INFECTION CONTROL AT A GLANCE

Topic	Content Summary	Page Number(s)
Infection Control	Scope of the problem, regulatory agencies	218–219
Microorganisms	Types of microorganisms	219–224
How Infections Spread and Preventing Infection	Breaking the chain of infection by using various methods, including standard and transmission precautions and asepsis	224–245
Procedures		
10–1 Handwashing	These procedures show step-by-step directions and rationales with accompanying figures to illustrate the steps.	227–228
10–2 Nonsterile Gloves		230–231
10–3 Applying and Removing PPE		232–235
10–4 Sterile Gloves		237–239
The Challenges	The most common contagions that health care professionals may encounter, including drug resistant organisms	245–253
Reporting Accidental Exposure	OSHA regulations that apply to all health care facilities	253

LIST OF VITAL SIGNS PROCEDURES

Procedure Number	Procedure	Purpose	Page Number(s)
20–1	Temperature	Measures how much heat is in the body. An elevation may indicate that an infection or other disease process is present	421–423
20–2	Radial Pulse	Measures how fast the heart is beating when felt at the wrist	424–425
20–3	Apical Pulse	Measures how fast the heart is beating by listening over the heart with a stethoscope	426–427
20–4	Respirations	Measures how fast the patient is breathing	428
20–5	Blood Pressure	Indicates how hard the heart is working to distribute blood to all parts of the body	431–432

LIST OF FIRST AID PROCEDURES

Procedure Number	First Aid Procedure	Page Number(s)
21–1	Allergic Reactions	445–447
21–2	Bleeding and Wounds	448–452
21–3	Bone, Joint, and Muscle Injuries	453–455
21–4	Facial Injuries	456–457
21–5	Burns	459–461
21–6	Drug-Related Problems	462
21–7	Poisonings	463
21–8	Temperature-Related Illnesses	464–465
21–9	Other Common Conditions	466–473
21–10	Applying a Triangular Sling	474–475
21–11	Applying a Spiral Wrap	475–476
21–12	Applying a Figure-Eight Wrap	476–477
21–13	Applying a Bandage to a Finger	478

About This Book

Objectives: Overview of chapter content and goals for learning. Review these before beginning to read the chapter and use the objectives to check your progress after completing the chapter.

Key Terms: List of important vocabulary and key concepts. Understanding vocabulary is critical to understanding the concepts presented in the chapter. Key terms are bolded and defined the first time they appear in the chapter. There is also a comprehensive glossary in the back of the book.

The Case of . . . : These health care scenarios introduce chapter content and show why the material in the chapter is important for the competent health care professional. An application exercise at the end of the chapter refers back to the case.

Fascinating Facts: Interesting information related to the chapter topics.

Tables: These provide summaries of related facts. Use them as study aids and for quick reference.

Boxes: These include special features and additional information that expand on and support the material presented in the chapter.

Colored photos and illustrations: These reinforce important concepts and topics. Use them to increase your understanding of the material.

FIGURE 1–5 As older nurses retire, there will be a great need for newly trained registered nurses.

Thinking It Through

Craig Oakley is a physical therapy assistant who does home visits for a rehabilitation service. One of his patients, Mr. Singh, suffers from rheumatoid arthritis and has asked Craig's opinion about taking Chinese herbal remedies that he has read help restore joint health.

1. How should Craig respond?
2. What are some of the resources he can consult in order to find out more about the treatment?
3. What precautions should Craig follow when speaking with Mr. Singh about complementary and alternative therapies?

Thinking It Through: Located throughout the chapter, these exercises are a very important part of this text. The health care scenarios require you to think about the concepts presented in the chapter and use them to resolve typical problems encountered by health care professionals. Use the exercises to develop the thinking skills necessary to be a successful health care professional.

PROCEDURE   10–1

HANDWASHING

Procedure	Rationale
1. Turn faucet on using a clean, dry paper towel. (See Figure 10–5a.)	Faucets are always considered contaminated.
2. Run warm water over hands and wrists.	Warm water helps remove superficial dirt and microorganisms.
3. Do not lean against the sink, and avoid splashing clothing with water.	The sink is always considered contaminated; water splashed from the sink is contaminated, and wet material easily conducts microorganisms.

Procedures: A step-by-step format that helps you master basic hands-on skills. Pay special attention to the rationales that explain the reasons for the actions.

SUGGESTED LEARNING ACTIVITIES

1. Create a personal plan for developing the core qualities demonstrated by health care professionals.
2. Determine if there are study skills you need to improve and create a plan to improve them.
3. Choose a problem in your life that you would like to work on and apply the five steps of the problem-solving process. Report on the results.
4. Seek opportunities to observe health care professionals at work. Report on the qualities they demonstrate that you believe make them effective.
5. Research an occupational area or specific career that interests you: interview a working professional, send for information or visit the Internet site of the appropriate professional organization (see Appendix 1), request a job description from a local facility, and/or read the job descriptions in the *Occupational Outlook Handbook*.

Suggested Learning Activities: Try these interesting projects that include doing research on the Internet, reporting on observations from daily life, and visiting health care facilities.

WEB ACTIVITIES

WikiHow
https://www.wikihow.com/Improve-Your-Study-Skills
How to Improve Your Study Skills
1. Read this illustrated guide.
2. Are there any suggestions you think might help you?
3. If so, try them for a couple of weeks and report on how they work for you.

Web Activities: Use these guided assignments to increase your research skills and learn more about the chapter content. The activities refer you to specific websites.

REVIEW QUESTIONS

1. What are the ten significant events that changed the way health care was delivered?
2. What are the definitions of the following terms: gene therapy and targeted drug therapy?
3. What is today's leading prevention and treatment option?
4. Explain the meaning of specialization and its impact on health care.
5. What are the effects of the aging population on health care?
6. What has happened with health care costs over the past few decades?

Review Questions: The questions are keyed to the chapter objectives to ensure your mastery of the chapter content. Use them to check your learning and identify areas that need more study.

PROBLEM-SOLVING PRACTICE

A growing number of children in Trueville, USA, are becoming overweight and obese. A group of concerned citizens has organized a committee to find ways to help children in the community attain normal weights and raise their levels of fitness. How might the committee use the five-step problem-solving process?

Problem-Solving Practice: Practice your skills with these typical, real-world problems encountered by students and health care professionals.

APPLICATION EXERCISES

1. Refer back to The Case of the Confused Student at the beginning of the chapter. Using the information in this chapter, list your recommendations for occupations that Kevin should investigate.
2. Juan has always been interested in helping people. He also likes science and has maintained good grades throughout high school in chemistry, biology, and physics. He has enrolled in the local community college and is taking "Introduction to Health Care." Juan thinks that a career in health care might be for him, but he doesn't feel that he knows enough to make a career decision at this time. He's not sure what's out there or what jobs would be appropriate for him.
   a. What does Juan need to know in order to conduct an effective career search?
   b. Describe how he can use the problem-solving process to help him make a tentative career decision.
   c. Explain methods that Juan can use to research and learn more about different career options.

Application Exercises: Opportunities to apply the chapter's major concepts to typical health care situations. Use these exercises to practice using your knowledge in ways similar to those you may encounter on the job.

I

Health Care Today

CHAPTER 1

Your Career in Health Care

KEY TERMS

assessment
biases
career ladders
certification
diagnostic
integrity
licensure
manual dexterity
objective data
opinions
problem-solving process
registration
reliable
scope of practice
signs
subjective data
symptoms
therapeutic

The Case of the Confused Student

Kevin Yang is a recent high school graduate who hopes to pursue a career in health care. He has enrolled to start classes in September at a local community college that offers many health care programs. Last spring Kevin attended two career fairs at local hospitals and learned about a variety of careers. He knows that he wants to combine his mechanical aptitude with his desire to work with people, but he feels

(continues)

OBJECTIVES

Studying and applying the material in this chapter will help you to:

1. Describe the current economic status of the health care industry.
2. Describe the general employment projections for the health care industry.
3. List the ten health care jobs expected to have the largest percentage increases between 2016 and 2026, according to the U.S. Department of Labor Statistics.
4. List the six health care jobs expected to have the highest numbers of openings between 2016 and 2026, according to the U.S. Department of Labor Statistics.
5. Explain why work in health care can be both satisfying and demanding.
6. Describe the essential core qualities demonstrated by effective health care professionals.
7. Give examples of how students can apply the essential core qualities while they are in school.
8. Explain the meaning of "learning for mastery."
9. Explain how students can use questions to master new subjects.
10. Give examples of suggestions to improve your note-taking, reading, writing, and test-taking skills.
11. Describe the advantages and challenges that may be experienced by adult students who are returning to school.
12. List the five techniques that adult students can use to develop their personal organization and time management skills.
13. Explain the meaning of "thinking like a health care professional."
14. Describe the five-step problem-solving process.
15. List the personal factors that should be considered when choosing a health care career.
16. List the five levels of education typical for health care career fields.
17. Explain the purpose of standards for health care professionals.
18. Give the meaning of the following terms as they pertain to health care professional standards: certification, registration, and licensure.
19. Explain the meaning of school accreditation and name the two major accreditation organizations for health care programs.
20. List the four requirements students typically must meet before taking professional exams.
21. Describe the four classifications of health care careers and give three examples of careers for each classification.
22. State the educational and certification requirements, major duties, and attributes necessary for success in occupations in which you are interested.
23. List the eight resources recommended for students to learn more about specific health care careers.

1

overwhelmed by the number of choices in the health care field. He is not sure how to learn more about the requirements and rewards of various occupations, what the daily duties would be, and how much education is necessary to enter them. He is also unsure how to best go about making a decision that will significantly affect his life. This chapter includes basic information about a variety of health care career areas and occupations, a problem-solving process that can be used to make effective personal and professional decisions, and tips on succeeding in a health care career program.

YOUR FUTURE IN HEALTH CARE

Health care is an exciting and growing field. The purpose of this text is to help you make an informed career choice and acquire the basic knowledge to continue the studies necessary for your chosen field.

The health care industry is the largest service employer in the United States, providing more than 18 million jobs and the need for health care professionals continues to grow (https://www.cdc.gov/niosh/topics/healthcare/default .html). According to the United States Bureau of Labor Statistics, the health care industry will increase by 18% and add 2.4 million new jobs between 2016 and 2020 (https:// www.bls.gov/ooh/healthcare/home.htm). This is faster than the average growth of all other occupations. Federal economists report that, in 2017, the amount spent on health care was $3.5 trillion. Further, it is projected that the cost of health care will continue to grow at least 4% annually.

Many health care occupations are projected to have employment increases of more than 25%. (See Table 1–1.) Ten of the 20 fastest-growing jobs in all industries are health care–related. At the same time, 6 of the 20 occupations with the largest numerical increases are in health care. (See Table 1–2.) It should be noted that various sources give different occupations as having the fastest growth and highest numbers of new hires; however, health care is included in all lists. The information provided here is from the U.S. Bureau of Labor Statistics.

Careers in health care can be sources of great satisfaction. Health care professionals perform valuable services that make a significant contribution to the community. Each day their work makes a difference in the quality of life of those they serve. Whether you choose to work directly with patients or provide support services, be assured that what you do is important and of benefit to others.

As well as providing satisfaction, health care work makes many demands on those who pursue it. The work must be taken seriously because it affects the well-being of others. All tasks must be performed thoughtfully and conscientiously. Nothing can be taken for granted or done automatically, not even routine assignments. Health care professionals must be willing to devote their full attention to everything they say and do. Potential problems must

Table 1–1 Examples of Growing Health Care Jobs

Job	Projected Percentage Increase in Employment, 2016–2026
Home Health Aide	47%
Personal Care Aide	39%
Physician Assistant	37%
Nurse Practitioner	36%
Physical Therapist Assistant	31%
Physical Therapist Aide	29%
Medical Assistant	29%
Occupational Therapy Assistant	29%
Physical Therapist	28%
Massage Therapist	26%

Source: Bureau of Labor Statistics. Occupational Outlook Handbook. Fastest Growing Occupations. https://www.bls.gov/ooh/fastest-growing.htm

Table 1–2 Occupations with the Largest Numerical Increases

Job	Numerical Increase in Positions, 2016–2026
Personal Care Aides	777,600
Registered Nurses	438,100
Home Health Aides	431,200
Medical Assistants	183,900
Nursing Assistants	173,400
Medical Secretaries	129,000

Source: https://www.bls.gov/ooh/most-new-jobs.htm/

be noted and addressed before they become critical. The consequences of mistakes can be devastating if, for example, a prescription for medication is incorrect or the wrong procedure is performed. The work can also be stressful. Depending on the chosen occupation, it can involve long hours, dealing with the death of patients, and working quickly under pressure. (See Figure 1–1.)

FIGURE 1–1 Successful health care professionals work hard. At the same time, they enjoy the satisfaction of helping others.

GETTING OFF TO A GOOD START

Health care educational programs are designed to prepare students to succeed in the workplace. Instructors dedicate themselves to helping students who put forth the necessary effort to graduate and become employed. Take advantage of the learning opportunities available in your school and commit yourself to doing your best toward becoming a competent, qualified health care professional.

Essential Core Qualities of Health Care Professionals

As a student, you have many opportunities in school to begin to practice good workplace habits. Work hard now to develop the skills that will make you a valuable employee. At the same time, you can be acquiring habits that also contribute to academic success. The qualities essential for health care professionals to be effective and successful can be applied in the classroom, in the lab, and at the clinical (externship/internship/fieldwork) site. Start now while you are in school to develop and apply them.

- Care about others: Have compassion. Apply knowledge and skills to decrease suffering and increase the well-being of others. When necessary, be willing to put the needs of patients ahead of your own. Have respect for all people and help them regardless of their race, nationality, economic status, religion, age, or lifestyle preferences. (See Figure 1–2.)
  - Start now: Show respect and consideration for instructors and classmates. Be kind to everyone, regardless of his or her background. Refrain from talking during lectures. Prepare for classes so the instructor does not need to take time to answer questions about material covered in the reading or study assignments. Practice courtesy in the classroom and throughout the school. Volunteer to help others, as needed or as possible.

- Have **integrity**: Be honest at all times. Respect the privacy of others. Be loyal to the employer. Accept responsibility for your actions.
  - Start now: Do your own work. Never copy the homework assignments of others or cheat on exams. Always tell the truth. Never share anything told to you in confidence.

- Be dependable: Be at work on time and as scheduled. Follow through and finish all assigned tasks. Perform work accurately and completely. Work without constant supervision and reminders.
  - Start now: Be at school on time and attend all classes. Complete assignments on time. Strive for accuracy in all written and practical assignments. Follow through on all obligations and anything you have volunteered to do.

- Work well with others: Strive to understand the feelings and needs of others. Be courteous and considerate. Practice good communication skills. Be a good team member by cooperating and contributing to the achievement of group goals. Take directions willingly from the supervisor.

Fascinating Facts

In 2016, there were 46 million persons aged 65 and over, representing 15% of the total population. By 2060, this number is projected to be 98 million persons, who will make up 24% of the population. This increase will have major implications for the health care industry, driving the need for more professionals.

Source: https://www.prb.org/aging-unitedstates-fact-sheet/

FIGURE 1–2 One of the most important qualities of the health care professional is compassion.

○ Start now: Be understanding of the needs of instructors and classmates. Participate in class. Do your share when working on group assignments.

- Be flexible: Be willing to adapt to changing conditions and emergencies. Do what is needed to carry out tasks. Acquire knowledge and skills necessary to keep up with advances in technology and changes in the way health care is delivered.

○ Start now: Accept instructional differences, changes in class schedules, and other unexpected occurrences. Be willing to cooperate as needed.

- Be willing to learn: Keep skills up to date. Ask questions, attend workshops, read professional publications, use the Internet, and continue to acquire new skills.

○ Start now: Be willing to learn: Take your studies seriously. Make school a high priority. Dedicate sufficient time to studying throughout the length of each course to ensure maximum learning.

Learning for Mastery

Health care professionals must know what they are doing. Mistakes on the job can result in serious consequences. Therefore, it is essential that students commit to learning the material presented in their courses. Learning means more than just memorizing facts. It means striving to understand and remember information so that it can be applied to new situations. This understanding provides a basis for thinking like a health care professional, which is discussed later in this chapter.

Students who do only the minimum necessary to pass tests may think they are learning, but in reality, they are not likely to have acquired the long-term knowledge necessary to perform on the job. Students who study to understand *and always search out the why of the subject* increase their chances of becoming highly competent health care professionals who can think on their feet and meet new challenges as they arise.

One effective way for students to master subjects is to ask themselves questions about what they are learning or doing. Questions serve to gather information, expand your view of a subject, and stimulate the mind. They help ensure that actions are not based on false assumptions or insufficient information.

Questions can be asked mentally (to oneself) or of others. Think of the five *W*s plus the one *H*: What, When, Where, Why, Who, and How. The following examples show how questions can be used to promote learning:

- When learning new information, ask *why* it is important and to *whom? How* does it relate to what is already known?

- When working with patients, ask *what* might work best for them and *when* it should be done.

- When sharing important information with a classmate or coworker, ask yourself *what* you know about this person that will help you communicate most effectively.

- When working in a health care facility, consider *how* your work habits might be changed to improve overall efficiency.

Some students believe that the role of their instructors is to *tell* them rather than *ask* them. In reality, instructors who continually ask questions that require students to explain their answers and actions are encouraging them to learn and to think like health care professionals. Some instructors even respond to a student's question with another question. Their intention is to teach students to begin to think for themselves and trust that they are capable of finding the answer. Instructors also use questioning to guide students in pulling known facts together, making connections, and applying what they know to new situations. For example, suppose that a respiratory therapy student is working with a hospitalized patient. He has studied the illness presented by the patient and knows how to perform the prescribed breathing treatments. Through questioning, the instructor guides this student to explain why these particular treatments have been prescribed. The student is encouraged to consider the nature of the illness and the properties of the treatments and medications, and draw conclusions about the relationships among these factors.

Getting the Most from Your Studies

If necessary, spend some time now working to improve your study skills: taking notes, reading, writing, and preparing for tests. Something to keep in mind is that these skills can also help you to get a job and succeed. For example, taking a patient history requires good note-taking skills; understanding the instructions for a piece of equipment requires the ability to read and understand technical material; preparing a letter asking about job openings requires good writing skills; and if you think about it, everything you do when working with a patient is a test, something you must do correctly "to pass."

The following suggestions may help you to:

- Take good notes: Concentrate on writing down the important points, rather than everything the instructor says. Listen for clues from instructors about what is important. Write in outline form to keep notes organized. Set up pages using the Cornell System format to leave space for adding notes and questions after class when you review your notes. (See Figure 1–3.) *For more detailed information about the*

Name Subject		Date Page #
study	notes column	
notes		
and		
questions		
to quiz		
self		
summary		

FIGURE 1–3 Page set-up for the Cornell note-taking system.

Cornell system, see http://lsc.cornell.edu/notes.html and http://www.openculture.com/2018/10/the-cornell-note-taking-system.html.

- Read for comprehension and learning: When reading textbooks or information on websites, start by skimming through the chapter or section. Then focus your attention by creating questions and reading for the answers. Create questions from articles or section titles and from the material itself. After reading a section of material, ask yourself the questions and try to answer without looking at the text. This has been shown to be one of the most effective ways to learn. *For more reading strategies, see https://www.educationcorner.com/textbook-strategies.html and https://learningcenter.unc.edu/tips-and-tools/reading-textbooks-effectively/.*

- Write: See Chapter 17 of this text. *Also, Purdue University's online writing lab has information on dozens of topics related to writing: https://owl.purdue.edu/owl/purdue_owl.html.*

- Prepare for tests: Plan to study every day, even for a short time. Reviewing material over time is much more effective than cramming at the last minute. Use the questions you create for reading and note-taking to practice. *For more information, see https://www.educationcorner.com/test-taking-strategies.html. Quizlet at https://quizlet.com/ that contains learning tools and flashcards on many subjects, and https://www.tests.com and http://www.testpreview.com that contains free practice tests for a number of health care subjects and occupations.*

Volunteering

If you have the time, volunteering is an excellent way to jump-start your career. Not only do you learn skills, such as working with others, you learn more about the health care field and acquire information that can help you choose a career that is right for you. Although work in a health care environment is optimal, volunteering for non profits, such as Habitat for Humanity, also provide good experience.

Some educational programs have an admission requirement that you have some experience in the field you are entering. For example, university veterinary medicine programs require applicants to have a minimum number of hours of experience. And when looking for a job, you can list on your résumé the skills you learned and applied through volunteering. This also shows potential employers that you have initiative and a sincere interest in helping others.

Professional Organizations

Joining a professional organization while you are a student gives you networking opportunities, a chance to learn how to be successful in your chosen field, and access to workshops and other learning activities. And, as with volunteering, putting a professional membership on your résumé demonstrates your interest and initiative. See Chapter 14 and Appendix 1 for more information about professional organizations.

Returning Adult Students

Many students who enroll in health care programs are adults returning to school after working in other fields, raising families, and/or handling other adult responsibilities. Some adults find the experience of attending classes stressful and wonder if they have what it takes to study and learn new information and skills.

These fears are natural, but the fact is that most adults have acquired life experiences and skills they can apply to their learning which, in many cases, will help them become excellent students. For example, holding down a job contributes to the ability to set priorities, communicate, demonstrate dependability, and apply practical skills such as math. The self-confidence developed as a result of handling adult responsibilities can be applied to reviewing one's study skills, including those that may not have been used for many years.

The most pressing problem for many adult students is finding the time to fulfill all their responsibilities: attending classes, studying, caring for the family, and perhaps holding down a full- or part-time job. Practicing good time management and personal organization skills, such as the following, can be helpful in handling the additional work of attending school:

- Start each day with a list of what needs to be accomplished, ranked from most to least important.
- Advise others of your study schedule. Plan care or activities for your children to allow you the time needed.
- Schedule time, even if for short periods, with family members. Some children enjoy doing homework with mom or dad.
- Create personal organization techniques, such as clustering errands, keeping things in repair, and planning backups to prevent wasting time and energy.
- Ask for help when you need it. Delegate tasks at home. Let another family member fix dinner once or twice a week.
- See the Time Management section in Chapter 12 for more suggestions.

LEARNING TO THINK LIKE A HEALTH CARE PROFESSIONAL

A common problem in health care today is that some graduates spend months, or even years, accumulating information, but are unable to apply it when they need it on the job. The lack of effective thinking skills is a primary reason for this unfortunate situation. Regardless of the health care area or occupational level chosen by students, it is essential that they learn to *think* like health care professionals. This type of thinking actually involves many skills and, in this text, has the following meanings:

- Learning for understanding, not simply to memorize facts
- Applying learned material to new situations
- Having an organized approach to problem-solving
- Basing decisions on facts, rather than on emotional reactions or biases (certain beliefs and feelings, usually negative, about a person because he or she belongs to a specific group or has certain characteristics)
- Drawing on many facts and creating relationships among them
- Locating reliable sources of information with which to make decisions
- Basing decisions on ethical principles (see Chapter 3)

- Practicing good communication skills when gathering and distributing information (see Chapters 16 and 17)
- Understanding exactly what one is legally allowed to do in one's profession, known as scope of practice

One of the major goals of this text is to provide students with opportunities to practice thinking like a health care professional. This discussion on thinking is being presented at the beginning of the text so that students will have maximum time to apply and practice thinking skills. The "Thinking It Through," "Application Exercises," and "Problem-Solving Practice" features, which appear in every chapter, encourage students to apply thinking skills to the topics presented.

Thinking proficiently can be applied to the personal, as well as professional, areas of your life. For example, buying a certain puppy simply because it is cute and seems the friendliest is an emotional decision. An informed, thinking decision involves learning about available breeds, physical and personality characteristics, common health problems, and methods of training. Knowing these facts will help ensure that the puppy selected best fits the new owner's lifestyle and will be a suitable companion.

Thinking like a health care professional can be described as an "examined process." This means not simply accepting situations without observing and considering the meaning of what is observed. Effective thinkers are aware of their thoughts and of why and how they are acting or making decisions.

As stated earlier, nothing in health care work can be done routinely and without thinking. Mindless actions occur as the result of not paying attention or basing decisions on ideas that have been accepted "just because." These ideas may come from family members, friends, personal experiences, television, movies, and magazines. Health care professionals must learn to think for themselves, gather facts, and use their own observations for making decisions.

Problem-Solving Process

Important applications of thinking skills are problem-solving and decision-making, two very important competencies for health care professionals. There are a variety of problem-solving and decision-making models. This book presents a five-step problem-solving process to help students and health care professionals approach problem-solving in an organized manner:

1. Identify the problem
2. Gather information
3. Create alternatives

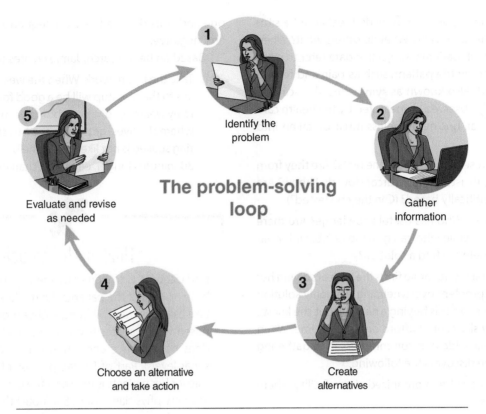

The problem-solving loop

1 Identify the problem

2 Gather information

3 Create alternatives

4 Choose an alternative and take action

5 Evaluate and revise as needed

FIGURE 1–4 Steps in the problem-solving process.

4. Choose an alternative and take action

5. Evaluate and revise as needed

(See Figure 1–4.)

Step One—Identify the Problem

Identifying problems is not always as simple as it sounds. Factors that are described as *the problem* are often only *symptoms* of the problem. For example, Jamie, a radiologic technologist, does not receive the high scores she had hoped for on her performance review at work. When she receives the rating "poor" in the dependability category, she feels upset and believes that her problem is "receiving a poor evaluation because her supervisor dislikes her."

Identifying the real nature of problems requires a willingness to observe, pay attention, and confront difficult issues. Problem-solvers must look beyond what seems obvious and use questions effectively to identify the real situation. Denying or ignoring problems does not make them go away. Problems that are not addressed tend to get worse, because no action is being taken to resolve them. In Jamie's case, she must be willing to speak frankly with her supervisor about her low rating. It turns out that the real problem is actually what *caused* the poor evaluation, not the evaluation itself. In Jamie's case, it is her frequent tardiness.

Jamie's first reaction is, "I can't help it. My car is old and breaks down a lot." When her car won't start, she must rely on family and friends to drop her off at work. Their schedules are not the same as Jamie's, so she often arrives late.

Taking the time to think about what she has said ("I can't help it"), Jamie realizes that being at work on time is her responsibility. She is now able to identify the real problem: lack of reliable transportation. This enables her to start seeking effective solutions. Accepting responsibility for a problem makes it possible to start doing something about it.

Step Two—Gather Information

Good problem-solving is based on having accurate and reliable information. Acting on assumptions (untested ideas), **opinions** (beliefs not based on facts or knowledge), and emotions can result in poor decisions. In health care, gathering information is also known as **assessment**. There are many methods for gathering information:

- Review what is already known: What knowledge do I have about the problem or situation? About the causes? About possible solutions?

- Collect **objective data**: What can be observed? Measured? Tested? What are the facts? When working with patients, objective data are called **signs**.

- Collect **subjective data**: How do I feel about a situation? What do I want? What do others want? When working with patients, subjective data refer to what is reported by the patient, such as pain and feeling nauseated. Also known as **symptoms**, they cannot be directly observed or measured by the health care professional, but nevertheless must be taken into account.
- Conduct research: What are the facts? Are they from a **reliable** (trustworthy) source? How do I know? Are they scientifically based? (Can they be tested?)
- Ask for help: Who has useful knowledge? Are there experts available who can give me reliable information and help me find a solution?

When she starts out, Jamie finds the idea of solving her transportation problem overwhelming. The only solution that makes sense to her is buying a new car, but she knows that most likely she cannot afford one at this time. When she puts her fear aside and commits herself to gathering information, she discovers the following:

- Carpools have been organized at the facility where she works.
- The most economical new car for sale in her area costs $14,795.
- There are many articles on the Internet about how to buy a car.
- *Consumer Reports* magazine has a recent article about purchasing used cars and publishes annual reports on the performance of most auto models manufactured over the past 10 years.
- Her credit union sponsors car sales to help buyers who have limited funds to spend. They also offer low-interest loans to buyers who qualify.
- A cousin has an older car that he wants to sell.
- There is a bus route within half a mile of her apartment.
- A local college offers a workshop that teaches people how to buy a car.
- The local high school has an auto-mechanic training program. For a small fee, students will check over used cars before they are purchased.

Step Three—Create Alternatives

The third step in problem-solving is to create a list of alternatives. Ideas for solutions and actions are generated based on the information collected. All possibilities should be considered before one is selected. Some alternatives may prove, on further investigation, to be impractical or unworkable. It is essential to think through each one and consider the likely consequences, both positive and negative.

Based on her research, Jamie creates the following list:

1. Take the bus to work. When the weather is nice, walking to the bus stop will be a good form of exercise. In rainy weather, common about five months of the year where she lives, getting to the bus stop without getting soaked is not likely. Also, the bus ride takes about 30 minutes longer, each way, than driving to work.

Thinking It Through

Linda Stevens, LPN, works on a medical floor at the local hospital. One of the patients she has been assigned to take care of is Frank Gibbons, a 72-year-old newly diagnosed with diabetes (a condition in which the body does not produce enough insulin to control blood sugar levels). Part of Linda's process of preparing to care for her patients is to review the patients' charts for any new physician orders. She notes that Dr. Romero was in the previous evening and ordered the patient's blood sugar to be checked at 8 a.m. According to the results, insulin is to be given. (The higher the level of blood sugar, the greater the amount of insulin that is given, based on a formula defined by the physician.) Linda is a "thinking nurse" and starts to question if this is an appropriate order. She realizes that breakfast trays arrive at 7:30 a.m. on her floor and that Mr. Gibbons will already have eaten when she checks his insulin level at 8 a.m. She knows that after eating, a person's blood sugar normally increases for a few hours. This is why blood sugar tests are usually ordered when the patient has not eaten for a number of hours. Linda reasons that if she calculates the amount of insulin based on the temporarily elevated blood sugar levels, Mr. Gibbons will receive too much insulin and may have a negative reaction. Linda calls Dr. Romero to clarify the order. Dr. Romero states that he believed the breakfast trays did not arrive until 8:30 a.m. He thanks Linda for catching the error and changes the order.

- What might have happened if Linda had simply performed the blood sugar test exactly as ordered?
- Do you think Linda should have been considered responsible for the error if she had followed the orders exactly?
- Review the five *Ws* and *How* questions in relation to this situation. Give examples of questions that Linda may have asked herself.

2. Take the workshop on how to buy a car, then purchase a used one through the credit union. The monthly car payments and higher insurance rates will mean having to budget carefully to meet all expenses. Chances of buying a "lemon" can be reduced by using the service offered at the high school.

3. Continue to rely on others for rides to work. (Nonaction is also an alternative.)

4. Ask her father for a loan to buy a new car. While Jamie would like to have a shiny new car, she has been financially independent for several years and prefers to remain that way.

Some potential alternatives do not appear on the previous list because of information acquired during step two:

1. Carpool participants must have a reliable vehicle of their own. This might be an alternative later, if she purchases a dependable car.

2. Her cousin's car has more than 175,000 miles and is not one of the more reliable models, according to the reports she studied.

Step Four—Choose an Alternative and Take Action

Step four is critical. A common difficulty in problem-solving and decision-making is failure to act. Opportunities are missed and accomplishments not realized when there is no follow-through.

Jamie decides to combine two alternatives. There are five months of dry weather ahead, so she decides to take the bus to work. She will use the extra riding time to read and keep up with advances in radiology. In October, she plans to buy a used car. In the meantime, she will create a personal budget to control expenses and save money, and will learn more about how to buy a car and which model is likely to give her the best value.

Step Five—Evaluate and Revise as Needed

Evaluation means reviewing the results of the actions taken. Even well-thought-out plans can prove to be ineffective or have unexpected, negative consequences. And circumstances can change. It is sometimes necessary to make adjustments or choose another alternative. It may even require going back to step two to gather additional information and go through the process again.

When applying the process to health care work, it is important to remember that the needs of patients and facilities may change and/or additional information may become available. This can affect the process and force revisions to be made before the entire process has been completed. Problem-solving is a continual process.

MAKING A CAREER DECISION

There are hundreds of job titles in health care and the number continues to grow. They require a wide range of skills and abilities. Students who are considering a career in health care should learn as much as possible about the requirements, responsibilities, and conditions of their areas of interest. This knowledge will help them to make good career choices that match their preferences and abilities. For example, some individuals interested in health care would find the emergency medical technician's (EMT) job to be interesting and exciting. EMTs have opportunities to apply their skills to help others in significant ways, sometimes even saving lives. At the same time, the work is physically and emotionally demanding. It is often performed under difficult circumstances. Emergencies do not happen at convenient times and places. The schedules for EMTs include nights, weekends, and holidays, and they are called out to work in all types of weather conditions. All aspects of an occupation must be considered to increase the chances of choosing a career that will provide long-term satisfaction.

When choosing an occupation, students should carefully consider the following factors about themselves:

- Educational background
- The amount of additional time they are willing to dedicate to their education
- Natural abilities
- Personality traits
- The type of activities they most enjoy
- Preferences for workplace environment and conditions

Educational Requirements

Each occupational area, such as radiology and physical therapy, has positions that require different amounts of education and training and involve varying amounts of responsibility. Collectively, these levels are known as **career ladders**. The following levels are typical for health care:

- Professional: requires 4 or more years of college. Many require advanced training and degrees, such as a doctorate. Examples of occupations: dentist, physical therapist
- Technologist or Therapist: 3–4 years of college. Many require graduate degrees and advanced training. Examples of occupations: speech therapist, occupational therapist
- Technician: associate's degree, vocational training, on-the-job training. Examples of occupations: pharmacy technician, veterinary technician

- Assistant: associate's degree, vocational training, or on-the-job training. Example of occupations: physical therapist assistant
- Aide: vocational training, on-the-job-training. Examples of occupations: home health aide, psychiatric aide.

It is important to note that in spite of these general categories, the occupational title does not necessarily indicate the level of education required. For example, most states require a physical therapist *assistant* to have a 2-year associate's degree. However, becoming a veterinary *assistant* does not require a degree. For this reason, it is necessary to investigate the educational and certification requirements for any job in which you are interested.

A current trend is that on-the-job training, in which individuals learn necessary job skills after being employed, is being replaced in many occupations by formal training. For example, aide-level positions are being assigned more responsibilities, and classroom training is becoming necessary. Today's health care facilities need individuals who have current skills, are able to think for themselves, and can start immediately as contributing members of the health care team.

Standards for Health Care Professionals

Standards for health care professionals have been established to protect the public from potential harm caused by incompetence. Testing, along with various approval and monitoring mechanisms, have been developed to determine whether professionals have met specific standards. The purpose of standards is to ensure that professionals master at least the minimum knowledge and skills necessary to safely and competently practice their professions. Students should be aware that in addition to knowledge and skill standards, some occupations require background checks and drug testing. Individuals who have been convicted of certain crimes are prohibited from taking certification exams or practicing certain occupations.

Standards may be set by state boards or national professional organizations. There are several terms that designate various types of approvals. **Certification** is a general term that means a person has met predetermined standards. The process of becoming certified usually involves completing certain educational requirements and passing a professional examination. Most individuals who work in health care go through a certification process, although their title might not include the term *certified*. Examples of occupations that do include this term in their title are certified occupational therapy assistant, certified medical assistant, and certified nursing assistant.

Some occupations require **registration**, which means being placed on an official list (registry) after meeting the educational and testing requirements for the profession.

Professionals who use this term in their title include registered nurse, registered respiratory therapist, and registered medical assistant. (A profession may require registration, but not include that term in the title.)

Licensure is a designation that means the person has been granted permission to legally perform certain acts. Licenses are granted by government agencies, often the state. The specific occupations that require licensure vary from state to state. Some occupations are licensed in most, but not all, states. The word *licensed* does not usually appear with the title of licensed professions. For example, in the following list of licensed professions, only one includes the term: dentist, dental hygienist, physician, registered nurse, and licensed practical/vocational nurse.

The various types of approvals can be confusing. Certification and registration are often, but not always, required to work legally. Even when not required by law, they provide credibility and are preferred by many employers when hiring. Medical assisting is an example of an occupation in which voluntary certification or registration enhances the graduate's chances of being hired. Licensure, if required for a profession, is never voluntary.

Some professions have more than one form of approval. Medical assistants, for example, can be either certified or registered. Both approvals require meeting specific educational requirements and passing a national exam. The American Association of Medical Assistants grants the title "certified." The American Medical Technologists grants the title "registered."

Certification and licensing exams vary by occupation. Some consist of multiple-choice questions that are presented in a computerized format. Others contain case studies and ask questions to test the candidates' knowledge about handling situations that may be encountered on the job. Still others have a practical component that requires candidates to demonstrate their ability to perform certain tasks. In addition to occupational questions, some states test the knowledge of the laws that apply to health care occupations.

Another point that can be confusing is that some professions are licensed but use the title "registered." Nurses take a national exam that, when passed, entitles them to apply for a license in the state where they want to work. They can become licensed in any state as long as they follow the proper application process. In addition, they are listed in a registry. Although "registered nurse" is the title for the occupation, it is also a licensed profession.

Study the contents of Tables 1–8 and 1–9. Note the variety of titles and educational levels within the nursing and occupational therapy careers. As you can see, professional titles and the types of approval granted do not necessarily indicate the level of education achieved. For example, the educational requirements for a certified nursing assistant can be less than 200 hours of instruction; a certified occupational therapy assistant, however, must earn an associate's degree. The titles given refer to the specific methods chosen by various organizations to ensure that their standards are met, rather than to the educational requirements. Furthermore, some titles may be acquired with varying amounts of education. Using the example of the registered nurse once again, we see that qualifying education can be either an associate's or bachelor's degree.

It is essential that students understand what is necessary for them to work in their chosen occupation. Most examining and licensing boards require attending an accredited school and/or program. The two common accrediting agencies for health care programs are as follows:

1. Commission on Accreditation of Allied Health Education Programs (CAAHEP). Find more information at www.caahep.org

2. Accrediting Bureau of Health Education Schools (ABHES). Find more information at www.abhes.org

Being accredited means that the school and/or program meets the standards set by a specific professional organization. To become accredited, a school or program must formally apply for approval. Once the application is accepted, a team from the organization visits the campus to ensure that all standards are being met. For some careers, such as paramedics, educational programs must be approved by the state. Others, such as occupational therapy assistant, require that programs be approved by the career's professional organization.

In addition to attending an accredited program, students must meet the following requirements before most professional exams can be taken:

- High school diploma or the equivalent
- Completion of specific courses
- Successful completion of the clinical portion of the training
- Not having been convicted of certain crimes

After being obtained, most certifications require specific amounts of continuing education. This is discussed further in Chapter 14. Individuals who fail to maintain the competency and conduct standards for their profession can lose their certification or license. The purpose of health care regulation is not to provide one-time approval. It is an ongoing effort to ensure that only qualified professionals are serving the public.

OCCUPATIONAL PROFILES

The occupations described in this section are organized into four categories:

1. **Therapeutic** and Treatment

2. **Diagnostic**

3. Health Information Management

4. Environmental

Note that there is overlap among the categories. For example, although listed in the therapeutic and treatment section, a major responsibility of dentists and physicians is to diagnose their patients' conditions. And although dietetics is listed in the environmental category, nutrition experts prescribe diets as part of the treatment of health conditions such as diabetes and heart disease.

Occupational titles are further divided into specific career areas, such as dental and mental health. The educational and certification, registration, and/or licensing requirements for various occupational levels are presented in Tables 1–3 through 1–20. (Note that the abbreviations given in the tables for job titles assume that the individual has achieved the required approval, such as certification. For example, RN stands for *registered nurse*.) Along with each table, occupations that generally require associate's degrees or vocational training are described in more detail.

It is important for students to keep in mind that the information in this chapter consists of brief overviews and contains only some of the hundreds of health care jobs available today. (See Box 1–1 for examples of additional occupations.) It is also important to note that there are more rungs on each career ladder than appear in the tables. For example, there are many nurse specialties, such as nurse anesthetist, clinical nurse specialist, and nurse practitioner, as well as doctoral degrees in nursing. Many health care providers earn advanced degrees beyond the basic requirements for their professions.

Job growth projections were taken from the Bureau of Labor Statistics for the period 2016 to 2026. Salaries, however, have not been included for the various occupations because it is difficult to provide accurate, up-to-date

Box 1–1

Examples of Health Care Occupations

Art Therapist

Athletic Trainer

Audiologist

Health Educator

Medical Illustrator

Medical Librarian

Medical Photographer

Medical Writer

Music Therapist

Speech and Language Pathologist

information that applies to all geographic areas, individual facilities, and current economic conditions. Students are encouraged to check the latest statistics provided by the Bureau of Labor to see current median salaries for occupations of interest. The median salary for a dentist means that half of all dentists earn less than that amount and half earn more. Students can also find sources on the Internet to learn about typical salaries in their states. For example, many professional organizations collect and report salary information.

It is also important to note that the education and certification requirements given in tables are subject to change. Students should check with professional organizations and their state's licensing board for the most up-to-date information.

Therapeutic and Treatment Occupations

Therapeutic and treatment occupations provide services that assist patients to regain or attain maximum wellness. They may involve direct patient care, such as nursing, or provide services that contribute to the patient's recovery, such as the pharmacy professions. The majority of health care occupations fall into this category.

Dental Occupations

Dental professionals treat diseases and conditions of the teeth and soft tissues of the mouth. They perform preventive measures, restore missing and defective teeth, diagnose and treat diseases of the gums, perform cosmetic dentistry, and provide patient education. (See Table 1–3.)

Dental Hygienist

The primary responsibility of a dental hygienist is to provide preventive dental care. This is accomplished by cleaning the teeth with special instruments and equipment, examining the mouth and taking X-rays, and providing patient education about dental care. Although hygienists perform their work independently, they are under the supervision of a dentist. Work schedules are often flexible, and many hygienists work part-time and/or for more than one dentist. The work involves prolonged patient contact, standing and reaching, and requires the ability to get along well with others. Good manual dexterity (skill working with the hands) and hand–eye coordination are essential. Jobs in dental hygiene are projected to grow by 20% from 2016, much faster than average among all occupations. *See https://www.bls.gov/ooh/healthcare/dental-hygienists.htm.*

Table 1–3 Dental Occupations

Career	Education	Testing and Approval
Dentist (DDS or DMD)	2–4 years college preprofessional education 4 years dental school 2–4 years additional education if seeking specialty	Licensed by states: 1. Graduate from accredited dental school 2. Pass written and practical exams
Dental Hygienist (RDH)	Associate's or bachelor's degree 2–4 years depending on program requirements	Licensed by states: 1. Graduate from accredited dental hygiene school 2. Pass national board exams administered by the American Dental Association Joint Commission on National Dental Examinations 3. Pass state and/or locally administered clinical exams 4. Pass state exam covering dental hygiene law
Dental Assistant (CDA or RDA)	1–2 year educational program (recommended) or on-the-job training	Requirements vary by state; voluntary certifications available through Dental Assisting National Board
Dental Laboratory Technician	On-the-job training or 2-year associate's degree program	Voluntary certification available from National Association of Dental Laboratories and/or National Board for Certification in Dental Laboratory Technology

Dental Assistant

Dental assistants are trained to perform a variety of duties in the dental office. They may work closely with the dentist by preparing patients for treatment, passing instruments, and suctioning the mouth during procedures performed by the dentist. Laboratory duties may include sterilizing and preparing instruments, creating casts of the teeth, and making temporary crowns. Administrative dental assistants greet patients, schedule appointments, keep patient records, send bills, and perform other clerical duties as needed. Dental assistants must have good manual dexterity, the ability and willingness to follow directions, and good interpersonal skills. This occupation is experiencing a 19% job growth, much faster than the average for all occupations. *See https://www.bls.gov/ooh/healthcare /dental-assistants.htm.*

Dental Laboratory Technician

Dental laboratory technicians make the items used by dentists to replace and restore teeth, such as crowns, bridges, and dentures. These are fabricated using models of the patient's mouth and involve working with plaster, wax, metal, and porcelain. Small handheld tools, grinding and polishing equipment, and heat sources for melting and baking are used. The work is precise and very delicate. Successful technicians are patient and steady-handed and have good vision, especially the ability to discriminate colors, needed for matching replacements to remaining teeth. Growth in the number of jobs is expected to be 13%, higher than average for all occupations. *See https://www .bls.gov/ooh/production/dental-and-ophthalmic-laboratory- technicians-and-medical-appliance-technicians.htm.*

Emergency Medical Occupations

Emergency medical technicians provide quick response service to victims of medical emergencies. All EMTs are qualified to give life support and immediate care such as restoring breathing, controlling bleeding, administering oxygen, bandaging wounds, and treating a person for shock. EMTs transport victims to health care facilities and provide necessary care en route. Intermediate EMTs have additional skills that include administering fluids intravenously and using a defibrillator to administer an electrical shock to a person whose heart has stopped. Paramedics, the highest level EMTs, are qualified to administer drugs, interpret electrocardiograms (measurements of the heart's electrical activity), and perform various invasive procedures (involving puncture or insertion of an instrument or material into the body). EMTs must be emotionally stable, able to deal calmly with stressful situations, physically coordinated, able to move quickly and easily, and able to lift and carry heavy loads. EMTs are employed by rescue squads, police departments, and fire departments, and employment is expected to grow 15% from 2016. (See Table 1–4.) *See https://www.bls.gov/ooh/healthcare/emts- and-paramedics.htm.*

Massage Therapy Occupations

Massage therapists use different types of massage, such as Swedish, deep tissue, and reflexology, to treat ailments and injuries; decompress tired muscles; reduce stress; and promote wellness. There are dozens of specialties, or types of massage, each designed to achieve specific results.

A large percentage of massage therapists are self-employed, with the remainder working in settings ranging from physician and chiropractors' offices to fitness centers to spas. Massage therapy is physically demanding, as it requires standing and repetitive movements. Working with clients requires good communication, empathy, and the ability to make clients feel comfortable with the personal nature of massage treatment. Job growth rate is excellent, projected to be 26%. (See Table 1–5.) *See https://www.bls .gov/ooh/healthcare/massage-therapists.htm.*

Medical Office Occupations

Medical office personnel treat patients who are seeking to maintain or improve their health or who need treatment for illnesses and injuries. Medical offices are staffed by a physician who may be either a medical doctor (MD) or a doctor of osteopathic medicine (DO). MDs and DOs receive similar training and perform similar functions. The major difference is that osteopathic physicians place more emphasis on the musculoskeletal system. Doctors of osteopathy also tend to approach medicine more holistically, meaning that they consider mental and emotional as well as physical health. Physicians may provide general care or they may specialize in what and who they treat. (For a list of medical specialties see Box 1–2.)

In addition to the physician, medical offices need support staff to assist with patient care and to perform clinical, laboratory, and administrative duties. (See Table 1–6.) (Note: Physicians and occupations designated as "medical office support staff" also work in other settings, such as large clinics, hospitals, rehabilitation centers, etc.)

Medical Assistant

Medical assistants must be prepared to carry out a wide variety of duties. They may work closely with the physician and/ or perform clinical tasks. Clinical, or "back office assistants'," duties include preparing patients, taking vital signs, helping the physician with exams and procedures, and performing a variety of tests and procedures on patients. Medical assistants may also choose to concentrate on administrative or "front office tasks," which include receiving patients,

Table 1–4 Emergency Medical Occupations

Career	Education	Testing and Certification
Paramedic	Typically 1–2 years; may result in a certificate or associate's degree	Licensed by states: Most states require certification from the National Registry of Emergency Medical Technicians, which includes the following: 1. Complete a state-approved paramedic course that meets or exceeds the U.S. Department of Transportation National Standard Curriculum 2. Pass written and practical exams 3. Pass a state-approved psychomotor exam
EMT-Intermediate/99 EMT-Intermediate/85 Note: Some states have only one level referred to as Advanced EMT	Training requirements vary by state Typically consist of 30–350 hours of training, depending on the scope of practice	Licensed by states: Most states require certification from the National Registry of Emergency Medical Technicians, which includes the following: 1. Complete a state-approved EMT-Intermediate/99 or EMT-Intermediate/85 course that meets or exceeds the U.S. Department of Transportation National Standard Curriculum 2. Pass written and practical exams 3. Pass a state-approved psychomotor exam
EMT-Basic	Training requirements vary by state, typically at least 120 hours over 6 to 15 weeks of training	Licensed by states: Most states require certification from the National Registry of Emergency Medical Technicians, which includes the following: 1. Complete a state-approved EMT-Basic course that meets or exceeds the U.S. Department of Transportation National Standard Curriculum 2. Pass written and practical exams 3. Pass a state-approved psychomotor exam
First Responder/Emergency Medical Responder	Training requirements vary by state	Licensed by states: Most states require certification from the National Registry of Emergency Medical Technicians, which includes the following: 1. Complete a state-approved first-responder course that meets or exceeds the U.S. Department of Transportation National Standard Curriculum 2. Pass written and practical exams 3. Pass a state-approved psychomotor exam

Note: Some states have their own certification programs and different names and titles for emergency service personnel.

Table 1–5 Massage Therapy Occupations

Career	Education	Testing and Certification
Massage Therapist	Requirements vary by state and locality; ranges from 3 to 24 months	Most states regulate and require formal education and national or state licensure or certification. In addition, some cities, towns, and counties have their own regulations and licensing requirements. Certification required for licensure in many states is offered by the National Certification Board for Therapeutic Massage and Bodywork (NCBTMB). Some states also require practical exams.

Box 1–2

Medical Specialists

Physicians who specialize in treating specific parts of the body:

Cardiologist	Heart and blood vessels
Dermatologist	Skin
Endocrinologist	Endocrine system (glands)
Gastroenterologist	Stomach and intestines
Gynecologist	Female reproductive organs
Internist	Internal organs, including the lungs, heart, glands, intestines, and kidneys
Nephrologist	Kidneys
Neurologist	Brain and nervous system
Ophthalmologist	Eyes
Orthopedist	Muscles and bones
Otolaryngologist or Otorhinolaryngologist	Ear, nose, and throat
Proctologist	Lower part of the large intestine
Psychiatrist	Mind
Urologist	Kidneys, bladder, and urinary system

Physicians who perform specific kinds of work:

Anesthesiologist	Administers medication to cause loss of sensation or feeling during surgery
Emergency Physician	Treats acute illnesses and injuries
Oncologist	Diagnoses and treats tumors (cancer)
Pathologist	Diagnoses disease by studying changes in organs, tissues, and cells
Physiatrist	Treats conditions associated with physical medicine and patients in need of rehabilitation
Plastic Surgeon	Performs corrective surgery to repair injured or malformed body parts
Radiologist	Uses X-rays and radiation to diagnose and treat diseases
Sports Medicine Physician	Prevents and treats injuries sustained in athletic events and physical activities
Surgeon	Performs surgery to correct deformities and treat injuries and diseases
Thoracic Surgeon	Performs surgery on the lungs, heart, and chest cavity

(continues)

Box 1-2

Physicians who work with specific populations:

Family Practice Physician	Promotes wellness and treats individuals in all age groups
Gerontologist	Promotes wellness and treats older persons
Obstetrician	Assists women with pregnancy and childbirth
Pediatrician	Promotes wellness and treats children

Table 1-6 Medical Office Occupations

Career	Education	Testing and Certification
Physician (MD, DO)	4 years college preprofessional education 4 years medical school MD: 3–8 years of graduate medical education (internship and residency) DO: 1-year internship and a 2- to 6-year residency	Licensed by states: 1. Graduate from accredited medical school 2. Complete graduate medical education 3. Pass written examination
Physician's Assistant (PA)	Varies. 2–4 years college + 24-month (minimum) PA program	Requirements vary by state; most require passing the exam administered by National Commission on Certification of Physician's Assistants
Medical Assistant Administrative and/or Clinical (MA, CMA, RMA) Certified Medical Assistant (CMA) Registered Medical Assistant (RMA)	Certificate program or associate's degree	Specific tasks, such as giving injections, regulated by some states. Optional certification through exam administered by the American Association of Medical Assistants. Optional registration through exam administered by the American Medical Technologists

answering the telephone, maintaining patient records, and handling insurance and billing duties. In small offices, the medical assistant may have both front and back office assignments. Medical assistants must be able to follow directions, work accurately, get along well with others, and have good manual dexterity. The occupation is expected to grow much faster than average for all occupations at 29%. *See https://www.bls.gov/ooh/healthcare/medical-assistants.htm.*

Mental Health Occupations

Mental health professionals provide care, treatment, counseling, and activities for patients with mental, emotional, and/or psychosocial (combination of mental and social) problems. These services are provided for patients in a wide variety of settings, including medical offices dedicated to the practice of psychiatry, psychiatric hospitals, halfway houses, general hospitals, clinics dedicated to

treating substance abuse problems, group homes, and prisons. Diagnoses encountered range from mild anxiety disorders, in which patients experience temporary feelings of distress, to serious conditions, such as schizophrenia, that result in behaviors that are unsafe for both the patient and the public. (See Table 1–7.)

Psychiatric/Mental Health Technician

Mental health technicians work with patients under the direction of a psychiatrist, a psychologist, or a registered nurse. They carry out care plans, assist with group activities, listen to patients and provide encouragement, and note behavior. The work requires a strong desire to help others, patience, understanding, excellent oral communication skills, and emotional stability. Employment growth is expected to be 6%, about average for all occupations. *See https://www.bls.gov/ooh/healthcare/psychiatric-technicians-and-aides.htm.*

Table 1–7 Mental Health Occupations

Career	Education	Testing and Certification
Psychiatrist (MD)	4 years college preprofessional education 4 years medical school 4–7 years of medical graduate education (internship and residency)	Licensed by states: 1. Graduate from accredited medical school 2. Complete specialized studies, internship, and residency 3. Pass written exam
Clinical Psychologist (PhD, PsyD)	4 years college 2–3 years graduate school (master's degree) Additional 3+ years (doctorate)	Licensed by states: Pass written exam
Clinical Social Worker	4 years college 2–3 years graduate school, including supervised experience (master's degree)	Licensed by states: Pass written exam
Psychiatric Clinical Nurse Specialist	Licensure as RN 2–3+ years graduate school (master's or doctoral degree)	Licensed by states: 1. Requirements vary by state but include passing a written exam
Mental Health Technician	Certificate or associate's degree in human services or mental health preferred	Licensed by some states
Psychiatric Aide	Some states require formal training program	Varies by state

Psychiatric Aide

Psychiatric aides assist other health care professionals and provide help with the physical needs of patients, such as hygiene and feeding. They provide companionship for patients and may help escort patients within or outside the care facility. Aides must be patient, caring, and responsible. (Note: Psychiatric aides generally have less formal education than mental health technicians. In some states, however, the two job titles refer to the same level of education and work duties.) Job growth is about the same as for mental health technicians at 6%. *See https://www.bls.gov /ooh/healthcare/psychiatric-technicians-and-aides.htm.*

Nursing Occupations

Nurses promote health and provide care and treatment for patients with all types of health problems. Nursing care is carried out through the application of a structured process to determine each patient's needs, develop individual care plans, implement the plans, and then evaluate their effectiveness. An important responsibility of the nurse is to provide education to patients and their families regarding self-care and health maintenance. (See Table 1–8.)

Registered Nurse

Registered nurses provide a wide variety of patient care services. They give direct patient care or supervise other personnel who do so, serve as patient advocates (support the interests of patients), and provide patient education. They are often the professionals who coordinate the overall care of patients by interacting with all other health care professionals involved. Registered nurses can achieve many educational levels and pursue a great number of specialties. Opportunities range from direct patient care to management of a hospital department. Specific day-to-day activities are determined by the work setting, which may be a hospital, clinic, long-term care facility, school, prison, or patients' homes. Registered nurses must be caring and responsible, have excellent assessment and communication skills, and be emotionally stable and able to both follow orders and supervise others. Registered nursing is one of the most versatile careers in any field. It is one of the occupations projected to have the largest number of job openings during the period 2016 to 2026. In fact, some areas of the United States are reporting shortages of qualified registered nurses. *See https://www.bls.gov/ooh /healthcare/registered-nurses.htm.* (See Figure 1–5.)

Table 1–8 Nursing Occupations

Career	Education	Testing and Certification
Certified Registered Nurse Anesthetist (CRNA)	Be a registered nurse Complete specialized education leading to a master's degree	Licensed by states: Pass a national certification exam
Nurse Practitioner (CRNP)	Be a registered nurse Complete additional educational and clinical practice requirements (most are master's or doctoral degree programs)	Licensed by states: Pass a national certification exam
Registered Nurse (RN)	4-year (bachelor's) college degree (preferred by most and required by many hospitals) or 2-year (associate's) degree	Licensed by states: 1. Graduate from approved program 2. Pass the National Council Licensing Examination for Nurses (N-CLEX)
Licensed Practical/Licensed Vocational Nurse (LPN/LVN)	1- or 2-year state-approved associate's degree or diploma program	Licensed by states: 1. Graduate from approved program 2. Pass national licensing exam
Certified Nursing Assistant (CNA)	States have various training requirements for classroom and clinical experience Programs must meet specific federal minimum standards Typical program is at least 8 weeks	All states require certification for work in long-term care facilities Requirements guided by federal regulations established by the Omnibus Budget Reconciliation Act of 1987 (OBRA) Certification requirements vary for other work environments
Patient Care Technician/Patient Care Assistant	Vocational training program	Certification required if nursing assistant duties are included. Voluntary certifications available: 1. National Health Association 2. National Center for Competency Testing
Home Health Aide	States have various training requirements for classroom and clinical experience. Some types of employers require formal training.	Approval requirements vary by state under guidance of OBRA Voluntary certification available from the National Association for Home Care and Hospice

Licensed Practical/Vocational Nurse

Licensed practical nurses (known as licensed vocational nurses in California and Texas) provide basic patient care under the direction of physicians and registered nurses. Most practical nurses carry out bedside tasks that include taking vital signs, administering medications, applying dressings and hot and cold packs, treating bedsores, and giving various comfort measures. They are also responsible for recording patient information. Practical nurses must be caring, responsible, emotionally stable, and able to follow directions and work under supervision. Job opportunities vary by region. Most new jobs are in residential care facilities and home health environments. Employment growth is expected to be faster than average for all occupations at 12%. *See https://www.bls.gov/ooh/healthcare/licensed-practical-and-licensed-vocational-nurses.htm.*

Certified Nursing Assistant

Nursing assistants work under the supervision of nursing staff to help care for patients' basic needs. They may take vital signs, assist patients with hygiene and feeding, give comfort measures, change bedding, and help transport

FIGURE 1–5 As older nurses retire, there will be a great need for newly trained registered nurses.

FIGURE 1–6 Home health aide is a fast-growing occupation. Aides must be compassionate, patient, and interested in helping older adults and people with disabilities.

patients. The variety and level of duties depend on state laws, the amount of training, and the needs of the facility. Assistants must be patient, caring, dependable, and able to follow directions. This is a fast-growing occupation, with an expected increase of 18%. This is especially true for individuals who are also qualified to work as home health aides. *See https://www.bls.gov/ooh/healthcare/nursing-assistants.htm.*

Patient Care Technician

The work of patient care technicians is similar to that of nursing assistants. They work under the supervision of physicians or nurses, taking vital signs, collecting specimens, and assisting patients with eating, hygiene, and grooming. Patient care technicians work in hospitals, clinics, and rehabilitation facilities. *See https://www.bls.gov/ooh/healthcare /nursing-assistants.htm.*

Home Health Aide

Home health aides help people with disabilities, older adults, and the chronically ill. Their work is similar to that of certified nursing assistants. In fact, many home health aides have nursing assistant certification. They may work in patients' homes or in a care facility, assisting with moving patients, providing personal care, and dressing. In the client's home, duties may include preparing meals, providing companionship, doing light housekeeping, and providing transportation. In some states, with the proper training and under the supervision of a nurse, they are allowed to give medications to clients, take vital signs, and assist patients with prescribed exercises. This is one of the fastest growing of all occupations, at 47%. (See Figure 1–6.) *See https://www.bls.gov/ooh /healthcare/home-health-aides-and-personal-care-aides.htm.*

Personal Care Aide

Personal care aides help residents and patients with daily tasks such as bathing, grooming, dressing, and eating. They cannot perform medically related tasks, such as giving medications. Because of the aging population, this is one of the fastest growing of all occupations, projected to be 39%. *See https://www.bls.gov/ooh/healthcare/home-health-aides-and-personal-care-aides.htm.*

Occupational Therapy Occupations

The purpose of occupational therapy is to help individuals attain the highest level of function and self-sufficiency possible. Difficulties in performing the activities of daily living can be the result of physical, mental, or emotional problems caused by disease, injury, or congenital (present at birth) conditions. Occupational therapists evaluate patients, set goals to increase their function and lessen their limitations, and create treatment plans to achieve these goals. Treatment may involve individual or group activities, exercise, providing adaptive equipment such as splints and special tools, and teaching patients new ways to perform daily tasks. Job growth rate for occupational therapists is projected at 24%, much faster than other occupations. (See Table 1–9.)

Occupational Therapy Assistant

Occupational therapy assistants work under the supervision of occupational therapists. They carry out rehabilitative activities and exercises prescribed in treatment plans prepared by occupational therapists. Other important duties include patient education, monitoring patient progress, and preparing reports for the therapist. Typical tasks include teaching a patient to use special devices that enable the performance of everyday tasks, such as reaching, dressing, and cooking; assisting with a stretching exercise; and making a hand splint. Occupational therapy assistants must have good communication skills, be patient and caring, and be sensitive to the needs of people who suffer from a variety of disabilities. The number of new positions is expected to grow rapidly at 29%. *See https://www.bls.gov/ooh /healthcare/occupational-therapy-assistants-and-aides.htm.*

Table 1–9 Occupational Therapy Occupations

Career	Education	Testing and Licensure
Occupational Therapist (OTR)	Master's degree (minimum) or doctorate	Licensed in all states National registration: 1. Graduate from program accredited by the American Occupational Therapy Association (AOTA) 2. Pass national exam administered by National Board for Certification in Occupational Therapy (NBCOT)
Occupational Therapy Assistant (COTA)	2-year (associate's) college degree	Licensure or certification required in most states National certification: 1. Graduate from program accredited by AOTA 2. Pass national exam administered by NBCOT
Occupational Therapy Aide	Certificate program or on-the-job training	None

Occupational Therapy Aide

Aides help therapists and assistants by performing supportive duties such as preparing supplies for activities, assisting with patient transfers, helping with patient treatments and activities, and cleaning activity areas. Some aides are cross-trained to assist other rehabilitation professionals such as physical therapists. Rehabilitation skills may be combined with nursing assistance training and certification. Aides must be responsible and able to follow directions. For aides who are also certified nursing assistants, the number of positions is expected to grow rapidly. *See https://www.bls.gov/ooh/healthcare/occupational-therapy-assistants-and-aides.htm.*

Pharmacy Occupations

Pharmacy professionals prepare and dispense medications to promote patient wellness and recovery, as well as pharmaceutical products used to diagnose health conditions. Important duties also include educating patients about the proper use of medications and ensuring that patients are not given drugs that will cause harm because of allergic reactions or negative interactions with other drugs. (See Table 1–10.)

Pharmacy Technician

Pharmacy technicians work under the supervision of a licensed pharmacist. They fill orders for drugs, stock medication carts, record and store incoming drug supplies, and reorder inventory as needed. They also assist in maintaining paperwork and records required for controlled drugs (drugs that have potential for abuse). Pharmacy technicians must be responsible, detail oriented, and able to follow directions exactly. Job opportunities are expected to grow

faster than average for all occupations, at 12% especially for technicians who are certified. *See https://www.bls.gov/ooh /healthcare/pharmacy-technicians.htm.*

Physical Therapy Occupations

The purpose of physical therapy is to help patients improve their physical functions by increasing muscle strength, range of motion, movement, and by decreasing pain. This is accomplished through assessment and the creation and implementation of treatment programs that may include exercise, massage, and the use of modalities such as heat, cold, and electrical stimulation. Physical therapists teach patients to perform exercises and use equipment, such as canes and crutches. (See Table 1–11 and Figure 1–7.)

Physical Therapist Assistant

Assistants work with patients under the supervision of a physical therapist to carry out treatment plans. They teach and supervise exercises, apply modalities, perform massages, assist patients with ambulatory devices such as walkers and canes, and document progress. Physical therapist assistants must be patient and encouraging and have the physical strength to assist patients with exercises. This occupation is projected to be among the fastest growing in the next several years at 29%. *See https://www.bls.gov/ooh/healthcare/physical-therapist-assistants-and-aides.htm.*

Physical Therapist Aide

Aides support the work of therapists and assistants by preparing and cleaning equipment and therapy areas, assisting with treatments, transporting patients, and ordering and maintaining supplies. Aides must be responsible and

Table 1–10 Pharmacy Occupations

Career	Education	Testing and Licensure
Pharmacist (PharmD)	2–3 years college 3–4 years pharmacy school (doctoral degree)	Licensed by states: 1. Graduate from college of pharmacy accredited by the American Council on Pharmaceutical Education 2. Pass the North American Pharmacist Licensure Exam (NAPLEX) 3. Most states also require passing the Multistate Pharmacy Jurisprudence Exam (MPJE) (Pharmacy law)
Pharmacy Technician	Up to 1 year on-the-job-training or 1- or 2-year college certificate program or associate's degree	A few states require licensure, certification, or registration Voluntary national certification available through examination administered by Pharmacy Technician Certification Board and the Institute for Certification of Pharmacy Technicians
Pharmacy Aide/Helper/Clerk	High school diploma and on-the-job-training or vocational training program	None

Table 1–11 Physical Therapy Occupations

Career	Education	Testing and Licensure
Physical Therapist (PT)	3–4 four years college (bachelor's degree) 3+ years graduate studies (doctorate)	Licensed by states: 1. Graduate from program accredited by the Commission on Accreditation in Physical Therapy Education (CAPTE) 2. Pass exam administered by the Federation of State Boards of Physical Therapy
Physical Therapist Assistant (PTA)	2-year (associate's) college degree	All states require licensure, certification, and/or registration: 1. Graduate from program accredited by CAPTE 2. Pass exam administered by the Federation of State Boards of Physical Therapy
Physical Therapist Aide	On-the-job-training or vocational training program	None

able to follow directions. Job growth is expected to be much faster than average. See https://www.bls.gov/ooh /healthcare/physical-therapist-assistants-and-aides.htm.

Respiratory Therapy Occupations

Respiratory therapy involves evaluating, treating, and caring for patients with breathing disorders. Respiratory therapists assist patients who have difficulty breathing or cannot breathe on their own because of conditions such as

heart disease, acute diseases (lasting a short time but are relatively severe) such as pneumonia, or chronic diseases (lasting a long time) such as emphysema. (See Table 1–12 and Figure 1–8.)

Respiratory Therapist

Respiratory therapists perform a variety of tasks to assist patients with breathing. These include using special instruments to measure lung capacity and drawing blood

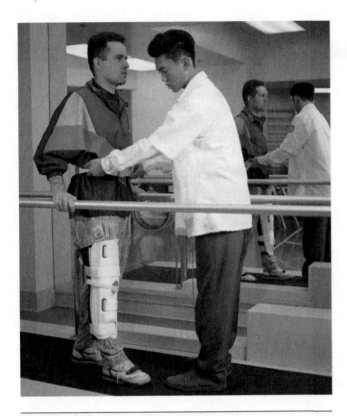

FIGURE 1–7 Physical therapist assistants help patients improve their physical function after accidents, surgery, and illness.

samples to test for levels of oxygen and other components. Therapists provide patients with oxygen and connect those who cannot breathe on their own to ventilators. The monitoring and maintenance of equipment are critical to a patient's well-being. Therapists also administer aerosol medications and perform chest physiotherapy, which involves thumping and vibrating the patient's chest cavity to remove mucus from the lungs. Respiratory therapists must have good technical aptitude and be attentive to detail and able to work under stress. Jobs are expected to grow much faster than average for all occupations at 23%. *See https://www.bls.gov/ooh/healthcare/respiratory-therapists.htm.*

Surgical Occupations

Surgical procedures vary from minor to extremely complex and from emergency to elective. The types of surgery available and their complexity are growing at a fast rate.

FIGURE 1–8 Respiratory therapists administer medications and treatments to patients who have lung and heart disorders.

Many people are alive today as a result of modern surgery. Surgical occupations involve the care of the patient before, during, and after surgery. (See Table 1–13 and Figure 1–9.)

Surgical Technologist/Surgical Technician/ Operating Room Technician

The health care professionals who are trained to perform important functions in the operating room may work under a variety of job titles. Duties include sterilizing and setting up instruments, preparing equipment and linens in the operating room, and preparing patients for surgery and transporting them to the operating room. During surgery, technicians may perform a variety of tasks: pass instruments to the surgeon, hold retractors (instruments that open or draw back tissue, bone, etc.), cut sutures, operate lights and equipment, and assist with the preparation of specimens. Work in surgery requires excellent manual dexterity, attention to detail, the stamina to stand for long hours, and the ability to respond quickly. Employment is expected to grow faster than average for all occupations at 12%. *See https://www.bls.gov/ooh/healthcare/surgical-technologists.htm.*

Table 1–12 **Respiratory Therapy Occupations**

Career	Education	Testing and Licensure
Respiratory Therapist (RRT, CRT)	Associate's or bachelor's degree	Licensed in all states except Alaska: 1. Graduate an accredited program (accepted approval agencies vary by state) 2. Pass exam administered by the National Board for Respiratory Care

Table 1–13 Surgical Occupations

Career	Education	Testing and Licensure
Surgeon (MD or DO)	4 years college preprofessional education 4 years medical school MD: Up to 6 years of graduate medical education (internship and residency) DO: 1-year internship and 3- to 5-year residency	Licensed by states: 1. Graduate from accredited medical school 2. Complete specialized studies, internship, and residency 3. Pass written exam
Surgical Physician Assistant	Varies; 4 years college (bachelor's degree) + 2-year PA program + 2-year surgical assistant master's degree program	State licensing requirements vary Must pass exams administered by the National Commission on Certification of Physician's Assistants
Certified Surgical Technician (CST), Operating Room Technician (ORT), Surgical Technologist	9-month to 2-year program leading to certificate or associate's degree Clinical experience	Some states require certification or registration by passing exam administered by National Board of Surgical Technology and Surgical Assisting

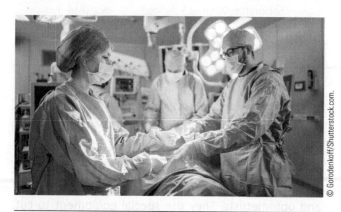

© Gorodenkoff/Shutterstock.com.

FIGURE 1–9 Surgical technologists prepare patients for surgery, set up instruments and supplies, and assist during surgery by passing instruments and supplies.

Veterinary Occupations

Veterinary professionals provide medical treatment and preventive care for many types of animals who fill a variety of roles: pets; food sources for humans; entertainment, such as zoo animals and racehorses; and animals used in laboratory experiments. Pet care has become a multibillion dollar industry in the United States as more people acquire pets as companions and consider them to be members of the family. Although most veterinary practices work with small animals, some work with livestock and other large animals. Others specialize in more exotic animals such as alpacas, ostriches, and lizards. Keeping livestock healthy contributes to human health by ensuring the health and safety of our meat, egg, and milk supply. (See Table 1–14 and Figure 1–10.)

Veterinary Technologists and Technicians

Veterinary technologists and technicians work under the supervision of a veterinarian in diagnosing and treating animals. Their duties are similar and include conducting laboratory tests, taking blood samples and X-rays, cleaning an animal's teeth, assisting in surgery, and educating animal owners. Individuals who work in veterinary careers must like animals and enjoy working with them. The work can be physically and emotionally demanding, as when large animals must be restrained or beloved pets are euthanized. Technologists and technicians must be able to work responsibly under supervision, communicate well, and demonstrate empathy for the owners of the animals they treat. The most common employment settings include private veterinary clinics, animal hospitals, and research facilities. These are expected to be very fast-growing occupations at 20%. *See https://www.bls.gov/ooh /healthcare/veterinary-technologists-and-technicians.htm.*

Vision Care Occupations

Vision care professionals perform the important work of assisting the up to 75% of Americans who use some form of corrective lens. In addition to working to correct vision problems, they identify and treat diseases of the eye, perform surgery, provide education and care to maintain good vision and eye health, and make eyeglasses. (See Table 1–15.)

Table 1–14 **Veterinary Occupations**

Career	Education	Testing and Licensure
Veterinarian (DVM or VMD)	3–4 years college preprofessional education 4 years veterinary college 2- to 5-year internship/residency required for specialties	Licensed by states: 1. Graduate from accredited veterinary school 2. Pass the North American Veterinary Licensing Exam (NAVLE) 3. Many states administer exam covering state laws and regulations
Veterinary Technologist	Bachelor's degree	Regulation varies by state All states require credentialing exam. Most use National Veterinary Technician (NVT) exam Voluntary certification for work in research facility is administered by the American Association for Laboratory Animal Science
Veterinary Technician	2-year associate's degree	Regulation differs by state Almost all states require credentialing exam Most use NVT exam Voluntary certification for work in research facility is administered by the American Association for Laboratory Animal Science
Veterinary Assistant	On-the-job training or college certificate program	No licensing required

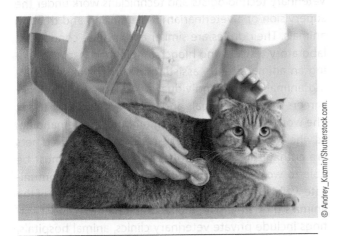
© Andrey_Kuzmin/Shutterstock.com.

FIGURE 1–10 Veterinary technologists and technicians assist veterinarians as they diagnose and treat various types of animals.

Ophthalmic Medical Technician

Ophthalmic medical technicians assist ophthalmologists in their work with patients. They take care of equipment, record patient histories, perform eye tests, assist with surgery, and carry out office maintenance duties. Good manual dexterity, observation skills, and attention to detail are important characteristics for success in this occupation.

Job growth is expected to be very good at 25%. *See https://www.bls.gov/oes/2017/may/oes292057.htm.*

Ophthalmic Laboratory Technician

Ophthalmic laboratory technicians make eyeglass lenses following prescriptions prepared by ophthalmologists and optometrists. They use special equipment to cut, grind, edge, and finish eyeglass lenses, which must then be checked for accuracy. The job sometimes includes inserting lenses into frames. Technicians must have good manual dexterity, attention to detail, and the ability to follow directions. Job growth is expected to be 13%, although the number working in this occupation is low. *See https://www.bls.gov/oes/2017/may/oes519083.htm and https://www.bls.gov/ooh/production/dental-and-ophthalmic-laboratory-technicians-and-medical-appliance-technicians.htm.*

Diagnostic Occupations

Professionals in diagnostic occupations help identify and/or determine the causes and extent of diseases and injuries so that proper treatment can be planned. They also monitor patient progress over time to determine if treatment is effective. Occupations may involve working directly with patients to perform tests and collect specimens, operating complex equipment, and carrying out tests in a laboratory setting.

Table 1–15 **Vision Care Occupations**

Career	Education	Testing and Licensure
Ophthalmologist (MD)	4 years college preprofessional education 4 years medical school 4–7 years graduate medical education (internship and residency)	Licensed by states: 1. Graduate from accredited medical school 2. Complete specialized studies, internship, and residency 3. Pass written exam
Optometrist (OD)	3–4 years college 4 years college of optometry 2+ years residency required to specialize in specific types of optometry	Licensed by states: 1. Graduate from accredited optometry school 2. Pass written and clinical state board exams or exam administered by National Board of Examiners in Optometry 3. Many states require exam on state law
Ophthalmic Medical Technologist	Associate's or bachelor's degree	Requirements vary among states Voluntary certification from the Joint Commission on Allied Health Personnel in Ophthalmology (JCAHPO)
Ophthalmic Technician	1-year certificate or diploma program	Requirements vary among states Voluntary certification from the JCAHPO
Optician	On-the-job training or 2- to 4-year apprenticeship or vocational or associate's degree program (apprenticeship means formal on-the-job training with specific conditions and goals). Some states require formal training to qualify to take certification exams.	Licensed or certified in 22 states; requirements vary Voluntary certification available through the American Board of Opticianry and National Contact Lens Examiners
Ophthalmic Assistant	On-the-job training or formal education ranging from 2 weeks to 2-year associate's degree	Optional certification: 1. Complete educational program 2. Clinical experience 3. Pass national exam administered by JCAHPO
Ophthalmic Laboratory Technician	On-the-job training or 6- to 12-month vocational training program	Voluntary certification available from the American Board of Opticianry and National Contact Lens Examiners: 1. Possess high school diploma 2. Pass examination
Optometric Assistant/ Technician	On-the-job training or vocational program	Voluntary certification available from the American Optometric Association, Commission on Paraoptometric Certification

Diagnostic Imaging Occupations

Diagnostic imaging involves the use of a variety of techniques and machines to view structures and functions inside the body. Many diseases and injuries can be diagnosed without carrying out invasive procedures. Equipment is used that employs X-rays, sound waves, magnetic fields, and radioactive substances. (See Chapter 18 for more information on imaging techniques.) The ongoing development of noninvasive diagnostic methods has resulted in new specialties and occupational areas, such as magnetic resonance imaging (MRI) technologist. (See Table 1–16.)

Radiologic Technologist/Radiographer

Radiographers perform X-ray procedures. They explain procedures to patients, position them properly, provide shielding against excessive exposure to X-rays, operate equipment, and develop film. This work requires great attention to safety factors, a high degree of technical aptitude, the ability to communicate well with patients, the stamina to stand for long periods, and the ability to work under emergency conditions. Faster than average employment growth is expected at 12%. Radiographers who learn a variety of specialties, such as skull X-rays and mammography, will have the best chances for employment. *See https://www.bls.gov/ooh/healthcare/radiologic-technologists.htm.*

Diagnostic Medical Sonographer

Sonographers operate equipment that uses sound waves (ultrasound) to produce images of soft tissue. This technology allows the movement of internal structures to be viewed on a screen, as well as the creation of images on film. Sonographers can specialize in cardiac, vascular, or

Table 1–16 Diagnostic Imaging Occupations

Career	Education	Testing and Licensure
Radiologist (MD or OD)	4 years college preprofessional education 4 years medical school 5–7 years of graduate medical education (internship and residency)	Licensed by states: 1. Graduate from accredited medical school 2. Complete specialized studies, internship, and residency 3. Pass written exam administered by the American Board of Radiology
Registered Radiologic Assistant	Bachelor's degree	Licensed in most states Voluntary registration from the American Registry of Radiologic Technologists (ARRT): 1. Graduate from accredited program or meet other specified requirements 2. Pass certification exam
Radiologic Technologist (RT)/Radiographer	Associate's or bachelor's degree	Licensed in most states Voluntary registration from ARRT: 1. Graduate from accredited program or meet other specified requirements 2. Pass certification exam
Computed Tomography Technologist	Associate's or bachelor's degree plus on-the-job training or training from manufacturer	Same as radiographer plus additional specialty exam
Magnetic Resonance Technologist	Be a registered radiographer Associate's or bachelor's degree plus on-the-job training or training from manufacturer	Same as radiographer plus additional specialty exam
Positron Emission Tomography Technologist	Be a registered radiographer Associate's or bachelor's degree plus on-the-job training or training from manufacturer	Same as radiographer plus additional specialty exam

(continues)

Table 1–16 Diagnostic Imaging Occupations *(continued)*

Career	Education	Testing and Licensure
Diagnostic Medical Sonographer	Certificate program or associate's or bachelor's degree (associate's degree most common)	Some states require licensure Voluntary certification available from the American Registry of Diagnostic Medical Sonographers (ARDMS): 1. Graduate from accredited program or meet other requirements 2. Pass national exam
Limited X-ray Machine Operator	Diploma or certificate program	Certification and title of position vary by state. Most states (32 currently) require licensure. Some require specific education from an accredited program and passing a certification exam
Cardiovascular Technologist/Diagnostic Vascular Technologist	Associate's or bachelor's degree	Some states require licensure Registration available with ARDMS Certification available from Cardiovascular Credentialing International
Electrocardiography Technician	On-the-job training or 6- to 12-month vocational education program	Certification available from the National Center for Competency Testing and the National Healthcareer Association
Neurodiagnostic Technologist/ Electroneurodiagnostic Technologist/ Electroencephalographic Technologist	Associate's degree (preferred) or formal training program of 1–2 years leading to a diploma or on-the-job training	Some states require certification Certification available from the American Board of Registration of Electroencephalographic and Evoked Potential Technologists

abdominal areas. A common use of ultrasound, because of its safety, is to observe the developing fetus. Sonographers must have good math and technical aptitude, the ability to communicate with patients, and accurate work habits. Employment growth is expected to be faster than for all occupations at 17%. *See https://www.bls.gov/ooh /healthcare/diagnostic-medical-sonographers.htm.*

Limited X-ray Machine Operator

Limited X-ray machine operators are licensed personnel whose duties are similar to those of a radiologic technologist, but more limited in scope. This position does not exist in all states and may have another title, such as radiologic technician or radiographic assistant.

Cardiovascular Technologist and Diagnostic Vascular Technologist

Cardiovascular and diagnostic vascular technologists assist physicians in the diagnosis and treatment of heart, vein, and artery disorders. They are qualified to perform

noninvasive tests using ultrasound as well as to assist with invasive procedures, such as cardiac catheterization, which is the insertion of a small tube through the blood vessels to the heart. Technologists prepare patients for procedures and monitor them throughout. They must work accurately, handle stress well, and have high technical aptitude. Employment growth is expected to be much faster than average at 17%, but the number of positions is not high because the occupation is small. *See https://www.bls.gov/ooh/healthcare/diagnostic-medical-sonographers.htm.*

Electrocardiography Technician

Electrocardiography records the electrical action of the heart. The electrocardiograph (ECG) technician attaches electrodes to specific points on the patient and manipulates switches on a machine to trace the electrical activity on graph paper. This skill is often included in the training of other patient care occupations, such as medical assisting. The number of jobs for ECG technicians who are not trained to perform other tasks in addition to this specialty is expected to grow at a slower-than-average rate.

Neurodiagnostic Technologist/ Electroneurodiagnostic Technologist/ Electroencephalographic Technologist

Electroneurodiagnostics is the monitoring, recording, interpreting, and study of the entire nervous system using various tests and instruments. Electroencephalic technology refers specifically to the recording and study of the brain's electrical activity. Technologists take patient histories, apply electrodes to the scalp, operate recording and monitoring instruments, and monitor patients during procedures.

They should have good manual dexterity and vision, technical aptitude, and excellent communication skills.

Medical Laboratory Occupations

Work in medical laboratory occupations involves collecting and studying specimens from the human body. These include blood and other body fluids, tissues, and cells. Many kinds of tests are available to detect the presence of disease and determine its cause. The work requires the use of specialized equipment, such as microscopes and cell counters, and various chemicals. (See Table 1–17 and Figure 1–11.)

Table 1–17 Medical Laboratory Occupations

Career	Education	Testing and Licensure
Pathologist (MD)	4 years college preprofessional education 4 years medical school 4 years of graduate medical education (internship and residency); 1 or 2 more years required for specialties	Licensed by states: 1. Graduate from accredited medical school 2. Complete specialized studies, internship, and residency 3. Pass written exam
Medical Laboratory Technologist (MT)	Bachelor's or master's degree	Licensed or registered in some states Certification available from: 1. American Medical Technologists 2. Board of Registry of the American Society for Clinical Pathology 3. Board of Registry of the American Association of Bioanalysts
Medical Laboratory Technician	Completion of certificate program or associate's degree	Licensing or registration required in some states Certification available from: 1. American Medical Technologists 2. Board of Certification of the American Society for Clinical Pathology
Medical Laboratory Assistant	1- to 2-year training program or specific work experience	Voluntary certification from the American Medical Technologists Association
Phlebotomist	On-the-job training or formal training program	Licensure required in California, Louisiana, Nevada, and Washington. (It is expected that more states will require in the future.) Certification is required by most employers and is available from: 1. National Phlebotomy Association 2. American Society for Clinical Pathology 3. Association of Phlebotomy Technicians 4. Several other organizations also test and certify phlebotomists

Note: All of the previously mentioned careers require completion of various amounts of training in order to take professional exams.

FIGURE 1–11 Medical laboratory workers perform manual and computerized tests to detect the presence of disease.

Medical Laboratory Technologists and Technicians

Laboratory technologists and technicians perform routine tests, which can require preparing slides, counting cells, and using sophisticated equipment. The work can also involve caring for and cleaning the equipment, maintaining supplies, and keeping records. Laboratory technicians must have good manual dexterity, great attention to detail and accuracy, and good observation skills. Employment projection is expected to be faster than for all occupations at 13%. *See https://www.bls.gov/ooh/ healthcare/medical-and-clinical-laboratory-technologists-and-technicians.htm.*

Medical Laboratory Assistant

Laboratory assistants perform routine tests and tasks that are less complex than those for which technologists and technicians are qualified. The necessary qualities and job outlook are similar to those of the technician. *See https://www.bls.gov/ooh/healthcare/medical-and-clinical-laboratory-technologists-and-technicians.htm.*

Phlebotomist

Phlebotomists draw blood from patients for medical testing and from blood donors. In addition to good manual dexterity, they must be calm and reassuring and able to work with individuals who fear blood and needles. Employment growth is expected to be much faster than for all occupations at 25%. *See https://www.bls.gov /ooh/healthcare/phlebotomists.htm.*

Health Information Management Occupations

Individuals who work in health information management occupations gather, analyze, organize, store, and document patient information. Consistent patient care, as well as regulatory compliance, and insurance requirements, depend on complete and accurate records. The increasing emphasis on monitoring the cost of health care delivery and the outcomes of patients who undergo treatment has increased the need for high-quality medical recordkeeping, with employment projections indicating much faster growth than average for all occupations. (See Table 1–18 and Figure 1–12.)

Table 1–18 **Health Information Management Occupations**

Career	Education	Testing and Licensure
Registered Health Information Administrator (RHIA)	Bachelor's or master's degree	Voluntary registration available from the American Health Information Management Association (AHIMA): 1. Complete educational program approved by the Commission on Accreditation for Health Informatics and Information Management Education (CAHIIM) 2. Pass national exam administered by AHIMA
Registered Health Information Technician (RHIT)	Associate's degree	Voluntary registration available from AHIMA: 1. Complete educational program accredited by CAHIIM 2. Pass national exam administered by AHIMA
Medical Transcriptionist (MT)	Certificate program or associate's degree	Voluntary certification available from Association for Healthcare Documentation Integrity

(continues)

Table 1–18 Health Information Management Occupations *(continued)*

Career	Education	Testing and Licensure
Certified Coding Specialist (CCS)	Associate's degree (preferred) or on-the-job training or coding seminars	Voluntary certification (Certified Coding Specialist [CCS]) available from AHIMA: 1. High-school diploma 2. Complete educational program accredited by CAHIIM 3. Written exam
Medical Records Clerk	On-the-job training	None

© Stocklite/Shutterstock.com.

FIGURE 1–12 Health information management professionals must have good computer skills and work accurately.

Registered Health Information Technician

Health information technicians perform a variety of tasks related to the collection and organization of patient data. They organize patient records, perform coding (the assignment of predetermined numbers that designate specific diagnoses and procedures), enter data from paper records into computerized recordkeeping systems, and compile data for reports. Good organizational skills, a high degree of accuracy with details, and good computer aptitude are necessary for success in this field. Job prospects are expected to be very good with an employment growth rate of 13%. *See https://www.bls.gov/ooh/healthcare/medical-records-and-health-information-technicians.htm.*

Medical Transcriptionist

Transcriptionists prepare written medical reports. A variety of reports are used in health care to describe all types of findings and procedures. They include topics ranging from descriptions of surgeries to reports documenting autopsies (examination of organs and tissues performed after death to determine cause of death). Transcriptionists must sit and concentrate for long periods; be able to hear and interpret spoken language that includes medical terms; have excellent grammar, spelling, and computer software skills; and

produce consistently accurate work. Employment prospects are expected to decline because of technological advances causing increases in productivity. *See https://www.bls.gov/ooh/healthcare/medical-transcriptionists.htm.*

Certified Coding Specialist

Medical coders classify medical data contained in patient records. Codes are assigned from the two major coding systems, the ICD-10-CM (diagnoses) and CPT (procedures). With experience and additional training, coders can achieve positions such as coding supervisor and compliance officer. A high level of accuracy and attention to detail is necessary for success as a coder. Job prospects are expected to be good. *See https://study.com/articles/Medical_Coding_Specialist_Job_Description_and_Requirements.html.*

Environmental Occupations

Individuals who work in environmental occupations develop and maintain therapeutic environments necessary to support patient care. Responsibilities include providing food services, cleaning and maintaining facilities and equipment, managing resources, and creating pleasant surroundings.

Nutrition and Dietary Service Occupations

Dietary service professionals support patients by planning and providing nutritious foods that are essential to the healing process. Therapeutic diets are sometimes prescribed by physicians for patients with specific health problems and conditions, such as high blood pressure and diabetes, and following abdominal surgery. (See Table 1–19.)

Dietetic Technician

Dietetic technicians work under the supervision of dietitians and perform tasks related to all aspects of food planning and preparation. They assist with creating menus, testing recipes, ordering food and supplies, and preparing meals. Some technicians work with patients to learn their food preferences and design special diets as ordered by a physician. Dietetic technicians must have good communication skills

Table 1–19 Dietary Service Occupations

Career	Education	Testing and Licensure
Dietitian (RD)	Bachelor's degree (minimum)	Licensure, certification, or registration required in most states. Registration available from Academy of Nutrition and Dietetics: 1. Complete educational program approved by the Academy 2. Complete supervised experience 3. Pass national exam administered by Commission on Dietetic Registration
Dietetic Technician (DTR)/Dietetic Assistant	Associate's degree	Complete educational program approved by the Academy Voluntary registration available from Commission on Dietetic Registration
Dietetic Aide	Certificate program in food services or on-the-job training	None

and be attentive to detail and able to follow specific directions. The projected employment rate is expected to be good. *See https://www.bls.gov/oes/2017/may/oes292051.htm.*

Biomedical Engineering

The application of engineering to health care has resulted in the creation of sophisticated medical equipment that helps in diagnosing, treating, and monitoring patient conditions. Life-enhancing and lifesaving inventions resulting from biomedical engineering include the heart-lung machine, cardiac pacemakers, surgical lasers, and ultrasound technology. All engineering specialties, including electrical, mechanical, computer, and chemical, have been applied to seeking improvements in health care. (See Table 1–20.)

Biomedical Equipment Technologist/Technician or Medical Equipment Repairer

Biomedical equipment technicians are specially trained to work on medical equipment that requires continual and competent maintenance to provide accurate diagnoses and reliable service to treat and monitor patients. Duties of the technician include installing, testing, servicing, and repairing all types of equipment. Technicians may specialize in one area, such as radiology or clinical laboratory equipment. Work in this area requires excellent manual dexterity, hand–eye coordination, mechanical aptitude, and interest in technology. Projected employment is expected to be much faster than average. *See https://www.bls.gov/ooh/installation-maintenance-and-repair/medical-equipment-repairers.htm.*

Table 1–20 Biomedical Engineering Occupations

Career	Education	Testing and Licensure
Biomedical Engineer	Bachelor's degree or higher	Licensed for some employment positions in some states Many states require passing exams administered by National Council of Examiners for Engineering and Surveying Certification also available from International Certification Commission for Clinical Engineering and Biomedical Technology (ICC): 1. Complete degree in engineering 2. Have at least 3 years of experience as hospital clinical engineer 3. Pass both written and oral exams
Biomedical Equipment Technician	Associate's degree	Certifications available from ICC: 1. Associate's degree in biomedical engineering or specific combinations of training and experience 2. Pass written exam

Sources of Additional Information

Students should use the tables and information in this text as a starting point and then thoroughly investigate all the career options in their areas of interest. Good starting points for collecting career information include the following:

1. The websites listed at the end of each paragraph describing a job title are from the U.S. Bureau of Labor's Occupational Outlook Handbook. They contain a summary of Quick Facts about the occupation, a short video that describes the work, median pay, educational requirements, personal attributes necessary for success in the occupation, and links to web pages that contain more detailed information.

2. The professional organizations for the various occupations. The contact information for these organizations is listed in Appendix 1.

3. Talking with and/or observing (shadowing) health care professionals about their work: your physician and dentist and his/her staffs; any other health care professionals you know.

4. Your instructors who work or have worked in the field may provide information.

5. Occupational Outlook Handbook from the Bureau of Labor Statistics: www.bls.gov/ooh /healthcare/.

6. Career One Stop, sponsored by the U.S. Department of Labor: https//careeronestop.org.

7. O*Net, sponsored by the U.S. Department of Labor: www.onetonline.org.

8. Explore Health Careers: https://explorehealthcareers .org.

SUGGESTED LEARNING ACTIVITIES

1. Create a personal plan for developing the core qualities demonstrated by health care professionals.

2. Determine if there are study skills you need to improve and create a plan to improve them.

3. Choose a problem in your life that you would like to work on and apply the five steps of the problem-solving process. Report on the results.

4. Seek opportunities to observe health care professionals at work. Report on the qualities they demonstrate that you believe make them effective.

5. Research an occupational area or specific career that interests you: interview a working professional, send for information or visit the Internet site of the appropriate professional organization (see Appendix 1), request a job description from a local facility, and/or read the job descriptions in the *Occupational Outlook Handbook*.

WEB ACTIVITIES

WikiHow

https://www.wikihow.com/Improve-Your-Study-Skills

How to Improve Your Study Skills

1. Read this illustrated guide.

2. Are there any suggestions you think might help you?

3. If so, try them for a couple of weeks and report on how they work for you.

Study Guides and Strategies

www.studygs.net

This is an excellent website with information on dozens of topics, including study habits, time management, writing effectively, and much more.

1. Choose any topics you think might help you improve your chance for success in school.

2. Select one or two to apply and report on the results.

Operation Self Reset

https://www.langspace.com/en/video/10560442669729526

Four "Study Tips" That Work

Careers in Government

https://www.careersingovernment.com/tools/gov-talk/career-advice/on-the-job/7-advantages-working-healthcare-industry/

Seven Advantages of Working in the Healthcare Industry

1. List the advantages described in the article.

2. Which one is most important to you? Why?

3. Are there advantages not listed that you believe are important?

Rasmussen College

https://www.rasmussen.edu/degrees/health-sciences/blog/working-in-the-healthcare-industry/

Seven Compelling Reasons to Consider Working in the Healthcare Industry

1. Compare the reasons listed here with those in the previous activity, Careers in Government. Which new ones are listed here?

2. Did this list add any information to help you make a career decision?

Open Colleges

https://www.opencolleges.edu.au/blog/2017/11/06/ca-6-qualities-truly-great-health-professionals/

Six Qualities of Truly Great Health and Community Care Professionals
    Here is a list that is different from the core qualities listed in this text.

1. Do you agree that these qualities are important?

2. If so, do you believe that you have these qualities?

3. If you don't, and you think they are important, how might you develop them?

Live Strong

https://www.livestrong.com/article/239565-what-are-the-benefits-of-volunteering-in-a-hospital/

What Are the Benefits of Volunteering in a Hospital?

1. What types of volunteer positions may be available in a hospital?

2. What are the benefits for volunteers?

3. What are the benefits for patients?

Nursing Times

https://www.nursingtimes.net/thinking-your-way-to-successful-problem-solving/200636.article

Thinking Your Way to Successful Problem-Solving
    Although written for nurses a number of years ago, this article shows how problem-solving is applied on the job in health care.

1. What are the two kinds of approaches nurses can use when approaching problems?

2. What are the three kinds of problems nurses are likely to encounter?

3. Why is perception important when addressing problems that deal with other people?

4. When should other people be involved in generating solutions to a problem?

5. What are some methods for generating ideas for solutions?

6. How does this information apply to the careers that interest you?

Rasmussen College

https://www.rasmussen.edu/resources/healthcare-careers/

The Healthcare Career Matchmaker

This tool matches your personality traits with various health care careers.

1. Take the matchmaker to see which careers are suggested.
2. Were you surprised by the results?
3. Are any of the suggestions for careers you have considered?

Note: This tool is only meant to give you some ideas about what to consider when choosing a career.

Occupational Outlook Handbook

https://www.bls.gov/ooh/healthcare/

1. Locate an occupation of interest in the list.
2. Using the information provided, write a description of the occupation that includes significant points, desirable personal qualities, job outlook, and typical earnings.

Health Care Professional Organizations

Explore the website of a professional organization from Appendix 1 for a career that interests you.

1. What information is provided by the organization that can help you make a career choice?
2. What information did you learn about the career?

Note: For example, the American Physical Therapy Association has information for prospective students at http://www.apta.org/ProspectiveStudents/.

Oregon Laws

https://www.oregonlaws.org/ors/688.515

This website contains information about the state requirements in Oregon for limited X-ray machine operators. Although you may live in another state and have a different career in mind, reviewing this page can give you an idea of how states regulate health care occupations.

1. What are the limitations of this occupation in Oregon?
2. What training is required?
3. Is an exam required?
4. Who supervises the work of limited X-ray operators?
5. Does your state have laws regulating this occupation? Does it regulate the occupation in which you are interested?

California Board of Registered Nursing

https://www.rn.ca.gov/

You may not be interested in a career in nursing—and don't live in California—but this website will give you an idea of the information provided by state licensing boards.

1. Skim the information available. Note that information about education, professional exams, and other topics of interest to students interested in pursuing a career in nursing are available.
2. Search for information provided by your state for your career of interest. Is there anything available? If so, what information is useful to you at this time?

REVIEW QUESTIONS

1. What is the current economic status of the health care industry?
2. What are the general employment projections in health care?

3. What are the ten health care jobs expected to have the largest percentage increases between 2016 and 2026, according to the U.S. Department of Labor Statistics?

4. What are the six health care jobs expected to have the highest numbers of openings between 2016 and 2026, according to the U.S. Department of Labor Statistics?

5. In what ways can work in health care be both satisfying and demanding?

6. What are the seven core qualities that every health care professional should demonstrate?

7. How can students apply the core qualities while still in school?

8. What is the meaning of "learning for mastery"?

9. How can students use questions to master new subjects?

10. What are ways students can improve their note-taking, reading, writing, and test-taking skills?

11. What are some skills that adult students bring from their life experience when they return to school to study a health care career?

12. What are five techniques that adult students can use to stay organized and manage their time efficiently?

13. What does it mean to "think like a health care professional"? Give two examples.

14. What are the five steps in the problem-solving process?

15. What are the personal factors that should be considered when choosing a health care career?

16. What are the five levels of education needed for various levels within a health care field?

17. What is the purpose of standards for health care professionals?

18. What is the meaning of the following terms as they apply to health care professionals: certification, registration, and licensure?

19. What is the meaning of school accreditation? What are the two major accreditation organizations for health care programs?

20. What are the four requirements that students must typically meet before taking professional exams?

21. What are the four classifications of health care careers? Give three examples of occupations for each.

22. What are the educational requirements, certification requirements, major duties, and attributes necessary for success in occupations in which you are interested?

23. What are the eight resources recommended for students to help them learn more about specific occupations?

APPLICATION EXERCISES

1. Refer back to The Case of the Confused Student at the beginning of the chapter. Using the information in this chapter, list your recommendations for occupations that Kevin should investigate.

2. Juan has always been interested in helping people. He also likes science and has maintained good grades throughout high school in chemistry, biology, and physics. He has enrolled in the local community college and is taking "Introduction to Health Care." Juan thinks that a career in health care might be for him, but he doesn't feel that he knows enough to make a career decision at this time. He's not sure what's out there or what jobs would be appropriate for him.

   a. What does Juan need to know in order to conduct an effective career search?

   b. Describe how he can use the problem-solving process to help him make a tentative career decision.

   c. Explain methods that Juan can use to research and learn more about different career options.

PROBLEM-SOLVING PRACTICE

Brenda has thought about being a dental assistant for a long time and has just enrolled in a one-year educational program. She wants to do well in school, but she is having trouble finding reliable day care for her two young children. Describe how she might use the five-step problem-solving process to ensure that she attends all her classes and that her children receive proper care.

CHAPTER 2

Health Care Yesterday, Today, and Tomorrow

KEY TERMS

acupuncture
adult foster home (also called adult foster care)
alternative medicine
Alzheimer's disease
ambulatory services
assisted living residence
chiropractic
complementary medicine
continuing care community
dementia
expanding consciousness
gene therapy
health disparities
Hippocrates
holistic medicine
homeopathy
hospice
implicit racism
inpatient
integrative medicine
intermediate nursing care facility (INCF)
massage therapy
Medicaid
medical malls
medication adherence
mutate
nursing homes
opioid pain medication
osteopathy
outpatient services
palliative
pandemic
personalized medicine

(continues)

OBJECTIVES

Studying and applying the material in this chapter will help you to:

1. Name ten significant events in the history of Western health care that changed the way care was delivered.
2. Define the following: gene therapy and targeted drug therapy.
3. State the leading prevention and treatment option in the health field today.
4. Explain the meaning of specialization and its impact on health care.
5. Explain the effect of our aging population on health care today.
6. Describe what has happened to health care costs over the past few decades.
7. List the factors that are changing how we approach health care today.
8. Explain the concept of "wellness," including how individuals can take responsibility for their own health.
9. Describe the theory of expanding consciousness.
10. Explain the concept of holistic medicine and list the aspects of the patient that it addresses and the factors emphasized by holistic providers.
11. Define the following approaches to medicine: Western, complementary, alternative, and integrative.
12. List the signs that a health care product may be fraudulent.
13. Explain the basis of osteopathy and chiropractic.
14. Describe the health benefits of massage therapy.
15. Explain the basis and uses of naturopathy, homeopathy, and acupuncture.
16. Explain the meaning and purpose of personalized medicine.
17. Describe the effect of health care costs on many Americans.
18. Describe the challenges of providing quality long-term care for older Americans.
19. List the six social problems that affect health care.
20. Define "health disparities."
21. Explain how racism affects health care.
22. Describe the difficulties of maintaining the quality of care in today's economic environment.
23. Define "preauthorization" and describe its potential effect on a patient's care.
24. List the problems associated with many of the nation's nursing homes.
25. Describe Alzheimer's disease and its effects now and in the future on the health care system.

KEY TERMS *(continued)*

preauthorization
precision medicine
psychiatric hospitals
psychosomatic
skilled nursing facility (SNF)
targeted drug therapy
vital statistics
wellness
Western medicine

26. Explain the difficulty in responding to infectious disease outbreaks.

27. Give the statistics that describe the problem of medication adherence among Americans.

28. Explain the extent and significance of the opioid crisis and list 11 strategies for fighting it.

29. Explain what it means when bacteria mutate and how this affects the use of antibiotics.

30. Give statistics that describe the increasing rate of suicide in the United States.

31. List the CDC's warning signs of potential suicide.

32. Explain why health care providers believe that prescription drugs should not be advertised.

33. List and describe the levels of care offered by the modern hospital.

34. List methods that hospitals are using to control costs.

35. List the ten ambulatory health care facilities and give examples of the type of services offered by each one.

36. Describe the major types of long-term care facilities.

37. Provide examples of health care services and care that can be provided in the patient's home.

38. Explain the purpose of hospice.

39. Explain why health care facilities are consolidating.

40. Give two examples of new types of health care facilities.

41. List the typical services offered by federal, state, and local health agencies.

The Case of the Confused Daughter

Until recently, Dora Freemont, age 87, lived alone in a small apartment. Last week she suffered a slight stroke. After several days in the hospital, she is ready to be discharged. Her daughter, Sally, is very concerned that her widowed mother is no longer capable of living alone and handling all her housekeeping and personal needs. She shares her concern with Angela Cisneros, one of the nurses who cared for her mother during her hospital stay. Sally is very worried and fears she will have to quit work in order to help take care of her mother. Angela knows that there are a variety of long-term care facilities and a number of options available for Mrs. Freemont. She refers Sally to the hospital social worker, who explains these options and discusses with her which might be most appropriate for her mother.

This chapter provides students with important information they can use to assist their future patients. It also helps learners understand the many settings in which they can seek employment.

THE HISTORY OF WESTERN HEALTH CARE

The long history of health care in the Western world was marked by gradual change until the beginning of the twentieth century. Table 2–1 contains a summary of significant events in the history of Western medicine. Starting about 100 years ago, the rate of discovery and change increased rapidly so that in the last few decades, medical technology and diagnostic and treatment methods advanced more than in the previous 100 years. At the beginning of the 1900s, the major killers were infectious diseases, the leading causes being influenza and pneumonia. Between 1918 and 1919, an influenza pandemic killed between 20 and 40 million people across the globe. Physicians at that time had a limited number of treatment techniques available. Because of the discovery of penicillin and antibiotics, along with the widespread use of immunizations, many infectious diseases are almost unheard of today.

Table 2–1 History of Western Medicine

Time Frame	Event	Impact
Ancient Times (???–A.D. 400)	Study of fossilized bones and Egyptian mummies indicates many modern health conditions, such as arthritis, infectious bone diseases, appendicitis, arteriosclerosis, and urinary and intestinal diseases.	Health care problems and diseases have been with us from the beginning of human life.
	Causes of disease were thought to be spirits, ghosts, or gods.	Home remedies were used and rituals performed to drive away the evil spirits. Examples of rituals are creating loud noises, beating the ill person, or bloodletting. Preventive medicine consisted of wearing amulets and mutilating or painting the body to ward off evil spirits.
	Life span was only 20–35 years.	Chronic illnesses were rare.
	Hippocrates of Cos (460–379 B.C.) was the most famous Greek physician of ancient times. He stressed observation and conservative treatment.	Called the "Father of Medicine," he used dietetics before resorting to drugs or surgery.
Medieval Times (A.D. 400–1350)	Two plagues (in A.D. 543 and 568) killed the majority of the people in Europe and led to breakdown in Western civilization.	Monks preserved written medical texts and monasteries served as centers of learning to maintain knowledge.
	Christianity became an increasing center of power. It was believed that disease was punishment for sins, possession by the devil, or a result of witchcraft.	Christians emphasized saving the soul, not the body. Treatment methods were prayer, penitence, and the assistance of saints. Any cure was considered a miracle.
	Black Plague of 1348 killed 30–50% of European population.	Concept of quarantine as preventive measure was recognized.
	Networks of hospitals were built.	Marked a new and more humane approach toward the ill. Hospitals were primarily a refuge for the sick, old, disabled, or homeless.
Renaissance (1350–1650)	Revival of learning and science. Tremendous growth in inquiry of how the body was structured and how it worked. Numerous autopsies were performed.	First attempts to connect autopsy results with clinical observations made during life. Accurate anatomical drawings were now available for study.
	Despite the new advances, it was still a time of tremendous filth in the cities and among their people, characterized by the spread of disease and extreme superstitions.	Criticisms of the old ways were frequently met with hatred.
	Printing press invented.	Allowed for widespread distribution of new information and books.
	Invention of gunpowder resulted in numerous gunshot wounds during frequent wars.	Need for surgical treatment of wounds elevated barber-surgeons to a higher status.
17th Century	William Harvey, an Englishman, stated that blood circulates throughout the body within a continuous network of vessels. Only the mechanical aspects of the system were addressed.	Vehemently opposed at first, this discovery led to the realization that medications could be injected into the circulatory system, and blood could be transfused. After many failed attempts, it fell out of favor for several centuries.

(continues)

Table 2–1 History of Western Medicine (continued)

Time Frame	Event	Impact
	In 1666, Anton van Leeuwenhoek invented the microscope.	Study of microscopic anatomy and visualization of organisms were now possible. Germs were only viewed under the microscope; the connection with disease came several centuries later.
	Quinine imported from Peru as a cure for malaria.	Separated malaria from other types of fevers. Confirmed the idea that specific diseases have specific cures.
	The study of the brain and psychology was of interest. (Prior to this time, a common belief was that the soul resided in the pineal gland and the rest of the body was purely mechanical in nature.)	Nervous system and stimulation of muscles discovered. The long-believed theory that mucus from a head cold was produced by the brain was disproved.
18th Century	Researchers and theorists still struggled with an explanation of how the body functioned.	Three theories were proposed. First, that the body functioned like a hydraulic pump that was run by an undefined fluid flowing through the nervous system. Second, that every disease was the result of overstimulation or inability to respond to stimulation. Treatment was then either a depressant or a stimulant (e.g., opium and alcohol). Third, that direct clinical observation should be used to define and categorize diseases. This led to the description of 2,400 different diseases. The same diseases were listed many times, just because the symptoms varied slightly between cases.
	Surgery became a respected form of treatment in France after the court physician successfully repaired an anal fistula for King Louis XIV.	Surgery was upgraded from a craft to an experimental science. Procedures were developed that could cure problems that were treatable only through surgery.
	Techniques for measuring blood pressure and temperature were developed.	Measurements of vital signs were used to monitor patient status.
	Science of chemistry came of age.	Digestion was now seen as a chemical process, rather than a purely mechanical process or one of putrefaction.
	The philosophy of "enlightenment" was developed, which stressed the rational approach to problems and dissemination of knowledge for others to study.	Numerous studies and experiments added rapidly to the expanding base of knowledge. Sharing of knowledge with others added to the increasing pace of progress.
	Focus went from belief in the devil and "possession" to recognition of mental illness as a disease. Previously, patients were locked up in filthy conditions, as mental illness was thought to be due to possession, sin, crime, or vice.	Mentally ill patients were released from their chains and treated in a more humane way.
	Preventive health came to the forefront in the form of public health.	Sanitary reform was initiated in hospitals, prisons, and military. Personal hygiene also improved dramatically.
	Interest in child health increased.	Decreased the appalling rate of deaths in infants and children.
	Edward Jenner (1749–1823) demonstrated that vaccination with cowpox provides immunity for smallpox.	Countless lives were saved. It opened the door into investigation for other vaccines to be developed.

(continues)

Table 2–1 **History of Western Medicine** *(continued)*

Time Frame	Event	Impact
19th Century	Advances in physiology continued.	Emphasis moved from individual organs to the identification of more specific tissues. For example, inflammation of the heart was now stated as endocarditis, pericarditis, or myocarditis (inflammation of one of the three layers of the heart).
	Tremendous increase in medical knowledge was acquired and documented. Physicians and surgeons were united into one profession.	Many first-time surgical operations were performed, such as tracheostomy and removal of thyroid and uterus. Medical profession started to develop specialty areas, such as pediatrics, psychiatry, dermatology (skin), public health, and preventive medicine.
	More powerful microscopes were developed.	Human tissue could now be seen at the cellular level.
	Advances were made in chemistry.	Laboratory tests for diagnostic purposes became common. Metabolism and dietetics came under scientific study. Pharmacology was established as a new science.
	Dentists introduced anesthesia, and this practice expanded to major surgical procedures.	Large-scale surgery could now be done. Death rate fell as anesthesia decreased shock and the need for speed in surgery.
	Elizabeth Blackwell (1821–1910) was the first woman MD in the United States. She opened the first nursing school in the United States in 1860.	Medical education opened for the first time to a female. Nursing was established as a profession in the United States.
	Louis Pasteur (1822–1895), a chemist, proved that specific microorganisms called bacteria are the cause of specific diseases in both humans and animals.	The results of his work led to the development of the germ theory.
	It was discovered that infectious microorganisms are carried by various means (e.g., humans, animals, mosquitoes, food). Specific identification of microorganisms led to the development of vaccines for prevention.	Revolutionized the ability to prevent, diagnose, and treat infectious diseases. In 1864, Lord Joseph Lister, MD, applied the germ theory to his surgical practice by reasoning that microorganisms could also fall into open surgical wounds.
	Anesthesia, asepsis, and invention of a variety of surgical instruments changed the face of medicine forever.	Previously the public viewed hospitals as a place one went to die. Now there was hope of recovery for the first time. Many more advanced surgeries could be performed (e.g., on joints, abdomen, head, spinal column).
20th Century	Preventive medicine made great strides as pasteurization, vaccination, asepsis, and sanitation were implemented.	Life expectancy increased from 47 years in 1900 to 70 years in 1950 due primarily to preventive, not curative, measures.
	In 1921, Karl Landsteiner of Vienna discovered blood groups.	Made transfusion of blood products safe for the first time in history.
	Insulin was extracted and tested for treatment of diabetes.	Diabetes was no longer considered a fatal disease, but could be managed with injections of insulin.
	Large-scale vaccination programs were conducted.	Many commonly feared infectious diseases were eradicated. But the influenza epidemic of 1918 that killed 20 million brought reality back after the euphoria of success.

(continues)

Table 2–1 History of Western Medicine *(continued)*

Time Frame	Event	Impact
	New diagnostic and therapeutic techniques were developed. The field of biomedical engineering was advanced with the invention of the computer.	X-rays, electrocardiograph (ECG), electroencephalograph (EEG), ultrasound, pacemakers, dialysis, and tomography provided physicians with more diagnostic and therapeutic tools.
	Vitamins were discovered; the United States took the leadership role in this research.	The belief that all diseases were caused by microbes was disproved when lack of certain vitamins was linked to various diseases (e.g., scurvy, beriberi).
	New synthetic drugs were developed to treat specific problems.	Chemotherapy was used to fight cancer. Antibiotics were developed to fight various infections caused by bacteria. Medications for treating allergies were developed.
	Mental illness became an increasing problem in modern society.	Shock treatment and psychosurgery were replaced with new drugs and psychotherapy. Tranquilizers, used to calm patients, changed the approach to and assessment of mental patients.
	Surgical techniques and anesthesia methods made great advancements. Transplantation of organs was now possible.	Heart, brain, and prosthetic joint replacements were performed. Definition of death was changed from cessation of heart and lung function to demonstration of brain death by EEG.
	People could be kept alive by mechanical means beyond the point of having any quality of life.	Emphasis was placed on people having written living wills to specify what they do and do not want done to prolong their lives. In 1975, the New Jersey Supreme Court ruled that the parents of a comatose woman could authorize the removal of life support systems.
	Patients with terminal illnesses publicly expressed the wish to die with dignity.	England opened the first hospice in 1967. Dr. Jack Kevorkian argued that patients should be allowed to request assistance to end their lives. Between 1990 and 1998, he participated in a number of physician-assisted suicides.
	Development of new and faster machines (e.g., automobiles, airplanes, various recreational vehicles) caused many accidental injuries.	Trauma medicine became a specialty.
	Genetic research into cause of certain diseases and conditions.	Identification of specific genes related to certain conditions, but how to alter to prevent condition was yet to be discovered.
	In 1978, the first "test tube" baby was born in England.	Opened up opportunity for couples previously unable to have children.
	In 1981, acquired immunodeficiency syndrome (AIDS) was identified as a disease.	Huge challenge to medical research that resulted in medications that prolonged life but did not cure the disease.
	First successful cloning of sheep in 1997.	Opened door for human cloning and growth of organs for transplantation.

(continues)

Table 2–1 History of Western Medicine *(continued)*

Time Frame	Event	Impact
21st Century and Beyond— What Is Possible?	Some of the hopes for the new millennium: • Vaccine to prevent human immunodeficiency virus (HIV) • Cure for AIDS • Cure for obesity • Cloning of organs for transplantation to overcome extreme difficulty in finding suitable organ donors • Development of medication specific to a person's genotype to optimize treatment • Cures for heart disease, hypertension, and cancer • More effective treatment and cure for mental illnesses • Preventive health and alternative therapies used in a complementary way with practice of traditional medicine • Life span of healthy living expanded to 100+ years • Less invasive diagnostic and therapeutic treatments and medications with fewer and less harmful side effects	When health care professionals several centuries into the future look back at the 21st century, they will be astounded. This reaction would be similar to ours when we look back to previous centuries and are mystified by the ignorance and resulting unnecessary human suffering.

TRENDS AND ISSUES IN HEALTH CARE TODAY

Modern discoveries and inventions build upon one another, increasing the rate of growth of new developments. There are now an amazing number of treatments, including organ transplantation, microscopic and robotic surgery, gene therapy (the transplantation of normal genes into cells in place of missing or defective ones in order to correct genetic disorders), and targeted drug therapy (treatment that uses drugs or other substances to identify and attack specific types of cancer cells with less harm to normal cells).

Pharmaceuticals are the leading prevention and treatment option today, and new drugs are being developed continuously. Keeping informed about these changes and learning to use and apply new equipment and techniques will be a continual and interesting challenge for the health care professional of the twenty-first century. (See Chapter 14 to learn more about continuing education in health care and Chapter 18 for discussions of technology now and in the future of health care.)

Specialization

At the beginning of the twentieth century, medicine and patient care became increasingly laboratory and science based. There was more emphasis on specialization which resulted in a loss of focus on the patient as a whole. Rather, he was broken down into various parts, each treated by a different physician. One patient might be seen by a cardiologist, gastroenterologist, and neurologist. And one physician might diagnose a problem and another do the surgery to take care of it.

In addition to the specialties of physicians, other health specialties were developed, such as physical, occupational, and speech therapy. This further increased the fragmentation of care and has had several effects on health care delivery:

- Diagnosis and treatment are improving as physicians and other practitioners concentrate on specific areas of expertise, such as endocrinology and cardiology.
- The cost of providing health care has increased.
- Long-term relationships between physicians and their patients are breaking down because one physician no longer provides all or most of the needed care.

Specialization has created many employment opportunities for health care professionals. At the same time, it has increased the need for caring attitudes and effective communication with patients. Lifelong relationships developed between physicians and their patients are rare today. Much of the care is provided to patients by professionals they do not know. Therefore, you may play an important part in helping patients understand and have confidence in the care they are receiving.

Aging Population

Improvements in medical care, especially the development of new drugs and surgical techniques, have lengthened the average life span. Life expectancy for individuals born in 1900 was 47 years. This has increased dramatically; current projected life expectancy for males is 76.1 years and 81.1 for females.

A second reason for the growing number of seniors is the continuing aging of the group known as the "baby boomers." An unusually large number of births occurred during the years following the end of World War II, starting in 1946 and lasting until 1964. These individuals have started and will continue entering their period of heaviest use of the health care system over the next 20 years. (See Figure 2–1.)

Older persons are the heaviest users of health care services. The tremendous growth of this segment of the population is putting increased demands on all types of facilities and services, including the following:

- Facilities that provide long-term care for older persons unable to live in their own homes
- Treatment and care devoted to chronic (persisting for a long time, not cured quickly) problems that develop in people who live longer
- Home care services ranging from housekeeping duties to high-level nursing care
- Care needed as a result of an increasing incidence of Alzheimer's disease (discussed later in this chapter)

FIGURE 2–1 Today's growing population of older patients is putting increasing demands on the modern health care system.

Fascinating Facts

It seems incredible that the importance of handwashing to prevent the spread of infection, a basic health care practice now taken for granted, was discovered less than 200 years ago. Ignaz Semmelweis, working in a hospital maternity ward in Vienna, became concerned about the high death rate of new mothers. He observed that it occurred most often among women who were assisted in childbirth by physicians who came directly from performing autopsies. Amazingly, his beliefs were rejected by colleagues. This is an example of how new ideas are often met with resistance and how being open to change can improve—and even save—the lives of many.

Cost of Health Care

The cost of providing health care has increased dramatically over the past few decades. While every type of product and service has steadily increased in price over the years, health care costs have grown at a faster rate than almost anything else. The affordability of health care has become a major social and political issue due to the increased literacy, availability of information, and global awareness that has increased the dissatisfaction of those unable to

Thinking It Through

Joseph Appleton's primary care physician has referred him to Dr. Nester, an oncologist (physician who specializes in diagnosis and treatment of cancer). Preliminary tests show that Mr. Appleton may have colon cancer. Mr. Appleton, age 77, is uncomfortable about visiting a specialist he has never met. He is especially distraught about the possibility of having a life-threatening illness and does not understand why the physician he has seen for many years cannot take care of the problem. Carmen Rodriguez, Dr. Nester's medical assistant, greets Mr. Appleton on his first visit to the office.

1. Discuss the changes in health care delivery that have led to the referral of patients to specialists.

2. What can Carmen do to help Mr. Appleton feel more comfortable?

access health care. The questions now being asked in the United States are, "Is health care a right or a privilege?" and "Does everyone have an equal right to health care?" (See Chapter 22, "Paying for Health Care" for more information. See Figure 2–2 to see how health care dollars are spent).

VARIETY OF APPROACHES TO HEALTH CARE

New approaches to health care are being developed due to a number of factors:

- Discoveries about the causes of disease and methods of treatment

- Access to information about the health care practices of other cultures

- Search for less invasive and less costly alternatives to surgery and drugs

- Growing interest in the use of natural products

- Belief that the mind and body are more closely connected than previously thought

- Emphasis on preventing rather than simply curing disease

- Increasing number of patients who want to assume more responsibility for their health by participating in preventive and self-care practices

- More patients conducting their own research and taking an active role in making decisions about their treatment and care through access to websites such as http://medlineplus.gov and www.mayoclinic.com

- Desire for increased humanization of medicine through touch, massage, and other hands-on methods

- Increased direct-to-consumer advertising of drugs and medical supplies and services

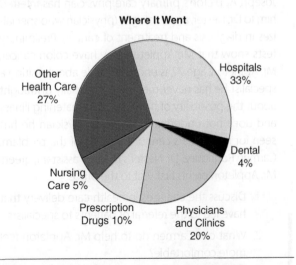

Where It Went

Hospitals 33%
Dental 4%
Physicians and Clinics 20%
Prescription Drugs 10%
Nursing Care 5%
Other Health Care 27%

FIGURE 2–2 Health care spending allocations in 2018.

Wellness

Wellness is the promotion of health through preventive measures and the practice of good health habits. There are a growing number of people who believe that more emphasis should be placed in health care on the maximization of good health. This goes beyond the traditional view of health as the absence of disease. Wellness centers have been established to offer services such as routine physicals, immunizations, nutrition and exercise classes, and educational programs on disease prevention.

An important part of the wellness concept is the emphasis on the need for patients to take responsibility for their own health. Encouraging patients and teaching them about the basic principles of health promotion and self-care are increasingly important tasks of health care professionals. This is especially important today as we find ourselves in a contradictory situation: We understand the importance of personal habits on health but at the same time are experiencing increasing rates of health risks such as obesity and lack of physical exercise. For example, heart disease, stroke, type 2 diabetes, and certain types of cancer are the leading causes of preventable, premature deaths related to obesity. Yet nearly 40% of adults in the United States are obese (https://www.cdc.gov/obesity/data/adult.html). Individuals must realize that modern medicine has limitations and that new technological advances do not guarantee that every disease can be cured and every injury repaired. On the other hand, nearly everyone can improve his or her own health and quality of life by making positive lifestyle choices. (See Chapter 12 for more information about lifestyle and health.)

Stephen Williams, a professor of public health, states it very well: "We cannot expect to be rescued from every source of morbidity [being diseased] and mortality [death] by the nation's health care system if we do not individually and collectively emphasize prevention of disease and illness in the first place" (Williams, 2005).

Some traditional health care providers are becoming more interested in extending the definition of health to mean more than the absence of disease. Margaret Newman, RN, developed a theory she calls **expanding consciousness**. She realized that many of her patients would never be "well" in the traditional sense. They would be living with an incurable disease or the results of an injury for the rest of their lives. Newman developed a nursing approach to assist patients in making their lives as meaningful as possible by focusing on their possibilities rather than on their limitations.

Holistic Medicine

Holistic medicine is a general term to designate the belief that the traditional view of medicine must be expanded. All aspects of the individual—physical, mental, emotional,

Fascinating Facts

Public health agencies were established early in our country's history, at the time of the colonies. Plymouth Colony collected vital statistics such as births and deaths. And Paul Revere, famous for his midnight ride at the beginning of the Revolutionary War, was the head of Boston's board of health in the late 1700s (Williams, 2005).

spiritual, and environmental—contribute to states of health and disease. In other words, the entire person must be considered when making therapeutic decisions. The prevention of disease, rather than simply the relief of symptoms, is emphasized. Patient education and participation in the healing process are encouraged.

There is a growing interest in holistic medicine today as evidence mounts that the mind has a powerful effect on physical health. Disorders caused by mental or emotional factors are known as **psychosomatic**. Researchers now know that these illnesses are not "all in one's head" but that physical symptoms can be the result of what is happening in the mind. It is believed that a high percentage of visits to physicians' offices are due to psychosomatic disorders.

Holistic medicine providers tend to combine traditional and nontraditional treatments and emphasize that:

- Prevention is preferable to treatment.
- Patients must accept responsibility for their own health.
- Stress is an important factor in health and should be reduced.
- Proper nutrition and exercise are essential.
- Attitude has a powerful effect, both positive and negative, on the body and its functioning.

Complementary, Alternative, and Integrative Medicine

To understand complementary and alternative medicine, we must start by differentiating it from **Western medicine** which is based on a scientific approach. A definition from the National Cancer Institute states that Western medicine is a "system in which medical doctors and other healthcare professionals (such as nurses, pharmacists, and therapists) treat symptoms and diseases using drugs, radiation, or surgery." Another broader definition is that Western medicine focuses on pathology and curing disease.

Complementary medicine comprises methods other than those traditionally used in Western medicine, but are used *together with* Western medicine. One example is using meditation, along with medication, to help patients lower their blood pressure. **Alternative medicine** refers to practices used *instead of* Western medicine. An example is when a patient chooses to use acupuncture rather than surgery to treat back pain. The National Center for Complementary and Integrative Health (NCCIH) reports that the use of true alternative medicine is not common; most people combine non-mainstream with conventional Western medical practices.

Integrative medicine is the term used when a health care provider offers a combination of Western medicine with complementary and alternative medicine. For example, a patient receiving chemotherapy for cancer may be prescribed meditation and nutritional supplements to manage symptoms and side effects (NCCIH, 2018). Table 2–2 lists the wide variety of nontraditional approaches to health care.

Complementary and alternative medicine (CAM) may provide a more holistic approach by treating not only the body, but also the mind, spirit, and emotions. Lifestyle changes to prevent and cure diseases are likely to be recommended, along with a wide range of practices such as using herbs and plants to treat symptoms, teaching patients meditation as a way to promote healing, and acknowledging the influence of the mind on physical symptoms. Although many health care providers do not accept the claims made for these techniques, a growing number of Western-style trained physicians, nurses, and others are conducting studies and adopting methods that were once considered to be unscientific and ineffective.

Nearly 40% of Americans use some form of complementary medicine. Table 2–3 lists the ten most common complementary methods used in 2012. Methods once considered to be alternative, such as massage, are increasingly being incorporated into treatment plans. Health care professionals are likely to come into contact with one or more forms of complementary or alternative medicine. Patients may ask opinions about something they have heard about; a friend or family member may seek these services; or their employer may be exploring the use of integrative medicine. Because the effectiveness and safety of many popular nontraditional therapies have not been proven, it is important for health care professionals to be aware of the various forms of complementary and alternative therapies so they can make intelligent decisions and direct patients to reliable sources of information where they can learn more for themselves. It is recommended that you inform yourself through reading, attending workshops and seminars, and asking questions. The NCCIH, part of the National Institutes of Health, is a reliable source of information and can be accessed at https://nccih.nih.gov.

Table 2–2 Complementary and Alternative Approaches to Health

Category	Examples
Whole Medical Systems *Complete systems of theory and practice*	• Homeopathic medicine: assist the body to heal itself of symptoms by giving very small quantities of a substance that produces the symptoms ("like cures like"). • Naturopathic medicine: assist the body to use its own healing power with methods such as exercise and medicinal plants. • Traditional Chinese medicine: ancient system based on balancing and maintaining the body's vital energy flow ("qi," pronounced "chee"); treatments include acupuncture and herbs. • Ayurveda: 5,000-year-old system practiced in India; treatments include herbs, massage, and yoga.
Mind–Body Medicine *Enhance the mind's influence on the body*	• Patient support groups • Meditation • Prayer • Guided imagery • Creative outlets, such as art and music • Yoga
Natural Products *Use substances found in nature*	• Aromatherapy: scent of essential oils from plants is inhaled • Herbs • Dietary supplements • Use of natural products, such as shark cartilage
Manipulative and Body-Based Practices *Move parts of the body to regain health and function* (Manipulation: controlled force to a joint beyond its normal range of motion)	• Chiropractic manipulation • Osteopathic manipulation • Massage • Reflexology: application of pressure to parts of the feet that are believed to be connected to specific parts of the body • Relaxation exercises

Energy Therapies
 	
Involve the use of energy fields and pathways
	• Biofield therapies: manipulate the fields of energy believed to surround and penetrate the body; practitioners use their hands to channel and balance this energy. Therapies include:
	   ◦ Qi gong: combines movement, meditation, and controlled breathing
	   ◦ Reiki: practitioners attempt to transmit universal energy to a person to heal the spirit and thus the body
	   ◦ Therapeutic (healing) touch: patient's energy field is altered when energy is passed from the practitioner's hands to the patient
	• Bioelectromagnetic-based therapies: unconventional use of electromagnetic fields, such as using magnets to relieve pain

CAM is particularly susceptible to health fraud, the deceptive sale or advertising of services and products that claim to be effective against various health conditions. The U.S. Food and Drug Administration (FDA) considers the following to be signs that a product may be fraudulent:

• Claims that the product is a quick, effective cure for a wide variety of health problems

• Suggests that the product is based on a "scientific breakthrough," "miraculous cure," or "secret ingredient"

• Uses text with impressive-sounding terms that are not defined elsewhere

• Provides undocumented case histories of amazing results

• Has limited availability and requires payment in advance

Table 2–3 Ten Most Common Complementary Health Approaches Among Adults—2012

Approach	Percentage of U.S. Adults Who Used
Natural Products (Includes vitamins, minerals, and probiotics)	17.7%
Deep Breathing	10.9%
Yoga, Tai Chi, Qi Gong	10.1%
Chiropractic and Osteopathic	8.4%
Meditation	8.0%
Massage	6.9%
Special Diets	3.0%
Homeopathy	2.2%
Progressive Relaxation	2.1%
Guided Imagery	1.7%

Source: https://nccih.nih.gov/health/integrative-health

Certain diseases and conditions are frequently the targets of false remedies. These include cancer, AIDS, arthritis, obesity and overweight, sexual dysfunction, and diabetes. Patients should be warned to check with their health care provider and to research the advice of government agencies, such as the FDA, before purchasing remedies online. Not only are many substances useless, some can be dangerous and cause serious health problems.

Osteopathy and Chiropractic

Osteopathy and chiropractic health care practices have become so widely accepted that they are no longer generally considered to be alternative. **Osteopathy** is based on the belief that the body can protect itself against disease if the musculoskeletal system, especially the spine, is in good order. The importance of good nutrition and favorable environmental conditions is also emphasized. Osteopathic physicians receive training that is similar to that of traditional doctors of medicine (MDs). They can prescribe drugs, perform surgeries, and have staff privileges at most hospitals. Osteopaths take the same state licensing examinations as MDs.

Chiropractic is based on the belief that pressure on the nerves leaving the spinal column causes pain or dysfunction of the body part served by that nerve. Treatment involves manipulation of the spine to correct misalignments. Chiropractors are not allowed to prescribe drugs, but may recommend nutritional and herbal remedies. Every state has licensure requirements for chiropractors. (See Figure 2–3.)

© SpeedKingz/Shutterstock.com.

FIGURE 2–3 Osteopaths, chiropractors, and physical therapists may include manipulation of the joints as part of a treatment plan.

Massage Therapy

Massage therapy is widely recognized, when administered by a trained practitioner, as a beneficial health practice. It involves using pressure or friction on the body. By enabling the muscles to relax, massage therapy promotes better blood circulation, faster healing of injuries, and pain relief. It is often recommended to supplement other forms of therapy and to provide an effective method of stress relief. Many types of formal training programs are available for people who wish to practice massage therapy. Most states and localities require therapists to be licensed.

Naturopathy

Naturopathic medicine is based on the belief that the human body has its own natural healing ability. Naturopathic doctors (NDs) teach their patients to use diet, exercise, lifestyle changes and cutting-edge natural therapies to enhance their bodies' ability to ward off and combat disease. They combine traditional medicine and natural remedies when developing treatment plans for their. Naturopathic physicians seek the causes of symptoms and believe the whole person, not just the symptoms, must be treated. Twenty states, the District of Columbia, and the U.S. territories of Puerto Rico, and the U.S. Virgin Islands have licensing laws for naturopathic doctors.

Homeopathy

Homeopathy is a method of treatment developed by a German physician in the early 1800s based on the idea of stimulating the body's own healing responses. Disorders are treated with very small amounts of the natural substances that cause the symptoms of the disorder in healthy people. For example, exposure to onions causes the same runny nose and eyes as are experienced with a head cold. Therefore, very diluted amounts of plants in the onion family are administered to treat cold symptoms. Belladonna,

secured from a poisonous European plant, is widely used in homeopathy to treat a variety of symptoms, including pain. It has been used in traditional medicine to dilate the pupils to facilitate examination of the eyes. Homeopathy has been practiced in Europe and India for more than 200 years and is used by some medical professionals in the United States. Three states—Arizona, Connecticut, and Nevada—require practitioners of homeopathy to be licensed by their states' homeopathic licensing boards.

Energy Theories

Theories about the existence and importance of body energy originated in Asia thousands of years ago. There is growing interest today in therapies that claim to encourage the free flow of energy throughout the body. This flow, it is believed, is necessary to promote and maintain good health. Acupuncture may be the oldest application of this theory. Developed by the Chinese more than 5,000 years ago, it involves the insertion of tiny needles into specific points in the body to relieve energy blocks. This treatment is becoming accepted in the United States as people who receive it find at least short-term relief from various health problems.

THE FUTURE OF HEALTH CARE

The most significant change predicted for the way health care is practiced is called personalized medicine or precision medicine. Rather than treating diseases and conditions based on standard treatments used on all patients for the specific *condition*, prevention, diagnosis, and treatment will be based on each patient's *own biochemical makeup*. This approach is being made possible by advances in genomic research or DNA sequencing that allow health care providers to see the biochemical variations that make every human body unique. So far, scientists have cataloged 665 million gene variants (Smith, 2019).

The implications of these findings are significant and provide hope for curing diseases such as cancer. Treatments traditionally have been based on the type of cancer, chosen because they have benefited some patients. In personalized medicine, the genes of the patient's tumors are analyzed to learn which treatments will be most effective. Already there have been success stories of advanced cancer being cured using this approach.

In 2015, President Obama launched the Precision Medicine Initiative to provide resources for further research. The Initiative's mission statement reads:

> To enable a new era of medicine through research, technology, and policies that empower patients, researchers, and providers to work together toward development of individualized care.

CHALLENGES IN HEALTH CARE TODAY

The tremendous medical progress made during the last century continues into the new millennium. At the same time, our country faces many challenges in effectively delivering the results of this progress to all who need it. These challenges represent complex problems that affect millions of people. Problems of this size are not easy to solve and finding solutions that satisfy the needs of everyone is very difficult. Some diseases, such as Alzheimer's, remain without a cure. Others, such as cancer, are sometimes curable and sometimes not, despite years of research and testing.

It is important for the health care professionals to be aware of major health care issues. They will affect where and how you perform your job, as well as influence your relationships with patients and other members of the health care team.

Providing Affordable Health Care

In response to the fact that millions of Americans lacked health insurance, the Patient Protection and Affordable Care Act was signed into law in 2010. (The law is discussed in more detail in Chapter 22.) However, the insurance that Americans can now purchase is sometimes expensive and may come with deductibles of several thousand dollars. This situation is especially challenging for the unemployed and the working poor (people who are employed but work part-time and do not qualify for employer-provided health insurance). It is even out of reach for many middle-class Americans, with reportedly one-third unable to afford required deductibles (Altman, 2015). Although government subsidies are available for millions of Americans, the high cost of health care still presents a problem for many individuals. The act is also politically controversial and the federal administration at the time of this writing has repealed parts of the act making it less economically feasible. Future administrations will continue to face the challenge of providing adequate health care.

Another group that struggles with health care costs are low-income seniors. Medicare, a government-run insurance program for persons age 65 and older and the disabled, pays for only 80% of certain costs and many seniors cannot afford to purchase supplemental insurance to cover the remaining 20%, which can be substantial for a major health event.

A potential problem with government subsidies is that when not enough taxes can be collected to support the costs, services must be cut. This is an especially serious concern when the economy is weak and unemployment is high, which results in decreased tax revenues. Many economists are warning that the Medicare trust fund is in danger of running out of funding; depending on the source, the years when this may happen range from 2026 to 2029.

Thinking It Through

Craig Oakley is a physical therapy assistant who does home visits for a rehabilitation service. One of his patients, Mr. Singh, suffers from rheumatoid arthritis and has asked Craig's opinion about taking Chinese herbal remedies that he has read help restore joint health.

1. How should Craig respond?
2. What are some of the resources he can consult in order to find out more about the treatment?
3. What precautions should Craig follow when speaking with Mr. Singh about complementary and alternative therapies?

The problem is worsened by fraudulent claims paid out by Medicare. Although sources vary widely in estimates ranging from $17 billion to more than $100 billion in losses, it is known that many false claims are paid out each year. The Federal Bureau of Investigation is the primary agency for exposing and investigating health care fraud and penalties have been increased recently. It is hoped that the combination of cutting fraudulent claims for Medicare reimbursement, raising taxes, and promoting efficiencies in the delivery of health care will support the future costs of the health care system. (See Chapter 22 for more information.)

Providing Long-Term Care

The increasing population of older persons, discussed previously, means that a growing number of people will need some sort of care as they age and experience health problems. As a result of medical advances, many people are living beyond their ability to care for themselves. Some suffer from chronic conditions and require 24-hour nursing care. (See Figure 2–4.)

The costs of nursing facilities and other long-term care housing are increasing as much as 5% annually. The cost varies widely from state to state. Table 2–4 gives the annual median costs in 2018 for various types of long-term care.

Covering these costs will be a challenge. Medicare currently covers only short-term stays in a nursing home following a hospitalization and provides no coverage for assisted living. Long-term care insurance is available, but because of the increasingly high expense of paying for care, many insurance companies no longer sell this type of policy, and those that do, charge more for coverage than many Americans can afford. The states' Medicaid programs cover nursing home care, but it is not known if there will be adequate funding to cover the projected rise in expenses. (Medicaid is a federally funded program for low-income individuals.)

Table 2–4 Annual Costs of Long-Term Care Services

Type of Service	Cost
Homemaker services	$48,048
Home health aide	$50,336
Adult day health care	$18,720
Assisted living facility	$48,000
Nursing home	
Semi-private room	$89,297
Private room	$100,375

Source: https://www.genworth.com/aging-and-you/finances/cost-of-care.html

FIGURE 2–4 Health care professionals can help seniors live the highest quality of life possible as they age.

Improving Social Conditions

Many social problems affect the country's health care delivery systems, resulting in health disparities, differences in the health status of different groups of people. For example, the 16% of Americans who do not graduate from high school have a higher rate of health problems than those who do finish high school. People living in poor neighborhoods that lack grocery stores, farmers' markets, and safe outdoor space for children to play and adults to walk experience higher rates of obesity, diabetes, and related health conditions.

Homelessness is a problem in many cities as people without other means of shelter erect tents on streets and in parks and in spaces such as bridge underpasses. Here they are exposed to inclement weather, lack of sanitation, and communicable diseases such as tuberculosis. Conditions such as diabetes, high blood pressure, and asthma worsen when treatment and medications are not available. In 2018, Los Angeles experienced an outbreak of typhus that originated in homeless camps infested by rats that carry infection-bearing fleas.

A sad result of poverty and other social problems is that those who most need health care services are the least able to pay for them, even when governmental and other services are available. People who do not seek preventive care and practice good health habits are more likely to develop serious conditions that result in more suffering as well as higher expenses for the health care system. Table 2–5 lists a number of social conditions that can result in negative consequences for individual health, as well as for health care delivery systems.

Eliminating Racism in Health Care

Racial and ethnic minority groups suffer more health problems and have shorter life expectancies compared with the overall population of the country. In addition to social factors, there is discrimination in the health care system that often results in a lower quality of care. This is due in part to racial discrimination as well as misperceptions about physical differences. One study revealed that some educated health care providers had false beliefs about biological differences between African Americans and Caucasians leading to systematically undertreating African Americans for pain (https://www.ncbi.nlm.nih.gov/pmc/articles /PMC4843483/). Although most health care professionals are not consciously racist, racism and discrimination are deeply ingrained in the social, political, and economic structures of our society (https://www.health.harvard. edu/blog/racism-discrimination-health-care-providers-patients-2017011611015). As a result, many Americans have limited access to good housing, livable wages, quality

schools, and other factors that contribute to good health. As discussed in Chapter 15, the first step in eliminating racism is to acknowledge that it exists, often in the form of **implicit racism** (outside of our consciousness). This is not easy, but it will be the first step in achieving health equity for all Americans.

Maintaining the Quality of Care

The skyrocketing costs of health care have prompted all levels of government, as well as providers of health care, to initiate cost controls. This has caused widespread concern that quality of care is being sacrificed to cut expenses. A related area of concern is that for-profit insurance and health care organizations may emphasize profits more than providing high-quality patient care. Complaints reported by residents in nursing homes, discussed later in this section, may be related to the growth of for-profit facilities.

Some current methods of paying physicians and other providers for their services encourage them to provide less rather than more care. Reviewers who work on behalf of insurance companies make many decisions about patient care. The purpose is to determine whether the proposed procedures are medically necessary and whether lower-cost alternatives are available. Permission is required in advance for certain procedures, a process called "**preauthorization**." Reviewers may or may not have the specific medical training needed to understand and approve the requested test or treatment. Many decisions are based on what is known about the "average patient"

Table 2–5 Social Conditions That Affect Health and Health Care Systems

Condition	Impact on Health and Health Care System
Breakdown of Family Unit and Children Born to Single Women	Poverty among women and children. Lack of access to prenatal care, immunizations for children, and other preventive measures
Homelessness	Lack of access to medical care. Malnutrition and poor hygiene. Difficult to contact patient for follow-up care. An increasing number of families and children now number among the homeless
Violence	Use of emergency and other health care services. Inability of many victims to pay
Substance Abuse	Increased violence and susceptibility to disease. Inability to care for self and family
Spousal and Child Abuse	Need for health and protective services. Use of emergency department services for injuries
Poverty and Malnutrition	Poor health and inability to access health care. Lack of prenatal care
An increasing Number of Americans Live Alone	Need outside assistance when ill or injured. Lack of emotional support

Sources: Adapted from Essentials of Health Services, *by S. J. Williams, 2005, Clifton Park, NY: Delmar Cengage Learning. U.S. Census Bureau, www.census.gov/Press-Release /www/releases/archives/families_households/006840.html* under the same or similar circumstances and reviewers can make a variety of decisions. For example, they can:

- Approve the procedure as recommended by the physician
- Deny the procedure
- Require surgery to be performed as an outpatient service (patient does not occupy a bed in the facility, such as a hospital)
- Approve a different, usually less-costly method
- Approve a limited number of treatments

Under the Patient Protection and Affordable Care Act, patients have the right to appeal a health insurance company's decision to deny payment for a claim or to terminate their health coverage. However, the process required may discourage many patients or, if they proceed, may result in delays before they can receive the care their provider believes they need.

Many physicians feel they have lost control of the practice of medicine to business interests or government agencies, such as the Centers for Medicare and Medicaid. Accustomed to having the authority to make decisions about the best care for their patients, they are frustrated by what they see as interference from inadequately trained personnel or those with financial interests.

Patients, in turn, believe the decisions of their physicians are being questioned and have concerns about the resulting quality of care. They worry that they are being denied needed procedures and treatments and that their health is being sacrificed for financial reasons.

At the same time, other health care experts point out that the number of unnecessary surgeries and other procedures, especially those used for diagnosis, have decreased. They believe that patient care has not suffered but has actually been improved by efforts to prevent the overuse of available techniques.

Another area of concern is the quality of the nation's nursing homes. Many for-profit facilities have been accused of providing inadequate care in order to raise profits. To address this issue, in 2015 the federal government raised its rating standards for more than 15,000 facilities providing nursing care, almost 11,000 of which are for-profit businesses. Criteria for these ratings include adequate staffing at appropriate professional levels, health and fire safety measures, and quality of care (lack of pressure sores in patients, etc.). The rate of turnover in nursing homes and other long-term care facilities tends to be very high. The public has access to the ratings of nursing homes nationwide at www.medicare.gov/NursingHomeCompare. Improvements are still needed as shown by the following statistic: In 2015, 21% of nursing homes received deficiencies for serious quality violations (https://www.kff.org/medicaid/issue-brief/key-issues-in-long-term-services-and-supports-quality/).

The health care professionals who fill the many future jobs in long-term care facilities need to be aware of the government oversight of these facilities. Restoring confidence in the system, while at the same time controlling costs, is a major challenge to ensuring good quality of care. As a health care professional, you can help restore confidence in long-term care by having respect for and providing the best care possible to America's elderly and disabled patients.

Treating Alzheimer's and Other Forms of Dementia

Dementia is a condition marked by a decline in memory and/or other thinking skills, caused by damage to the nerve cells in the brain. **Alzheimer's disease** is the most common dementia, accounting for 60% to 80% of cases. Alzheimer's is a progressive disease that eventually affects basic body functions and results in death. It is now ranked as the sixth leading cause of death in the United States.

Alzheimer's is increasingly challenging the health care system's ability to handle the growing number of cases. As the population ages and people live longer because of advances in treating other diseases, more and more Americans are being diagnosed with this disease: one in nine individuals age 65 and over and one in three people age 85 and over. In 2018, an estimated 5.7 million Americans had Alzheimer's and this number is expected to grow to 8.4 million in 2030 and 16 million in 2050 (https://www.cdc.gov/features/alzheimers-disease-deaths/index.html).

The need for care of dementia patients in terms of appropriate facilities and cost is of concern. Two-thirds of patients with Alzheimer's live their last years or months in a nursing home. At the same time, few can afford the cost of this care so payment is made by government programs, such as Medicare and Medicaid. When last reported, Medicare and Medicaid paid $175 billion for Alzheimer's care. According to the Alzheimer's Association, it is "one of the costliest chronic diseases to society," going so far as to say that treating the disease could eventually bankrupt Medicare. The cost of treating Alzheimer's in 2018 may have reached $277 billion.

There is a growing need for trained caregivers to work with patients suffering from dementia. Patience, understanding, and the knowledge to safeguard individuals who have difficulty communicating and are experiencing changing patterns of behavior are required. These changes can include the inability to recognize themselves or others, fear and anxiety, and paranoia. While the work can be challenging, it can also be very satisfying to help provide the best possible quality of life for some of our society's most vulnerable members.

Addressing Public Health Concerns

The United States faces challenges in its efforts to safeguard the health of the public. Monitoring and researching health issues must be ongoing. For example, although most infectious diseases are under control in this country, there are increasing concerns about a pandemic occurring in the near future. The global outbreak in 2009 of influenza caused by the H1N1 virus demonstrated how difficult it can be to respond quickly as the United States encountered slow-downs in its efforts to develop an effective vaccine. More recently, the 2017–2018 flu season was reported as the worst on record with an estimated 900,000 hospitalizations and 80,000 deaths. (See Chapter 10 for information about infection control.)

Encouraging Medication Adherence

Medication adherence means taking medications correctly: the right dosage at the right time and as often as prescribed. Approximately two-thirds of Americans have prescribed medications but as many as 50% do not take their medications as directed. The failure of medication adherence in the United States accounts for up to $300 billion in annual preventable medical costs and 125,000 deaths annually. Recent studies show that although the high cost of medications and a fear of their side effects account for nonadherence, for 69% it was inattention: Patients forget to take them or procrastinate getting prescriptions refilled, thus failing to get them on time. An underlying problem may be related to communication: Patients do not understand the purpose and importance of their medications and/or how to take them. As the CDC states, "Communication is the key!" (CDC, 2013). Chapters 15 and 16 contain information about how health care professionals can better communicate with patients and help them to understand why it is important for them to take their medications and the possible negative consequences of failing to take them. (See Figure 2–5.)

Managing the Opioid Crisis

A health care challenge that is the opposite of nonadherence is the overuse of painkillers. Starting in the late 1990s, pharmaceutical companies heavily promoted **opioid pain medications** (drugs that contain addictive substances, such as heroin), reassuring health care providers that they were not addictive. Believing the drug companies and to help their patients, providers increased the number of prescriptions for painkillers. Unfortunately, opioid painkillers turned out to be extremely addictive and have resulted in what the U.S. Department of Health and Human Services (HHS) is calling a public health emergency.

FIGURE 2–5 Prescription medications are the most used treatment in the United States, but must be used as directed—no more and no less.

Millions of Americans are now addicted, experiencing overdoses, and dying. In 2017, 47,600 people died from opioid overdoses, an average of 130 each day.

The HHS has identified five specific strategies to fight the crisis:

- Improving access to treatment and recovery services;
- Promoting the use of overdose-reversing drugs;
- Strengthening our understanding of the epidemic through better public health surveillance;
- Providing support for cutting edge research on pain and addiction; and
- Advancing better practices for pain management.

Other measures being taken to prevent overdoses and death include the following:

- Creating safe prescribing guidelines for providers
- Regulating pain clinics
- Identifying fraudulent prescriptions
- Teaching patients other methods for controlling pain
- Educating patients about the risks of opioid pain medications
- Improving access to naloxone, the antidote to opioid overdose

Preventing Antibiotic Resistance

Antibiotics are drugs that fight infections caused by bacteria. They are not effective against viruses, the microorganisms that cause colds and flu as well as other illnesses.

Antibiotic resistance occurs when the bacteria the drugs target mutate, which means they change in ways that reduce or eliminate the effectiveness of antibiotics to destroy them. Antibiotic resistance is one of our most serious health threats, causing 2 million illnesses and 23,000 deaths each year (https://medlineplus.gov/magazine/issues/winter18/articles/winter18pg8-11.html). This is because as bacteria become resistant, they are increasingly difficult or even impossible to treat. Drug-resistant organisms are discussed in more detail in Chapter 10.

Preventing Suicides

Since 1999, the suicide rate in the United States has increased by 30%. In 2016, there were almost 45,000 suicides. These occurred among all ages and economic and social groups and rank as the tenth leading cause of death overall and the second leading cause among young people, aged 10 to 34. In addition to the emotional cost to family and friends, a recent study reported that suicides and suicide attempts cost $93.5 billion in medical and work and productivity costs (https://www.sprc.org/about-suicide/costs). Other statistics with implications for health care providers:

- In a study of 5,000 people who died by suicide, 83% had a health care visit within the previous year.
- About 2,500 of these people did not have a documented mental health diagnosis.
- About 50% had a health care visit within 30 days of death, most without a mental health diagnosis (https://acpinternist.org/archives/2018/10/preventing-suicide-in-primary-care.htm).

In spite of these numbers, according to some researchers, suicide prevention has not been a core priority in health care. There have been strategies developed recently, but they are not yet widely used. To help prevent these tragedies, a program called Zero Suicide has been developed as a model for better identification and treatment by health care providers (https://www.healthaffairs.org/doi/full/10.1377/hlthaff.2015.1672).

The CDC advises that suicide is often preventable and lists the following warning signs: expressing hopelessness, threatening to hurt oneself or talking about wanting to die, increasing alcohol and drug use, and withdrawing from friends and family. If a patient speaks to you about suicide or you suspect that a patient may be contemplating suicide, report this to your supervisor immediately. You may be the link that can save a life.

Dealing with TV Prescription Drug Ads

Television ads for prescription drugs have greatly increased in number over the past several years. One source reports that average viewers may see up to 30 hours of drug ads annually, while spending as little as 20 minutes during that same period with their primary care physicians (https://www.sciencedaily.com/releases/2013/09/130916140455.htm). Health care providers, including physicians and pharmacists, believe that drugs should not be advertised, especially on television. In 2015, the American Medical Association called for a ban because many physicians believe the ads are dangerous: The information is not complete and/or accurate and the medications advertised may not be the most appropriate for a patient's condition. Another problem is that medical conditions are often complex and the simple solutions presented do not give patients all the information they need. When urged to "ask your doctor about drug X," patients may assume that it is right for them and feel short changed if their physicians recommend something else.

Drug advertising also adds to the burdensome cost of health care in the United States, discussed previously. In 2016, advertising costs were $6.4 billion, which adds to the already high cost of prescription drugs in the United States.

As a result of these concerns, all but two developing countries—the United States and New Zealand—ban drug ads. In the United States, two factors may account for the ads remaining on television: a broad interpretation of free speech laws and the efforts of the multibillion-dollar pharmaceutical industry.

HEALTH CARE FACILITIES AND SERVICES

A wide variety of health care facilities are available that offer many services for patients with all types of needs. They range in size from a private physician's office to nationwide health care systems that include hospitals, clinics, and long-term care facilities. (See Figure 2–6.) Health care facilities offer many kinds of services, ranging from preventive care to emergency treatment; from routine physical exams to in-home assistance for dying patients. There are many kinds of employment settings for today's health care professional.

Hospitals

Hospitals are the traditional facilities for the care of the ill and injured. The following conditions accounted for the majority of hospital admissions in 2015: births, pneumonia, osteoarthritis (fractures), heart attack and congestive heart failure, septicemia, mood disorders, cardiac dysrhythmias (abnormal heart beat), and chronic obstructive pulmonary disease (COPD) (https://www.hcup-us.ahrq.gov/faststats/NationalDiagnosesServlet). In the past, most patients remained in the hospital for all care needed until they were

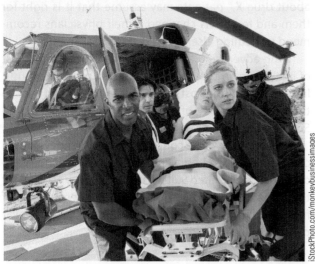

FIGURE 2–6 Health care professionals are employed in a wide variety of settings.

able to return home. However, the cost of hospital care has increased so dramatically that other means of patient care have been developed to limit the number and length of patient stays. Hospitals are now just one of many facilities that provide patient care.

The trend is for hospitals to be high-tech facilities that specialize in serving patients who need sophisticated treatment and 24-hour nursing care. The various levels of care offered by hospitals include the following:

- **Trauma center:** Offers comprehensive services for life-threatening injuries. Specific criteria must be met to qualify as a trauma center, such as having certain sophisticated diagnostic equipment and trauma surgeons available.

- **Emergency department:** Treats conditions that occur suddenly and require immediate attention. Examples include serious injuries from accidents and heart attacks.

- **Intensive care unit (ICU):** Provides specialized equipment and continuous care and monitoring for patients with serious illnesses or injuries. Offers continuous nursing care with one or two patients per nurse.

- **Cardiac care unit (CCU):** Provides specialized equipment and continuous care and monitoring for patients with serious heart conditions. Offers continuous nursing care with one or two patients per nurse.

- **Definitive observation unit or step-down unit:** Offers continuous nursing care for patients who are less critical than ICU patients.

- **General unit:** Provides care for patients who are seriously ill but do not need a high level of specialized equipment and continuous nursing care. There may be ten or more patients per nurse.

  ○ Surgical floor: Provides care for patients recovering from surgery.

  ○ Medical floor: Provides care for patients with conditions such as infections and diabetes.

- **Transitional care unit (TCU):** Provides lower-level care while patients' needs are assessed and arrangements made to release patients to return home or enter another care facility.

Some hospitals also have rehabilitation units, which provide treatment for musculoskeletal, neurological, and orthopedic conditions. Rehabilitation focuses on helping patients regain as high a level of normal function as possible.

Other hospitals offer specialized care for certain populations, such as children, or specific conditions, such as burns or psychiatric conditions. **Psychiatric hospitals** offer treatment to individuals with psychiatric and behavioral disorders, including assistance with crises, medication management, counseling, and monitoring of activities of daily living. Patients may be treated on an outpatient or **inpatient** (hospitalized) basis, depending on their needs.

The modern hospital faces the challenge of controlling expenses and at the same time maintaining a certain occupancy rate (number of patients) in order to meet its operating costs. A variety of approaches have been developed to resolve this conflict:

- Diversification of services. Examples include offering rehabilitation, outpatient surgery, and long-term care in lower-tech wings or separate buildings.
- Elimination of services that duplicate those offered at nearby hospitals.
- Merging with other hospitals to share expenses and avoid duplication of services.
- Joining a large health care system that also operates clinics, nursing homes, diagnostic centers, home health agencies, and so on.
- Being purchased by a national corporation that owns and manages many hospitals.

A problem faced by some hospitals is the number of insured individuals who use emergency departments to receive care that could be provided by a clinic, physician, or other less costly provider. By law, emergency departments must give basic needed care. In many cases, patients who cannot afford routine care wait until their condition is critical before seeking help. What might be a $250 visit to a physician becomes a $2,500 emergency-department expense for which the hospital is not reimbursed. Some hospitals, unable to afford the burden of providing free care, have closed their emergency departments. Others have set up hospital clinics that offer basic care to walk-in patients. This problem is being somewhat relieved by the Patient Protection and Affordable Care Act (discussed in Chapter 22) that has helped millions of Americans obtain health insurance. A remaining problem, however, is educating patients who have never had health insurance to seek primary care physicians and not rely on emergency departments for routine and nonemergency care.

Changes will continue to be made as hospitals seek ways to control costs and at the same time provide adequate services for the communities they serve. Maintaining quality of care is another concern, and 82% of hospitals are accredited by the Joint Commission, the private, nonprofit organization whose purpose is to encourage the attainment of high standards of institutional medical care. It establishes guidelines for the operation of hospitals and other facilities, such as ambulatory surgery centers, long-term care facilities, and laboratories, and conducts inspections to ensure that standards are being met.

Health care professionals who are employed at facilities approved by the Joint Commission should become familiar with the standards that regulate the duties and areas for which they are responsible. Being accredited is very important because Medicare and many insurance companies will not pay for services provided at nonaccredited facilities.

Ambulatory Services

Ambulatory services are for patients who do not require hospitalization. Also known as outpatient services, they are provided by the many diagnostic, treatment, and rehabilitation facilities that account for most patient care activities. Many procedures that were previously performed in hospitals are now done on an outpatient basis. For example, a growing number of surgeries are now performed in ambulatory surgery centers with some patients being discharged 1–3 hours after surgery.

The physician's office is the location of the majority of ambulatory services. Ambulatory care is also provided by comprehensive facilities that offer a variety of services. A large clinic, for example, may have on-site radiographic and laboratory services. Other freestanding facilities offer one type of specialized service, such as an imaging center that only performs X-rays, ultrasound, and other imaging procedures. These facilities accept patients on a referral basis from professionals, such as physicians and nurse practitioners. Table 2–6 lists common ambulatory settings and their services.

Long-Term Care Facilities

Various forms of long-term care are available for people who do not need to be hospitalized but are unable to live at home. This is one of the fastest growing areas in health care and offers an increasing number of services for patients and employment opportunities for health care professionals. There are many types of long-term care:

- Nursing homes: There are two types of facilities commonly referred to as nursing homes:
  - Skilled nursing facility (SNF): Provides nursing and rehabilitation services on a 24-hour basis. Includes regular medical care for patients with long-term illnesses and those recovering from illness, injury, or surgery.
  - Intermediate nursing care facility (INCF): Provides personal care, social services, and nursing supervision for at least 8 hours per day. It provides care for individuals who do not require 24-hour nursing, but are unable to care for themselves.
- Adult foster home: Provides 24-hour personal care and supervision for a small number of residents (five is typically allowed by state regulations) in a family-type home or similar setting.
- Assisted living residence: Provides housing, meals, and personal care to individuals who need help with

Table 2–6 Ambulatory Facilities

Facility	Services Offered
Adult Day Care	Activities, meals, and supervision for adults who need assistance, such as older persons and persons who are developmentally disabled
Dental Offices	Prevention, diagnosis, and treatment of problems with the teeth
Diagnostic Centers	Procedures, such as radiography, to determine the cause and nature of diseases and injuries
Emergency and Urgent Care Centers	Care for conditions that need immediate attention
Health Care Services in Companies, Schools, and Prisons	Basic and preventive care for employees, students, and prisoners
Laboratories	Clinical labs draw blood and collect urine and other samples, and perform tests that provide information needed to diagnose, treat, or prevent disease. Dental labs make false teeth, crowns, and corrective devices for the mouth
Medical Offices	Prevention, diagnosis, and treatment of all types of health conditions
Rehabilitation Centers	Therapies to help patients regain maximum physical and mental function; types include physical, occupational, speech, and hearing. Specialized centers help patients overcome problems with substance abuse
Specialty Clinics and Offices	Treatment for specific conditions such as cancer and venereal disease; rehabilitative services such as hand therapy, psychological counseling, and many others
Surgical Centers	Outpatient surgeries that do not require hospitalization
Wellness Centers	Routine physicals; preventive measures such as immunizations; educational programs about nutrition, exercise, and so on

daily living activities but do not need daily nursing care. The level of assistance provided depends on individual needs. This type of residence is also known by other names, such as supportive housing, residential long-term care facilities, adult residential care facilities, board-and-care, and rest homes.

- **Continuing care community:** Provides a variety of living arrangements that support lifestyles as they change from independent living to the need for regular medical and nursing care. Additional services, such as meals and daily nurse visits, can be contracted for as required.

Providing quality care for an aging population will be one of society's biggest challenges in the coming decades. The expense of such care is not covered by Medicare, except for short periods of time in a nursing home under certain conditions. The burden on individuals can be heavy, as the average cost of a skilled nursing home ranges from $82,128 to $92,376 annually; in some states, the cost is as high as $138,000. Long-term care insurance policies are available, but many people do not purchase these because of the relatively high cost or their inability to qualify for a

policy. Other challenges include improving and maintaining the quality of care in long-term care facilities so that older Americans can live out their lives in a supportive, non-warehousing environment.

Home Health Care Providers

The provision of home health services is growing rapidly with various levels of services and care being provided to patients in their homes. Several factors have caused this need:

- Shorter hospital stays
- Increase in the older population
- Advances in equipment that allow more technical procedures to be carried out in the home
- Desire of individuals to remain in their homes as they age

A wide range of professionals deliver care to patients in their homes:

- **Registered and practical/licensed vocational nurses:** Educate patients about self-care; administer medications, including intravenous (IV) therapy (administered through the veins); check progress; and change dressings, check the healing of wounds, and remove sutures following surgery.

- Physical therapists and physical therapist assistants: Recommend and teach physical exercises, work with patients to increase physical stamina and movement, monitor progress following injury or surgery.
- Occupational therapists and occupational therapy assistants: Assist patients in attaining maximum function and performing activities of daily living (ADLs), such as eating, bathing, and toileting, as independently as possible.
- Speech therapists: Help patients recover speech and ability to swallow.
- Medical social workers: Provide supportive counseling, assist with financial planning and arranging for in-home help or placement in the appropriate facility.
- Certified nursing assistants/home health aides: Provide personal care, such as bathing and grooming, and follow care plans developed and monitored by a registered nurse or other designated professional.

Medicare pays for medically related home health services only when it is expected that the person who is homebound will improve and recover. Although nonmedical services are also available to help individuals with shopping, cooking, cleaning, and other housekeeping tasks, these are not considered medical in nature and are not usually covered by health insurance plans.

Some of the occupations showing the largest numerical increase in employment involve home health care. At the same time, quality of care becomes a concern when health care providers work in off-site locations without direct supervision. In response to these concerns, states require the licensing of home health agencies. The types of care that may be performed in the home by various health care personnel are strictly regulated by both state law and insurance reimbursement guidelines. Medicare and most insurance companies will cover only those services provided by specific personnel.

Hospice

Hospice provides **palliative** (relieves but does not cure) care and support to patients who are expected to die within 6 months and their families. It involves a team of professionals and volunteers who provide medical, emotional, and spiritual assistance and is covered by Medicare. The emphasis of hospice is to make the patient's last days as pain-free and meaningful as possible. Care may be provided in a special facility, known as a hospice, in a care facility, or in the patient's home. After the patient dies, continuing support is available for the family.

Consolidation of Health Care Services

Mainly due to efforts to control costs, many health care facilities are combining under the same ownership. In this way they enjoy a number of advantages:

- Buy supplies in large quantities, thus negotiating for better prices
- Share expensive equipment
- Avoid duplication of laboratory and diagnostic services
- Share knowledge and management expertise
- Consolidate services and prevent duplication

Multiservice systems offer patients more coordinated health care, a sort of "one-stop shopping." For example, following a hospital stay, a patient can be transferred to the system's skilled nursing facility and at the same time be referred to its rehabilitation services. Some systems include a home health division.

An advantage of consolidation for patients is that they may experience more consistent care and better follow-through when dealing with one system. A disadvantage to consolidation is that there are fewer choices for health care consumers. There is the danger, too, that the lack of competition will result in higher prices and lower quality. Government regulation and patient demands help prevent these problems and ensure that large health care systems are accountable and maintain good patient care as their first priority.

New Types of Health Care Facilities

The high cost of health care, in terms of both facilities' and physicians' fees, has encouraged the development of alternative sites to provide medical care. Pharmacies, for example, now offer immunizations. Going a step further, the CVS chain of drugstores opened MinuteClinics in which nurse practitioners diagnose patients, decide on treatments, and then prescribe the needed medication. The typical cost for the patient runs from $60 to $100, but also accepts most insurance plans. When necessary, patients are referred to a physician or the local emergency department. CVS predicts that this service not only can save the lives of patients who do not have a primary care physician or are unable to pay for medical care, but can also save hundreds of billions of dollars in annual health care costs.

Some areas of the country have more hospitals than necessary to service their communities, leading in some cases to overutilization and higher health care costs. At the same time, many shopping malls are becoming vacant as Americans change their shopping habits. To take advantage of the vacated buildings and provide truly needed services, health care providers and investors are developing **medical malls**, facilities that provide a variety of outpatient services, some of which were previously provided by the hospitals. Box 2–1 lists examples of typical services.

Box 2-1

What Might You Find in a Medical Mall?

- Physicians' offices
- Same-day surgery
- Adult day care
- Urgent care
- Substance abuse treatment
- Medical lab
- Home health care agency

This grouping of services, especially those previously provided by high-cost hospitals, in one location is believed to reduce costs in addition to making needed health care more convenient for patients, especially the elderly. Several medical malls in New Jersey have adult day care centers whose employees can take seniors out for services located nearby, such as physician visits and eye exams. This type of all-inclusive care may be a less expensive alternative to nursing home stays for some patients.

Government Health Services

Federal, state, and local governments provide a variety of important services to protect and promote the health of the American public. Supported by taxpayers, agencies have been created that concentrate on conducting research, creating and enforcing regulations, and providing educational materials and activities. Four of the major federal health-related agencies are shown in Table 2–7. Other U.S. Department of Health and Human Services agencies include the Administration on Aging, the Agency for Toxic Substances and Disease, the Indian Health Service, and the Substance Abuse and Mental Health Services Administration.

State and local health departments receive monetary and administrative support from the federal government. The following lists include examples of typical services offered.

State Health Departments

- License health care personnel, hospitals, and nursing homes
- Monitor chronic and communicable (contagious) diseases
- Provide laboratory services
- Provide emergency medical services
- Establish health data systems
- Conduct public health planning
- Provide mental health services

Local Health Departments

- Collect **vital statistics** (births and deaths)
- Conduct sanitation inspections
- Provide health education
- Screen for diseases such as cancer and diabetes
- Carry out insect control measures
- Supervise water and sewage systems
- Provide immunizations
- Operate venereal disease clinics
- Provide mental health and substance abuse counseling
  (Adapted from Williams, 2005)

Government services provide a variety of employment opportunities for health care professionals. Everyone who works in health care, whether public or private, must understand the regulations of these agencies and how they affect their occupation. For example, the Centers for Disease Control and Prevention (CDC) developed standard precautions for the safe handling of body fluids. These are essential for health care professionals who have contact with patients and are explained in Chapter 10.

Table 2–7 Health-Related Agencies of the Federal Government

National Institutes of Health (NIH)	Centers for Disease Control and Prevention (CDC)
Twenty-seven institutes and centers that conduct and support all types of medical research	Research ways to control the spread of diseases that are contagious, caused by environmental conditions, or spread by animals and insects
U.S. Department of Labor Occupational Safety and Health Administration (OSHA)	**Food and Drug Administration (FDA)**
Develops and enforces minimum health and safety standards (which employers must follow) for all of America's workers	Ensures that foods are safe, pure, and wholesome; that therapeutic drugs are safe and effective; and that cosmetics are harmless

SUGGESTED LEARNING ACTIVITIES

1. Look for articles about health care trends and challenges on the Internet, and in newspapers and magazines. Which trends are mentioned most frequently? How do you think they will affect your future career as a health care professional?

2. Visit some of the health care facilities described in this chapter. What services do they offer? What types of volunteer and employment opportunities are available?

3. Conduct a search of websites for major hospitals and health care systems in your area. What kind of information is available?

4. Investigate the services provided by your local public health department.

5. Learn about complementary and alternative therapies practiced in your area. Interview a practitioner about the theory on which his or her therapy is based.

6. Learn more about the factors that contribute to cancer, heart disease, chronic lower respiratory disease, and stroke. Explore the websites of the American Cancer Society, the American Heart Association, the American Lung Association, and the National Stroke Association. Explore other sources on the Internet using the key words "cancer prevention," "heart disease prevention," "chronic lower respiratory disease prevention," and "stroke prevention."

WEB ACTIVITIES

Ancient History Encyclopedia

Justinian's Plague

https://www.ancient.eu/article/782/justinians-plague-541-542-ce/

1. When did Justinian's plague epidemic take place?

2. How was the disease transmitted?

3. How many were killed during a later plague, known as the Black Death, in the 1300s?

4. How did war contribute to the spread of the disease?

5. What home remedies were used?

Student's Choice

Choose one the following leaders in Western medicine to learn more about and answer the questions that follow.

- Hippocrates
- William Harvey
- Edward Jenner
- Elizabeth Blackwell
- Louis Pasteur

1. When did this person live?

2. What was his or her contribution to Western medicine?

3. What was the impact of the contribution? That is, how did it change the way medicine was practiced?

Medium Lifestyle

The 8 Pillars of Holistic Wellness: What It Truly Means to Be Well

https://medium.com/@alexandra.baker/the-8-pillars-of-holistic-wellness-what-it-truly-means-to-be-well-b0d0b8e55bd1

1. Do you agree with the eight types of wellness?

2. Which ones do you think are most related to maintaining physical wellness?

3. Are there any you feel you would like to work on improving for yourself?

National Public Radio

Results of At-Home Genetic Tests for Health Can Be Hard to Interpret

https://www.npr.org/sections/health-shots/2018/06/18/609750963/results-of-at-home-genetic-tests-for-health-can-be-hard-to-interpret

Kaiser Family Foundation

www.kff.org

1. Choose a topic to read about.
2. Based on what you learned, what changes do you think might take place in health care in the next 10 years?
3. What might be done to control health care costs in the United States?

National Institutes of Health—National Center for Complementary and Integrative Health

https://nccih.nih.gov

1. Click on the tab Health Info, then on Topics A-Z.
2. Choose five therapies to explore and write a paragraph about each.

U.S. Food and Drug Administration

Health Fraud Scams . . . Are Everywhere: Get the Facts

https://www.fda.gov/media/84561/download

1. Download the pdf file.
2. List the reasons why the FDA recommends not using the products described for various illnesses and conditions.
3. How and where are fraudulent products sold?
4. What are the three ways recommended to avoid health care frauds?
5. How can you report what you believe to be a fraudulent product?

National Library of Medicine—Medline Plus

www.medlineplus.gov

1. Click on (a) Drugs and Supplements, (b) Herbs and Supplements, (c) All About Herbs and Supplements
2. Choose five from the list to read about and write a paragraph about each.

Zero Suicide

https://zerosuicide.sprc.org/

1. Explore this organization's website.
2. Write a short paper describing its goals.
3. What do you think health care professionals can do to help prevent suicides?

Mayo Clinic

https://www.mayoclinic.org/diseases-conditions/suicide/in-depth/suicide/art-20044707

Suicide: What to do when someone is suicidal

Read the very practical information given and think about how you might use it in your future work in health care.

National Institute on Drug Abuse

https://www.drugabuse.gov/drugs-abuse/opioids/opioid-overdose-crisis

Opioid Overdose Crisis

1. What contributing factors are included in the $78.5 billion cost of the opioid crisis in the United States?
2. How did the opioid crisis start?
3. What are the seven statistical facts about the crisis listed on the web page?

Your Choice

Choose five of the following websites to explore and learn more about issues in health care.

American Association of Naturopathic Physicians. www.naturopathic.org

American Cancer Society. www.cancer.org

American Heart Association. www.americanheart.org

American Hospital Association. www.aha.org

American Stroke Association. www.strokeassociation.org

Centers for Disease Control and Prevention. www.cdc.gov

Centers for Disease Control and Prevention. Antibiotic resistance threats in the United States, 2013. www.cdc.gov/drugresistance/threat-report-2013/

Centers for Medicare and Medicaid. www.medicare.gov

Expanding Consciousness. www.healthasexpandingconsciousness.org

Food and Drug Administration. www.fda.gov

The Joint Commission. www.jointcommission.org

Medline Plus. http://www.nlm.nih.gov

National Association for Home Care and Hospice. www.nahc.org

National Center for Complementary and Alternative Medicine. https://nccih.nih.gov

National Center for Health Statistics. www.cdc.gov/nchs

National Hospice and Palliative Care Organization. www.nho.org

National Institutes of Health. www.nih.gov

Occupational Safety and Health Administration. www.osha.gov

The Commonwealth Fund

https://www.commonwealthfund.org/publications/newsletter-article/2018/sep/focus-reducing-racial-disparities-health-care-confronting

In Focus: Reducing Racial Disparities in Health Care by Confronting Racism

1. Write a report or discuss the continuing problem of racial discrimination in health: Who are the racial minorities affected and how?

2. What has the federal government done to investigate and reduce health disparities due to discrimination?

REVIEW QUESTIONS

1. What are ten significant events that changed the way health care was delivered?

2. What are the definitions of the following terms: gene therapy and targeted drug therapy?

3. What is today's leading prevention and treatment option?

4. Explain the meaning of specialization and its impact on health care.

5. What are the effects of the aging population on health care?

6. What has happened with health care costs over the past few decades?

7. What are the factors changing how we approach health care today?

8. What is the meaning of "wellness"?

9. What is the theory of expanding consciousness?

10. What is the meaning of holistic medicine? What are the aspects of the patient that it addresses and the factors that holistic providers emphasize?

11. What are the definitions of the following approaches to medicine: Western, complementary, alternative, and integrative?

12. What are the warning signs that a health care product may be fraudulent?

13. What are the bases of osteopathy and chiropractic?

14. What are the health benefits of massage therapy?

15. What are the bases and uses of naturopathy, homeopathy, and acupuncture?

16. What is the meaning and purpose of personalized medicine?

17. What is the effect of health care costs on many Americans?

18. What are the challenges of providing quality long-term care to older Americans?

19. What are six social problems that affect health care?

20. What is the meaning of "health disparities"?

21. How is racism a problem in health care?

22. What are the difficulties in maintaining high-quality health care?

23. What is the meaning of "preauthorization" and what is its potential effect on a patient's health care?

24. What are the problems encountered in many of the nation's nursing homes?

25. What is Alzheimer's disease and what are its effects on the health care system?

26. Why is it difficult to respond quickly to infectious disease outbreaks?

27. What are the statistics that describe the problem of medication adherence?

28. What are the statistics that describe the extent of the opioid crisis? What are 11 strategies for fighting this crisis?

29. What does it mean when bacteria mutate and how does this affect the use of antibiotics?

30. What are the statistics that describe the increasing rate of suicide in the United States?

31. What are the CDC's four warning signs of a potential suicide?

32. Why do many health care providers believe that prescription drugs should not be advertised?

33. What levels of care may be provided in a modern general hospital?

34. What are examples of methods hospitals are using to control costs?

35. What are the ten common ambulatory health care facilities? What type of services does each one offer?

36. What are the major types of long-term care facilities? What type of care is offered by each?

37. What types of health care services can be provided in a patient's home?

38. What is the purpose of hospice?

39. Why are many health care facilities consolidating?

40. What are two new types of health care facilities?

41. Give examples of typical services provided by federal, state, and local health agencies.

APPLICATION EXERCISES

1. Refer to The Case of the Confused Daughter at the beginning of the chapter. Put yourself in the place of the social worker. What information would you give Mrs. Freemont and her daughter?

2. Jim Parker has been working as a licensed practical nurse for 7 years. Most of his career has been spent working in a community hospital providing direct patient care. Jim has been thinking about other settings in which he can apply his nursing skills.

    a. Describe at least five facilities that might offer employment opportunities for Jim.

    b. What type of patients should he expect to work with in each one?

PROBLEM-SOLVING PRACTICE

A growing number of children in Trueville, USA, are becoming overweight and obese. A group of concerned citizens has organized a committee to find ways to help children in the community attain normal weights and raise their levels of fitness. How might the committee use the five-step problem-solving process?

CHAPTER 3

Ethical and Legal Responsibilities

KEY TERMS

adult
advance directives
agent
assault
autonomy
battery
breach of contract
codes of ethics
confidentiality
consent
contracts
damages
defamation of character
discreet
durable power of attorney for
    health care
emancipated minors
ethical dilemma
ethics
euthanasia
express consent
express contract
false imprisonment
fraud
implied consent
implied contracts
informed consent
invasive procedures
justice
legislation
libel
living will
malpractice
mercy killing

(continues)

OBJECTIVES

Studying and applying the material in this chapter will help you to:

1. Explain the meaning of ethics and its importance in the practice of health care.
2. Explain how ethics and laws are related.
3. Explain how the use of medical marijuana is an example of an ethical conflict.
4. List four current health care ethical dilemmas.
5. State the purpose of professional codes of ethics.
6. Explain the meaning of values and how they influence personal and professional behavior.
7. List the eight major ethical principles that apply to health care.
8. Explain how each of the following presents ethical challenges to the health care community: euthanasia, organ transplants, and rationing of care.
9. Define "consent," "informed consent," and "express consent."
10. Explain the importance of patient consent and the possible consequences when actions are taken without the patient's consent.
11. State the conditions under which a minor may be emancipated.
12. Define "battery" and "assault" as they relate to health care.
13. Explain the meaning of "false imprisonment" as it relates to health care.
14. Describe the two main types of advance directives.
15. List eight signs of child abuse.
16. State the actions that health care professionals should take in cases of suspected child abuse.
17. List six forms of elder abuse.
18. Explain the purpose of the federal schedule of controlled substances.
19. Define "fraud" and give three examples of health care fraud.
20. Explain the importance of patient confidentiality and the possible legal consequences when it is breached.
21. Describe the Health Insurance Portability and Accountability Act (HIPAA) and its implications for health care professionals.
22. Define "contract" and list the three components that make a contract enforceable.
23. Explain the difference between an "implied contract" and an "express contract."

KEY TERMS (continued)

negligence
principles
protocols
respondeat superior
slander
values

24. Explain the meanings of "agent" and "respondeat superior."
25. Explain the meaning of "malpractice," including the leading causes of these lawsuits.
26. Describe ways by which malpractice lawsuits can be avoided.
27. Explain the purpose of patients' bills of rights.
28. Give three patients' bills of rights that are currently in place.
29. List six ways that decisions regarding ethics are made by health care facilities.

The Case of the Missing Consent Form

Mrs. McChesney is bringing her 3-year-old son, Sammy, to Dr. Michaels for a minor surgery to be performed in the physician's office. Medical assistant Gretchen Mills scheduled the surgery in the appointment book. Last night she checked to be sure that the necessary instruments and supplies were prepared and that an appropriate room was ready. When checking Sammy's file on the day of the surgery, she cannot find a consent form, signed by Mrs. McChesney, to authorize the surgery. Proceeding with the procedure without this having been completed could have serious legal implications.

Health care professionals must understand and help their facilities follow ethical principles and meet legal requirements.

THE PURPOSE OF ETHICS

Over the centuries human beings have struggled to answer questions about the meaning of life and how to properly conduct themselves. Ethics is a system of principles (fundamental truths that serve as the foundation for a system of beliefs) a society develops to guide decisions about what is right and wrong. Ethics helps people make daily decisions as well as deal with difficult and complex problems that lack easy answers.

The ethical principles adopted by a society are influenced by religion, history, and the collective experiences of the people in the group. The United States has one of the most diverse populations of any country on earth, made up of many cultures and religions. People here are guided by a variety of ethical principles and beliefs about right and wrong. This accounts for many of the disagreements that occur when the government tries to pass laws and make policy decisions that affect all citizens. The ongoing debate about abortion is an example of strongly held opposing beliefs in which each side believes it is right.

Even within a single ethical system, following one principle may appear to contradict another. The result is an ethical dilemma, a situation in which there is no clear answer. Table 3–1 contains examples of ethical dilemmas faced by Americans today.

Often, there simply is not a clear right answer that will satisfy everyone. Right behavior for some people results in wrong effects for others. Flight (2004), who writes about health care ethics, points out that realizing there may not be a "perfect" answer can prevent some of the agonizing that occurs when trying to make the "correct" decision.

ETHICS AND THE LAW

Ethics provides the general principles on which laws are based. Put another way, laws are a means of enforcing ethical principles. For example, if a society agrees that life is precious, its members pass laws that make murder a crime. The American legal system is based on the belief that everyone must take responsibility for his or her actions (Flight, 2004). Its purpose is to require people to act in the best interest of society as a whole. For example, the Occupational Safety and Health Administration (OSHA) was created to protect the health and safety of all workers. OSHA regulations require employers to follow our society's ethical principle that human life and health are precious and should be safeguarded.

Laws, however, can conflict with the ethical and moral principles held by some members of society. The use of marijuana for medical purposes is an example. Marijuana has been found to relieve the nausea experienced by patients

Table 3–1 Ethical Dilemmas Faced by Americans

Values	Action	Contradiction
Criminals should be punished for their crimes. ("An eye for an eye.") "Thou shall not kill."	Capital punishment for convicted murderers	If it is wrong to kill, can society justify killing anyone, even a criminal?
Freedom of speech is a human right. All people should be treated equally and be protected under the law.	Speeches on public grounds that contain hate messages directed toward minority groups	Should free speech be allowed if the messages encourage unequal treatment?
Citizens should have the right to own guns and protect themselves. Society must protect itself against criminals.	Criminals use guns to harm others.	Should gun sales be controlled if it results in limiting the rights of law-abiding citizens?

undergoing chemotherapy. It is also believed by many to relieve joint pain and help with neurological disorders. However, it has not been approved by the U.S. Food and Drug Administration and its sale, distribution, and use are against federal law. In spite of this, 33 states and the District of Columbia have approved the medical use of marijuana, asserting that it is unethical to allow human suffering when it can be prevented. Opponents to its legalization believe that its use encourages inappropriate drug use and is a gateway to stronger drugs, such as heroin. Both groups believe they are doing the "right thing" for society.

Some well-intentioned laws do not result in their intended purpose. Others have harmful consequences that are not recognized until after the laws are in effect—unintended consequences. For example, federal legislation requires hospital emergency departments to evaluate and treat all patients who require emergency care, regardless of their ability to pay. Many hospitals could not afford the financial losses of treating every patient who came for care. This resulted in many emergency departments closing down, thus denying the entire community an important health care resource.

The third principle of the American Medical Association Principles of Medical Ethics addresses the issue of problematic laws:

A physician shall respect the law and also recognize a responsibility to seek changes in those requirements, which are contrary to the best interests of the patient. (https://www.ama -assn.org/about/publications-newsletters/ama -principles-medical-ethics)

It is *never* appropriate, however, to undermine a patient's trust in the care being given by discussing what the health care professional believes to be problems with the system. It is proper to listen to patients' concerns and then work to promote positive changes in laws or the health care system.

Professional organizations often provide opportunities to discuss these issues. Many groups represent their members in promoting legislation and policies that are beneficial for both patients and health care professionals.

ETHICS AND HEALTH CARE

The importance of ethics in the practice of health care has been recognized for thousands of years. The practice of health care involves life-and-death issues and health care professionals have a significant impact on human life. Recognition of the important role of health care professionals has existed since ancient times. Hippocrates, a Greek physician who lived about 2,500 years ago, was concerned with the ethical considerations of medicine. The Hippocratic Oath, taken by physicians over the centuries, contains issues and ideas that are still being debated today. Read the Oath in Box 3–1 and look for the references to mercy killing, abortion, and sexual harassment. At the same time, the practice of medicine has changed over time—as with the use of surgery, which for centuries was not practiced by physicians.

Health care professionals today are confronted by more ethical problems than at any other time in history. Flight (2011) notes: "Technology has progressed beyond society's readiness to deal with the ethical and legal issues it presents" (p. 235). Today we are able to prevent conception, prolong life, transplant organs, and perform lifesaving procedures to an extent never before imagined. In some cases, cures seem miraculous and add to human happiness. In others, society is confronted with difficult questions like the following:

- Anencephalic babies are born with only a partial brain. Most die shortly after birth. When this condition is diagnosed, usually at 18 weeks of pregnancy, should the mother be allowed to abort the child?

Personal Values

Values reflect what we care about most and guide our decisions and behavior. Individuals develop their personal values as they grow and mature. Values are influenced by factors such as family, religious teachings, education, and personal experience. For example, one person may place great importance on having material possessions, while another believes that enjoying close relationships with friends is most important. The first individual *values* possessions; the second *values* relationships.

Values are not necessarily right or wrong, but it is important to be clear about personal values. They may conflict with situations encountered on the job. Health care professionals, however, must support the decisions and practices of the facilities where they work. If this is impossible, it may be best to seek employment elsewhere. The following example illustrates this type of situation:

> Hannah is one of eight children in a Catholic family. She attended Catholic elementary and high school and continues to attend Mass every Sunday. She believes that abortion is wrong and cannot be justified under any circumstances. Hannah recently graduated from a medical assisting program and is ready to seek employment. She realizes that she must support the desires and well-being of her patients and never judge them in any way. Therefore, Hannah has decided not to work in any facility where abortions are performed. In this way, she can avoid ethical conflicts between her personal beliefs and the needs of the patients.

Cultural background and personal values may influence the choice of a specific type of work, as in the following case:

> Karen Chin's parents emigrated from China to the United States in 1980. Her mother's parents came with the family and have always played an important part in Karen's life. She respects her grandparents' knowledge and experience and often turned to them for advice while she was growing up. Today, in spite of health problems and the inability to handle their daily needs, they remain in the family home, cared for by younger family members.
>
> Inspired by her home experience, Karen decided to do volunteer work in a nursing home. Karen's interest in caring for older patients increased. She has decided to specialize in geriatric nursing and devote her career to working with older patients. She wants to offer them the care and compassion that she believes older persons deserve.

Professional Values

Professions have values that reflect the work they do and what their members believe to be the guiding principles for their work. The values of a profession may be expressed in its code of ethics, or they may be stated separately as in the following example from the American Association of Medical Assistants:

CMA (AAMA) Core Values

Actively participate in the delivery of quality health care.
Promote patient safety and well-being.
Contribute to a positive health care experience for patients.
Demonstrate integrity and respect, and protect patient confidentiality.
Advocate the essential value of certification and continuing education.
Embrace change, growth, and learning.

GUIDING PRINCIPLES OF HEALTH CARE ETHICS

In this chapter, the discussion of ethics that apply to all health care occupations is organized around eight guiding principles:

1. Preserve life
2. Do good
3. Respect autonomy
4. Uphold justice
5. Be honest
6. Be discreet
7. Keep promises
8. Do no harm

These principles are discussed in the following sections, along with examples of corresponding laws that support them. Refer to Table 3–2 for examples of how health care professionals apply ethical principles on the job.

Preserve Life

The basic guiding principle for health care professionals states that life is precious and that all possible means should be taken to preserve it. The Hippocratic Oath, which has influenced medical ethics for more than 2,000 years, states: "I will neither give a deadly drug to anybody if asked for it, nor will I make a suggestion to this effect."

Difficulties arise when there is disagreement about the definition of "life." Advances in technology such as ventilators and feeding tubes have made it possible to maintain life by artificial means. The argument has been made that

Table 3–2 Applying Ethics on the Job

Ethical Principle	Examples of Health Care Professional Responsibilities
Preserve Life	• Provide all patients, including the terminally ill, with caring attention. • Become familiar with your state laws regarding organ donations.
Do Good	• Practice good communication skills. (See Chapters 15, 16, and 17.) • Treat every patient with respect and courtesy. • Serve as a positive role model and promote healthy living. • Learn about the stages of dying and grieving. (See Chapter 8.)
Respect Autonomy	• Be sure that patients have consented to all treatment and procedures. • Become familiar with the state laws and facility policies dealing with advance directives. • Respect the beliefs and values of various cultural groups.
Uphold Justice	• Treat all patients equally, regardless of economic or social background. • Know the rules for handling all categories of controlled substances. • Learn the state laws and your facility's policies and procedures for handling and reporting suspected abuse. • Follow all safety rules and OSHA guidelines to ensure the safety of yourself and others.
Be Honest	• Admit mistakes promptly. Offer to do what is necessary to correct them. • Refuse to participate in any form of fraud. • Document all procedures accurately. Perform coding accurately, if this is part of your responsibilities. • Give an "honest day's work" every day.
Be Discreet	• Never release patient information of any kind unless there is a signed release. • Do not discuss patients with anyone who is not professionally involved in their care. • Conduct necessary conversations about patients with other health care professionals in private areas. • Keep documentation out of the view of people who are not authorized to see it. (See Figure 3–2.) • Do not leave records or patient registers on the reception desk in plain sight of anyone who approaches the desk. • Keep phone conversations with or about patients private. • Protect the physical privacy of patients.
Keep Promises	• Be sure that necessary contracts have been completed. • Be very careful about what you say to patients. They may only hear the "good news." • Complete all tasks assigned by your employer.
Do No Harm	• Focus on providing excellent customer service. (See Chapter 23.) • Always work within your scope of practice. Never give information or perform duties you are not qualified to do. • Observe all safety rules and precautions. Keep areas safe from hazards and make the safety of patients a top priority. (See Figure 3–3.) • Perform procedures according to facility **protocols** (standard methods for performing tasks) listed in the policy and procedure manual or the employee handbook. Never take shortcuts. • Ask an appropriate person about anything you are unsure about. • Keep your skills up to date. See Chapter 14 for more information about continuing education. • Keep certifications current (cardiopulmonary resuscitation [CPR], first aid, professional certifications and/or licenses). • Stay informed about new laws that affect health care.

FIGURE 3–2 Always take care to protect the confidentiality of medical records.

© GagliardiPhotography/Shutterstock.com.

FIGURE 3–3 Ensuring patient safety must be a high priority for health care professionals.

patients suffering from terminal diseases and injuries are being forced to exist under cruel and unnatural conditions. Some suggest that a better description would take the quality of life into consideration. Is it worth prolonging a life, they ask, when the patient is:

- In severe pain that cannot be relieved?
- Suffering from a terminal condition?
- In a coma with no reasonable hope of regaining consciousness?
- Without brain function?
- Requesting that treatment be discontinued?
- Asking that life be terminated?

Thinking It Through

Juan Ruiz is a physical therapy assistant working in a skilled nursing facility. He loves his work and enjoys helping patients regain strength and range of motion through exercise. The amount of rehabilitation that patients may receive is limited by their insurance companies and Medicare. Juan is concerned that patients who could be regaining the full use of their limbs are not being given an adequate number of sessions. One of Juan's patients, on learning that he has only one more session with Juan, asks him if he has received "enough therapy." Juan believes that this person would benefit from at least five more sessions.

1. How should Juan respond?
2. What can he do to help the patient progress toward his full potential?
3. What can Juan do to help increase the funding allocated for rehabilitation services?

Withdrawing artificial means of supporting life has become widely accepted, as long as this is the desire of the patient or those who are authorized to make this decision. Withholding life support can be justified, some argue, because it simply allows an existing fatal condition to take its course. That is, artificial support merely delays a death that cannot be avoided. Others believe that life support should be sustained as long as possible. If a patient has not given instructions to the contrary through an advance directive (discussed later in this chapter), it may be impossible for health care providers to discontinue this support.

Right to Die

Euthanasia, also called mercy killing, is performing an action that results in the death of a patient to alleviate suffering or when it is believed that there is no hope for recovery. According to a recent survey, most physicians and health care professionals believe this to be contrary to their stated professional purpose and oppose assisted suicide (https://www.medicinenet.com/script/main/art.asp?articlekey=173522). A well-known exception is Dr. Jack Kevorkian, a Michigan physician who assisted more than 100 patients to end their lives, believing that helping patients achieve a painless death is the kindest act a physician can perform. His actions were deemed illegal and in 1999, a jury convicted him of second-degree murder and he spent 8 years in prison.

As of January 1, 2019, eight states have passed a physician-assisted life termination law: California, Colorado, Hawaii, Montana, New Mexico, Oregon, Vermont, and Washington. The Oregon law was the first, passed in 1997. After its passage, it was successfully challenged by the U.S. Justice Department. However, in 2006, the U.S. Supreme Court upheld the law and it remains in force today. Due to opposing opinions about assisted life termination (also called "assisted suicide"), state laws have been challenged in court. Some judges in the previously listed states have overturned the laws, but as of this writing, all appeals to reinstate the laws have been successful.

Regardless of their personal beliefs about assisted dying laws, it is the duty of health care professionals to follow their state laws and dedicate themselves to maintaining as high a quality of life as possible for all patients. Respecting life means giving people attention during every phase of life, even in their final days.

Organ Transplantation

The ability of surgeons to successfully transplant organs has saved the lives of many who, without the procedure, had limited hopes for survival. At the same time, it created an ethical dilemma because not everyone agrees to have their own organs, or those of family members, donated at the time of their death. The following statistics show the extent of the problem:

- 115,000 people are currently on the waiting list for an organ transplant.
- 36,500 transplants were performed in 2018.
- 10,721 people were donors in 2018.
- 20 people die each day while waiting (https://www.americantransplantfoundation.org/about-transplant/facts-and-myths/).

While the organs from one person can save the lives of as many as eight others, it is illegal to take organs without the prior permission of the patient or, following death, his family members. Payment cannot be given to donors or to their survivors. To further prevent abuse, it is illegal for the physician who pronounces the donor's death to participate on the transplant surgical team.

Individuals who wish to be organ donors should make their wishes known to family members. Many states place symbols on driver's licenses indicating that the driver has consented to being a donor. Although signed donor cards and driver's licenses with an "organ donor" designation are legal documents, organ and tissue donation is always discussed with family members prior to the donation.

The allocation of donated organs is another ethical consideration. Who should get priority? People who are the sickest or those who have the greatest chance of surviving and achieving a long life? Should personal behavior, such as drug abuse, heavy smoking, or alcoholism that contributed to the organ failure, be considered? At present, the following are common considerations when choosing an organ recipient:

- Medical urgency
- Blood, tissue, and size match
- Time on the waiting list
- Proximity to the donor
- Age of the patient (children are sometimes given priority)

Organ transplantation presents difficult questions for which there are no easy answers (https://optn.transplant.hrsa.gov/learn/about-transplantation/how-organ-allocation-works/).

Rationing Care and Resources

Rationing care has become an increasingly serious concern as the cost of health care rises. Some have argued that rationing has always existed because insurance carriers make decisions about which diagnostic tests and recommended treatments they will and will not cover. As a result, certain types of care are not available to patients who cannot pay for it themselves. Access is also rationed, in a sense, when patients are unable to afford insurance, co-pays, and/or deductibles and therefore do not receive care. (See Chapter 22, Paying for Health Care.)

Medicare and Medicaid, like private insurance companies, also have limitations on which services they cover. Medicaid, which helps low-income individuals and families pay for health care, is funded by the federal and state governments. Many states, dealing with thousands of new Medicaid recipients as a result of the Patient Protection and Affordable Care Act, are cutting benefits to prevent running out of funds. Examples of cuts include limiting hospital stays, not covering certain drugs, and not paying for vision and chiropractic care. There is continuing debate about how to offer expanded coverage to help low-income individuals without raising taxes or taking money from other state programs.

Access to health care itself is rationed to some degree. Because of low reimbursement rates to physicians, especially for Medicaid patients, many doctors do not accept new patients who have Medicare or Medicaid. Some Americans believe that doctors who do not accept Medicaid patients "breach their contract with society" (https://www.statnews.com/2017/12/28/medicaid-physicians-social-contract/). On the other hand, doctors argue that they cannot afford to run their practices if they have too many patients in these categories.

Do Good

Helping and promoting the welfare of others is a basic duty of the health care professional. The reasonable needs of a patient must be considered before the needs of self, making personal convenience secondary to patient welfare.

Working in the best interest of patients means the following:

- Listening carefully to what they say
- Making an effort to understand their ethnic and cultural backgrounds
- Carefully assessing their needs
- Being aware of their ethical beliefs
- Explaining what you are doing as you perform tests, treatments, and other procedures
- Providing appropriate instruction
- Allowing the patient to feel comfortable enough to ask questions
- Answering all patient questions, or finding the answers if necessary (See also Chapters 15 and 16.)

Part of the appeal of health care work is the potential to promote the well-being of the community. Health care professionals should serve as role models by being examples of healthy living practices. (See Chapter 12.)

Health care professionals are paid by their employer for their services and should never accept monetary tips from patients. "Doing good" includes the idea of performing one's job without the expectation of receiving anything extra.

Respect Autonomy

Americans value **autonomy**, which means self-determination. Patients have the right to make decisions about their health care, including whether or not they choose to receive treatment. They can choose who, if anyone, will treat them and what treatments they will receive. As much as possible, based on their physical and mental capabilities and age, patients should be involved in their own care.

Consent

Medical treatment cannot be carried out unless the patient gives his or her **consent** (permission). **Informed consent** is the process in which the patient receives information about treatment and gives his or her permission. Full informed consent consists of several elements:

- Explanation of the procedure
- Information about any alternatives
- Risks, benefits, and uncertainties of each alternative

- Assessment of patient understanding
- Acceptance of treatment by the patient (De Bord, 2014)

There are two types of informed consent: implied and express. **Implied consent** is indicated by the patient's actions: showing up for a medical appointment, opening the mouth for the dentist to administer an injection, or participating in therapeutic exercises. **Express consent** is more formal, either oral or in writing, in which a patient gives permission directly to the provider to receive treatment. Express consent is required for many procedures, especially those that are invasive. (**Invasive procedures** involve punctures or incisions of the skin or insertion of instruments or foreign material into the body.) See Box 3–3 for a sample of a written consent form. Consent forms for complicated procedures, such as surgeries, will contain more information.

The conditions under which a consent form is signed are important. It is not sufficient that patients be given full information. They must understand it as well. If necessary, a translated written form or an interpreter, or both, must be provided. If patients do not understand English or are hearing impaired, means must be arranged to ensure that they completely understand all the required items listed previously for informed consent.

A written consent form does not protect the health care provider if the patient claims to have signed under pressure. It is essential that patients understand it is their right to refuse treatment and that signing is completely voluntary. It is legal for patients to refuse treatment, even if doing so may damage their health.

Consent forms can be signed legally by mentally competent adults if they are not impaired by medication. In most states, **adult** is defined as someone 18 years of age or older. **Emancipated minors** are individuals younger than age 18 who are financially independent, married, in the military, or have been emancipated by a court. They are considered to be legal adults and can sign consent forms on their own behalf for treatment. Individuals younger than age 18 who are not emancipated minors may require a consent form signed by a parent or guardian before a procedure is performed. Many states allow non-emancipated minors as young as 14 to make decisions regarding their health care. Some states do not require parental permission for minors to receive birth control information, abortions, or drug counseling. It is essential that health care professionals learn the laws in the state where they work and keep up with changes to them.

Touching a patient or performing a procedure without his or her permission can result in being charged with the crime of **battery**, the unauthorized touching of another person. If a patient feels threatened about receiving unwanted

Box 3-3

Sample Consent for Treatment

Date _____ Time _____

I authorize the performance of the following procedure(s) _____ on _____ (name of patient) _____ to be performed by (name of physician) _____, MD.

The following have been explained to _____ by Dr. _____ (name of physician) _____

Nature of the procedure _____ (describe procedure) _____

For the purpose of _____

_____

The possible alternative methods of treatment are _____

The risks involve the possibility of _____

The possible complications of this procedure are _____

I have been advised of the serious nature of this procedure and have been further advised that if I desire a more detailed explanation of any of the foregoing or further information about the possible risks or complications, it will be given to me.

I do not request a more detailed listing and explanation of the above information.

Signed _____ Date _____
(Patient/Parent/Guardian)

Witnessed by: _____ Date _____

Thinking It Through

Dr. C. Everett Koop, formerly Surgeon General of the United States, presents the following situation. It involves a 5-year-old girl who has a type of childhood brain tumor that Dr. Koop has studied for many years. The child's original tumor was removed, but it has recurred in spite of all known treatment. Dr. Koop writes: "I know her days are limited and that the longer she lives the more likely she is to have considerable pain. She might also become both blind and deaf." He goes on to explain that the child is severely anemic and this causes her to be unaware of what is happening to her. If he treats the anemia, this may prolong her life. At the same time, it will increase her awareness of pain and ability to understand her situation. Anticancer drugs can be prescribed, but he knows these have no chance of curing the child. Dr. Koop poses the question "Would it be better to let this little girl slip into death quietly . . . or should we prolong her life?"

1. It can be argued that it is Dr. Koop's responsibility as a physician to treat all aspects of the child's condition, including the anemia. Do you agree? Explain your answer.

2. Should anyone else be involved in making the decision about how to treat this child? Explain why.

3. Discuss what you think should be done for this child.

treatment, even if it is not performed, this can result in the crime of **assault**. Assault, in this case, is any threatened or implied act, whether carried out or not. (This use of the word should not be confused with an alternate definition of "assault" meaning a violent, physical attack.) It does not matter if the patient benefits from the treatment. The only difference between proper medical treatment and the crimes of assault and battery is whether the patient gives permission. An exception is emergency care administered when the patient is physically unable to give consent. This is discussed in Chapter 21.

Battery can also be charged if patients are handled more roughly than necessary. Flight (2004) describes a case in which a physician spanked a 4-year-old child who refused to lie still while he was removing her sutures (stitches). The spanking caused bruises that lasted for 3 weeks. The mother successfully sued the physician for assault and battery.

The patient's full consent must be obtained before performing any procedure. An action that the patient resists, done "for his or her own good," may be illegal and result in criminal charges or a lawsuit. Particular care should be taken when using any type of restraint, especially with an uncooperative patient. The health care professional must always use proper techniques when moving patients to prevent pulling on limbs or other unintended roughness.

Excessive persuasion is also a form of assault. A patient who feels "talked into" a procedure may charge assault and battery. For example, a woman who believes she was pressured into being sterilized by having her tubes tied, against her true wishes, may successfully sue. Patients who are

worried about health problems or financial matters often feel afraid and confused. They may accept the advice of a health care provider, only to change their minds later. In some cases, this is because they did not understand what they were told. (See Chapter 16 for more information about health literacy, patients' ability to understand what they are told by physicians and other providers.)

A claim of **false imprisonment** can be charged if patients are held against their will, unless they are mentally incompetent or a danger to themselves. For example, a person cannot be kept in a hospital or clinic "for his own good" because he needs medical attention. Without the patient's consent, release is the only option. Patients may be asked to sign a statement that they are discontinuing care against medical advice. This may protect the facility and professional staff from damages (financial responsibility) if the patient suffers harm as a result of refusing treatment.

Advance Directives

Self-determination about health care decisions is possible through the use of **advance directives**. These are written instructions that outline individuals' desires regarding care should they become unable, as the result of illness or injury, to make these decisions. There are two main types of advance directives:

1. **Living Will**. (Health care instructions.) This document outlines an individual's wishes regarding the type and extent of care to be given. Some living wills allow the inclusion of specific directions about whether the individual consents to certain procedures, such as cardiac resuscitation, mechanical respiration, and feeding tubes. A "do not resuscitate" (DNR) request can be included. This means that CPR is not to be administered if the individual stops breathing. An exception is if the individual is not in a health care facility and emergency personnel cannot locate a DNR request. Living wills are regulated by state laws.

2. **Durable Power of Attorney for Health Care.** (Designation of health care surrogate/representative.) In this document, sometimes called a "health care power of attorney," individuals designate specific people to act on their behalf if they become unable to make health care decisions. An individual can select anyone to be a surrogate; it is not necessary for the surrogate to be related. Each state has specific requirements and designation forms. (See Figure 3–4.)

The Patient Self-Determination Act passed in 1991 is federal **legislation** (law) that requires hospitals, nursing homes, rehabilitation facilities, and hospices to have written policies regarding advance directives. They must provide

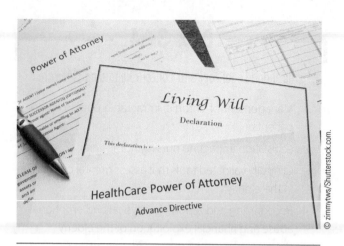

© zimmytws/Shutterstock.com.

FIGURE 3–4 Advance directives help ensure that the wishes of patients about their health care are followed.

adult patients with information about advance health directives upon their admission to the facility. Patients are not legally required to prepare advance directives, but they must be informed of their right to have them.

Problems can arise when patients do not indicate their wishes while they are competent to do so. Family members and physicians may disagree about the proper course of action. In some cases, the courts are called on to make the final decision. A well-publicized and very controversial case involved Terri Schiavo, a woman who, most physicians believed, was in a nonreversible vegetative state for 15 years. Her parents and husband disagreed about her state of awareness and wishes for care. After years of court battles, her husband's request to remove her feeding tube was granted and she died within 2 weeks. There are still many similar cases in the court system. Sometimes the conflict involves family members and health care providers. In March 2009, a New Jersey judge rejected a hospital's decision to remove the life support of a patient who had been in an unconscious state since suffering complications from surgery in January 2008. The family contested the hospital's decision and the hospital was required to reconnect a feeding tube, ventilator, and dialysis machine.

The growing number of older Americans has presented an increasing number of situations in which health care providers become involved in determining competency. Giving up one's home and independence can be extremely difficult and in many cases, individuals do not recognize that their safety and well-being are threatened by their living alone. Home care professionals are often faced with clients who do not use their walkers, as advised by their physicians; do not eat the meals delivered to their homes; and are unable to properly take their medications. In these cases, the need to provide additional care or to move the older adult to assisted living or a care facility conflicts with the principle of autonomy if the older adult is adamant

---

Box 3-4

Ethical and Legal Topics of Concern Regarding Eldercare

- Management of chronic, intractable pain in aging patients
- Legislation impacting nursing home care
- Clinically validated tools that assess mental capacity in the elderly
- Recognizing and reporting physical and emotional abuse and financial exploitation of the elderly
- Management of geriatric patients with advanced illness when further active treatment is no longer desirable or feasible or not likely to improve the patient's quality of life

---

about living alone or staying in the home. Sometimes a team approach that includes the physician, nurse, social worker, and family members must make difficult, but necessary, decisions regarding the client's welfare. Box 3–4 contains a list of other ethical issues that concern the care and welfare of older adults.

Uphold Justice

Justice refers to fairness. Justice requires that all patients, regardless of race, economic status, religion, nationality, or personal characteristics, receive the same level of care and consideration.

Illness and injury do not always bring out the best in human nature. Patients may experience fear and anxiety. Health problems shake self-confidence and upset otherwise stable lives. Patients can be unreasonable, unpleasant, and uncooperative. It is these very patients who are most in need of respect and consideration. To disregard or take advantage of them in any way is highly unethical.

Reporting Abuse

Justice also refers to the use of authority or power to uphold what is right or lawful. Our society encourages us to protect each other from harm. This principle supports the laws that require health care professionals, among others, to report suspected abuse.

Child Abuse

The Federal Child Abuse Prevention and Treatment Act was passed to require the reporting of physical, sexual, and mental abuse of children and to protect those who do the reporting. Patient confidentiality does not exist in cases of suspected abuse. Signs of abuse may be physical or behavioral and include the following:

- Bruises and welts
- Burns
- Lacerations and abrasions
- Skeletal injuries
- Head injuries
- Repeated injuries at a higher rate than normal for a child of the same age
- Different explanations for the cause of an injury given by the child and the parent
- Unusually compliant, fearful, or aggressive behavior of the child

Any suspected cases of child abuse should be reported immediately to the supervisor. In cases where this is not possible, most state laws have broad statutes that require "any person" to report, therefore enabling health care professionals themselves to report.

Elder Abuse

With the increasing number of older citizens, elder abuse and neglect are growing problems. It is estimated that 1 in 10 or up to 5 million Americans have suffered some form of abuse. Two-thirds of perpetrators are spouses or adult children and it is reported that only 1 in 14 cases is reported (https://www.ncoa.org/public-policy-action/elder-justice/elder-abuse-facts/). Others, such as paid caregivers may be perpetrators and the abuse can occur in various forms:

- Neglect and lack of proper physical care
- Taking financial and other resources without the permission or understanding of the older person
- Physical mistreatment
- Mental and emotional abuse
- Sexual abuse
- Abandonment

All states have reporting systems for elder abuse. The principal public agencies responsible for investigating elder abuse and providing treatment and protective services are Adult Protective Services, the area agency on aging, or the county department of social services. Most states have an elder abuse hotline. Abuse is reported in a small percentage of cases. An elderly person may not report abuse for fear of retaliation, because of a lack of physical or cognitive ability to report, or because they do not want to get the abuser into trouble. Even if not

required by law, it is the ethical duty of health care professionals to report suspected cases of elder abuse to their supervisors.

Domestic Violence

Most states have mandatory reporting laws for health care providers when they know or reasonably suspect that their patient has been injured as a result of domestic violence or abuse. These laws are different from those covering child and elder abuse. Some states list specific injuries and wounds that require reporting, such as firearm injury, battery, stabbing, and rape. A negative consequence of mandatory reporting is that some victims will not seek medical care for fear that the report to law enforcement will cause the abuser to retaliate. In these cases, health facilities are encouraged to address safety concerns and guide victims of violence through available options.

Health care professionals must be familiar with their state laws and the reporting procedures for their facility. (See Table 3–3 for a list of resources.)

Laws That Protect

Americans believe that government has an ethical obligation to protect all citizens. For example, employers may not take advantage of employees by exposing them to dangerous working conditions. The Occupational Safety and Health Act was established in 1970 by the federal government. The act requires employers to accept responsibility for the safety and health of their employees in the workplace. Health care employers are directed under OSHA to take measures to prevent employees from contracting contagious diseases. Specifically, there must be a written plan that includes waste management procedures, personal protection methods, and employee

training programs. (See Chapter 26 for a description of employment laws.)

Preventing behaviors that lead to individual and social harm is another responsibility that the government believes it has an ethical obligation to uphold. Drug abuse is an example of a behavior considered to be harmful to not only the individual, but also society as a whole. The Controlled Substances Act is a federal law regulated by the U.S. Drug Enforcement Administration (DEA) to help prevent the misuse of addictive substances. Drugs that have addictive potential are classified into five categories called schedules. (See Box 3–5.) Each group has specific guidelines for medical use, including prescribing and handling. Examples of drugs that fall under each of the five groups can be found at the Office of Diversion Control's website at www.deadiversion.usdoj.gov/schedules/. Violations of these laws are criminal acts and can result in fines and imprisonment. Not only is the illegal or overuse of drugs a criminal offense, it can lead to death as discussed in Chapter 2.

Be Honest

Patients' trust in the health care professional is an important factor in their well-being, and trust is built on honesty. Truth-telling is also important among coworkers and with supervisors. This is not always easy. For example, if you make a mistake in performing a lab test, it is tempting to "forget" to mention it. Mistakes, however, can have serious consequences and must be admitted and corrected as quickly as possible.

At the same time, it can be argued that telling a patient the truth may not be in his own best interest, leading to an ethical dilemma. For example, should a clinically depressed patient be told he has terminal cancer if it is believed this

Table 3–3 Abuse Resources for Health Care Providers

Resource	Contact Information
Child Welfare Information Gateway	www.childwelfare.gov
The National Child Abuse Hotline	1-800-4-A-CHILD (1-800-422-4453)
Child Welfare Information Gateway List of state child abuse reporting phone numbers	https://www.childwelfare.gov/organizations/?CWIGFunctionsaction=rols:main.dspList&rolType=Custom&RS_ID=%205
Child Welfare Information Gateway Links to laws for each state	www.childwelfare.gov/topics/systemwide/laws-policies/state/
Eldercare Locator (referrals and information)	1-800-677-1116; https://eldercare.acl.gov/Public/index.aspx
Links to state domestic abuse laws	www.womenslaw.org/laws/general

Box 3–5

Schedules of Controlled Substances

1. Schedule I.
   A. The drug or other substance has a high potential for abuse.
   B. The drug or other substance has no currently accepted medical use in treatment in the United States.
   C. There is a lack of accepted safety for use of the drug or other substance under medical supervision.

2. Schedule II.
   A. The drug or other substance has a high potential for abuse.
   B. The drug or other substance has a currently accepted medical use in treatment in the United States or a currently accepted medical use with severe restrictions.
   C. Abuse of the drug or other substances may lead to severe psychological or physical dependence.

3. Schedule III.
   A. The drug or other substance has a potential for abuse less than the drugs or other substances in Schedules I and II.
   B. The drug or other substance has a currently accepted medical use in treatment in the United States.

C. Abuse of the drug or other substance may lead to moderate or low physical dependence or high psychological dependence.

4. Schedule IV.
   A. The drug or other substance has a low potential for abuse relative to the drugs or other substances in Schedule III.
   B. The drug or other substance has a currently accepted medical use in treatment in the United States.
   C. Abuse of the drug or other substance may lead to limited physical dependence or psychological dependence relative to the drugs or other substances in Schedule III.

5. Schedule V.
   A. The drug or other substance has a low potential for abuse relative to the drugs or other substances in Schedule IV.
   B. The drug or other substance has a currently accepted medical use in treatment in the United States.
   C. Abuse of the drug or other substance may lead to limited physical dependence or psychological dependence relative to the drugs or other substances in Schedule IV.

Source: U.S. Department of Justice, Diversion Control Division. https://www.deadiversion.usdoj.gov/schedules/

---

might lead him to attempt suicide? Or should a physician tell a critically ill patient that he might not survive and should arrange his personal affairs and prepare his will? Or is it better to let the patient have hope and optimism, factors that may help him overcome his illness?

Fraud is a form of dishonesty that involves cheating or trickery. Medical fraud can result in severe penalties, ranging from losing the right to bill Medicare to imprisonment. Here are examples of health care fraud:

- Submitting insurance claims for services not performed
- Charging different rates for insured and uninsured patients
- Selling treatments, drugs, and devices that have not been proven effective
- Claiming to have a degree, experience, or credentials that one does not have

The health care professional who dedicates time on the job serving the employer and patients is behaving honestly. Arriving late, using paid time to perform personal tasks, and socializing with coworkers rather than attending to patients are forms of dishonesty. Accepting payment to work in a health care position indicates agreement to do the tasks expected for that occupation. Conducting yourself honestly and ethically on the job means making work a priority and striving to do your best every day.

Be Discreet

Being **discreet** means being careful about what you say, preserving confidences, and respecting privacy. In health care, not only this is one of the most important ethical principles, but it is the law. Patients have a legal right to privacy concerning their medical affairs. This is referred to as **confidentiality**. Violating that right, even if well intentioned, can result in a lawsuit.

Thinking It Through

The Patient Protection and Affordable Care Act extends Medicaid coverage to millions of Americans, which may result in both physician and funding shortages. One way to deal with this problem is to ration care.

1. Do you agree or disagree with the concept of basic coverage for everyone, if some treatments and procedures cannot be covered? Explain your reasons.

2. Who should decide which procedures will be paid for and which will not?

3. How would you rank medical procedures? Which ones should never be denied? Are there any that you believe patients should be required to pay for themselves?

Patient information cannot be released to anyone without the patient's written approval. (See Box 3–6.) This includes relatives, friends, insurance companies, and others who may claim to have the "right to know." The only exceptions are disclosures and reports allowed or required by law, such as births, deaths, certain infectious and communicable diseases, abuse, and life-threatening injuries caused by violence. The exact requirements and methods for reporting vary, so health care professionals should become familiar with the laws in their location.

In 1996, Congress passed the Health Insurance Portability and Accountability Act, commonly referred to as HIPAA. Implemented in 2003, an important part of this law was to promote the creation of national standards

Thinking It Through

Carin is a medical assistant for Dr. Allen, a dermatologist who has been in practice for many years. During his first 20 years in practice, Dr. Allen had a registered nurse assisting him in the office. When speaking with patients, he often refers to Carin as "my nurse."

1. Do you believe that Dr. Allen is misleading his patients?
2. Why or why not?
3. What could be the consequences?
4. How should Carin handle this situation?

Box 3–6

Sample Authorization to Release Health Care Information

Patient _____ Date of Birth _____

SSN _____ Previous name _____

I request and authorize _____ to release health care information of the patient named above to:

Name _____

Address _____

This request and authorization applies to: (Please initial the appropriate box)

_____ Health care information **EXCLUDING** specific information relating to sexually transmitted diseases (including HIV/AIDS), alcohol or drug use, or visits related to psychiatric disorders or mental health.

_____ All health care information **INCLUDING** specific information relating to sexually transmitted diseases (including HIV/AIDS), alcohol or drug use, or visits related to psychiatric disorders or mental health. _____ Other: _____

I understand that my express consent is required to release any health care information relating to testing, diagnosis, and/or treatment of HIV (AIDS virus), sexually transmitted diseases, psychiatric disorders/mental health, or drug and/or alcohol use. If I have been tested, diagnosed, or treated for HIV (AIDS virus), sexually transmitted diseases, psychiatric disorders/mental health, or drug and/or alcohol use, you are specifically authorized to release all health care information relating to such diagnosis, testing, or treatment. _____ / _____

_____ _____
Signature of patient or patient   Relationship to patient
authorized representative

_____
Date

to protect patient privacy and personal health information, which many people believed could be compromised by the use of electronic medical records. Health care facilities have formulated policies to comply with HIPAA. (Requirements regarding medical records are discussed in detail in Chapter 19.) The following paragraphs contain general guidelines for maintaining confidentiality, but it is essential that new health care professionals learn the specific policies of the facilities in which they work. (See Figure 3–5.)

Health care professionals should not talk about patients with coworkers where they might be overheard by other people. They must remember that hospital cafeterias and clinic elevators are used by the public and are inappropriate locations for such discussions. Reports to friends and family about your work that include the mention of patients must be avoided. Even without giving the names of patients, there may be enough details revealed so that others can guess their identities. Friendly conversations that seem innocent may be serious breaches of confidentiality.

Disclosing unauthorized information can result in being charged with harming the reputation of another. This is known as **defamation of character**. When disclosed in written form it is called **libel**. In spoken form it is called **slander**. These are serious offenses and can result from innocent but careless behavior. For example, reporting a patient's acquired immunodeficiency syndrome (AIDS) test results within the hearing of others could result in charges of slander.

When working directly with patients, take care to protect their physical privacy. Shut the doors of occupied examination rooms, close curtains around hospital beds when performing procedures, and drape patients properly to ensure that there is no more exposure than necessary. If patients must move from one area to another, be sure they are covered properly and do not have to pass through a public area.

Individual rights to privacy sometimes conflict with the public's right to be informed about matters concerning its safety. An incident in Baltimore illustrates this dilemma. Firefighters assisted an injured woman and took her to the

FIGURE 3–5 Federal law requires that health care facilities comply with HIPPA to protect confidential patient information.

Thinking It Through

A nurse who worked at the Baltimore hospital, in the example referred to in the text, decided to tell the firefighters that they had been exposed to AIDS.

1. Do you believe that she did the right thing? Explain your answer.
2. Do you think that breaking the rules of confidentiality was justified in this case?
3. Do you think this nurse should be fired for her actions?
4. Did the nurse commit slander against the woman?
5. What might you do in a similar situation?
6. What consequences would you be willing to accept in order to carry out what you believe to be your ethical responsibilities?

hospital. The hospital staff was aware that the woman had AIDS, but was forbidden by physician–patient confidentiality laws to inform the firefighters that they had been exposed to the virus (Flight, 2004). A more recent example is the arrival in the United States of patients from West Africa who had contracted the Ebola virus. HIPPA regulations prevented hospitals from reporting the names of patients who had been transferred for treatment. However, there were many who believed the public had a right to know because they viewed Ebola as a threat to public health.

Another difficult situation occurs when patients tell health care professionals information in confidence that, if not revealed, may result in harm to the patients themselves or to others. For example, if a patient discloses that she plans to use prescription drugs to end her life after her release from the hospital, the health care professional has a duty to inform the patient's physician. Health care professionals must reveal patient confidences to their supervisors *if* they believe serious harm is likely to result if they do not reveal the information.

Keep Promises

In everyday life, promises are an important part of our relationships with others. **Contracts** are formalized promises that are enforceable by law. They contain the agreements of people to do certain specified things. For example, a contract is formed when an orthopedic surgeon agrees to perform a knee replacement and the patient agrees to pay for the procedure. If one of the parties fails to fulfill his part of the agreement, this can result

in a **breach of contract**. If this failure results in a loss for the other party, a court may award money to make up for this loss.

In order for a contract to be enforceable, it must contain three components:

1. *Offer*: This is the action that starts the process of forming a contract. Examples:

   • Mr. Nguyen visits the dentist because of a toothache. His attendance is considered a request for the dentist to enter into a contract to provide treatment.

   • Marcia Parsons is referred to a physical therapist. By making an appointment with the therapist, she initiates a contract.

2. *Acceptance*: This means that both parties—the patient and the health care provider—agree to enter into the contract. They each agree to do something. Examples:

   • The dentist agrees to treat Mr. Nguyen.

   • The physical therapist sets a time to see Ms. Parsons.

3. *Consideration*: Something of value must be exchanged by the parties. In health care this generally means that the professional provides a service and the patient pays for the service. Examples:

   • The dentist examines Mr. Nguyen, takes X-rays, and fills a cavity. The patient pays for the service before leaving the office.

   • The physical therapist teaches Ms. Parsons to perform a series of leg-strengthening exercises. The patient provides information about her medical insurance coverage and also agrees to pay for any portion not covered by the insurance plan.

In order for a contract to be enforceable, the people who enter it must be competent. The law defines competency by age and mental condition, as it does with consent. State laws govern who may legally enter into a contract. In addition, the actions agreed to must be legal. Suppose that a patient requests his physician to assist him in ending his life (committing suicide). In spite of the action being illegal in their state, the physician agrees. If the drug given does not end the life of the patient as promised, he cannot legally sue the physician for breach of contract because the action agreed to was illegal. (The physician might be charged with a criminal action, however.)

Most contracts between health care providers and patients are **implied contracts**. This means that the actions of the parties create the contract. In the dental example earlier, the actions of visiting the dentist, filling the tooth, and paying for the service fulfill the requirements of an implied contract. Giving emergency treatment is also a form of implied contract.

An **express contract** is created when the parties discuss clearly and in detail what is to take place and agree on specific terms and conditions. The contract can be either written or oral.

It is important for health care professionals to avoid making statements that might be interpreted as a contract. Although it is natural to want to reassure and encourage patients, this should never be confused with giving what might be understood as a guarantee or false hope. Being "too nice" as the result of good intentions can cause legal difficulties, as illustrated in the following example:

A middle-aged man was worried after a consultation with a surgeon. "Looks like I'll have to have a heart bypass," the patient remarked to the assistant at the front desk.

"Don't worry," she assured him, "the doctor is very good at that procedure. You won't have any trouble. I can promise you that."

There were several complications during the surgery, and the patient died several weeks later. His family successfully sued the surgeon on the grounds that his assistant had made a promise that amounted to a warranty. (Flight, 1998, p. 82)

The surgeon in this case was sued because the assistant was acting as his **agent**. An agent is someone who has the authority to represent another person. This case occurred a number of years ago. However, the fact that health care professionals are generally considered to be agents of the licensed professionals for whom they work remains true today and the principles still apply. Employers can be held liable (legally responsible) for the behavior and actions of their employees. This concept is known as **respondeat superior**, which means "let the master answer." The following examples illustrate this concept:

• A physician could be held liable for the consequences of a medical assistant administering the wrong medication.

• A patient suffering injuries from a fall caused by the incompetence of a physical therapist assistant could be awarded **damages** (money to compensate for an injury or loss). The supervising therapist could be financially responsible.

Do No Harm

An essential responsibility of health care professionals is to *do no harm*. They must work within their scope of practice, performing only those duties that they have been trained to do. It is critical that safety rules be followed and that medical advice never be given by a person who is not qualified to do so.

Harm can result from **negligence**. This is failure to meet the standard of care that can be reasonably expected from a person with certain training and experience. Negligence can result from an action performed incorrectly or from the failure to take a necessary action. People who are trained in health care are expected to have special knowledge and skills. Thus they are held to a higher standard of care than those who are untrained. There are various levels of standards within the health care professions:

- A physical therapist (PT) is held to a higher standard of care than a physical therapist assistant (PTA).

- The PTA is held to a higher standard than the PT aide.

- The PT aide is held to a higher standard than an untrained person.

Malpractice is the term for improper, illegal, or negligent professional activity or treatment. Examples of actions the health care professional can take to prevent negligence include the following:

- Always check medications three times before administering. (See Box 3–7).

- Do not perform any procedures you are not trained to do.

- Double-check your documentation.

Malpractice lawsuits are filed by patients who believe they have received improper care. It is important to understand, however, that not all lawsuits are the result of actual malpractice. Leading causes of lawsuits are patient anger and the lack of a satisfactory personal relationship with the health care provider. Good interpersonal relationships are a key factor in preventing malpractice lawsuits. Most patients understand that positive treatment results cannot be guaranteed. But they want to be treated with dignity and to feel that everything possible has been done to help them. Patients who perceive a lack of attention, care, and respect are much more likely to sue than those who feel positive about their care. As Flight (2004) states, "anger is the thread running through the entire malpractice saga" (p. 113). Communicating well, especially listening, and treating patients with kindness and respect are the most effective ways to reduce the risk of being sued. (See Figure 3–6.) (See Chapters 15 and 16 for information about effective communication and Chapter 23 for information about providing good customer service.)

Good Samaritan Laws

Good Samaritan laws have been passed by states to protect individuals, including health care professionals, from liability when they volunteer to give care in emergency situations. In order to be held liable, further injury must be caused intentionally or from extreme carelessness. Even in an emergency, it is important for health care professionals not to offer aid beyond their scope of training. Good Samaritan laws are discussed further in Chapter 21.

PATIENT RIGHTS

In 1973, the American Hospital Association (AHA) developed the Patient's Bill of Rights. The AHA has since updated the rights and renamed it The Patient Care Partnership. This

---

Box 3–7

Don't Forget the Three Checks in Medication Administration

Before administering medication, it is critical to have five areas of information correct: patient identification, medication, dosage, time, and route. But, it's not only critical to ensure this information is correct, you should check three times:

1. The first check occurs when the medications are pulled or retrieved from the automated dispensing machine, the medication drawer, or whatever system is in place at a given institution.

2. The second check occurs when preparation of the medications for administration takes place.

3. The final check occurs at the patient's bedside just before medications are given. This is also an outstanding opportunity to teach the patient about the medications.

Source: http://www.hcpro.com/NRS-251960-4931/In-the-know-Dont-forget-the-three-checks-in-medication-administration.html

---

FIGURE 3–6 Communicating a sincere, caring attitude toward patients is the best defense against malpractice lawsuits.

Partnership states that a hospital's first priority is to treat patients with skill, compassion, and respect. The AHA has published a brochure to help patients and hospitals understand expectations, rights, and responsibilities of both parties. The outlined statement of what patients can expect during their hospital stay is as follows:

- High-quality hospital care
- A clean and safe environment
- Involvement in your care
- Protection of your privacy
- Help when leaving the hospital
- Help with your billing claims

More specifically, the responsibilities of hospitals include giving each patient a Notice of Privacy Practices that describes the way patient information is used and safeguarded, as well as how patients can obtain copies of their medical records; giving patients a general consent for treatment plan to sign; explaining and requesting consent for specific treatment such as surgery; and explaining hospital bills that may be confusing and filing insurance claims. Other important rights of patients are being able to refuse treatment and/or participate in a research study.

Patients, in turn, have certain responsibilities that include supplying the following information:

- Past illnesses, surgeries, or hospital stays
- Allergic reactions
- Medications or supplements being taken
- Network or admission requirements under the patient's health plan

Patients should also advise the hospital about any religious or spiritual beliefs that might affect their care. Hospitals will take these into account as much as possible. Finally, patients should give the hospital copies of their advance directive and/or living will.

In 2010, a Patient's Bill of Rights was created as part of the Affordable Care Act. Its purpose is to protect patients when they are dealing with health insurance companies. Here are examples of the protections now provided by federal law:

- No lifetime dollar limit for coverage of defined essential benefits
- No denial of coverage because of pre existing medical conditions
- Young adult meeting certain requirements can stay on parent's policy until age 26
- Certain preventive health screenings without extra charge
- 30 days' notice if your health insurance is canceled

Other specialized patient rights have been developed for mental health and hospice patients. Historically, mental health patients have suffered discrimination and abuse which may have included restraints, lobotomies, and isolation. A U.S. code (42 U.S. Code § 9501. Bill of Rights) protects patients with mental health and substance use conditions. A few examples of the rights include the following:

- Personal liberty protection
- Protection from seclusion and restraint
- The right to participate, as capable, in planning services and treatment
- The right to an individual, written treatment plan
- The right to refuse treatment

Thinking It Through

Medical errors are a cause for growing concern. According to a recent Johns Hopkins study, more than 250,000 people in the United States die every year from medical errors. Other reports claim the number to be as high as 440,000. In 2000, President Clinton made an unsuccessful request for a law to require the public reporting of medical errors. Congress addressed the issue again in 2005, but no legislation was passed. People in favor of a reporting law believe it will improve the overall quality of health care. Those who are opposed, argue that it will result in increased attempts to cover up errors and thus prevent the follow-up needed to correct them. The Health Care Reform Act of 2010 reportedly does not require the reporting of medical errors. However, some states have begun to require reporting.

1. Do you believe that medical errors should be reported publicly? Explain your answer.
2. How serious should errors be to require reporting them within the organization? Outside the organization?
3. Who should be responsible for tracking and handling medical errors?
4. What do you think might be the consequences if a law that required the reporting of medical errors were passed?

Source: https:www.cnbc.com/2018/02/22/medical-errors-third-leading-cause-of-death-in-america.html

The National Hospice and Palliative Care Organization has developed an extensive list of Hospice Patient Rights that include what hospice must provide to a person receiving hospice care. Examples of these rights and services include the following:

- Be treated with respect
- Receive quality end-of-life care
- Receive pain management and symptom control
- Be allowed to refuse care or treatment
- Choose his or her attending physician

HANDLING ETHICAL DILEMMAS

The first consideration of the ethical health care professional is the well-being of patients. Illegal and unethical behavior can endanger patient welfare and cannot be tolerated. Observations of this behavior in others must not be ignored. Although it is difficult to confront a wrongdoer or "tell on" a coworker, doing what is right must override short-term discomfort. Accepting responsibility for making difficult decisions is part of health care work.

If the behavior observed in a coworker is illegal, it should be reported to the supervisor. For example, if a nurse observes a coworker using an illegal substance at the workplace, it should be reported immediately to the supervisor. If the behavior involves legal but ethically questionable behavior, such as "badmouthing" an employer, it may be best to first speak directly to the coworker.

WHO DECIDES?

When an individual or an organization is faced with a case that presents special ethical difficulties, there are several sources of help:

- The American Medical Association Council on Ethical and Judicial Affairs promotes standards of ethical professionalism, reviews situations, and publishes opinions about current issues to provide guidelines for physicians.
- Hospitals and other large health care facilities have ethics committees composed of health care professionals and members of the community. These committees review individual cases and make recommendations.
- Clergy and counselors provide assistance to health care professionals in making decisions and dealing with personal feelings when coping with difficult situations.
- Conferences are held among the health care team members, the patient, and family members to explore possible actions.
- Many universities and medical colleges study ethical issues and share their findings.
- Some hospitals and clinics have a risk management department. Lawyers and specially trained health care professionals are charged with making ethical and legal decisions on behalf of the organization.

SUGGESTED LEARNING ACTIVITIES

1. Locate articles on the Internet, in the newspaper, or in news magazines about ethical issues. Do you agree with the points of view presented?

2. Secure a copy of the code of ethics for your occupational area of interest. Can you find statements that correspond to the ethical principles presented in this chapter?

3. Explore your personal beliefs about ethical issues such as abortion, euthanasia, and individual privacy versus the public's right to know.

4. Contact the child protective unit of your state's department of social services (or their website) for information about reporting child abuse.

5. Visit the website of the National Center on Elder Abuse to learn more about this growing problem. Think about your role as a future health care provider working with elderly patients.

6. Contact a local health care facility and ask for a copy of their patient consent form.

WEB ACTIVITIES

Medscape

Physicians' Top 20 Ethical Dilemmas—Survey Results Slideshow

https://www.medscape.com/features/slideshow/public/ethical-dilemmas major

1. Slide #4: Do you agree with the decision made by the majority of physicians in using placebos? Why or why not?

2. Slide #5: How does this question relate to the current opioid crisis and the difficult position of physicians in controlling pain?

3. Slide #6: What are some of the circumstances given in which doctors believe patients should not be told they have a terminal condition?

4. Slides #7 and #8: Discuss the opposing arguments given for covering up a mistake.

5. Slide #9: Why would physicians want to perform defensive medicine?

6. Slide #11: How do you feel about reporting an impaired coworker?

7. Slides #13, #14, and #15: Discuss the problem of retaining patients versus dealing with the financial issues of maintaining a health care practice.

8. Slide #16: Physicians see two sides to HIPAA. Do you think it is ethical for physicians to consult colleagues not involved in their patients' care if they believe the colleague can help with the patients' diagnoses or treatments?

9. Do you believe, as 53% of doctors surveyed do, that it is acceptable to break patient confidentiality if the patient's condition might harm others?

Myrko Thum

https://www.myrkothum.com/personal-values/

Do You Know Your Personal Values?

1. What does the author mean when stating that values are on "auto-pilot"?

2. Why is it good to know and be aware of your personal values?

3. Try creating your own value hierarchy as suggested in the article.

4. Now try creating a list of your top ten negative values.

5. Did these exercises help you learn more about yourself?

Health Law & Policy Brief

http://www.healthlawpolicy.org/the-debate-surrounding-the-right-to-die/

The Debate Surrounding the Right to Die

Choose a side of the debate and present your arguments.

STAT

https://www.statnews.com/2017/12/28/medicaid-physicians-social-contract/

Doctors Who Don't Accept Medicaid Breach Contract with Society

1. Do you agree with the author's arguments?

2. What do you think about the arguments of physicians who say they can't remain in business with low reimbursements from Medicaid?

3. Is there anything our society or government can do to solve this problem?

Help Guide

https://www.helpguide.org/articles/abuse/elder-abuse-and-neglect.htm

Elder Abuse and Neglect: Spotting the Warning Signs and Getting Help

1. What factors of aging contribute to elder abuse?

2. What are the warning signs of the six types of elder abuse?

3. What are the reasons that many victims of elder abuse won't report the abuse?

U.S. Department of Health and Human Services

https://www.hhs.gov/hipaa/for-individuals/guidance-materials-for-consumers/index.html

1. Watch the video entitled, "Your Rights Under HIPAA"

2. What are the basic patient rights under HIPAA?

3. What is the Notice of Privacy Practices?

4. What can patients do if they believe their rights under HIPAA have been violated?

Mental Health America

http://www.mentalhealthamerica.net/issues/mental-health-rights

Mental Health Rights

1. Why do people with mental health problems need protection of their rights? Include information about the history of abuse in the treatment of mental illness.

2. According to the article, what percent of Americans will have a diagnosable mental health problem sometime in their lifetime?

3. What are five policy changes called for by Mental Health America?

REVIEW QUESTIONS

1. What is the meaning and importance of ethics in health care?

2. How are ethics and laws related?

3. How is the use of medical marijuana an example of an ethical conflict?

4. What are four current health care dilemmas?

5. What is the purpose of a professional code of ethics?

6. What are values and how do they influence personal and professional behavior?

7. What are the eight major ethical principles that apply to health care?

8. How do each of the following present an ethical challenge to the health care community: euthanasia, organ transplants, and rationing of care?

9. What is the meaning of the following types of consent: informed, implied, and express?

10. What is the importance of consent and the possible consequences if actions are taken without the patient's consent?

11. Under what conditions can a minor be emancipated?

12. What are the meanings of "battery" and "assault" as they relate to health care?

13. What is the meaning of "false imprisonment" as it relates to health care?

14. What are the names and contents of the two types of advance directives?

15. What are the eight signs of child abuse?

16. What action should health care professionals take if they suspect child abuse?

17. What are the six forms of elder abuse?

18. What is the purpose of the federal schedule of controlled substances?

19. What is the definition of "fraud" and what are three examples of health care fraud?

20. Why is patient confidentiality important and what are the possible legal consequences if it is breached?

21. What is the Health Insurance Portability and Accountability Act and what are its implications for health care professionals?

22. What is a "contract" and what are its three components?

23. What is the difference between an implied contract and an express contract?

24. What are the meanings of "agent" and "respondeat superior"?

25. What is "malpractice" and the leading causes of this type of lawsuit?

26. What are ways by which malpractice lawsuits can be avoided?

27. What is the purpose of patients' bills of rights?

28. What are three patients' bills of rights that are currently in place?

29. What are six ways that decisions regarding ethics are made by health care facilities?

APPLICATION EXERCISES

1. Refer to the Case of the Missing Consent Form at the beginning of this chapter. Put together a list of the legal implications that might have resulted if the consent form was not signed.

2. You are working as a licensed practical nurse in a small urgent care center. You love the work. The physicians are excellent, and you have the opportunity to work with a variety of patients. You have become good friends with your coworkers and enjoy an especially close relationship with the administrative medical assistant, Amy. One day you observe Amy removing medication from the drug cabinet. You find this to be unusual because the administrative staff do not normally work with medications. While performing a routine inventory check later that day, you discover a shortage of a drug that is classified as a controlled substance. Explain what you would do in this situation.

PROBLEM-SOLVING PRACTICE

Maria has been working for a few weeks as a licensed practical nurse in a hospital. She has heard the other staff talking a lot about HIPAA and the many new rules, but she does not feel that she knows enough about these regulations. How can she use the five-step problem-solving process to become more informed?

Unit **2** The Language of Health Care

CHAPTER 4

Medical Terminology

KEY TERMS

acronyms
combining forms
combining vowel
consonant
eponyms
medical terminology
prefixes
suffixes
word parts
word root

OBJECTIVES

Studying and applying the material in this chapter will help you to:

1. Explain why it is important for health care professionals to use medical terminology correctly when reading, writing, and speaking.
2. Explain when and with whom medical terminology should be used.
3. Define and give an example for each of the following: word root, combining form, suffix, and prefix.
4. List the steps for breaking down medical terms into their component parts and interpreting the terms correctly.
5. Provide five examples of medical terms that include a prefix and a suffix. Give their meanings.
6. Give five examples of medical eponyms and explain their origin.
7. Give three examples of everyday words that have other meanings when used as medical terms.
8. State the four types of names given to approved prescription drugs.
9. List the guidelines for medical terms that are spelled differently from the way they are pronounced.
10. Give the meaning of eight common abbreviations and five symbols presented in this chapter.
11. Explain the importance of using abbreviations correctly, including the use of the do-not-use list.
12. Describe the features that should be considered when selecting a medical dictionary.
13. Describe five study techniques designed to help students master medical terminology.

The Case of Where Is the Pain?

Dr. Chen states that Ms. Mitchell called yesterday complaining of *epigastric* (ep ih GAS trick) pain and requests that LaTonya, the medical receptionist, call her to follow up and find out if she is feeling any better. LaTonya calls Ms. Mitchell and says, "Dr. Chen has asked me to call and ask how the epigastric pain is today." Ms. Mitchell is confused and says, "I'm not sure what you mean. What is epigastric?" LaTonya does not know what "epigastric" means, and this has prevented her from restating the question in terms that the patient can understand.

Health care professionals must know medical terminology, such as this term (which means "over the stomach"). Failure to learn medical language prevents them from communicating effectively with other health care professionals and with patients. This chapter will help students learn this new language.

IMPORTANCE OF MEDICAL TERMINOLOGY

Understanding and correctly using **medical terminology** is essential to your career in health care. The study of medical terminology includes learning not only medical terms but also the associated abbreviations and symbols. Medical terminology is used during conversations with other health professionals, in medical charting and documentation, and in professional journals and texts. It adds necessary preciseness to professional communications. For example, when directions for procedures are described using exact language, there is less chance for confusion and error.

Patients can receive ineffective or even harmful treatment if words or abbreviations are misunderstood. For example, if the physician orders medication to be taken "a.c." (before a meal), a medication error will result if the health care professional interprets this to mean after a meal, which is written "p.c."

It is not always appropriate to use medical language. Most patients find the use of technical words confusing. They may be intimidated and will hesitate to ask for an explanation. When communicating with patients it is essential to first determine their level of understanding. Appropriate language can then be chosen to ensure clear communication. Patients cannot benefit from, and may even be harmed by, information they do not understand.

THE BUILDING BLOCKS OF MEDICAL LANGUAGE

Many health care programs include a more in-depth study of medical terminology than will be presented in this chapter. For those students with no prior study of

Fascinating Fact

Many of today's medical terms have been used for more than 2,000 years. The ancient Greek physician, Hippocrates, developed many medical words. When the Romans conquered the Greeks in the year 400, the Greek terms were merged with those developed by the legendary Roman physician, Claudius Galen. This is how we ended up with a combination of words that seem strange to us, but were actually related to everyday words in ancient Greek and Latin.

medical terminology, this material will serve as an introduction to the subject. For other students, it will serve as a review.

Medical terms are composed of several parts, referred to as **word parts**. Each word part has its own meaning and location in the term. Like building blocks, they can be combined to create thousands of different words. Learning the meaning of commonly used word parts and applying this knowledge to decipher medical terms is much more efficient than trying to memorize each new word as it is encountered.

The four word parts that make up medical terms are a word root, combining form, prefix, and suffix.

Word Roots and Combining Forms

The **word root** is the part of the medical term that gives the main meaning. It usually, but not always, refers to a structure or function of the body. All medical terms have at least one word root. The following are examples of word roots:

1. *gastr*—stomach
2. *enter*—small intestine
3. *cardi*—heart

Combining forms consist of word roots plus a vowel, usually the letter "o," separated from the word root with a slash mark:

1. gastr/o
2. enter/o
3. cardi/o

The letter "o" is called the **combining vowel**. It links the word root to the next word part in the term, known as the suffix, if the suffix begins with a **consonant** (any letter *except* a, e, i, o, or u). (Suffixes are explained in the next section.) The combining vowel is always used when linking two word roots, even if the second one starts with a vowel. For example, *gastr/o* and *enter/o* are often combined when referring to both the stomach and the intestines. The combining form *gastr/o* is used even though *enter/o* begins with a vowel to form the word *gastroenterology*, which means "the study of the stomach and intestines." Note the word root *enter* is used because the next word part, the suffix, *ology*, starts with a vowel. Medical word roots, when listed in the dictionary, appear as combining forms, and it is recommended that students learn them in this form.

The vocabulary used by health care professionals usually differs from everyday language because, like the language of other sciences, many medical terms have their origins in Greek and Latin. Table 4–1 contains several examples.

There are thousands of word roots and combining forms that make up medical language. The complete list of combining forms each student must learn depends on

Table 4–1 Origins of Medical Word Root Words

Original Word	Meaning	Modern Medical Combining Form
kardia (Greek)	heart	cardi/o
derm (Greek)	skin	derm/o
enteron (Greek)	small intestines	enter/o
bucca (Latin)	cheek	bucc/o
lumbus (Latin)	loin (lower part of the back)	lumb/o
mykes	mushroom, fungus	Myc/o
vivere (Latin)	life	viv/o

his or her chosen occupation. Table 4–2 contains a list of commonly used combining forms that refer to the parts of the body and Table 4–3 lists combining forms that indicate color.

Diagrams can be helpful when learning a new language. Many students find that illustrations provide visual clues for remembering new terms. Figure 4–1 illustrates some of the terms contained in Table 4–2.

Table 4–2 Common Combining Forms That Refer to Body Parts

Combining Form	Meaning	Combining Form	Meaning
adip/o; lip/o; steat/o	fat	lapar/o	abdominal wall
arteri/o	artery	laryng/o	voice box, larynx
arthr/o	joint	myel/o	spinal cord
axill/o	armpit	my/o; muscul/o	muscle
blephar/o	eyelid	nas/o; rhin/o	nose
cardi/o	heart	neur/o	nerve
cephal/o	head	ophthalm/o; ocul/o	eye
cerebr/o; encephal/o	cerebrum, brain	or/o; stomat/o	mouth
cervic/o	neck	oste/o	bone
cholecyst/o	gallbladder	ot/o	ear
col/o	large intestine	pancreat/o	pancreas
cost/o	rib	pharyng/o	throat
crani/o	skull	pneum/o; pneumon/o	lung
cyst/o	urinary bladder	ren/o; nephr/o	kidneys
cyt/o	cell	splen/o	spleen
derm/o; dermat/o	skin	thorac/o	chest
enter/o	small intestine	thyroid/o	thyroid gland
esophag/o	esophagus	trache/o	windpipe, trachea
gastr/o	stomach	ven/o; phleb/o	vein
hem/o; hemat/o	blood	vertebr/o	vertebra
hepat/o	liver		

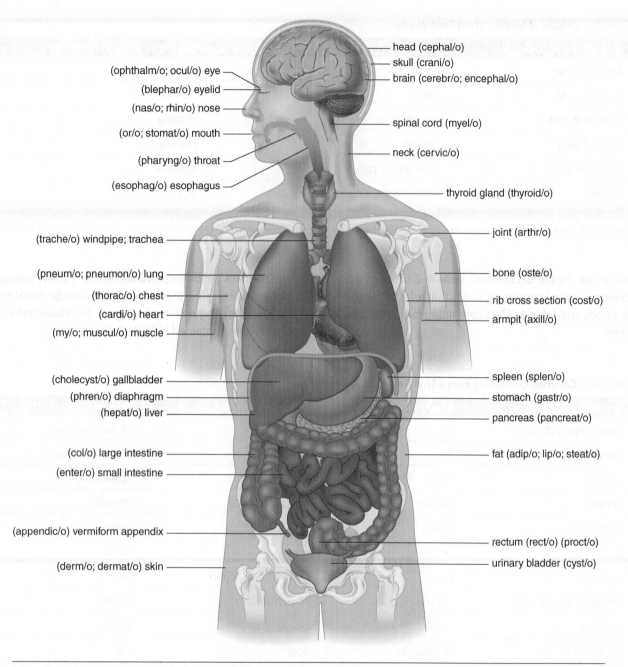

head (cephal/o)
skull (crani/o)
brain (cerebr/o; encephal/o)
(ophthalm/o; ocul/o) eye
(blephar/o) eyelid
(nas/o; rhin/o) nose
spinal cord (myel/o)
(or/o; stomat/o) mouth
neck (cervic/o)
(pharyng/o) throat
(esophag/o) esophagus
thyroid gland (thyroid/o)
(trache/o) windpipe; trachea
joint (arthr/o)
(pneum/o; pneumon/o) lung
bone (oste/o)
(thorac/o) chest
rib cross section (cost/o)
(cardi/o) heart
armpit (axill/o)
(my/o; muscul/o) muscle
(cholecyst/o) gallbladder
spleen (splen/o)
(phren/o) diaphragm
stomach (gastr/o)
(hepat/o) liver
pancreas (pancreat/o)
(col/o) large intestine
fat (adip/o; lip/o; steat/o)
(enter/o) small intestine
(appendic/o) vermiform appendix
rectum (rect/o) (proct/o)
(derm/o; dermat/o) skin
urinary bladder (cyst/o)

FIGURE 4–1 Medical terminology for body parts.

Table 4–3 Color Word Roots

Word Root	Meaning	Example
cyan/o	blue	cyanosis (sigh us NOH sis)
		blueish discoloration of the skin
erythr/o	red	erythrocyte (eh RITH roh sight)
		red blood cell
leuk/o	white	leukocyte (LOO koh sight)
melan/o	black	melanoma (mel uh NO muh)
		tumor of melanin-forming cells (melanin is a dark brown or black pigment)
poli/o	gray	poliomyelitis (poh lee oh my eh LIE tis)
		infection of the gray nerve tissue of the spinal cord

Suffixes

Suffixes are word parts that are attached to the end of word roots and combining forms to add to or change their meaning. All medical terms have an ending, or suffix, unless the word root is a complete word by itself. Some common meanings of suffixes include the following:

1. Pathological (disease) conditions
2. Diagnostic procedures
3. Surgical procedures
4. Pertaining to
5. Produced by
6. Resembling

Recall that the combining form is used when the suffix begins with a consonant, as in the following example:

| cardi/o | + | megaly | = | cardiomegaly |
| heart | + | enlarged | = | enlarged heart |

Notice that the slash mark is dropped when the suffix is attached to the combining form.

When the suffix begins with a vowel, it is attached to the word root, as in the following example:

| gastr | + | itis | = | gastritis |
| stomach | + | inflammation | = | inflammation of the stomach |

Each suffix can be added to many different word roots. Knowing that -*itis* means "inflammation" enables the student to know that the following words all indicate an inflammation of the body part indicated in the word root:

1. Appendic**itis**: Inflammation of the appendix
2. Arthr**itis**: Inflammation of the joint
3. Gastr**itis**: Inflammation of the stomach

Another common suffix is -*ectomy*, which means "surgical removal." Like -*itis*, it can be combined with many word roots. In each case, it means removal of the part indicated by the word root:

1. Append**ectomy**: Removal of the appendix
2. Gastr**ectomy**: Removal of all or part of the stomach
3. Lump**ectomy**: Removal of a lump

When suffixes are listed in medical dictionaries and word lists, they are positioned alphabetically with other entries, preceded by a hyphen, and identified as a word part. Dictionary entries typically include the language of origin, as in the following sample dictionary entries:

1. -*megaly* word part (Gr.) enlargement
2. -*itis* word part (Gr.) inflammation
3. -*ectomy* word part (Gr.) surgical removal

See Table 4–4 for a list of commonly used suffixes.

Table 4–4 Common Suffixes

Suffix	Meaning	Term	Meaning
-ac, -al, -ar, -ary, -eal, -ia, -iac, -ic, -ical, -ose, -ous, -tic	All of these mean "pertaining to"	cardi**ac** cellul**ar** psych**otic**	pertaining to the heart pertaining to the cell pertaining to psychosis
-algia	Pain, painful condition	neur**algia** (new RAL jee ah)	pain along a nerve
-centesis	surgical puncture to remove fluid	amnio**centesis** (am nee oh sin TEE sis)	insertion of needle to withdraw sample of amniotic fluid
-cide	to kill, destroy	germi**cide** (JER mih side)	chemical substance that kills germs
-cyte	cell	leuko**cyte** (LOO koh cite)	white blood cell
-ectomy	surgical removal of	gastr**ectomy** (gas TREK toh me)	removal of part or all of the stomach
-emia	blood; blood condition	bacter**emia** (back ter EE mee ah)	bacteria in the blood
-gram	record	electrocardio**gram** (ee lek troh KAR dee oh gram)	record of the electrical activity of the heart

(continues)

Table 4–4 Common Suffixes *(continued)*

Suffix	Meaning	Term	Meaning
-graph	an instrument used to record	electrocardio**graph** (ee lek troh KAR dee ah graf)	instrument that records electrical variations in cardiac muscle activity
-graphy	process of recording	electrocardio**graphy** (ee-lek-troh-kar-dee-AH-graf-ee)	the making and study of electrocardiograms
-ia	condition, especially an abnormal state	tachycard**ia** (tak ee KAR dee ah)	condition of abnormal rapid heart rate
-ion	condition	hypertens**ion** (high per TEN tion)	high blood pressure
-ism	condition	hypothyroid**ism** (high poh THIGH roid izm)	condition created by less than normal levels of thyroid hormones
-itis	inflammation of	card**itis** (kar DYE tis)	inflammation of the heart
-lithiasis	presence of or formation of stones	chole**lithiasis** (koh lee lih THIGH ah sis)	presence of stones in the gallbladder
-logy	study of	cardio**logy** (kar dee OL oh jee)	study of the heart
-megaly	enlargement	hepato**megaly** (hep ah toh MEG ah lee)	enlargement of the liver
-oid	resembling	rheumat**oid** (ROO mah toyd)	resembling rheumatism
-oma	tumor	my**oma** (my OH mah)	tumor containing muscle tissue
-osis	abnormal condition or disease	nephr**osis** (nef ROH sis)	kidney disease
-otomy	surgical incision	trache**otomy** (tray kee OT oh mee)	incision into trachea
-pathy	disease	encephalo**pathy** (en sef ah LOP ah thee)	disease of the brain
-plasty	surgical or plastic repair	rhino**plasty** (RYE no plas tee)	plastic surgery of the nose
-plegia	paralysis	hemi**plegia** (hem ee PLEE jee ah)	paralysis of one side (half) of the body
-pnea	breathing, respiration	a**pnea** (ap NEE ah)	temporary cessation of breathing
-rrhaphy	surgical suturing	gastro**rrhaphy** (gas TROR uh fee)	suturing a perforation of the stomach
-rrhea	drainage, flow, discharge	rhino**rrhea** (rye no REE ah)	drainage from the nose
-rrhexis	rupture	cardio**rrhexis** (car dee oh REX is)	rupture of the heart wall
-scope	instrument used to view	oto**scope** (OH toh skope)	instrument used to examine the ear
-scopy	examination using a scope	sigmoido**scopy** (sig moy DOS koh pee)	examination of the sigmoid colon using a scope
-sis	action, process, state, condition	myco**sis** (my COH sis)	disease caused by a fungus
-stasis	stoppage, controlling, standing	veno**stasis** (vee no STAY sis)	stoppage of blood in a vein
-stomy	surgically create an artificial mouth or stoma (opening)	colo**stomy** (koh LOSS toh me)	surgical opening into the colon to create a stoma

Prefixes

Prefixes are word parts that are attached to the beginning of word roots and combining forms to add to or change their meaning. Many, but not all, medical terms have a prefix. Some common meanings of prefixes include the following:

1. Location
2. Position
3. Direction
4. Time
5. Number
6. Negation, absence of
7. Color

Just as with suffixes, the same prefixes can be attached to many word roots, resulting in thousands of variations. Knowing that the prefix *hyper-* means "abnormally increased" or "excessive" gives a clue to the meaning of the hundreds of words that contain this word part, including the following examples:

1. **Hyper**acid: Abnormally or excessively acidic
2. **Hyper**active: Exhibiting abnormally increased activity

3. **Hyper**tension: Persistently high blood pressure

In the same way, knowing that *poly-* means "many" or "much" helps decipher the following examples:

1. **Poly**atomic: Made up of many atoms
2. **Poly**glandular: Pertaining to or affecting many glands
3. **Poly**phobia: Irrational fear of many things

Prefixes can dramatically change the meaning of a word. For example, *systole* (SIS toh lee) means "contraction of the heart." The addition of the one-letter prefix *a*, which means "without," creates the word ***a**systole* (a SIS toh lee), meaning *without* contractions. This is a very different condition! Careful spelling is critical when using medical language. Illegible handwriting can also lead to errors. *Always make sure your spelling is correct and your writing is legible to others.*

When prefixes are listed in medical dictionaries and word lists, they are arranged alphabetically, followed by a hyphen, and identified as a word part, as in the following sample dictionary entries:

1. *epi-* word part (Gr.) over; above; upon
2. *hyper-* word part (Gr.) abnormally increased; excessive
3. *poly-* word part (Gr.) many; much

See Table 4–5 for a list of commonly used prefixes.

Table 4–5 Common Prefixes

Prefix	Meaning	Term	Meaning
a-/an-	without, not, absence of	**an**uria (an YOU ree ah)	absence of urine formation
anti-	against	**an**tibiotic (an tie buy AHT ick)	substance that inhibits growth of or destroys microorganisms
auto-	self	**auto**immune (aw toh ih MYOON)	disease that results in immune response to one's own body
bi-	two, double	**bi**furcate (BUY fur kate)	having two branches or divisions
brady-	slow	**brady**cardia (brad ee KAR dee ah)	slow heart rate
dys-	bad, difficult, painful, abnormal	**dys**pnea (disp NEE ah)	difficulty breathing
epi-	over, above, upon	**epi**gastric (ep ih GAS trik)	over the stomach
eu-	good, normal	**eu**pnea (oop NEE ah)	normal breathing
hemi-	half	**hemi**plegia (hem ee PLEE jee ah)	paralysis of one side or half of the body
hyper-	above, excessive	**hyper**tension (high per TEN shun)	high blood pressure
hypo-	less than, under	**hypo**tension (high poh TEN shun)	low blood pressure
inter-	between	**inter**costal (in ter COS tahl)	between the ribs
intra-	within	**intra**venous (in trah VEE nus)	within a vein
multi-	many	**multi**nodal (mul tih NO dahl)	having many nodes or knots
non-	not	**non**toxic (non TOK sik)	not poisonous

(continues)

Table 4–5 **Common Prefixes** *(continued)*

Prefix	Meaning	Term	Meaning
peri-	around, surrounding	**peri**anal (per ee A nal)	around the anus
poly-	many, much	**poly**uria (pol ee YOU ree ah)	excretion of large amounts of urine
post-	after, behind	**post**operative (post OP er ah tiv)	following a surgical procedure
pre-	before, in front	**pre**operative (pree OP er ah tiv)	before a surgical procedure
pseudo-	false	**pseudo**hematuria (sue doh hee mah TOO ree ah)	red pigment in the urine that makes the urine "falsely" appear to have blood in it
quadri-	four	**quadri**plegia (kwad rih PLEE jee ah)	paralysis of all four extremities
semi-	half	**semi**permeable (sem ee PER mee ah bull)	half permeable—a membrane that allows fluids but not the dissolved substance to pass through
sub-	under, below	**sub**sternal (sub STIR nuhl)	below the sternum
supra-	above, over	**supra**pubic (sue prah PEW bik)	above the pubic area
tachy-	fast, rapid	**tachy**cardia (tak ee KAR dee ah)	rapid heart rate
tri-	three	**tri**chotomy (try COT oh me)	division into three parts

DECIPHERING MEDICAL TERMS

Learning the meanings of commonly used word parts and understanding how they combine enable the health care professional to decipher thousands of medical terms. When confronted with a new term, start at the far right, with the suffix. Think of each word as a combination of building blocks, fitted together to create a precise meaning. (See Figure 4–2.) Work from right to left, identifying and defining each word part, as in the following examples:

Example # 1 cardiology

1. Starting from the right, find word part -*logy*
2. Determine meaning: study of

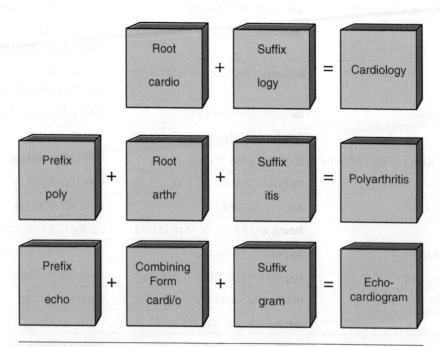

FIGURE 4–2 Think of the elements of medical terms as building blocks that can be used to construct new words.

3. Moving left, find word part *cardio*

4. Determine meaning: heart

5. Combine word parts: study of the heart

Example # 2 polyarthritis

1. Starting from the right, find word part *-itis*

2. Determine meaning: inflammation

3. Moving left, find word part *arthr*

4. Determine meaning: joint

5. Moving left, find word part *poly*

6. Determine meaning: many, much

7. Combine word parts: inflammation of many joints

Example # 3 echocardiogram

1. Starting from the right, find word part *-gram*

2. Determine meaning: written, record

3. Moving left, find word part *cardi/o*

4. Determine meaning: heart

5. Moving left, find word part *echo*

6. Determine meaning: echo (reflections of sounds)

7. Combine word parts: recording of the heart using echoes (to determine position and motion)

EPONYMS

Many medical terms that identify diseases, body structures, and procedures are named for the person who identified or discovered them. These are called **eponyms**. Examples of diseases include Alzheimer's disease, Hodgkin's disease, and Munchausen syndrome. The Heimlich maneuver is an example of a medical treatment. The well-known Pap test is short for Papanicolaou, the surname of the physician who discovered that uterine cancer can be detected in vaginal fluids.

WORDS WITH SPECIAL MEANINGS IN MEDICINE

Some everyday words have special meanings when used in medicine. For example, a "sign" is observable or measurable evidence of a patient's condition. "Acute" describes a condition that comes on quickly, progresses rapidly, and requires urgent care. And "benign" means not malignant, usually referring to cancer.

NAMES OF DRUGS

Drug names can be confusing because each drug approved by the Federal Drug Administration has four different names:

1. Generic name: the common name assigned by the United States Adopted Name Council

2. Trade name: the brand name

3. Chemical name: the molecular formula of the drug

4. Official name: name as it appears in the United States Pharmacopia/National Formulary (usually the same as the generic name)

For example, the generic name for the brand Tylenol is *acetaminophen* and the chemical name is $C8H9NO2$.

SPELLING AND PRONUNCIATION

Accurate spelling is critical when using medical language. Some words look and/or sound similar and can be easily confused. (See Figure 4–3.) It is important to pay attention to the context (the surrounding words and facts) to determine the correct meaning. The following examples contain words that are often confused:

1. Ilium (ILL ee um): Part of the hipbone

   Ileum (ILL ee um): Part of the intestine

2. Alveoli (al VEE oh lie): Tiny air sacs in the lungs

   Areola (ah RE oh lah): Brown pigmented area around the nipple

3. Palpation: examination technique in which examiner's hands are used to feel the texture, size, and location of a body part

4. Palpitations: pounding of the heart

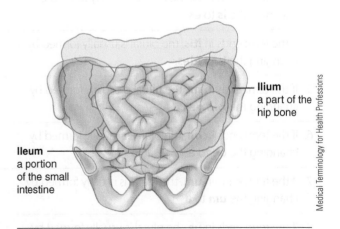

Ilium
a part of the hip bone

Ileum
a portion
of the small
intestine

Medical Terminology for Health Professions

FIGURE 4–3 There is only one letter difference between ileum and ilium, but they are very different parts of the body.

As with nontechnical English words, which have their origin in many different languages, some medical terms are spelled differently from the way they are pronounced. Table 4–6 contains common examples. Many of the guidelines apply to familiar words as well and are taken for granted in everyday speech. For example, "ph" used as "f" in the words *philosophy*, *Philadelphia*, and *Phoenix*.

The plural forms of many medical words are created with the original Greek and Latin endings, instead of the familiar "s" used for many English words. (See Figure 4–4.) Table 4–7 contains guidelines for creating the plural forms of many medical terms.

Misspelled words can lead to treatment and medication errors. Take the time to learn the correct spelling when learning new word parts. Health care professionals cannot take the chance that others will guess correctly what they intended to write.

Table 4–6 Spelling and Pronunciation Guidelines

Letter	Sounds Like	Examples
c when followed by e, i, or y	S	cell, circulatory, cyst
Ch	K	chronic
g when followed by e, i, or y	J	genetic, gingivitis, gyration
i when used to create plural	eye	bacilli (sing. bacillus)
Ph	F	pharmacist
Pn	N	pneumonia
Ps	S	psychiatrist
X	Z	Xylocaine (pronounced "ZIE loh cane," this is an anesthetic applied to the skin)

Table 4–7 Guidelines to Plural Forms

Guideline	Singular	Plural
1. If the term ends in **a**, the plural is usually formed by adding an **e**.	bursa	bursae
	vertebra	vertebrae
2. If the term ends in **ex** or **ix**, the plural is usually formed by changing the **ex** or **ix** to **ices**.	appendix	appendices
	index	indices
3. If the term ends in **is**, the plural is usually formed by changing the **is** to **es**.	diagnosis	diagnoses
	metastasis	metastases
4. If the term ends in **itis**, the plural is usually formed by changing the **is** to **ides**.	arthritis	arthritides
	meningitis	meningitides
5. If the term ends in **nx**, the plural is usually formed by changing the **x** to **ges**.	phalanx	phalanges
	meninx	meninges
6. If the term ends in **on**, the plural is usually formed by changing the **on** to **a**.	criterion	criteria
	ganglion	ganglia
7. If the term ends in **um**, the plural is usually formed by changing the **um** to **a**.	diverticulum	diverticula
	ovum	ova
8. If the term ends in **us**, the plural is usually formed by changing the **us** to **i**.	alveolus	alveoli
	malleolus	malleoli

If you are in doubt as to how a plural is formed, look it up in a medical dictionary!

Source: Medical Terminology for Health Professions (7th ed.), by A. Ehrlich & C. L. Schroeder, 2013, Clifton Park, NY: Delmar Cengage Learning.

Phalanges
(plural)

Phalanx
(singular)

Medical Terminology for Health Professions

FIGURE 4–4 Singular and plural endings. A phalanx is one finger or toe bone. Phalanges are more than one finger or toe bone.

MEDICAL ABBREVIATIONS AND SYMBOLS

Medical abbreviations and symbols are the shorthand of medical language. Many of them have been standardized and are universally accepted. In addition, each health care profession, agency, and facility has its own list of approved abbreviations and symbols. Each medical office or facility should have a policy and procedure manual or an employee handbook that includes this information. It is important that the health care professional ask for a copy of and become familiar with the list. *Never* substitute personal versions of abbreviations and symbols for those on the list when preparing any type of written documentation that will be used by the facility. Using abbreviations or symbols not on the approved list is against state and federal regulatory guidelines. If misuse is discovered during an accreditation or licensing survey visit, the agency or facility can be cited for not following the guidelines. If there are common abbreviations or symbols missing from the list, the supervisor should be notified. Common abbreviations used in texting, such as LMK ("let me know") and OFC ("of course") should never be used with medical correspondence.

There are dozens of medical abbreviations. Refer to Table 4–8 and Table 4–9 for some examples of frequently used abbreviations and symbols. Additional abbreviations and symbols will be encountered as students take health care specialty courses. For example, a dental assistant will learn the standardized numbering system used for identifying each tooth.

Some abbreviations are acronyms, groups of letters taken from the first letter of a phrase. Examples include MRI for "magnetic resonance image," ACL for "anterior cruciate ligament" (a main ligament of the knee), and LASER for "light amplification by stimulated emission of radiation."

Certain abbreviations, symbols, and dose designations have led to frequent errors due to misinterpretations. As a result of these reported errors, the Institute for Safe Medication Practices has created a list that is recommended never to be used in any medical communications (https://www.ismp.org/recommendations/error-prone-abbreviations-list). The Institute also recommends that the names of drugs not be abbreviated. The Joint Commission also has developed a requirement that certain abbreviations must appear on an accredited organization's do-not-use list. (See Table 4–10.)

Table 4–8 Examples of Abbreviations

ad lib	freely, at will, as necessary	P	pulse
a.c.	before a meal	p.c.	after meals
ASAP	as soon as possible	PO, p.o.	by mouth
b.i.d., bid	twice a day	p.r.n.	as needed
BM	bowel movement	q.h., qh	every hour
BP	blood pressure	q.i.d., QID, qid	four times a day

(continues)

Table 4–8 Examples of Abbreviations *(continued)*

c̄	with	R	respiration
CDC	Centers for Disease Control and Prevention	s̄	without
c/o, C/O	complains of	stat	immediately
h	hour	T	temperature
H₂O	water	t.i.d., TID, tid	three times a day
HTN	hypertension	TPR	temperature, pulse, and respiration
I&O	intake and output	Tx	traction or treatment
Lab	laboratory	URI	upper respiratory infection
NPO	nothing by mouth	UTI	urinary tract infection
N&V	nausea and vomiting	VS, vs	vital signs
O₂	oxygen	wt.	weight
p̄	after	x	multiplied by, times

Table 4–9 Examples of Symbols

↑	higher, elevate, or up	°	degree
↓	lower or down	♀	female
#	pound or number	♂	male
′	foot or minute	Δ	change
″	inch or second		

Table 4–10 Examples of Abbreviations Not to Be Used

IU	International unit	Write "units." Could be mistaken as IV (intravenous) or 10 (ten).
q.d. or QD	every day	Write "daily." The period after q or the tail of the Q is mistaken for an "I", which is qid (four times a day).
q.o.d. or QOD	every other day	Write "every other day." Could be mistaken for "q.d." (daily) or "q.i.d." (four times a day) if the "o" is poorly written.
U or u	unit	Write "unit." Could be mistaken as the number 0 or 4 (e.g., 4U seen as "40" or 4u seen as "44." Also can be mistaken as "cc" (e.g., 4u seen as 4cc).

Source: The Joint Commission. http://www.jointcommission.org/facts_about_do_not_use_list. Accessed 4/12/18

Thinking It Through

Mr. Fiacco is complaining of an irritation on his left arm where he had been applying a cream prescribed by the provider. You know that Mr. Fiacco has a skin condition and he was given a prescription for a cream he was to apply to his left arm q.d. for 10 days. You examine Mr. Fiacco's arm and note that the skin condition is gone, but now there is a red, irritated-looking area. You check the instructions on the prescription packaging and it says to apply the cream four times a day.

1. Is the patient applying the cream as originally intended?
2. What does q.d. mean?
3. What might be the reason for the newly reddened area on his left arm?
4. What is the abbreviation for four times a day?
5. What are some reasons for this problem occurring?
6. What can you do to correct each of the different possible causes of the problem?

Thinking It Through

Charles Grant, LVN, is given Mr. Grover's chart and asked to take the BP and P stat. Charles reviews the notes and sees that Mr. Grover has hypertension and tachycardia and that the physician has ordered the patient to be NPO. The chart also states that he has polyuria, rhinorrhea, eupnea, and a history of cholelithiasis. When Charles greets Mr. Grover and informs him that he is going to take his BP and P, Mr. Grover requests a drink of water first, as he is feeling quite thirsty.

1. What are BP and P? Is there any urgency in doing these?
2. Noting that Mr. Grover has hypertension and tachycardia, do you expect the readings to be too high, normal, or too low? Explain.
3. What do polyuria, rhinorrhea, eupnea, and cholelithiasis mean?
4. Is it appropriate to give Mr. Grover a glass of water? Why or why not?

MEDICAL DICTIONARY

Students are encouraged to purchase a medical or specialty dictionary, now available in both print and electronic versions. It is a valuable resource not only when taking health care courses but also as a handy reference in the work setting. The following features should be considered when selecting a dictionary:

- Clear, easy-to-understand definitions
- Explanations of medical procedures, conditions, disorders, and diseases
- Pronunciation hints
- Abbreviations and symbols
- Reference tables containing information such as laboratory values, units of measurement with conversion values, nutritional values of foods, and emergency resources
- Useful diagrams, charts, and tables
- Expanded explanations of topics of interest to the student
- Application of information to patient care
- Extent of vocabulary coverage specific to student's occupational area

It is very important to check the coverage of terms in the student's specialty area. Some dictionaries are more inclusive than others.

MASTERING MEDICAL TERMINOLOGY

Learning to use medical language is challenging for many students. Many words come from languages, such as Latin, that are no longer spoken. The words look and sound strange and seem long and complex. Medical terminology, however, can be mastered. The keys are *study* and *practice*. The following suggestions have helped many students:

- Study a few words each day. Avoid having to learn entire lists at the last minute just before test time.
- As word parts are learned, practice using them in new combinations.
- Use study techniques designed for mastering medical terminology. See the list of ideas in Table 4–11.
- Practice both the written and spoken forms as much as possible and in as many settings as possible.
- Learn new medical terms as they appear in this and other textbooks.
- Use a medical dictionary when unsure about how to spell or pronounce a word correctly.

- When working in a health care environment, accept help as needed from coworkers and supervisors to correct pronunciation and usage.

Having a strong understanding of the key concepts presented in this chapter will serve as a foundation for learning the material in subsequent chapters and throughout the entire health care educational program. The following are just a few of the subjects that depend heavily on knowledge of medical terminology:

- Anatomy (structure of the body)
- Physiology (function of the body)

- Pathophysiology (study of diseases and abnormal conditions)
- Medical insurance coding (assigning standardized codes to specific diagnoses and procedures)
- Pharmacology (therapeutic drugs)

The time initially spent learning the correct meaning, spelling, and pronunciation of medical word parts will save time later and prevent frustration when learning future subjects. Being proficient in the use of medical terminology is a mark of a competent health care professional. (See Box 4–1 for a list of useful resources for learning and using medical terminology.)

Table 4–11 Suggested Study Techniques

Suggestions
• Write down medical terms that you hear during lectures.
• Ask the instructor to write words on the board.
• Create cartoons using medical terms.
• Prepare flashcards with a word or picture on one side and the definition on the back.
• Study word roots that refer to the body by studying drawings of the body parts.
• Write words many times, using colored ink.
• Visualize familiar images along with the new terms. For example, visualize the Queen of Hearts playing cards for *cardi/o,* a rhinoceros with its big horn for *rhin/o,* and a gas tank for *gastr/o,* a part of the body that sometimes produces gas.
• Concentrate on terms when you hear them presented in lectures.
• Read medical terms aloud to yourself.
• Watch medical terminology YouTube videos that feature the pronunciation of medical terms.
• Take turns quizzing each other with another student.
• Create verbal rhythms; try setting them to music.
• Create audio, "sounds-like" cues to remember definitions.
• Draw images, and even color them.
• Create pairs of flashcards with the medical term on one card and the definition on the other. Then lay them out on a large table and move them around until you have them all matched correctly.
• Touch the part of your body referred to in the term or point to where it is located if it is not on the surface.
• Study the models of the body systems or build them from kits.

Box 4–1

Suggested Resources for Learning and Using Medical Terminology

ONLINE

Dictionaries of medical terms

www.medilexicon.com/

https://medlineplus.gov/appendixa.html

https://www.merriam-webster.com/medical/

Lists of medical abbreviations

https://medlineplus.gov/appendixb.html

www.upstate.edu/gch/patients-families/socialwork/glossary.php

Facts about the Official "Do Not Use" List of Abbreviations

www.jointcommission.org/facts_about_do_not_use_list/

Medical Acronyms

https://www.acronymslist.com/cat/medical-acronyms.html

(continues)

Box 4-1

PRINT

Dorland's illustrated medical dictionary (32nd ed.). (2011). Philadelphia: W. B. Saunders Company.

Ehrlich, A., & Schroeder, C. L. (2017). *Medical terminology for health professions* (8th ed.). Clifton Park, NY: Cengage Learning.

Miller-Keane encyclopedia & dictionary of medicine, nursing, & allied health (7th ed.). (2013). Philadelphia: W. B. Saunders Company.

Stedman's medical dictionary for health professionals and nursing (7th ed.). (2011). Baltimore: Lippincott Williams & Wilkins.

Taber's cyclopedic medical dictionary (22nd ed.). (2013). Philadelphia: F. A. Davis.

SUGGESTED LEARNING ACTIVITIES

1. Start a list of new medical terms, with their definitions, as you encounter them. This can be a list written in your notebook or created on your computer.

2. Watch television programs and/or videos on YouTube that portray medical settings and listen for medical terms. Do the professionals on these programs use a different level of language when speaking among themselves than when speaking with patients? Do you recognize any of the terms used?

3. Watch and listen for "medical" prefixes and suffixes that are also used in everyday English (or Spanish!).

4. Using the examples of terms provided in Figure 4–5, create ten medical terms for other body parts. Use the charts in this chapter and a medical dictionary.

5. Choose three study techniques from the list in Table 4–11 to use for a week as you study medical terminology. Did you find them helpful?

cardi/o

cardiac
cardiology
cardiologist
cardiogram
cardiopathy
postcardiopathy
tachycardia

derm/o
dermat/o

dermatology
dermatologist
dermatitis
dermatoplasty
epidermis
intradermal

FIGURE 4–5 The combining form for each body part is the basis for many terms.

WEB ACTIVITIES

American Institute of Medical Sciences & Education

http://www.aimseducation.edu/blog/how-to-learn-medical-terminology/

Super Easy Tips to Learn Medical Terminology

This website is an excellent resource. It contains short descriptions of study methods, links to helpful videos, lists of apps, and more. Choose techniques to try and report on the results.

Medlineplus

http://medlineplus.gov/medicalwords.html

Understanding Medical Words: A Tutorial from the National Library of Medicine

Review frequently used medical terms, including root words, suffixes, and prefixes with this interactive tutorial.

MediLexicon International Ltd.

www.medilexicon.com/

MediLexicon is an online database of medical vocabulary and abbreviations. Use the search field to find definitions for five abbreviations and five medical terms. Record your findings.

Institute for Safe Medical Practices

https://www.ismp.org/recommendations/error-prone-abbreviations-list

Review the "Error-Prone Abbreviation List" and list ten examples other than those presented in Table 4–10.

National Library of Medicine

https://www.ncbi.nlm.nih.gov/pmc/articles/PMC4120137/

Read the article about medical eponyms and list the ten conditions described, along with a sentence about the physician/scientist associated with each.

Study Stack

https://www.studystack.com/flashcard-137287

Make online flashcards to practice medical word parts.

REVIEW QUESTIONS

1. Why is it important to use medical terminology correctly when reading, writing, and speaking?
2. When and with whom should medical terminology be used?
3. What do the following terms mean: word roots, combining forms, suffixes, and prefixes? Give an example of each.
4. What are the steps for breaking medical terms into their component parts and interpreting them correctly?
5. Provide five examples of medical terms that include a prefix and a suffix. Give their meanings.
6. Provide five examples of medical eponyms and explain their origin.
7. What are three examples of everyday words that have different meanings when used as medical terms?
8. What are the four types of names given to approved prescription drugs?
9. What are the guidelines for medical terms when the pronunciation differs from the spelling?
10. Provide eight examples of abbreviations and five examples of symbols presented in this chapter.
11. Why is it important to use medical abbreviations correctly? What is the do-not-use list?
12. What are the features of a medical dictionary that should be considered when choosing one?
13. What are five study techniques designed to help students mastering medical terminology?

APPLICATION EXERCISES

1. Refer to The Case of Where Is the Pain? presented at the beginning of this chapter. What does *epigastric* mean? How would you respond to Ms. Mitchell's question, "What is epigastric?"

2. Kelly Cordeiro is a recent medical assisting graduate who is hired by a prominent ophthalmologist. She is excited about having the opportunity to work in this area. However, Kelly quickly discovers that there are many terms related to the anatomy of the eye, special procedures, eye surgery, and medications with which she is not familiar. She feels a little lost and is concerned about her ability to communicate effectively with the physician and maintain patient records appropriately.

   a. What references would you suggest for Kelly to learn the vocabulary she needs?

   b. Suggest study techniques she can use to quickly learn the new vocabulary.

PROBLEM-SOLVING PRACTICE

Jason Lopez is currently taking a class in medical terminology. He studies hard and feels he knows the material well, but when he gets his test results back, there are several marked wrong that he says are correct. The instructor states that she could not read it clearly enough to be absolutely sure it was correct and refuses to change his score. Using the five-step problem-solving process, determine what Jason can do about his problem on the test.

CHAPTER 5

Medical Math

KEY TERMS

angles
apothecary system
basic formula
Celsius (C)
decimals
degrees
estimating
Fahrenheit (F)
fractional equation
fractions
gram
household system
improper fractions
liter
math anxiety
meter
metric system
military time
mixed number
nomenclature
percentages
proportion
ratios
reciprocal
reducing the fraction
reference plane
Roman numerals
rounding numbers
sample
simplifying the fraction
statistics
whole numbers

OBJECTIVES

Studying and applying the material in this chapter will help you to:

1. List examples of how math is used by health care professionals.
2. Explain why accuracy is essential when using math in health care.
3. Describe the signs of math anxiety and explain how it prevents confidence and competence in the study and application of math.
4. List ways that students can review or learn the concepts of basic math.
5. Define the meaning of a whole number.
6. Describe a decimal and define the term decimal point.
7. List the steps for performing basic math calculations with decimals.
8. Describe a fraction.
9. List the steps for performing basic math calculations with fractions.
10. Describe a percentage.
11. List the steps for converting among the following numerical forms: decimals, fractions, percentages, and ratios.
12. Describe how to round off numbers correctly.
13. Demonstrate how to set up and use an equation to solve a proportion problem.
14. Demonstrate how to use the basic formula to calculate drug dosages.
15. Explain the purpose of estimating and describe the guidelines for its use.
16. Give examples of how statistics are used in health care.
17. Explain how military time differs from the traditional system and list its advantages.
18. Describe how to convert Arabic numerals into Roman numerals
19. Give examples of how angles are used in health care.
20. Describe how to estimate angles from a reference plane.
21. Describe the household, metric, and apothecary units used to express length, volume, and weight.
22. Explain how to convert among the household, metric, and apothecary units of measurement.
23. Give the formula for converting between the Fahrenheit and Celsius temperature scales.

The Case of Exactly How Much Does My Baby Weigh?

During a well-baby checkup, Jamie Brown weighs Jessica Munoz and reports to the mother that her baby weighs 10 kilograms. The mother states her daughter weighed 20 pounds on the last visit and asks how much 10 kilograms is in pounds. Jamie explains that 10 kilograms is the same as 22 pounds, so there has been a 2-pound increase in weight.

Not knowing how to convert between kilograms and pounds would have prevented Jamie from answering the mother's question. This chapter will cover the math needed by the health care professional, including information about converting between commonly used systems of measurement.

IMPORTANCE OF MATH IN HEALTH CARE

Work in health care requires the use of math skills to measure and perform various types of calculations. There are applications in all types of occupations:

- Calculating medication dosages
- Taking height and weight readings
- Measuring the amount of intake (fluids consumed or infused) and output (urine, vomit)
- Performing billing and bookkeeping tasks
- Performing lab tests
- Mixing solutions
- Processing medical bills
- Handling insurance claims
- Collecting payments

Errors in math can have negative effects on patients. For example, administering the wrong dosage of medication is a serious mistake and can harm or even result in the death of a patient. Health care professionals must strive for 100% accuracy. *If there is any doubt, it is essential to ask your supervisor or a qualified coworker to double-check calculations.*

MATH ANXIETY

Millions of people experience feelings of intimidation and fear when confronted with mathematics. This condition is called **math anxiety**, math avoidance, or math phobia. A person experiencing math anxiety may be afraid of making mistakes, freezing up and going blank, or being judged as a failure.

Math anxiety may be based on a past unpleasant experience that interferes with learning. The good news is that a positive experience learning math can overcome these past feelings so that success with future achievement in math can be achieved.

Students who suffer from math anxiety may be feeling dread at just the thought of reading this chapter. If you are unsure whether you suffer from math anxiety, take the math anxiety test listed in the Web Activities at the end of this chapter.

When students are experiencing math anxiety, it is difficult to test them for math ability because the test-takers' anxiety can negatively affect the results. Math anxiety can be felt so strongly that it prevents memorization, concentration, and the ability to pay attention, all of which are required for solving math problems.

The first step to overcoming math anxiety is to recognize that it exists and be willing to do something about it. Many people who think they have a learning disability or just "can never do math" have found that it is the anxiety that causes the mental block and interferes with their ability to learn. After this block is overcome, they are able to learn and perform the math necessary for their work. Table 5–1 addresses some common negative beliefs about math that can set up mental blocks to learning. These blocks can be overcome by applying the suggestions listed in Table 5–2. Keep in mind that it is never too late to catch up on your math skills.

BASIC CALCULATIONS

The information presented on whole numbers, decimals, fractions, percentages, and ratios is included in this chapter as a review of the basics needed to perform

Table 5–1 False Beliefs about Math

The Fear Thought	The Reality
I don't get math, never have and never will.	Math is a learned skill and requires practice.
Males are better at math than females.	Research has proven this to be false.
I am better with words than with numbers and you can't be good at both. I just will not ever get math.	People commonly show high capability on both mathematical and verbal testing.
There is only one right way to solve a problem.	The best way to do a math problem is the method that works for you.
It's bad to count on your fingers.	Most people find counting on their fingers helpful, and there is no reason to feel guilty. The Chinese have used an "abacus" for centuries. This is a sophisticated finger-counting machine that is fast and accurate.
Mathematicians do problems quickly, in their heads.	If anyone performs a skill quickly, it is because they have done it many times. Any unfamiliar process takes time and practice.
I don't have a good memory.	Understanding is superior to memorization. If you truly understand something, you will use reason to naturally arrive at the answer.
It is hopeless, and much too hard for the average person.	After you overcome your emotional blocks and develop self-confidence by practicing, you will be happy to find that you also can do math.
There is a magic key to doing math.	There is no magic or any one approach you need to learn to do math well.

Table 5–2 Overcoming Math Anxiety

What to Do	How This Helps
The first step is to identify that you have math anxiety.	Overcoming math anxiety calls for experiencing and being aware of your emotional responses to math.
Identify what you already know and what you need to learn.	This is less overwhelming than simply saying "I can't do math." It provides a starting point for learning.
Do not delay identifying and working on your weak areas in math.	Procrastination increases anxiety.
Say "I will keep trying" rather than "I can't do it."	As long as there is the willingness to continue trying, the mind will work on mastering new material.
Take breaks as needed to clear your mind.	When the mind lacks clarity, you will start going in circles. A break allows for a fresh start.
Maintain a positive and confident manner.	Doing math requires confidence and concentration; panic and anxiety make this impossible. Expecting the worst makes it hard to concentrate.
Accept that there are no secrets to be handed out.	Participation and engagement in the process is what is needed for success.
As with any new material, many repetitions will be needed to master the new material.	Some topics have to be read, heard, and/or discussed many times before they become clear. There is nothing wrong with this and it is part of the normal process of learning.

(continues)

Table 5–2 Overcoming Math Anxiety (continued)

What to Do	How This Helps
Monitor your thoughts and replace negativity with productive thoughts. For example, instead of thinking "This is just the kind of problem I can never solve," change it to "What is making this problem difficult for me, and what can I do to make it easier for myself?"	Those who do well in math are not necessarily smarter, but they seem to know themselves better. They can anticipate the difficulties they will have and know what questions and actions will give them the power and confidence to continue.
If you come across a formula or process that seems too complex, break it down into small parts: write down what you know and what you are being asked to solve.	This will help you to overcome the fear of complexity and being overwhelmed.

many medical math applications. The purpose is to jog the student's memory: "Yes, that's right, now I remember." For students who cannot easily follow the review or believe they never learned the concepts, a refresher course or more extensive review is recommended. There are many excellent books and computer programs on basic arithmetic. Another option is to find out if your campus has a resource center that offers assistance to students who need to review math.

To work safely in health care, it is essential to accurately add, subtract, multiply, and divide whole numbers, decimals, fractions, and percentages. Students also need to understand equivalents when using decimals, fractions, and percentages. (See Figure 5–1.)

Many health care professionals use small calculators, also available on cell phones, to assist them with calculations. During your health care studies, some instructors will allow the use of calculators and others will not. It is always best to know how to do the basic functions by "longhand" (without a calculator), because calculators can quit working at any time during a test or at the workplace. Some professional exams required for licensure or certification do not allow the use of calculators.

FIGURE 5–1 An easy way to remember how to convert decimals, percentages, and fractions is to think of this humorous cartoon.

Whole Numbers

Whole numbers are what we traditionally use to count (1, 2, 3, . . .). They do not contain fractions or decimals. For example, 30 is a whole number, whereas 30½ and 30.5 are not. Students must be able to accurately add, subtract, multiply, and divide whole numbers.

- Add: $15 + 24 = 39$ (verbal: fifteen plus twenty-four equals thirty-nine)
- Subtract: $54 - 15 = 39$ (verbal: fifty-four minus fifteen equals thirty-nine)
- Multiply: $14 \times 8 = 112$ (verbal: fourteen times eight equals one hundred and twelve)
- Divide: $60 \div 12 = 5$ (verbal: sixty divided by twelve equals five)

Decimals

Decimals are one way of expressing parts of numbers or anything else that has been divided into parts. The parts are expressed in units of 10. That is, decimals represent the

Fascinating Facts

Quote from Albert Einstein (1879–1955):

"Do not worry about your difficulties in mathematics, I assure you that mine are greater."

number of tenths, hundredths, thousandths, and so on that are available. For example, 0.7 represents 7 of the 10 parts into which something has been divided. When reading decimals verbally, it is necessary to know the placement values for the decimals (digits to the right of the decimal point) and that the decimal point may be read as "and." (See Figure 5–2.) For example:

- 0.5 is read "five tenths"
- 1.5 is read "one and five tenths"
- 1.50 is read "one and fifty hundredths"

An alternative method for verbalizing these numbers is as follows:

- 0.5 is read "zero point five"
- 1.5 is read "one point five"
- 1.50 is read "one point five zero"
- 1.500 is read "one and five hundred thousandths"
- 1.5000 is read "one and five thousand ten thousandths"

Decimal points are so small, they can be missed when reading numbers. This can lead to medication errors, so guidelines have been developed to help prevent these

Thinking It Through

Ms. Cree is a new graduate and has just been hired as a medical assistant in Dr. Albright's office. She is anxious about learning the new routines and doing a good job. She has always struggled with math calculations, but was able to develop her skills to pass her courses in school. However, when Dr. Albright orders a medication that needs to be calculated, Ms. Cree panics. She is unable to find her calculator, and even though she has been able to manually solve this type of problem in the classroom setting, she now becomes too afraid to trust her own skills. Where *is* that calculator? Ms. Cree is afraid of losing her job if she admits the problem, and yet she knows that if she makes a mistake, she could jeopardize the health of the patient.

1. What job-related factors are contributing to Ms. Cree's anxiety and panic?
2. What suggestions would you recommend to her?
3. What thoughts are going through her mind that may be adding to the problem?

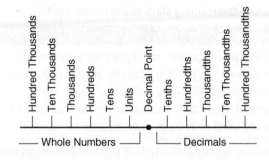

FIGURE 5–2 The position of the number to the left or the right of the decimal point is its place value. The value of each place to the *left* of the decimal point is *10 times* that of the place to its right. The value of each place to the *right* of the decimal point is *one-tenth* the value of the place to its left.

errors. The Joint Commission requires the following practices when writing decimals:

- Never use a trailing zero (e.g., write 1 mg, *not* 1.0 mg because the decimal point can be missed and it could be read as 10 mg. This would result in a tenfold error in dosage.).
- Always use a leading zero if less than 1 (e.g., write 0.1 mg, *not* .1 mg because the decimal point can be missed and the number read as 1 mg. This would result in a tenfold error in dosage.).

Decimals are added, subtracted, multiplied, and divided in the same way as whole numbers. (See Table 5–3 for examples.) The most common mistake when working with decimals is incorrect placement of the decimal point.

Fractions

Fractions are another way of expressing numbers that represent parts of a whole. A fraction has a numerator (top number) and a denominator (bottom number). An example of a fraction is ³⁄₁₀, where the 3 is the numerator and 10 is the denominator. One way of looking at it is that the denominator (bottom number) defines how many parts make a whole and the numerator (top number) is the number of parts of this whole that are represented by the fraction. See Figure 5–3 for an illustration of this concept. The fraction ³⁄₁₀ is read as "three tenths."

Although performing calculations with fractions is not difficult, it does require following a series of steps. These are described in Table 5–4. There are a few special considerations to remember when working with fractions. When adding and subtracting fractions, it is necessary to change all the denominators to the same number in order to perform the calculations. This is known as "converting the fractions." To do this, find a number that each denominator can divide into evenly and then adjust the numerators

Table 5–3 Working with Decimals

Function	Example	Steps to Follow
Add (+):	$\begin{array}{r}1.5\\+\ 2.25\\\hline 3.75\end{array}$	1. Line up the decimal points. 2. Add the numbers. 3. Bring the decimal point straight down.
Subtract (−):	$\begin{array}{r}3.75\\-1.25\\\hline 2.50\end{array}$	1. Line up the decimal points. 2. Subtract the numbers. 3. Bring the decimal point straight down.
Multiply (×):	$\begin{array}{r}2.5\\\times\ 2.5\\\hline 125\\+\ 50\\\hline 6.25\end{array}$	1. Multiply the numbers. 2. Count the total number of digits to the right of the decimal points in the numbers you are multiplying. 3. Count the same number of places in your answer. Start to the right of the last digit in your answer and move left that number of places. This is where the decimal point is placed.
Divide (÷):	$2.5\overline{)50.5} = 25\overline{)50.5}$ $= 25\overline{)505.0}$ $\begin{array}{r}20\\50\\\hline 5\end{array}$ $= 25\overline{)505.0}$ $\begin{array}{r}20.2\\50\\\hline 50\\50\\\hline 0\end{array}$	1. Move the decimal point to the right in the number you are dividing by (to make it a whole number). 2. Move the decimal point the same number of places to the right in the number being divided. Add zeros if necessary. 3. Divide the numbers. 4. Place the decimal point in the answer by moving it straight up from the number that was divided.

to maintain an equivalent fraction. For example, to add $\frac{1}{2} + \frac{1}{3}$, convert both fractions to sixths: $\frac{3}{6} + \frac{2}{6} = \frac{5}{6}$ (The denominators 2 and 3 both divide into 6 evenly; then the numerator is multiplied by the number of times the old denominator divides into the new denominator [2 divides into 6 three times, so 1×3 creates the new fraction $\frac{3}{6}$; 3 divides into 6 two times, so 1×2 then creates the new fraction $\frac{2}{6}$].)

Multiplying fractions is straightforward. First multiply the two numerators and then the two denominators. For example, $\frac{1}{2} \times \frac{1}{2} = \frac{1}{4}$ ($1 \times 1 = 1$ and $2 \times 2 = 4$).

Dividing fractions requires the dividing fraction to be inverted (turned upside-down). The new, upside-down fraction is called the **reciprocal**. The numerators and denominators are then multiplied to get the answer. For example, $\frac{1}{2} \div \frac{1}{2} = \frac{1}{2} \times \frac{2}{1} = \frac{2}{2}$ or 1.

Two processes are frequently used when working with fractions. **Reducing the fraction** to its lowest terms means finding a number that can be divided evenly into both the numerator and the denominator. For example, the fraction $\frac{2}{4}$ can be reduced to the lower equivalent fraction of $\frac{1}{2}$ by dividing both the numerator and the denominator

by 2 ($2 \div 2 = 1$ and $4 \div 2 = 2$). This process is also known as **simplifying the fraction**.

Improper fractions have numerators that are larger than the denominators. To reduce these fractions, divide the denominator into the numerator. The result will be a whole number or a **mixed number** (whole number and a fraction). For example, the fraction $\frac{12}{4}$ would be reduced to the whole number 3 ($12 \div 4 = 3$); the fraction $\frac{11}{4}$ would be reduced to the mixed number $2\frac{3}{4}$ ($11 \div 4 = 2\frac{3}{4}$).

Percentages

Percentages are used to express either a whole or part of a whole. The whole is expressed as 100% (percent). Refer back to Figure 5–3 and imagine this as a hot apple pie sliced into 10 equal pieces. The 10 slices together equal the whole, or 100%, of the pie. One hundred divided by ten equals ten. Therefore, each slice represents 10% of the pie. If each slice is 10%, then three slices represent 30% of the pie.

When working with percentages, it is easier to convert the percentage to a decimal and then to perform the addition, subtraction, multiplication, and division. Converting percentages to decimals is explained later in this chapter.

Table 5–4 Working with Fractions

Function	Example	Steps to Follow
Add (+):	$\dfrac{1}{5} = \dfrac{6}{30}$ $+\dfrac{1}{6} = +\dfrac{5}{30}$ $\dfrac{11}{30}$	1. If the denominators are not the same, find a number both denominators divide evenly into. In these examples, the number that divides evenly into both denominators is 6. 2. Multiply the numerators by the number of times the old denominators divide into the new denominator. 3. Add the numerators. 4. Place the new numerator over the denominator. 5. Reduce the fraction, if necessary.
Subtract (−):	$\dfrac{1}{5} = \dfrac{6}{30}$ $-\dfrac{1}{6} = \dfrac{5}{30}$ $\dfrac{1}{30}$	1. If the denominators are not the same, find a number both denominators divide evenly into. 2. Multiply the numerators by the number of times the old denominators divide into the new denominator. 3. Subtract the numerators. 4. Place the new numerator over the denominator. 5. Reduce the fraction, if necessary.
Multiply (×):	$\dfrac{1}{5} \times \dfrac{1}{6} = \dfrac{1}{30}$	1. Multiply numerators. 2. Multiply denominators. 3. Reduce the fraction, if necessary.
Divide (÷)	$\dfrac{1}{5} \div \dfrac{1}{6} = \dfrac{1}{5} \times \dfrac{6}{1} = \dfrac{6}{5} = 1\frac{1}{5}$	1. Invert the dividing fraction. 2. Multiply numerators. 3. Multiply denominators. 4. Reduce the fraction, if necessary.

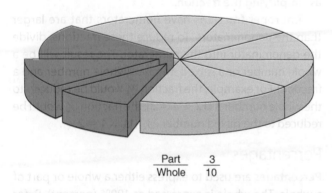

$$\frac{\text{Part}}{\text{Whole}} \quad \frac{3}{10}$$

FIGURE 5–3 A fraction is a comparison of parts (numerator) to a whole (denominator).

Ratios

Ratios show relationships between numbers or like values: How many of one number or value is present compared to the other. Converting between ratios and percentages is explained in the next section.

When working with liquids, it is necessary to look at the part compared to the whole quantity. For example, a

1:3 bleach to water solution contains one part of bleach and three parts of water. The whole quantity in this case is four parts. To determine the strength of the bleach solution, the amount of bleach (1 part) is divided by the whole (4 parts): 1 ÷ 4 = 0.25 or 25%. Therefore, it can be stated that this is a 25% bleach solution.

Converting Decimals, Fractions, Percentages, and Ratios

Decimals, fractions, and percentages all express parts of a whole. The cartoon in Figure 5–1 humorously portrays how they are related: The fraction $\frac{1}{2}$, the decimal 0.5, and the percentage 50% all represent the same amount of the sandwich. The steps involved in converting among these numerical forms are shown in Table 5–5.

Rounding Numbers

Rounding numbers means changing them to the nearest ten, hundred, thousand, and so on. Deciding which to use depends on the size of the original number and the degree of accuracy required. Deciding whether to round

Table 5–5 Converting Decimals, Fractions, and Percentages

Converting	Example	Steps to Follow
Decimals to fractions	$\dfrac{0.075}{1}$ $\dfrac{0.075}{1} \times \dfrac{1000}{1000} = \dfrac{75}{1000} = \dfrac{3}{40}$	1. Write down the number to be converted (0.075) divided by 1, as shown. 2. Multiply the numerator and the denominator by 10 for each number after the decimal point (in this case, there are three numbers after the decimal point, so multiply by 10×10×10 which is the same as 1000). If appropriate, reduce the resulting fraction.
Decimals to percentages	$5.275 \times 100 = 527.5$ 527.5%	1. Multiply the number to be converted (5.275) by 100 (this is equivalent to moving the decimal point two places to the right, because percentages are based on 100). 2. Add the percent sign.
Fractions to decimals	3/5 $3 \div 5 = 0.6$	1. Write down the fraction to be converted (3/5). 2. Divide the numerator by the denominator.
Fractions to percentages	7/8 $7 \div 8 = 0.875$ $0.875 \times 100 = 87.5$ 87.5%	1. Write down the fraction to be converted (7/8). 2. Divide the numerator by the denominator. 3. Multiply by 100 (this is equivalent to moving the decimal point two places to the right, because percentages are based on 100). 4. Add the percent sign.
Percentages to decimals	125.5% 125.5 $125.5 \div 100 = 1.255$	1. Write down the percentage to be converted (125.5%). 2. Remove the percent sign. 3. Divide by 100 (this is equivalent to moving decimal point two places to the left, because percentages are based on 100).
Percentages to fractions	5% 5 $5/100 = 1/25$	1. Write down the percentage to be converted (5%). 2. Remove the percent sign. 3. Divide the number (5) by 100 and if appropriate, reduce the fraction.

up or round down depends on the digits (numbers) located to the right of the value chosen for rounding. The following examples illustrate how these rules are applied:

Example 1 When rounding to the nearest 10, look at the digit in the units place which is just to the right of the tens place. If the number is 5 or above, round up. If it is less than 5, round down.

88 rounds up to 90

83 rounds down to 80

Example 2 When rounding to the nearest 100, look at the digit in the tens place which is just to the right of the hundreds place. If the number is 5 or above, round up. If it is less than 5, round down.

67 rounds up to 100

133 rounds down to 100

668 rounds up to 700

621 rounds down to 600

Example 3 When rounding to the nearest 1000, look at the digit in the hundreds place, just to the right of the thousands place. If the number is 5 or above, round up. If it is less than 5, round down.

7777 rounds up to 8000

7355 rounds down to 7000

Numbers of all sizes can be rounded. Review Figure 5–2 and study the examples in Table 5–6.

Table 5–6 Rounding Numbers

Round the Number 1234.5678 to the Nearest:	Result	Comments
Whole number	1235	The digit to the right of the whole number (1234) is 5, so you round up one number.
Tens	1230	The digit to the right of the tens place is 4, so you round down.
Hundreds	1200	The digit to the right of the hundreds place is 3, so you round down.
Thousands	1000	The digit to the right of the thousands place is 2, so you round down.
Tenths	1234.6	The digit to the right of the tenths place is 6, so you round up.
Hundredths	1234.57	The digit to the right of the hundredths place is 7, so you round up.
Thousandths	1234.568	The digit to the right of the thousandths place is 8, so you round up.
Ten thousandths	1234.5678	No change.

Solving Problems with Proportions

A **proportion** is a mathematical statement that two ratios are equal. For example, the proportion 2:6 = 3:9 means that 2 is related to 6 in the same way that 3 is related to 9. Stated another way, 2 = 1/3 of 6 and 3 = 1/3 of 9. This proportion is verbalized as "two is to six as three is to nine."

Note that proportions have four parts or terms. They are useful for finding an unknown when you know three of the terms. Here is an example:

- You need $32.50 to make a payment, but you have only quarters. How many quarters do you need?

- Three terms are known:

  1. $32.50—the amount you need

  2. 4—the number of quarters that are in $1.00

  3. $1.00—the unit of measurement, dollars, in this proportion

- Unknown: number of quarters in $32.50. This is represented by the letter "x"

- Set up an equation to answer the question: "If four quarters equal $1.00, how many quarters are there in $32.50?" Stated in the language of proportions, this would be: "4 quarters are to $1.00 as 'x' quarters are to $32.50."

- With this information, you can set up the proportion as follows:

$$\frac{4 \text{ quarters}}{x \text{ quarters}} = \frac{\$1.00}{\$32.50}$$

- This is verbalized as "4 quarters are to $1.00 as x quarters are to $32.50." (*Note that the two unit measurements on each side of the equation are the same:* quarters on the left and dollars on the right.)

There is more than one way to solve a proportion problem. One way, illustrated here, is called the **fractional equation** method. In spite of its name, it is not difficult. Use the following steps:

1. Cross multiply the terms in the fractions:

$$\frac{4 \text{ quarters}}{x \text{ quarters}} \times \frac{\$1.00}{\$32.50}$$

$$1 \times x = 4 \times 32.50$$

Therefore, 1x = 130.

2. Divide each side of the equation by the number in front of "x." (In this case, each number is divided by one, so this does not change the number. This number will not always be one.)

$$1x \div 1 = x \text{ and } 130 \div 1 = 130$$

$$x = 130 \text{ quarters}$$

3. Answer: 130 quarters are needed to make a payment of $32.50.

4. The completed proportion is

$$\frac{4 \text{ quarters}}{130 \text{ quarters}} = \frac{\$1.00}{\$32.50}$$

Here is a health-related example of using a fractional equation:

- You need to give medication to a patient who weighs 165 pounds. How many milligrams (mg), a unit of measurement discussed later in this chapter, of the medication should you give if the dosage is 20 mg per 10 pounds of the patient's weight?

- Three terms are known:

  1. 20 mg—the amount required per every 10 pounds

  2. 10 pounds—the number of pounds for each mg

3. 165 pounds—the patient's weight

4. Unknown: the number of milligrams of medication to give the patient. This is represented by the letter "x."

- Set up an equation to answer the question: "If 20 mg are required for each 10 pounds of a patient's weight, how many milligrams are required for a 165-pound patient?"

- Set up the proportion:

1. $\dfrac{20 \text{ mg}}{x \text{ mg}} = \dfrac{10 \text{ lb}}{165 \text{ lb}}$

2. Cross multiply the terms in the fractions:

$\dfrac{20 \text{ mg}}{x \text{ mg}} \diagup\diagdown \dfrac{10 \text{ lb}}{165 \text{ lb}}$

$10 \times x = 20 \times 165$

Therefore, $10x = 3{,}300$.

- Divide each side of the equation by the number in front of "x."

$10x \div 10 = x$ and $3{,}300 \div 10 = 330$

- Answer: 330 mg of medication is needed for a 165-pound patient.

- The completed proportion is:

$\dfrac{20 \text{ mg}}{330 \text{ mg}} = \dfrac{10 \text{ lb}}{165 \text{ lb}}$

Converting units of measure is another common application of proportions. For example, you want to know how many feet are in 29 inches. Again, three of the terms in the proportion are known:

1. 29 inches

2. 12 (the number of inches in 1 foot)

3. 1 foot (the unit of measure desired)

The proportion is set up as follows:

$\dfrac{1 \text{ foot}}{x \text{ feet}} = \dfrac{12 \text{ inches}}{29 \text{ inches}}$

To solve this problem, follow these steps:

1. Cross multiply:

$\dfrac{1 \text{ foot}}{x \text{ feet}} \diagup\diagdown \dfrac{12 \text{ inches}}{29 \text{ inches}}$

$12 \times x = 1 \times 29$

Therefore, $12x = 29$.

2. Divide each side of the equation by the number in front of "x":

$12x \div 12 = x$ and $29 \div 12 = 2.42$

$x = 2.42$ feet (rounded to nearest hundredth)

3. The completed proportion is

$\dfrac{1 \text{ foot}}{2.42 \text{ feet}} = \dfrac{12 \text{ inches}}{29 \text{ inches}}$

Converting Medications

A common application of proportions in health care is to find the value of an unknown when converting medications from one form to another. For example, a physician orders a patient to have 50 grams, a unit of measurement explained later in this chapter, of a medication. When the nurse checks, she notes that the medication is available only in 12.5-gram tablets. How many tablets should she give the patient?

To solve this problem:

- Three terms are known:

1. 50 grams (medication ordered for patient)

2. 12.5-gram tablets (form in which medication is available)

3. 1 tablet (form in which medication comes)

- Set up the proportion

$\dfrac{1 \text{ tablet}}{x \text{ tablets}} = \dfrac{12.5 \text{ grams}}{50 \text{ grams}}$

- Cross multiply:

$\dfrac{1 \text{ tablet}}{x \text{ tablets}} \diagup\diagdown \dfrac{12.5 \text{ grams}}{50 \text{ grams}}$

$12.5 \times x = 1 \times 50$

Therefore, $12.5x = 50$.

- Divide each side by the number in front of "x":

$12.5x \div 12.5 = x$ and $50 \div 12.5 = 4$

$x = 4$ tablets

- Answer: 4 tablets are needed to equal 50 grams. This is the amount to be given to the patient.

- The completed proportion is

$\dfrac{1 \text{ tablet}}{4 \text{ tablets}} = \dfrac{12.5 \text{ grams}}{50 \text{ grams}}$

While you can use the cross multiplication method for calculating medication dosages, some health care professionals prefer to use the **basic formula** method. It is based on the following:

$$\dfrac{D}{H} \times Q = x$$

in which D = desired dosage; H = the dosage strength that is available/on hand; Q = the form and amount in which the medication comes.

Here is an example:

- A patient is to receive 50 mg of Demerol. Tablets are available in 25-mg tablets. How many tablets should the patient be given?
- Determine what is known:
  - D (dosage) = 50 mg
  - H (on hand) = 25 mg
  - Q (form) = 25-mg tablets (1 tablet/25 mg)
- Set up the formula:
- $\dfrac{50}{25} \times 1 = x$

  $50 \div 25 \times 1 = 2$

- Answer: The patient should be given 2 tablets of Demerol.

ESTIMATING

Health care professionals must work carefully and thoughtfully when performing calculations. An important skill to help check work is anticipating the results. This involves estimating—calculating the approximate answer—and then judging if the calculated results seem reasonable. If calculations are performed without thought and answers simply accepted, errors can go unnoticed. It is easy for mistakes to occur when you are working in a hurry. Numbers can be placed in the wrong order, decimal points misplaced, or operations carried out incorrectly. Knowing when an answer "just doesn't look right" serves as an alert to double-check the results. Working on "automatic pilot" is not acceptable when using math in the workplace. *Health care professionals must use their thinking skills at all times.*

Learning to estimate and detect incorrect answers takes practice and thought. Here are a few guidelines to make estimating useful:

- First, use rounding to get numbers that are easier to mentally compute. For example, when multiplying 47 times 83, round 47 up to 50 and 83 down to 80. 50 times 80 is much easier to mentally multiply than the original numbers.
- Second, watch place values carefully. In the 50 times 80 example, if 5 is multiplied times 8, two zeros must be added to the quick result of 40.
- Third, look at the size of the answer. Does it make sense? For example, when multiplying whole numbers, the answer should be larger than either of the numbers in the problem. When dividing, it should be smaller.

- Fourth, be careful about placing decimal points. Remember that everything to the right of the point is a fraction. Even 0.99999 does not equal 1.0.

STATISTICS

Statistics is the collection and analysis of large amounts of numerical data and, when organized, are commonly presented as percentages and averages. Statistics help health care providers, insurance companies, health care administrators, researchers, pharmaceutical companies, and others make decisions about providing care and services to patients. Here are a few examples of health care statistics:

- Percentage of overweight or obese patients who develop diabetes
- Percentage of smokers who develop lung cancer
- Average age of death of a female born in 1945
- Increase in number of patients using the emergency room of the local hospital
- Success rate of heart transplant surgery in New York
- Percent of patients in a clinical trial whose condition is improved by taking a particular drug

It is not possible to collect the data from every person in a given group, such as all smokers in the United States, so a large, but manageable, group is used. This is called a sample, and is used to represent everyone in the group. A gerontologist may want to know how many of his patients over the age of 80 develop signs of dementia. Rather than going through the records of all his patients in that age group, he may randomly select 30 as a sample and calculate the percentage. He can also use the sample to calculate the average age at which the signs appear.

MILITARY TIME

Military time is often used in health care to avoid the confusion created by the a.m. and p.m. used in the traditional system to designate the correct time. The problem with the traditional system is that if the a.m. or p.m. is omitted or misread, an error of 12 hours is made. Errors in recording times are unacceptable in health care. For example, accuracy is critical when entering data on a patient chart, reporting when medications are given, or signing off on physician orders.

When military time is the standard used, all time designations are made with the 24-hour clock. The twelfth hour is at 12 noon and the twenty-fourth hour is at 12 midnight.

FIGURE 5–4 The military clock is based on a 24-hour day.

(See Figure 5–4.) When using the 24-hour clock, remember the following key points:

- Time is always expressed using four digits (e.g., 0030, 0200, 1200, 1700).

- The a.m. hours are expressed with the same numbers as the traditional clock, except that for times earlier than 10 a.m., you add a zero in front of them:

  1:00 a.m. is 0100

5:30 a.m. is 0530

But 10:00 a.m. is 1000

- An easy way to convert the p.m. hours from traditional to military time is to add the time to 1200. For example:

  1 p.m.: 1200 + 0100 (1:00 p.m. expressed in four digits) = 1300

  5:30 p.m.: 1200 + 0530 (5:30 p.m. expressed in four digits) = 1730

  10 p.m.: 1200 + 1000 (10:00 p.m. expressed in four digits) = 2200

- When times are verbalized, there is a specific way in which they are expressed:

  0400 = zero four hundred hours

  1300 = thirteen hundred hours

  1301 = thirteen zero one

  1730 = seventeen thirty hours

  2200 = twenty-two hundred hours

  For a.m. hours, think of "hundred" as replacing "o'clock."

Study Table 5–7 to practice converting between traditional and military times.

Table 5–7 Military (24-Hour Clock) and Traditional Time Conversion Chart

Traditional	24-Hour Time	Traditional	24-Hour Time
12:01 a.m.	0001	12:01 p.m.	1201
12:30 a.m.	0030	12:30 p.m.	1230
1:00 a.m.	0100	1:00 p.m.	1300
2:00 a.m.	0200	2:00 p.m.	1400
3:00 a.m.	0300	3:00 p.m.	1500
4:00 a.m.	0400	4:00 p.m.	1600
5:00 a.m.	0500	5:00 p.m.	1700
6:00 a.m.	0600	6:00 p.m.	1800
7:00 a.m.	0700	7:00 p.m.	1900
8:00 a.m.	0800	8:00 p.m.	2000
9:00 a.m.	0900	9:00 p.m.	2100
10:00 a.m.	1000	10:00 p.m.	2200
11:00 a.m.	1100	11:00 p.m.	2300
12:00 noon	1200	12:00 midnight	2400

ROMAN NUMERALS

The traditional numbering system we use every day is referred to as Arabic numerals (1, 2, 3, ...). In health care, it is necessary to know **Roman numerals** because they are used for some medications, solutions, and ordering systems. You may also see some files or materials organized using Roman numerals. When using Roman numerals, remember the following key points:

- All numbers can be expressed by using seven key numerals:

  I = 1

  V = 5

  X = 10

  L = 50

  C = 100

  D = 500

  M = 1000

- If a smaller numeral is placed in front of a larger numeral, the smaller numeral is *subtracted* from the larger numeral. For example: In IV, the 1 is placed before the 5, so it is subtracted (5 − 1 = 4).

- If a smaller numeral is placed after a larger numeral, the smaller numeral is *added* to the larger numeral. For example: In VI, the 1 is placed after the 5, so it is added (5 + 1 = 6).

- When the same numeral is placed next to itself, it is added. For example:

  III = 1 + 1 + 1 = 3

  XX = 10 + 10 = 20

  IXX: this has two of the same numeral preceded by a smaller numeral, but the rules still apply (10 + 10 − 1 = 19 *or* 10 − 1 + 10 = 19)

- The same numeral is not placed next to itself more than three times. For example:

  XXX = 30

  XL = 40 (XXXX is not correct)

- When Roman numerals are used with medication dosages, the lowercase (i, v, x, l, c, d, m) may be used rather than uppercase (capital letters). For example:

  ii = 2

  iv = 4

  ixx = 19

Study Table 5–8 to practice converting between Arabic and Roman numerals.

Table 5–8 Arabic and Roman Numeral Conversion Chart

Arabic	Roman	Arabic	Roman
1	I	23	XXIII
2	II	24	XXIV
3	III	25	XXV
4	IV	26	XXVI
5	V	27	XXVII
6	VI	28	XXVIII
7	VII	29	XXIX
8	VIII	30	XXX
9	IX	40	XL
10	X	50	L
20	XX	100	C
21	XXI	500	D
22	XXII	1000	M

Fascinating Facts

Roman numerals were developed in ancient Rome, as their name implies, and used in Europe for almost 1,000 years. Starting about 1500, they were gradually replaced with the number system we use today. Imagine having to multiply and divide with Roman numerals—and without a calculator!

ANGLES

Angles are used in health care when injecting medications, describing joint movement, and indicating bed positions. **Angles** are always defined by comparison to a **reference plane**, a real or imaginary flat surface from which the angle is measured. The distance between the plane and the line of the angle is measured in units called **degrees**. For example, if a flat stick is placed on a table (the reference plane), the angle is at 0 degrees. There is no distance between the plane and the stick. If the stick is lifted to stand straight up (perpendicular to the table), there is a 90-degree angle to the table. Moving the stick halfway between these two positions creates a 45-degree angle. Rotating the stick all the way around the arc and returning to the reference point creates a complete circle and represents 360 degrees. (See Figure 5–5.) The following examples illustrate how angles are used in health care:

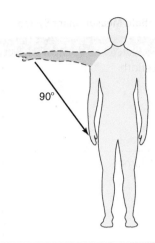

FIGURE 5–7 Body in full upright position with right arm lifted to 90-degree angle.

FIGURE 5–5 All angles are expressed in relation to a real or imaginary reference plane.

Example 1 Angles for injecting needles vary, depending on the type of medication or procedure being performed. (See Figure 5–6.) Note that in this case the reference plane is the skin surface.

Example 2 When describing the angle of extremities (arms and legs), the body in a full upright position is the reference plane. (See Figure 5–7.) Each joint (e.g., elbow, knee, hip) in the body has a normal range it is intended to move within. Physicians assess the range of a patient's joint compared to this normal range to chart loss of function or progress of recovery.

Example 3 After surgery on a joint (e.g., hip or knee replacement), the physician will order that the joint not be moved more than a certain number of degrees to prevent the new joint from "popping" out of place.

Example 4 Sometimes the physician will order that the head of the bed be kept elevated by 30 to 45 degrees at all times. This is usually ordered to aid in respiration or to prevent aspiration (stomach contents entering the lungs). In this situation, the bed in the flat position is the reference plane.

SYSTEMS OF MEASUREMENT

Basic skills in calculation are applied when learning and using the various systems of measurement used in health care. Each system has its own terminology for designating distance (length), capacity (volume), and mass (weight). Converting between these systems requires the use of the skills presented in this chapter. The three systems used in health care are household, metric, and apothecary. Each system has its own nomenclature (method of naming).

Household System

The **household system** is probably the method of measurement most familiar to students who are educated in the United States. (See Table 5–9.) Note that "ounce" is used as both a measurement of capacity and volume and mass and weight. Health care professionals use both. Liquids, such as an 8-ounce glass of water, are measured in terms of capacity or volume. Determining mass or weight, such as with a 6-pound 12-ounce infant, is done by weighing with a scale. The various units of measurement in the household system relate to each other and conversions can be made within the system. For example, volume and capacity is measured in drops, teaspoons, tablespoons, ounces, cups, pints, quarts, and gallons. Knowing the equivalencies of these units enables you to calculate each one in terms of the others. (See Figure 5–8.)

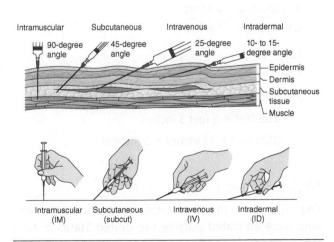

FIGURE 5–6 The correct angle must be used when inserting needles for administration of injections.

Table 5–9 Household Measurement System

Type of Measurement	Nomenclature	Common Equivalents
Distance and Length	inch (" or in)	12 in = 1 ft
	foot (' or ft)	3 ft = 1 yd
	yard (yd)	1,760 yds = 1 mi
	mile (mi)	
Capacity and Volume	drop (gtt)	60 gtt = 1 t
	teaspoon (t or tsp)	3 t = 1 T
	tablespoon (T or tbsp)	2 T = 1 oz
	ounce (oz)	8 oz = 1 C
	cup (C)	2 C = 1 pt
	pint (pt)	2 pt = 1 qt
	quart (qt)	4 qt = 1 gal
	gallon (gal)	
Mass and Weight	ounce (oz)	16 oz = 1 lb
	pound (lb)	

1 gtt

60 gtt = 1 tsp

3 tsp = 1 tbsp

2 tbsp = 1 oz

8 oz = 1 cup

FIGURE 5–8 Common household measurements used in health care.

When the basic equivalents are known, unknown measurements can be determined using proportions. Suppose that three tablespoons of a liquid are needed, but the only measuring device available is a cup marked in ounces (oz). How many ounces are in three tablespoons (3 T)? Knowing that 2T = 1 oz, the proportion would be set up as follows:

$$\frac{2T}{3T} \times \frac{1\,oz}{x\,oz}$$

$$2x = 3\,oz$$

$$2x \div 2 = 3\,oz \div 2$$

$$x = 1.5\,oz$$

The next example involves measurement of height. If a patient is 63 inches tall and asks how many feet that is, the calculation would use the following proportion:

$$\frac{12\,inches}{63\,inches} \times \frac{1\,feet}{x\,feet}$$

$$12x = 63$$

$$12x \div 12 = 63 \div 12$$

$$x = 5.25\,feet$$

$$x = 5.25\,feet = 5\,feet\,3\,inches$$

$$(0.25\,feet \times 12\,inches = 3\,inches)$$

Metric System

The **metric system** will probably be familiar to students who were educated outside the United States or have taken science classes. It is a more accurate system than the household system and also is easier to convert between numbers because everything is based on a unit of ten. The base units for the metric system are as follows:

- Distance and Length: **meter** (m)
- Capacity and Volume: **liter** (l or L)
- Mass and Weight: **gram** (g)

The meter, liter, and gram are modified by adding the appropriate prefix to express larger or smaller units. (See Table 5–10).

Being based on multiples of ten, conversions within the decimal system are calculated by multiplying by 10, 100, 1,000, and so on:

- 1 *kilo*liter = 1,000 × 1 liter = 1,000 liters
- 1 *hecto*liter = 100 × 1 liter = 100 liters
- 1 *deca*liter = 10 × 1 liter = 10 liters
- 1 *deci*liter = 0.1 × 1 liter = 0.1 liter
- 1 *centi*liter = 0.01 × 1 liter = 0.01 liter
- 1 *milli*liter = 0.001 × 1 liter = 0.001 liter

A shortcut for performing these operations is to move the decimal point the number of places indicated by the prefix. Here are three examples:

Example 1 Multiplying 1 by 10 means moving the decimal point one place to the right. This may require adding one or more zeros. With whole numbers, it is understood that there is a decimal point following the number. 10 × 1 is the same as 10 × 1.0, so moving the decimal point one place to the right results in 10 × 1.0 = 10

Example 2 Multiplying 4.2 by 10 = 42

Example 3 Multiplying 4.2 by 100 = 420

The ability to convert units within the metric system is often needed in health care. For example, if the physician orders 2,000 milligrams of a medication and this needs to be converted to grams, the conversion is made as follows:

1. *Milli* is in the third place to the right of gram. Move the decimal point three spaces to the left *toward gram*: 2,000 = 2.000, or 2.
2. Change unit name to grams: 2 grams.
3. The proper dose would be 2 grams, or two 1-gram tablets.

A second example involves converting 1,000 centimeters to kilometers:

1. *Centi* is five decimal places to the right of *kilo*, so move the decimal point five spaces to the left *toward kilo*. Add zeros as needed: 1,000 = 0.01.
2. Change unit name to kilometers: 0.01 kilometers.

See Figure 5–9 for a visual representation of decimal placement.

In addition to moving the decimal point the correct number of places, it is critical that it be moved in the correct direction. This can be confusing. The easiest way is to determine if the answer should be a larger or smaller number and then just move the decimal point accordingly:

1. If converting from a larger to a smaller unit (prefix) (e.g., kilo to milli), the answer will be larger. It takes more of the smaller units to equal the larger units.
2. If converting from a smaller to a larger prefix (e.g., milli to kilo), the answer will be smaller. It takes fewer of the larger units to equal the smaller units.

Table 5–10 Common Prefixes of the Metric System

Prefix	Meaning	Examples	Meaning of Examples
Kilo	1,000 times	kilogram	1,000 grams
		kilometer	1,000 meters
		kiloliter	1,000 liters
Hecto	100 times	hectogram	100 grams
deca (also "deka")	10 times	decaliter	10 liters
meter, liter, gram	Whole units of measurement		
Deci	1/10	decigram	1/10 of a gram
Centi	1/100	centimeter	1/100 of a meter
Milli	1/1,000	milliliter	1/1,000 of a liter
Micro	1/1,000,000	microgram	1/1,000,000 of a gram

PREFIX	KILO-	HECTO-	DEKA-	BASE	DECI-	CENTI-	MILLI-	DECIMILLI-	CENTIMILLI-	MICROMILLI-
Common Units	kilogram			gram liter meter		centimeter	milligram milliliter millimeter			microgram
Value to Base	1000	100	10	1.0	0.1	0.01	0.001	0.0001	0.00001	0.000001

FIGURE 5–9 Comparison of common metric units used in health care.

Thinking It Through

Part of Mrs. Cabinos's job as an admitting assistant in an ambulatory clinic is to ask all patients their height and weight and record it on a graph. When she asks Mr. Summerton, he reports that he is 6 feet tall and weighs 160 pounds and 8 ounces. The graph used at this clinic is in inches and pounds.

1. How many inches are in 6 feet?
2. How do you convert 160 pounds and 8 ounces to pounds only?

Apothecary System

The **apothecary system** is the oldest and least used of the three systems of measurement presented. (See Table 5–11.) This system is seldom seen in the modern health care environment, although it is sometimes seen with pharmaceutical products. The Joint Commission has advised that the apothecary symbols and measurements should no longer be used, but has not yet added this system to its official "do-not-use" list.

Roman numerals can be used in conjunction with the apothecary system, and may be seen in uppercase or lowercase formats. If lowercase is used, the Roman numeral for "1" is written with a line and a dot. For example, "2" would be written as ïï. A commonly used abbreviation that originated with the apothecary system is s̄s̄ which means "half." For example 2½ would be written as īīss̄.

Converting Systems of Measurement

Health care work sometimes requires that units from one system of measurement be converted to those of another. This requires knowledge of the equivalencies between the units of the systems. There are frequently no exact equivalents, so when converting between systems the answer is considered to be a close approximation. (See Table 5–12.)

Table 5–11 **Apothecary Measurement System**

Type of Measurement	Nomenclature	Common Equivalents
Distance and Length	N/A	N/A
Capacity and Volume	minim (♏)	1 minim = 1 drop
	fluid dram (fl dr or ℨ)	60 minims = 1 fl dr
	fluid ounce (fl oz or ℥)	8 fl dr = 1 fl oz
	pint (pt)	16 fl oz = 1 pt
	quart (qt)	2 pt = 1 qt
Mass and Weight	grain (gr)	
	dram (dr or ℨ)	60 gr = 1 dr
	ounce (oz or ℥)	480 gr = 1 oz

Table 5–12 Approximate Equivalents between Measuring Systems

Distance and Length	Capacity and Volume	Mass and Weight
1 in = 2.5 cm	1 tsp = 5 mL	2.2 lb = 1 kg
39.4 in = 1 m	1 oz = 30 mL	1 grain = 60 mg
	1 qt = 1,000 mL	15 grains = 1 g

Using the appropriate equivalencies, a proportion is set up to identify and solve for the unknown quantity. The following steps are used for performing conversions:

1. Identify an equivalent between the two systems.
2. Set up a proportion so unit measurements on each side of the equation are the same.
3. Use "x" for the unknown value being calculated.
4. Cross multiply.
5. Solve for "x."
6. Verify if the answer is reasonable.

   a. If converting from a smaller unit to a larger unit, the answer will be smaller. For example, when converting 2 quarters to dollars, the result will be smaller than 2 because a quarter is a smaller unit than a dollar. Because there are 4 quarters in 1 dollar, 2 quarters = 0.5 dollar.

   b. If converting from a larger unit to a smaller unit, the answer will be larger. For example, when converting 2 dollars to quarters, the result will be a larger unit than 2 because a dollar is a larger unit than a quarter. Because there is 1 dollar for every 4 quarters, 2 dollars = 8 quarters.

The following examples illustrate how to perform conversions:

Example 1 Convert 19 inches to centimeters:

1. Identify equivalency: 1 inch = 2.5 centimeters.
2. Set up a proportion with same units on each side of equation. Use "x" for the unknown.

$$\frac{1 \text{ inch}}{19 \text{ inches}} = \frac{2.5 \text{ cm}}{x \text{ cm}}$$

3. Cross multiply:

   1x = 47.5 cm

4. Solve for x:

   1x ÷ 1 = 47.5 ÷ 1

   x = 47.5 cm

5. Verify if the answer is reasonable: It takes a larger number of centimeters (2½ times) to measure the same distance as 1 inch. Therefore, it makes sense that the answer is larger than 19.

Example 2 Convert 1.5 meters to inches:

1. Identify equivalency: 39.4 inches = 1 meter.
2. Set up a proportion with the same units on each side of equation. Use "x" for the unknown.

$$\frac{39.4 \text{ inches}}{x \text{ inches}} = \frac{1 \text{ m}}{1.5 \text{ m}}$$

3. Cross multiply:

   1x = 59.1 inches

4. Solve for x:

   1x ÷ 1 = 59.1 ÷ 1

   x = 59.1 inches

5. Verify if the answer is reasonable: It takes many inches to measure the distance designated by 1 meter. Therefore, the answer 59.1 makes sense.

Example 3 Convert 5 teaspoons to milliliters:

$$\frac{1 \text{ tsp}}{5 \text{ tsp}} = \frac{5 \text{ mL}}{x \text{ mL}}$$

x = 25 mL

Example 4 Convert 75 milliliters to ounces:

$$\frac{1 \text{ oz}}{x \text{ oz}} = \frac{30 \text{ mL}}{75 \text{ mL}}$$

30x = 75 (note that in solving for x, each side is divided by 30)

x = 2.5 oz

Example 5 Convert 120 pounds to kilograms:

$$\frac{2.2 \text{ lb}}{120 \text{ lb}} = \frac{1 \text{ kg}}{x \text{ kg}}$$

2.2x = 120 (note that in solving for "x," each side is divided by 2.2)

x = 54.5 kg (rounded to nearest tenth)

Example 6 Convert 60 kilograms to ounces:

$$\frac{2.2\,lb}{x\,oz} = \frac{1\,kg}{60\,kg}$$

This problem cannot be solved using this proportion, because the unit measurements on the left side of the equation are not the same size (pound and ounce). To solve this problem, pounds must first be converted to ounces. Refer back to the household system and Table 5–9: 16 ounces = 1 pound.

$$\frac{16\,oz}{x\,oz} = \frac{1\,lb}{2.2\,lb}$$

$$x = 35.2\,oz$$

Knowing that 2.2 pounds = 35.2 ounces = 1 kilogram allows the appropriate proportion to be set up:

$$\frac{35.2\,oz}{x\,oz} = \frac{1\,kg}{60\,kg}$$

$$x = 2,112\,oz$$

Example 7 Convert 15 grains to milligrams:

$$\frac{1\,gr}{15\,gr} = \frac{60\,mg}{x\,mg}$$

$$x = 900\,mg$$

Example 8 Convert 2 g to grains:

$$\frac{15\,gr}{x\,gr} = \frac{1\,gm}{2\,gm}$$

$$x = 30\,gr$$

MEDICATION SAFETY

The misidentification of alphanumeric characters in hand-written orders has been a long-standing problem and has led to medication errors resulting in severe problems and, in some cases, death. Fortunately, computerized physician order entry can overcome most problems with poor handwriting. However, even typed or computerized physician orders does not prevent all of them. Anyone familiar with email knows how easy it is to misidentify a computer-generated lowercase letter L (l) in an email address as the numeral one (1), or the letter O as zero (0)! It is also easy to confuse the uppercase letter Z with the number 2. In fact, the Institute for Safe Medication Practices reports that these characters (l/1, O/0, and Z/2), plus the number 1, which can look like a 7, account for over 50% of the errors caused by character misidenti-fication. More about medication safety is discussed in Chapter 23. (See Table 5–13.)

TEMPERATURE CONVERSION

Thermometers using Fahrenheit (F) as the measuring unit are more familiar to people living in the United States, though the Celsius (C) system (also known as centigrade) of measurement is frequently seen in medical practice. One way to start understanding the difference between the two systems is to compare how each one expresses the boiling and freezing points of water.

Boiling points: 212°F = 100°C

Freezing points: 32°F = 0°C

See Figure 5–10 for a comparison of Fahrenheit (F) and Celsius (C) thermometers, and Table 5–14 for a conversion chart. Health care professionals may have to convert between the F and C systems when a conversion chart is not available. Table 5–15 contains the formulas for conversion. A fraction and a decimal approach give the same results. Deciding which to use depends on whether you have stronger skills working with fractions or decimals. All the formulas include parentheses. These are used

Table 5–13 Tips to Reduce Medication Errors

Avoid	Preferred Method	Rationale
U	units	Always write "units" not "u." The handwritten "u" after the dose is often read as zero, causing a potential tenfold overdose.
10 mg	1 mg	Never use a trailing zero. Do not follow a whole number with a decimal point and a zero. The decimal point is often not seen, causing a potential tenfold overdose.
.5 mg	0.5 mg	Always use a leading zero. Use a leading zero before a number with a decimal point. The leading decimal point alone is often not seen, causing a potential tenfold overdose.
cc	mL	Always write "mL" or "milliliter," not "cc." When handwritten, the abbreviation "cc" has been mistaken as "00" causing a potential one hundred-fold overdose.

FIGURE 5–10 Comparison of Fahrenheit and Celsius temperature scales.

Table 5–14 Fahrenheit–Celsius Conversion Chart

Fahrenheit	Celsius
32 (freezing point)	0 (freezing point)
95	35
96	35.6
97	36.1
97.4	36.3
98	36.7
98.6	37
99	37.2
99.4	37.4
100	37.8
101	38.3
102	38.9
103	39.4
104	40
212 (boiling point)	100 (boiling point)

to indicate that the enclosed calculation must be performed first. For example the steps to solve the formula $(°F - 32) \times 5/9 = °C$ are to first subtract 32 from the value for F and *then* multiply that value by 5/9.

Table 5–15 Temperature Scale Conversion Formulas

Convert From:	Fraction Formula	Decimal Formula
Celsius to Fahrenheit	$(°C \times 9/5) + 32 = °F$	$(°C \times 1.8) + 32 = °F$
	Example: 37°C	Example: 37°C
	$(37 \times 9/5) + 32 = °F$	$(37 \times 1.8) + 32 = °F$
	$333/5 + 32 = 98.6°F$	$66.6 + 32 = 98.6°F$
Fahrenheit to Celsius	$(°F - 32) \times 5/9 = °C$	$(°F - 32) \div 1.8 = °C$
	Example: 101°F	Example: 101°F
	$(101 - 32) \times 5/9 = °C$	$(101 - 32) \div 1.8 = °C$
	$69 \times 5/9 = °C$	$69 \div 1.8 = 38.3°C$
	$345/9 = 38.3°C$ (rounded to nearest tenth)	(rounded to nearest tenth)

SUGGESTED LEARNING ACTIVITIES

1. Cut a whole pie, cake, or paper plate into slices (you determine how many). Then practice by separating out some of the slices and expressing them as part of the whole in decimals, fractions, percentages, and ratios.

2. If you have a large wall clock, attach numbers cut out of paper to it to indicate military time. Or make a paper clock and put it up where you see it frequently. Practice telling time using the 24-hour format.

3. When you see numbers on street signs, practice converting them to Roman numerals.

4. Stand in front of a mirror and as you move your extremities try to estimate the degree of movement.

5. Practice, practice, practice using the systems of measurement until you can consistently use them accurately:

   - Weigh yourself in pounds and convert to kilograms.

   - Measure your height in inches and convert to meters.

   - Find various household measurement items (teaspoon, tablespoon, measuring cup) and convert them to the metric system.

   - Look at the strength of any medications you currently have in the house and convert them to another system of measurement (e.g., if the Tylenol or aspirin bottle has the strength listed in grains, convert to milligrams, or if listed as milligrams, convert to grains).

   - Take your temperature in Fahrenheit and convert to Celsius.

   - Exchange handwriting samples containing both alphabetic and numeric characters with another student. Look for any characters that are unclear or difficult to interpret. Exchange feedback.

WEB ACTIVITIES

Math Anxiety

http://mathpower.com

1. Take the Math Anxiety Test and record your score.

2. If you scored 20 points or higher, review the Ten Ways to Reduce Math Anxiety and develop a plan to decrease your math anxiety.

Math.com

www.math.com/

1. Go to this site for a good review of math principles and examples.

2. Review the information on fractions, decimals, and percents.

3. Work with a buddy and each of you create five examples of fractions, decimals, and percents. When both of you have completed the math problems, compare your answers to see if they are the same.

4. If you have any questions, ask your instructor or another student to help solve the problems.

Khan Academy

www.khanacademy.org

The Khan Academy contains lessons on many math topics, including conversions of measurements within each system. Choose one or more topics to review.

National Center for Health Statistics

https://www.cdc.gov/nchs/

1. Choose a subject listed under Topics and list the type of statistics collected.

2. What new facts did you learn about the status of health in the United States?

Statistics and Health Care

https://www.livestrong.com/article/186334-why-are-statistics-important-in-the-health-care-field/

"Why Are Statistics Important in the Health Care Field"

1. Read the article and list the ways that statistics are used in health care.

2. Which do you think apply to your chosen occupation?

Using Math in Medicine

http://mathcentral.uregina.ca/beyond/articles/medicine/med1.html

"Medicine and Math" is an interesting article about practical math applications in health care. After reading the article, write a short summary.

Military Time

https://bestlifeonline.com/military-time/

"Military Time Made Easy: The Best Ways to Use a 24-Hour Clock: Learn Everything You Need to Know about the Metric-System-For-Clocks"

Learn more about using the 24-hour clock.

Calculating Dosages

https://basicmedicalkey.com/dosage-calculation-using-the-formula-method/

"Dosage Calculation Using the Formula Method"

1. Study the information and examples to increase your understanding of the formula method.

2. Why shouldn't health care professionals rely solely on the answers to their formula calculations?

REVIEW QUESTIONS

1. Give five examples of how math is used by health care professionals.

2. If a health care professional makes a math error at work, what is the most serious potential consequence?

3. What are the signs and consequences of math anxiety?

4. What are three ways that students can review or learn basic math?

5. What is the definition of a "whole number"?

6. What are the definitions of "decimal" and "decimal point"?

7. What are the steps to follow when adding, subtracting, multiplying, and dividing decimals?

8. What is the definition of a fraction?

9. What are the steps to follow when adding, subtracting, multiplying, and dividing fractions?

10. What is a percentage?

11. What are the steps to follow when converting decimals, fractions, percentages, and ratios?

12. What are the guidelines for rounding off numbers?

13. Give an example of an equation set up to solve a proportion problem.

14. Give an example of using the basic formula to calculate a drug dosage.

15. What is the purpose of estimating when performing calculations and what are the guidelines for using it.

16. What are three examples of how statistics are used in health care?

17. How does military time differ from the traditional system and what are its advantages?

18. How do Roman numerals differ from the traditional numbering system? What are the key points to remember when using Roman numerals?

19. What are three examples of how angles are used in health care?

20. How are angles estimated from a reference plane?

21. What are the three systems of measurement currently used in health care? Within each system, what are the names of the basic units used for length, volume, and weight?

22. What are the steps to follow when converting among the three systems of measurement?

23. What are the equations for converting Fahrenheit to Celsius? Celsius to Fahrenheit?

APPLICATION EXERCISES

1. Refer to The Case of Exactly How Much Does My Baby Weigh? at the beginning of this chapter. Jamie explains that the baby also grew 2 inches. How many centimeters would this be?

2. Maria is working in the hospital and when taking vital signs, she discovers that a patient has a temperature of 37.6°C. When she checks the orders, she finds the physician has ordered Tylenol gr x to be given every four hours as needed for a temperature above 101°F. Maria notes it is 4 p.m. and the last dose was given at 1300 hours. The Tylenol tablets she has available are marked as 525 mg/tablet. She gives the patient two tablets and charts the time given as 1500.

   a. Assuming the last dose was given at 1300 hours, when would the next dose of Tylenol be due? If it is now 4 p.m., how much time has elapsed since the medication was given?

   b. Did Maria note the time correctly? If not, how is 4 p.m. expressed in military time?

   c. What would be the equivalent of 101°F in the Celsius system? Was the temperature elevated high enough to give the Tylenol as ordered?

   d. Was the correct amount of medication given? If not, was too much or too little given?

PROBLEM-SOLVING PRACTICE

Genevieve Foust has always dreamed of working in health care, but she is scared to death of taking Math for Health Care Professionals next semester. She has always struggled with math and when she spoke with her parents about her fears they said, "It must be genetic as neither of us can do math either." Using the five-step problem-solving process, determine what Genevieve can do about her fear of the upcoming math course.

CHAPTER 6

Organization of the Human Body

KEY TERMS

abdominal cavity
anatomical position
anterior (ventral)
anterior body cavity
apex
base
body systems
caudal
cell
cephalic (cranial)
cranial cavity
deep
distal
frontal plane
homeostasis
inferior
lateral
medial
midsagittal plane
organism
organs
pelvic cavity
peripheral
posterior (dorsal)
posterior body cavity
proximal
spinal cavity
superficial
superior
thoracic cavity
tissues
transverse plane

OBJECTIVES

Studying and applying the material in this chapter will help you to:

1. Explain the meaning of homeostasis.
2. Name the levels in the structural organization of the body.
3. Name and explain the functions of the major components of a typical human cell.
4. Name and state the function of the four primary types of tissues.
5. Describe the anatomical position.
6. Identify and state the location of the three directional body planes.
7. Use directional terms to describe various locations on the body.
8. Name the main body cavities and what structures are found in each.
9. Identify the abdominal regions and quadrants.

The Case of the Exact Location

Paula Holland is seen in the urgent care center with complaints of pain in the left lower arm. Several bruises and cuts are also noted on the upper and lower areas of the same arm. Arlene Dealy is working at the center and charts: "Mrs. Holland has lower arm pain, with multiple bruises and cuts on the arm."

When the patient returns the following week because of complaints of pain in both her arms, Gary Heinz reads the notes made by Arlene and is unable to determine if the original visit was for pain in the left or right arm. He also questions how many, what size, and exactly where the bruises and cuts were located.

The material in this chapter will give the health care professional the medical language that is used to describe body locations, so that other health care professionals will know where to check when they see the patient.

THE BASIS OF LIFE

The processes that maintain life are remarkable in their complexity and effectiveness. They can only be truly appreciated by studying all the structures and functions that make up the human body. Sormunen and Moisio (2009) express it well:

> Our bodies are marvelously intricate, delicate, and unique. Each part of the body has a purpose and function that fits into the total. Cells, tissues, organs, and systems are all part of the human anatomy.

The body is constantly working to keep itself in what is called a state of homeostasis. **Homeostasis** is the tendency of a cell or the whole organism to maintain a state of balance. To maintain this balance numerous tiny adjustments are made every second throughout the body. For example, when the temperature outside rises, the body works to maintain a steady internal temperature by perspiring. Most adjustments occur without our conscious awareness.

The structural organization of the body can be described as a series of levels organized from the smallest to the largest. This text will not cover atoms, ions, and molecules. Our study will start at the smallest living structure in the body which is at the cellular level and will progress to the largest which is the human body as a whole. It can be summarized in the following order:

1. **Cells**: Smallest living structures in the body
2. **Tissues**: Cells with similar function grouped together
3. **Organs**: Two or more types of tissues combined to work together (e.g., kidneys, lungs, heart, and liver)
4. **Body** (organ) **systems**: Two or more organs combined to provide a major body function (e.g., respiratory, nervous, and urinary systems)
5. **Organism** (human body as a whole)

The human body is an amazing and complex organism. The cells themselves are complex living structures (see next section) that group together to form tissues. Different types of tissues work together to create body organs. When two or more of these body organs work together, they create the major body systems that work in harmony to maintain a state of homeostasis for the human body.

The cells and tissues will be presented in this chapter and the organs and body systems in the next. (See Figure 6–1.)

Cells

Cells are the smallest structures that carry on all the fundamental functions of life. Many of them perform specialized

functions, such as support (bone cells), communication (nerve cells), oxygen transportation (red blood cells), movement (muscle cells), and protection (skin cells). (See Figure 6–2.) Cells can reproduce, grow, and repair themselves. To perform these functions, they take in nutrients (food) and oxygen to create heat and energy. Cells can move, adapt to their environment, and eliminate waste products.

Human cells contain the following components (see Figure 6–3):

1. Cell membrane: The outer covering; it controls which substances enter and leave the cell
2. Cytoplasm (protoplasm): Gel-like liquid inside the cell that consists of water, proteins, carbohydrates, nucleic acids, lipids (fats), and salts
3. Organelles: Structures that have specialized functions

   - Nucleus: Controls the activity of the cell, reproduction; contains the 23 (normally) chromosomes that contain the genes that transmit hereditary characteristics
   - Mitochondrion: Produces energy used for cellular processes; called the "powerhouse"
   - Lysosome: Contains various enzymes that help to digest (break down) molecules
   - Ribosomes: Produce protein for the cell structures
   - Golgi apparatus: Produces, stores, and packages products for discharge from the cell (e.g., transports proteins made by the ribosomes)
   - Centrioles: Play a role in the division of the cell (reproduction)
   - Endoplasmic reticulum: Network of tubular structures to facilitate transport of materials in and out of the nucleus
   - Vesicles: Storage and transportation unit

LEVEL

EXAMPLES

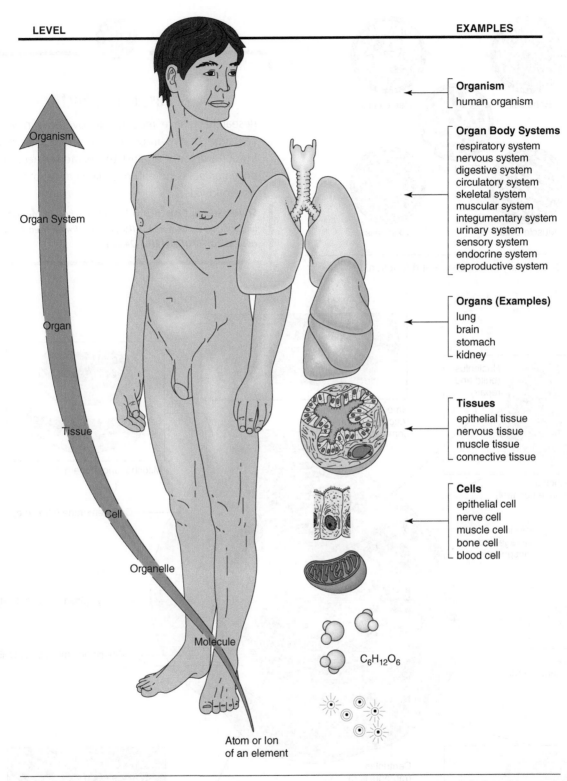

Organism

Organ System

Organ

Tissue

Cell

Organelle

Molecule

Atom or Ion
of an element

Organism
human organism

Organ Body Systems
respiratory system
nervous system
digestive system
circulatory system
skeletal system
muscular system
integumentary system
urinary system
sensory system
endocrine system
reproductive system

Organs (Examples)
lung
brain
stomach
kidney

Tissues
epithelial tissue
nervous tissue
muscle tissue
connective tissue

Cells
epithelial cell
nerve cell
muscle cell
bone cell
blood cell

$C_6H_{12}O_6$

FIGURE 6–1 The structural organization of the body progresses from cells to the body as a whole.

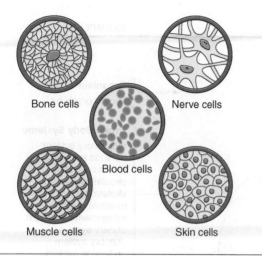

Bone cells

Nerve cells

Blood cells

Muscle cells

Skin cells

FIGURE 6-2 Cells vary in size, shape, and function.

Fascinating Fact

Researchers have recently discovered a new lung cell type that is implicated in the body's natural immune defense against the bacteria *Streptococcus pneumoniae*—one of the leading causes of pneumonia worldwide.

Source: Science Daily, Boston University School of Medicine, New lung cell type discovered, 9/18/17, https://www.sciencedaily.com/ releases/2017/09/170918163424.htm

Nucleolus (build and repair)

Nucleus (master control)

vesicle (storage and transportation)

Lysosome (environmental control)

Golgi apparatus (environmental control)

Centrioles (reproduction)

Smooth endoplasmic reticulum (intracellular communication)

Mitochondrion (energy)

Cell membrane (structure)

Vesicle

Cytoplasm (cellular fluid)

Ribosomes (build and repair)

Rough endoplasmic reticulum (intracellular communication)

FIGURE 6-3 Major components of a typical human cell.

Epithelium tissue

Connective tissue

Nerve tissue

Muscle tissue

FIGURE 6–4 The four primary types of tissues found in the human body.

Tissues

Tissues are categorized into four primary types (Figure 6–4):

1. Epithelial: Covers the internal and external organs of the body; lines body cavities, vessels, glands, and body organs

2. Connective: Holds parts of the body in place; can be liquid (blood), fibrous (tendons and ligaments), solid (bone), fatty (protective padding), or cartilage (rings of the trachea)

3. Nervous: Transmits impulses throughout the body to activate, coordinate, and control many functions

4. Muscular: Contracts and relaxes to cause or allow movement; the three types are as follows:

   • Skeletal: Attached to bone and enables movement of the skeleton

   • Smooth (visceral): Found in the walls of the hollow internal organs of the body (e.g., stomach and intestines), blood vessels, and lung airways

   • Cardiac: Makes up the muscular wall of the heart

DESCRIBING THE BODY

Health care professionals need a specialized language to use when speaking or writing about a particular location of a structure or an area of the body. This language and special vocabulary describes body planes, directional terms, body cavities, and abdominal regions.

A mastery of these terms will allow you to accurately interpret descriptions written by other personnel and also to chart (document in writing) your findings in a way that others can understand.

The descriptive terms refer to the body as viewed in a full upright position (standing), with the arms relaxed at the side of the body, palms facing forward, feet pointed forward, and eyes directed straight ahead. This is called the anatomical position. (See Figure 6–5.)

Fascinating Facts

There are approximately 75 trillion cells in the human body. They vary in shape and size, but most are microscopic and range from 1/3 to 1/13 the size of the period at the end of this sentence. Every human started the first half hour of life as a single cell.

FIGURE 6–5 The anatomical position.

Body Planes

A body plane is an imaginary flat surface that cuts through the body either horizontally or vertically. Imagine the body divided up by a large pane of window glass. There are three primary planes (Figures 6–6a and 6–6b):

1. **Midsagittal** (median or midline) **plane**: Passes from top to bottom through the center of the body and divides it into equal right and left sides
2. **Frontal plane** (coronal): Divides the body from top to bottom through the center and divides the body into front and back portions
3. **Transverse plane**: Divides the body horizontally (crosswise) into top and bottom portions

Directional Terms

Using east, west, north, and south works well for traditional directions, but would be of no value when referring to the body. Directional terms for medical descriptions were

FIGURE 6–6a Sagittal plane. The midsagittal (median or midline) plane divides the body from top to bottom into equal left and right halves.

created to solve this problem and are listed in Table 6–1. Also refer to Figures 6–6a and 6–6b.

The Body Cavities

Within the body there are interior spaces called cavities that contain and protect the internal organs. (See Figure 6–7.) The **posterior** (dorsal) **body cavity** protects the structures of the nervous system and has two parts (although the space is continuous):

1. **Cranial cavity**: Located in the skull and contains the brain
2. **Spinal cavity**: Located within the spinal column and contains the spinal cord

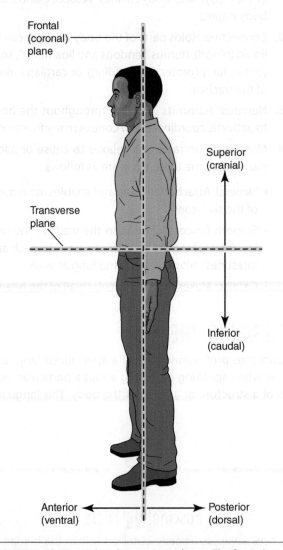

FIGURE 6–6b Frontal and transverse planes. The frontal (coronal) plane divides the body into front (anterior) and back (posterior) portions. It is located at right angles to the sagittal plane. The transverse plane divides the body horizontally into top (superior) and bottom (inferior) portions. This division can be at the waist or any other level across the body.

Table 6–1 Directional Terms

Term	Meaning	Example
Lateral	Away from center of body (toward the sides)	The lateral ligament of the knee is located on the outer side of the knee.
Medial	Toward midline or center of body	The navel is on the medial line.
Anterior (ventral)	Toward the front of body	The breasts are on the anterior surface of the body.
Posterior (dorsal)	Toward the back of the body	The buttocks are on the posterior surface of the body.
Inferior	Below	The lungs are inferior to the head.
Superior	Above	The nose is superior to the mouth.
Caudal	Closer to the coccyx (lower back)	The hips are caudal to the waist.
Cephalic (cranial)	Closer to the head	The neck is cephalic to the shoulders.
Deep	Farther from the body surface	The accident victim had a deep laceration (wound or irregular tear) that exposed the muscle.
Superficial	Near or close to the body surface	There were only superficial scrapes on the skin.
Distal	Farther from the reference base point	The hand is distal to the elbow.
Peripheral	Away from the center	The patient had peripheral edema (excess fluid in the extremities—arms and legs).
Proximal	Closer to the reference point	The shoulder is proximal to the elbow.
Apex	At the top (highest point)	The top of the lung is called the apex.
Base	At the bottom (lowest point)	The bottom of the lung is called the base.

Source: Adapted from Essentials of Anatomy and Physiology *(4th ed.) by F. H. Martini & E. F. Bartholomew, 2008, San Francisco, CA: Benjamin Cummings Publishing*

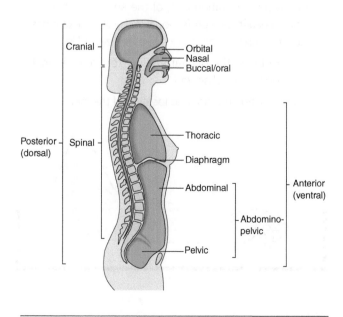

FIGURE 6–7 Cavities of the body.

The **anterior** (ventral) **body cavity** protects the internal organs and has three parts:

1. **Thoracic cavity**: Located in the chest and contains the heart, lungs, and major blood vessels; the diaphragm separates this cavity from the abdominal cavity
2. **Abdominal cavity**: Located in the abdomen and contains the stomach, intestines, liver, gallbladder, pancreas, and spleen (the kidneys are located behind the abdominal cavity); the abdominal and pelvic cavities are continuous
3. **Pelvic cavity**: Located in the lower abdomen and contains the urinary bladder, rectum, and reproductive organs

Smaller cavities include the orbital, which contains the eyes and associated muscles, nerves, and ducts; the nasal, which contains the structures of the nose; and the buccal, which contains the teeth and tongue.

Abdominal Descriptions

The abdominal area is so large that it has been divided into nine regions so that specific areas can be described with greater accuracy. The nine regions include the lower portion of the thoracic cavity and the abdominal and pelvic cavities. (See Figure 6–8.)

These regions are as follows:

- Epigastric ("over the stomach"): Located just below the sternum (breastbone)
- Right and left hypochondriac regions: Located below the ribs on either side of the epigastric region
- Umbilical: Located around the umbilicus (navel)
- Right and left lumbar regions: Extend anterior to posterior on either side of the umbilical region (a person will complain of lumbar or back pain)
- Hypogastric ("below the stomach"): Located over the pubic area
- Right and left iliac (hip bone) regions: Located on either side of the hypogastric region (also called right and left inguinal areas)

Another approach used in health care for describing the abdomen divides the region into quadrants. Imaginary lines are used to create four quadrants (Figure 6–9) that divide the abdominal area. All the quadrants contain part of the large and small intestines, but some of the other internal organs can be identified within a particular quadrant.

1. Right upper quadrant (RUQ): Liver and gallbladder
2. Right lower quadrant (RLQ): Appendix and some of the female reproductive organs

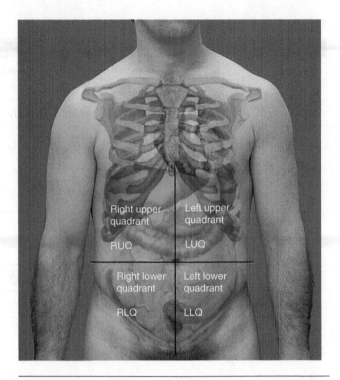

Right upper quadrant

RUQ

Left upper quadrant

LUQ

Right lower quadrant

RLQ

Left lower quadrant

LLQ

FIGURE 6–9 The abdomen is divided into quadrants (fourths).

3. Left upper quadrant (LUQ): Pancreas, stomach, and spleen
4. Left lower quadrant (LLQ): Some of the female reproductive organs

Thinking It Through

A patient arrives at the urgent care center to be seen for a recent laceration (cut) of the arm. Miss Heather Jones, a health care professional at the clinic, examines the arm and describes the injury as to size and location.

1. Examine the diagram below to visualize what Miss Jones observed.
2. Describe the size and location of the injury.

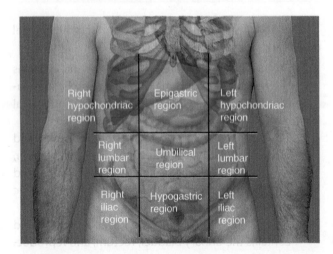

Right hypochondriac region

Epigastric region

Left hypochondriac region

Right lumbar region

Umbilical region

Left lumbar region

Right iliac region

Hypogastric region

Left iliac region

FIGURE 6–8 Nine abdominal regions.

Thinking It Through

Esteban Valdez is a patient on a medical-surgical floor of a community hospital. He is experiencing some discomfort in the right buttock area and reports it to Martha Duarte, a licensed vocational (practical) nurse. The patient points to the area of discomfort, and Martha can see a small red dot but no other abnormalities. Martha notes that the location identified by the patient is on the upper lateral side of the right buttock and inferior to the waist. She thinks it may be tenderness due to a recent injection (shot) that was given to the patient and checks the medication record. The record shows that Mr. Valdez had an injection into the RUOQ (right upper outer quadrant) of the buttock.

1. RUQ, RLQ, LUQ, and LLQ do not apply only to the abdomen, but can be used to divide any area into four equal parts (see Figure 6–10). When giving an injection into the buttocks, the only correct sites would be into the upper outer quadrant of either buttock. Based on the description given, where was the small red dot located?

2. Do you agree with Martha's conclusion?

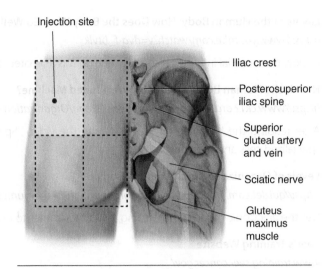

FIGURE 6–10 The buttocks divided into quadrants.

SUGGESTED LEARNING ACTIVITIES

1. Draw and label the structures of the cell from memory.

2. Stand in front of a mirror in the anatomical position and visualize the midsagittal, frontal, and transverse planes of the body.

3. Point to any area of your body and describe its position using the directional terms.

4. Stand in front of a mirror and identify the abdominal regions and quadrants.

WEB ACTIVITIES

Homeostasis

https://www.khanacademy.org/science/biology/principles-of-physiology/body-structure-and-homeostasis/a/homeostasis

Read the article and study the diagrams, then write a short paper describing how the human body maintains homeostasis.

Biology: Cell Structure

https://www.youtube.com/watch?v=URUJD5NEXC8

Watch this excellent video to learn more about cells and their structure.

Levels of the Human Body: How Does the Body Work So Well?

https://www.youtube.com/watch?v=dva-f_btvlk

Review the material in this chapter by watching this animated description of the various body levels.

How Is the Human Body Similar to a Well-Tuned Machine?

https://www.ck12.org/biology/human-body/lesson/Organization-of-the-Human-Body-BIO

After reading the text material and watching the video "Specialized Cells and Tissues," write a short paper describing the specialized cells and their purpose.

Levels of Organization in the Human Body

https://quizlet.com/14302204/levels-of-organization-in-the-human-body-flash-cards/

Use the electronic flashcards, matching, and other games to review and quiz yourself on the content of this chapter.

Seer's Training Website

www.training.seer.cancer.gov/

Enter the key words "anatomical terminology" in the search box. List the body cavities and which organs are located in each one. Then click on "Directional Terms" and "Planes of the Body" to review these topics.

REVIEW QUESTIONS

1. What is homeostasis?
2. What are the levels in the structural organization of the body?
3. What are the components of the cell, and what are their functions?
4. What are the four primary types of tissues?
5. What is the anatomical position?
6. What are the three body planes and how do they divide the body?
7. What are the main directional terms used for medical descriptions?
8. What are the primary body cavities and what structures are in each one?
9. What are the two methods used for describing the abdominal area?

APPLICATION EXERCISES

1. Refer to The Case of the Exact Location. If Arlene had used anatomical descriptions to identify Mrs. Holland's site of original pain, bruises, and cuts, what words would she have used?

2. A patient comes into the physician's office complaining of a lot of abdominal pain. You ask her to show you where the pain is located. She points to an area between her breasts and to another area to the right of the pelvic area. You then leave to report your findings to the physician.

   a. What abdominal descriptor would you use to describe the first location?

   b. What abdominal descriptor would you use to describe the second location?

PROBLEM-SOLVING PRACTICE

Moses Johnson is taking a course titled Introduction to Health Care. He has been studying hard and really pushing himself to learn each chapter completely. His goal is to get 100% on his tests and he has met this goal thus far. But when he starts to study the body planes, he finds himself feeling angry and discouraged. He cannot understand why top/bottom, back/front, and right side/left side cannot be used instead of learning more new terms that mean nothing to him. Every time he tries to memorize the new terms, he gets frustrated and continually confuses them. He fears he will not get them right on the upcoming exam. Using the five-step problem-solving process, determine what Moses can do about his problem.

CHAPTER 7

Structure and Function of the Human Body

KEY TERMS

anatomy
diagnosis
diagnostic procedures
diseases
etiology
genetics
hypertension
illness
integumentary
objective
pathophysiology
physiology
prevention (of disease)
prognosis
signs and symptoms
subjective
syndrome
treatment

OBJECTIVES

Studying and applying the material in this chapter will help you to:

1. Explain the difference between anatomy, physiology, and pathophysiology.
2. Define what determines a state of wellness as opposed to illness.
3. Name and describe the primary anatomical features and explain the physiological actions of the systems for movement and protection of the body.
4. Name and demonstrate the movements made possible by joints.
5. Name and describe the primary anatomical features and explain the physiological actions of the systems for providing energy and for removing waste from the body.
6. Name and describe the primary anatomical features and explain the physiological actions of the systems for sensing and for coordinating and controlling the body.
7. Name and describe the primary anatomical features and explain the physiological actions of the systems for producing new life.
8. Name common diseases and disorders associated with each system.
9. Give three examples of behaviors and actions for each body system that promote health and help prevent major diseases and disorders.

The Case of the Unfamiliar Diagnosis

Janet Waring is an X-ray technician who works in a large medical center. Mr. Petersen is admitted with a diagnosis of red cedar disease, and a lung X-ray is ordered. Janet has never heard of this disease and decides to do some independent research. The reference she uses explains why and how this disease damages the lungs, what to watch for when caring for the patient, and what tests may be ordered. By understanding how to properly use reference materials, Janet is able to learn that this condition is a type of occupational asthma and can occur in loggers and sawmill workers when a high concentration of sawdust is inhaled, causing damage to the lungs. Janet knows the normal structure and function of the lungs and can now apply this new knowledge to determine what consequences the damaged lungs may have for her patient. The information she has accessed also clarifies why the chest X-ray was ordered. Learning the material in this chapter will provide the health care student with a foundation for understanding the structure and function of the body.

THE IMPORTANCE OF ANATOMY AND PHYSIOLOGY

Many health care programs include a more in-depth study of anatomy and physiology than will be presented in this chapter. For those students with no prior study of anatomy and physiology, this material will serve as an introduction to the subject. For other students, it will serve as a review.

The study of anatomy and physiology (A&P) is fundamental to understanding the normal structure and function of the body. **Anatomy** is the study of the *form and structure* of an organism, such as the names and locations of the bones, muscles, and organs. **Physiology** is the study of the *functions* (how and why something works) of these structures. Examples include how bones and muscles produce movement, how organs assist in digestion, and how nerve impulses from the brain trigger the eyelids to blink.

Understanding the normal structure and function of the body provides a base to help the health care professional recognize abnormal conditions. These abnormal conditions are called **diseases**. When an abnormality occurs it is referred to as a pathophysiological finding (*patho* means disease). **Pathophysiology** is the study of why diseases occur and how the body changes its function in reaction to the diseases. When studying pathophysiology, several other terms are used to provide a complete description of the disease process and related information. These terms are as follows:

- **Etiology**: Study of the causes of diseases. Diseases have a variety of causes. Examples include bacteria, viruses, hazardous materials, and personal habits.

- **Signs and symptoms**: Signs and symptoms (S/S) are usually used as one phrase, but actually have separate meanings. Signs are **objective** evidence of an illness. This means that the health care professional can observe or measure them. Signs include patient behaviors, visible marks on the body, and test results. Symptoms are **subjective**. They cannot be directly observed by the health care professional, but are reported by the patient. For example, a patient may report pain (subjective data), which cannot be observed directly. However, a behavior (objective data) such as a facial grimace or limp could be present that is an indication of pain. Another example is a patient who states that he has **hypertension** (high blood pressure). This is subjective data and must be verified by taking the blood pressure to obtain objective data. Signs and symptoms serve as clues to the nature of underlying diseases or **syndromes** (not a precise disease, but a group of related signs and symptoms).

- **Diagnostic procedures**: Tests performed to determine the **diagnosis** (determination of a disease or syndrome). To arrive at a diagnosis, the signs and symptoms are evaluated by taking a thorough patient history, doing a physical exam, and ordering laboratory tests, X-rays, or other special tests. An accurate diagnosis is necessary to determine the correct treatment and predict the outcome of the problem.

- **Treatment**: Medications or procedures used to control or cure the disease. Common treatments include surgery, exercise, and special diets.

- **Prognosis**: Prediction of the possible outcome of the disease and potential for recovery.

- **Prevention**: Behaviors that promote health and prevent diseases.

The state of wellness or illness of individuals is directly related to their body structure (anatomy), function (physiology), and underlying disease processes (pathophysiology). A state of wellness is experienced when the body maintains homeostasis. As explained in Chapter 6, homeostasis is the tendency of a cell or the whole organism to maintain a state of balance. A state of **illness** occurs when one or more of the body's control systems loses the ability to maintain homeostasis. All the cells of the body suffer when this occurs. A moderate dysfunction causes illness, and a severe dysfunction can lead to death.

There is an increasing focus on preventive measures as researchers learn more about the causes of diseases and injuries. Prevention is organized into three levels:

1. Primary: Prevent the initial occurrence of the disease or injury by maintaining homeostasis. Practicing good lifestyle habits (Chapter 12) and avoiding exposure to bacteria and viruses (Chapter 10) are examples of preventive measures.

2. Secondary: Treat conditions that do occur as quickly as possible to prevent further damage.

3. Tertiary: Rehabilitate to allow the person to regain as much function as possible and prevent further disability.

GENETICS

Genetics determines one's inherited characteristics, such as eye and hair color, height, and skin tone. The focus in this chapter is related to the impact of genetics on medical disorders that can be passed from parent to child. These inherited conditions can affect any of the body systems and are too numerous to include in this text. In the Web Activities section at the end of the chapter, a website is listed that describes various inherited conditions of each body system (www.genome.gov). A review of this site will provide an awareness of the prevalence of these conditions and the impact of disorders related to heredity.

THE SYSTEMS OF THE BODY

Chapter 6 included information about the function of cells and how cells that perform a similar function group together to form tissues. Recall that when two or more of the four primary types of tissues (epithelial, connective, nervous, and muscular) combine to work together, they form organs. When two or more organs combine to perform a major body function, it is called a body system. Examples of body systems include respiratory, nervous, and urinary. See Table 7–1 for an overview of the organ systems covered in this chapter.

The systems work together in a very complex manner to maintain the body in a state of homeostasis or wellness. They are all interrelated and changes in one will affect others. A good practice when studying each system is to ask, "How does the function of this system affect all the other systems?" Some systems have a wide range of functions, and there are organs that actually belong to several systems and have more than one role.

SYSTEMS FOR MOVEMENT AND PROTECTION

The skeletal, muscular, and **integumentary** (skin) systems provide support, allow movement, and protect the body. Without bones and muscles, the body would be like an empty sack of skin without shape or the ability to move. The skin plays a critical role because it protects the body from hazards, prevents fluid loss, and helps control temperature.

Skeletal

The *skeletal system* is composed of the bones that provide a framework that:

- Gives shape to the body
- Provides places to which muscles can attach to produce movement
- Protects the internal organs
- Stores minerals
- Manufactures blood cells

Table 7-1 Organ Systems of the Body

Organ Systems	Major Functions
Systems for Movement and Protection	
Skeletal	• Provide framework to support muscles, fat, soft tissues, and skin • Furnish locations for attachment of skeletal muscles • Protect internal organs • Store minerals • Help in the formation of red and white blood cells
Muscular	• Enable locomotion (movement) • Give support to the body • Produce heat
Integumentary	• Protect from environmental hazards • Control temperature

(continues)

Table 7-1 Organ Systems of the Body (continued)

Organ Systems	Major Functions
Systems for Providing Energy and Removing Waste	
Circulatory (cardiovascular and lymphatic)	• Transport cells and dissolved materials, including nutrients, wastes, and gases • Provide defense against infection and disease • Maintain fluid balance • Remove waste products
Respiratory (pulmonary)	• Deliver gases to sites where gas exchange occurs
Digestive (gastrointestinal)	• Process food and absorb nutrients, minerals, vitamins, and water • Eliminate undigested food from the body
Urinary	• Eliminate excess water, salts, and waste products
Systems for Sensing, Coordinating, and Controlling	

Sensory (eyes, ears)	• Collect visual and auditory information; note that the organs for the other three senses are covered in other systems:
	  ° Smell (olfactory)—nose, discussed in respiratory
	  ° Taste (gustatory)—tongue, discussed in digestive
	  ° Touch—skin, discussed in integumentary

Nervous	• Direct immediate responses to stimuli, usually by coordinating the activities of other organ systems
Endocrine	• Direct changes in the activities of other organ systems
Systems for Producing New Life	
Female reproductive	• Produce sex cells and hormones necessary for female characteristics to develop and for pregnancy, delivery, and breastfeeding to occur
Male reproductive	• Produce sex cells and hormones necessary for male characteristics to develop and for production of semen for impregnation of female

Source: Adapted from Essentials of Anatomy and Physiology *(5th ed.), by F. H. Martini & E. F. Bartholomew, 2009, San Francisco, CA: Benjamin Cummings.*

Newborns have 270 bones. But as children grow, some of the bones fuse together, so adults have only about 206 bones. (The number of bones in the hands and feet can vary among individuals.)

Bones vary in shape and are classified as follows (Figure 7–1):

- Long bones: Longer than they are wide (arms: humerus, radius, ulna; legs: femur, tibia, fibula; fingers and toes: metacarpals, metatarsals, phalanges)

- Short bones: Similar in length and width (bones of the wrist and ankles, which are called carpals and tarsals, respectively)

- Flat bones: Two layers with space between them (cranium, ribs, shoulder blade [scapula], breastbone [sternum], pelvis)

- Irregular bones: Those that do not fit into the other categories (spinal column [vertebrae], facial bones, patella)

Bone Structure

It may be difficult to think of bones as organs, but they take in nutrients and oxygen and perform functions just like other organs. Bones do not consist of solid material,

FIGURE 7–1 Bone shapes.

FIGURE 7–2 Structures of a long bone.

but contain layers that have different functions. The long bones have the following structure (Figure 7–2):

- Medullary cavity (canal): Center cavity containing *yellow marrow* (primarily fat cells); covered by a layer called *endosteum*

- Diaphysis: Portion that runs between the ends of the bone; also called the "shaft"

- Epiphyses: Ends of bone (proximal and distal)

- Periosteum: White, fibrous layer that covers the outside of bone; contains blood, lymph vessels, and nerves. Bone growth, repair, and nutrition occur in the periosteum. It also serves as an attachment for muscles, tendons, and ligaments.

- Red marrow: Manufactures the red blood cells (RBCs), which carry oxygen, and the white blood cells (WBCs), which protect the body from infections.

Red bone marrow is also found in other types of bones such as ribs (flat) and vertebrae (irregular).

- Cartilage: Elastic connective tissue that covers the end of the bones and functions as a cushion between bones. Cartilage also covers the surface of joints and forms the flexible parts of the skeleton, such as the ear lobes and the tip of the nose.

The skeletal system is divided into two major parts, known as the axial and the appendicular skeletons. The *axial skeleton* includes the bones of the:

- Skull
- Inner ear
- Hyoid (U-shaped bone lying at base of tongue)

- Spinal column
- Ribs
- Sternum (breastbone)

The *appendicular skeleton* includes the bones of the:

- Shoulders
- Arms
- Hands
- Pelvis
- Legs
- Feet

See Figure 7–3.

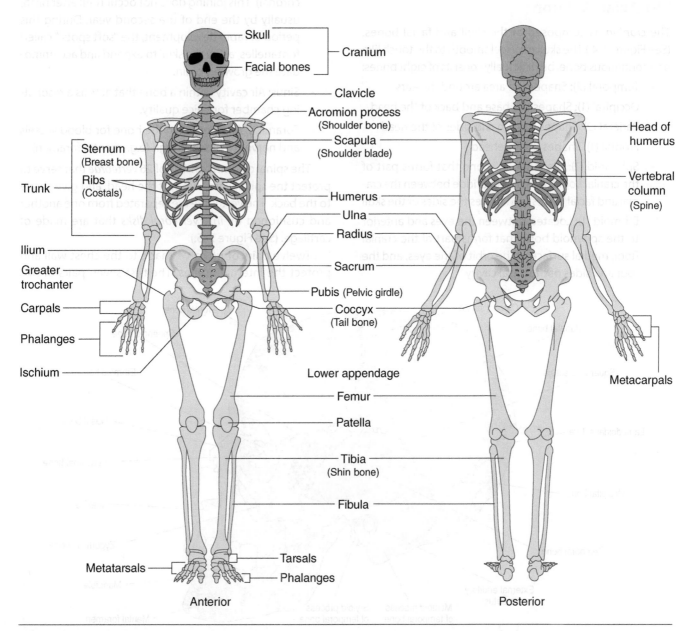

FIGURE 7–3 Bones of the skeleton (axial in blue, appendicular in tan).

The 206 bones in the adult can be divided as follows into those of the axial skeleton and the appendicular skeleton.

Axial skeleton:

- Head: 29 bones (22 in the cranium, 3 in each inner ear, and 1 hyoid)
- Trunk: 51 bones (26 vertebrae in spine, 24 ribs, and 1 sternum)

Appendicular skeleton:

- Upper extremities: 64 bones in shoulders, arms, wrists, and hands
- Lower extremities: 62 bones in pelvis, legs, ankles, and feet

The Axial Skeleton

The *cranium* is composed of the skull and facial bones. (See Figure 7–4.) The skull may feel smooth to the touch like one continuous bone, but it actually consists of eight bones:

- Temporal (2): Shapes the area around the ears
- Occipital (1): Shapes the base and back of the head
- Parietal (2): Shapes the top and sides of the head
- Frontal (1): Shapes the forehead
- Sphenoid (1): "Bat-shaped" bone that forms part of the cranial floor that acts as a bridge between the cranial and facial bones, and braces the sides of the skull
- Ethmoid (1): Located between the eyes and anterior to the sphenoid bone that forms part of the cranial floor, medial surface of the orbit of the eyes, and the roof and sides of the nasal cavity.

The face consists of 14 bones:

- Nasal (5): Shapes the nose
- Lacrimal (2): Located in the inner corner of the eye (tear duct)
- Maxilla (2): Shapes the upper jaw
- Zygomatic (2): Shapes the cheeks
- Mandible (1): Shapes the lower jaw (the only movable bone in the face)
- Palatine (2): Shapes the hard palate of the mouth

Other structures that are related to the cranium include the following:

- Suture lines: Areas where the cranial bones have joined together (e.g., lambdoidal, squamous, and coronal). This joining does not occur until after birth, usually by the end of the second year. During this period of rapid development, the "soft spots," called fontanelles, allow the skull to expand and accommodate the growing brain.
- Sinus: Air cavity within a bone that acts as a resonating chamber for voice quality.
- Foramina: An opening in the bone for blood vessels and nerves to pass through (e.g., mental foramen).

The spinal column consists of 26 *vertebrae* that serve to protect the spinal cord, support the head, and give shape to the back. The vertebrae are separated from one another and cushioned by *intervertebral disks* that are made of cartilage. (See Figure 7–5.)

Twelve pairs of *ribs* give shape to the chest wall and protect the internal organs. The first seven pairs of ribs

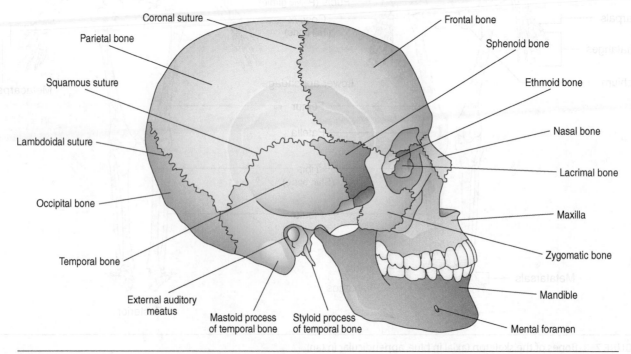

FIGURE 7–4 Bones of the cranium (skull and facial bones).

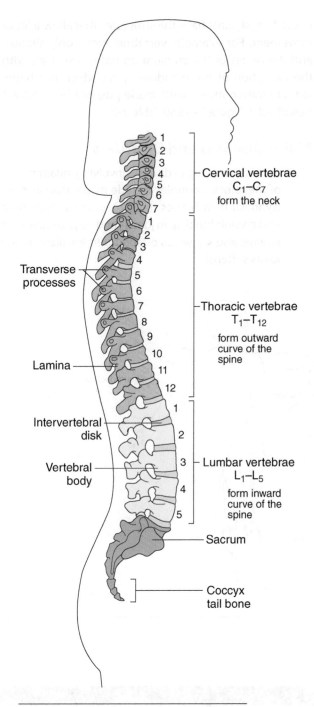

FIGURE 7–5 Lateral view of the spinal column.

Cervical vertebrae
C_1–C_7
form the neck

Transverse processes

Thoracic vertebrae
T_1–T_{12}
form outward
curve of the
spine

Lamina

Intervertebral disk

Vertebral body

Lumbar vertebrae
L_1–L_5
form inward
curve of the
spine

Sacrum

Coccyx
tail bone

Appendicular Skeleton

The upper extremities include the shoulder girdle, arms, wrists, and hands:

- Shoulder girdle: Two curved *clavicles* (shoulder bones) and the two triangular *scapulae* (shoulder blades).

- Arm: The long bone of the upper arm is the *humerus*, which is connected to the scapula by muscles and ligaments. The two long bones of the forearm are the *radius* (runs up thumb side) and *ulna* (proximal end forms the elbow that connects to the humerus).

- Wrist and hand: Eight bones in the wrist (*carpals*) form two rows of bones. The hands have five *metacarpal* bones (palm), and the five fingers have 14 *phalanges* (each finger has three except for the thumb, which has two). The hand, with its many bones, is truly an engineering marvel.

The lower extremities include the pelvic (hip) girdle, legs, ankles, and feet:

- Pelvic girdle: Serves as an area of attachment for the leg and to protect the internal organs of the lower abdomen. The girdle starts out as three bones (*ilium, ischium,* and *pubis*), which allows for growth. In adulthood these fuse to form the girdle. The bones fuse on the posterior side with the sacrum and in front by forming the *symphysis pubis*. The pelvis and pelvic inlet of the female are wider than those of the male to allow for childbirth.

- Leg: The long bone of the upper leg (thigh) is the *femur;* the femur is the longest bone in the body and fits into a cavity of the ilium known as the *acetabulum*. The two long bones of the calf are the *fibula* and *tibia*. The *patella* (kneecap) is found in front of the knee joint.

- Ankle and foot: Seven bones in the ankle (*tarsals*) provide a connection between the foot and leg bones. The foot has five *metatarsal* bones (forming the arch of the foot), and the five toes have 14 *phalanges* (each toe has three except for the big toe, which has two).

are called "true ribs" because they attach to the sternum (breastbone) in the front of the body. The next five pairs are called "false ribs." The first three pairs of false ribs attach to the cartilage of the rib above. The last two pairs are called "floating ribs" because they do not attach to the front of the body. The small piece of cartilage at the bottom edge of the sternum is called the *xiphoid process*. Health care professionals become very familiar with the xiphoid process when they learn to perform cardiopulmonary resuscitation (CPR).

Fascinating Facts

The ankles and feet account for one-quarter of all the bones in the human body.

Joints

A joint (articulation) is the connection between bones that allows for movement. Joints are covered by a synovial membrane that produces a lubricating fluid called *synovial fluid*. This enables them to move freely and without discomfort. Ligaments, the fibrous connective tissues that connect one bone to another, create the stability of the joint. Another structure that some joints (elbow, knee, and shoulder) have is a *bursa*, a small fluid-filled sac or cavity. A bursa serves as a cushion and prevents friction between moving parts, such as tendons and bones.

Joint types that enable a wide range of mobility are ball-and-socket (shoulder and hip) and hinge (elbow and knee). Not all joints have the structures that allow a lot of movement. For example, vertebrae move only slightly, and the bones of the cranium do not move at all, with the exception of the mandible (jaw), which is a hinge joint. Common movements made possible by joints are described in Figure 7–6 and Table 7–2.

Major Diseases and Disorders

- *Arthritis* is a group of diseases involving inflammation of the joints. Examples include *rheumatoid arthritis* (synovial membranes thicken), *gouty arthritis* (uric acid crystals build up in joints), and *degenerative joint disease*, also known as *osteoarthritis* (cartilage in the joints softens).

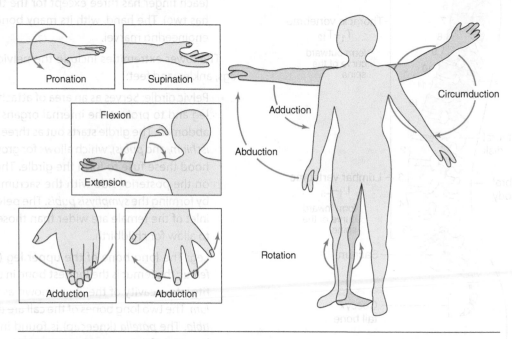

FIGURE 7–6 Movements of joints.

Table 7–2 **Movement of Joints**

Movement	Description
Abduction	Movement away from the median plane of the body
Adduction	Movement toward the median plane of the body
Circumduction	Movement in a circular direction
Extension	To straighten (increase the angle between the bones forming a joint)
Flexion	To bend (decrease the angle between the bones forming a joint)
Pronation	Turning the hand so the palm faces downward or backward (also refers to lying facedown)
Rotation	Motion around a central axis
Supination	Turning the palm or foot upward (also refers to lying face up)

- *Back pain* is a common complaint, affecting more than 80% of Americans and costing $100 million annually. It has many causes, including intervertebral disks pressing against nerves. Pain that runs down the leg is usually due to pressure on the sciatic nerve.

- *Carpal tunnel syndrome* is caused by pressure on a nerve in the wrist as a result of repetitive movement or trauma. This diagnosis has become quite common with the increased use of computers. (See Chapter 9 for ways to prevent this.)

- *Dislocation* occurs when excessive force is exerted on a joint causing a bone to slip out of the joint.

- Excessive *curvature of the spine* can occur in three directions.

  1. *Scoliosis* is a lateral (to the side) curvature.

  2. *Lordosis*, sometimes referred to as "swayback," is an inward curvature of the lumbar area.

  3. *Kyphosis*, sometimes referred to as "hunchback," is rounded bowing of the thoracic area. (See Figure 7–7.)

- *Fractures* (broken bones) usually occur from some external injury to the body, but can also occur without injury if the bone is thin and brittle as a result of a disease (e.g., osteoporosis, Paget's disease). The fracture may be closed (skin not broken) or open (bone breaks through skin). The different types of fractures are shown in Figure 7–8.

- *Osteomyelitis* is an infection of the bone.

- *Osteoporosis* is a weakening of the bones caused by the loss of calcium in the bones.

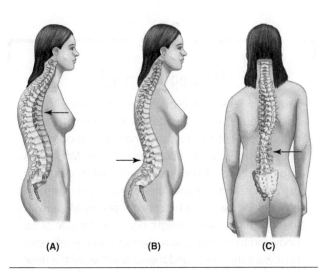

FIGURE 7–7 Abnormal curvatures of the spinal column: (A) kyphosis, (B) lordosis, and (C) scoliosis.

Preventive Measures

- Get adequate exercise, especially weight-bearing activities such as walking.

- Avoid overextension of joints.

- Eat properly and take in sufficient calcium and vitamin C.

- Do stretching exercises, especially before participating in other forms of physical activity.

- Maintain good posture (Chapter 9).

- Position the body properly when using a computer and other types of equipment (Chapter 9).

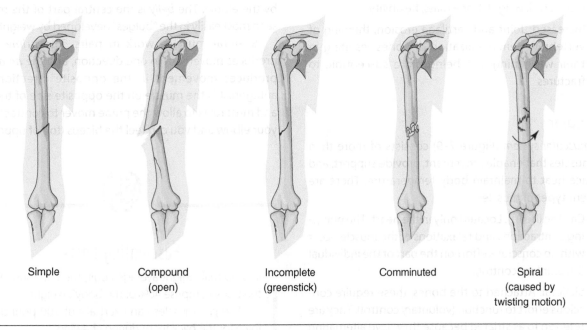

| Simple | Compound (open) | Incomplete (greenstick) | Comminuted | Spiral (caused by twisting motion) |

FIGURE 7–8 Types of fractures.

Thinking It Through

Randolph Jenkins is brought by ambulance to the hospital emergency department after a serious automobile accident. His right arm and leg are broken, and he has a skull fracture above his right ear. Mr. Jenkins also complains of pain in the left upper and lower extremities, and Dr. Printz, the emergency department physician, is assessing function by asking Mr. Jenkins to move his left arm straight out from the side of his body and then back down, then to turn the left palm up toward the ceiling and then down toward the floor.

1. Does Mr. Jenkins have injuries to the axial or appendicular skeleton, or both?

2. What are the medical terms for the four movements the patient is requested to do with his left arm and hand?

3. From the description given for the location of the skull fracture, which cranial bone is most likely involved?

- Use proper lifting techniques (Chapter 9).
- Use protective equipment, such as seat belts when in a vehicle or kneepads and helmets when cycling and skateboarding.

Age-Related Changes: Skeletal System

- Decreased: Height, bone mass, flexibility
- Increased: Joint and cartilage erosion, thinning of vertebrae, demineralization of bones resulting in their weakening and being more susceptible to fractures

Muscular

The *muscular system* (Figure 7–9) consists of more than 600 muscles that enable movement, provide support, and produce heat to maintain body temperature. There are different types of muscles:

- Cardiac (heart): Located only in the heart. The pumping contractions and relaxations of the muscle occur with no conscious effort on the part of the individual (involuntary control).
- Skeletal: Attached to the bones, these require conscious effort to function (voluntary control). They are referred to as striated because they have alternating light and dark bands circling the muscle fibers. Any

movement that is self-generated involves skeletal muscles (e.g., walking, chewing, and talking).

- Smooth (visceral): Located in the walls of internal organs (e.g., stomach, intestines, uterus, and blood vessels). Their movement is involuntary, they are nonstriated (no markings), and controlled by the autonomic (automatic) nervous system.
- Sphincter (dilator): A circular muscle that controls the opening and closing of a passageway, such as in the digestive (food passing into and out of the stomach) and urinary (urine passing out of the bladder) systems.

All muscles have the following four characteristics:

- Contractibility: Ability to be tightened, which makes the muscles shorter and thicker
- Excitability (irritability): Readiness to respond to various types of stimuli
- Extensibility: Ability to be stretched
- Elasticity: Ability to return to their original length when relaxing

Skeletal muscles are attached to the bones by bands of strong, tough connective tissues known as *tendons* or by a sheet-like membrane that covers, supports, and separates the muscles known as *fascia*. Tendons are like *ligaments* in being tough, flexible cords. But tendons differ from ligaments in that tendons extend from muscle to bone whereas ligaments go from bone to bone as at a joint. Skeletal muscles are attached to bones at two points: the *origin* and the *insertion*. The origin is the less movable bone; the insertion is attached to a more movable bone that will be affected by the action of the muscle. For example, the origin of the triceps muscle is toward the shoulder and the insertion is by the elbow. The *belly* is the central part of the muscle, seen most easily in the "bulges" developed by weightlifters.

Skeletal muscles work in pairs. The *prime mover* produces movement in one direction, and the *antagonist* produces movement in the opposite direction. The antagonist is the muscle on the opposite side of the joint and must relax to allow the prime mover to contract. Bend your elbow and you can feel the biceps (top of upper arm)

Fascinating Facts

In a normal-weight average adult, the 600 muscles of the body comprise 40% of the body's weight.

The jaw muscles can exert about 200 pounds of force for the back teeth during chewing.

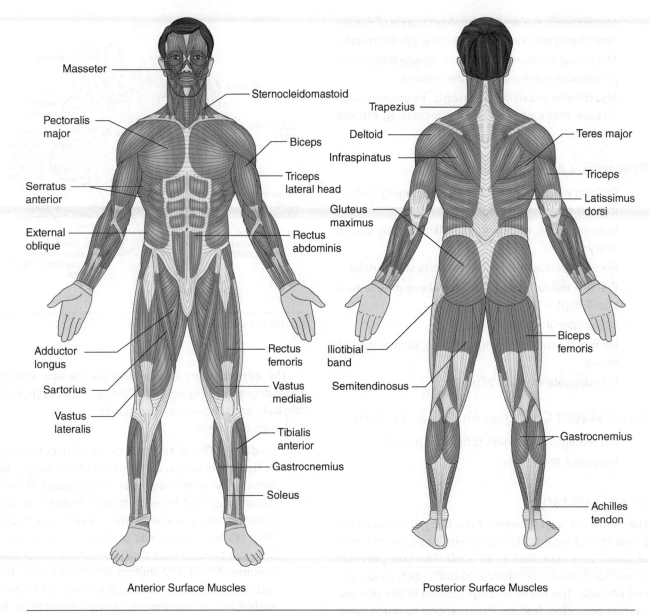

Anterior Surface Muscles

Posterior Surface Muscles

FIGURE 7–9 Muscles of the body.

contract and the triceps (back of upper arm) relax. Now extend your forearm and feel the biceps relax and the triceps contract. To demonstrate the need for opposing pairs of muscles, extend your arm partway, contract both the biceps and the triceps, and you will discover that movement is no longer possible.

Muscle tone is a muscle's normal resistance to stretching caused by always being in a state of slight contraction. Loss of muscle tone can occur from illness, injury, or from lack of use. Too much tone is called *spasticity*. This, too, can be caused by illness or injury. Spastic muscles are too tight to move smoothly.

When the muscles are not used, they can *atrophy* (shrink in size and become weak) and appear floppy. Lack of use can also result in *contracture*, in which a shortened muscle holds the joint in a flexed position.

Major Diseases and Disorders

- *Contractures* occur when the muscle stays in a short-ened position. If the joint is not moved regularly, it will lose its flexibility as ligaments and tendons shorten.

- *Fibromyalgia* is a disorder characterized by chronic widespread musculoskeletal pain accompanied by fatigue and issues with sleep, memory, and mood.

- *Gangrene* is caused by *Clostridium* bacteria, which kills muscle tissue.

- *Muscle spasms* (cramps) are sudden and painful invol-untary muscle contractions.

- *Muscle sprain* is the result of torn ligament fibers that results in loosening of the joint.

- *Muscle strain* is the result of a sudden tearing of muscle fibers during exertion; also referred to as a pulled muscle.
- *Muscular dystrophy* is an inherited disease that causes progressive deterioration of the muscles.
- *Myasthenia gravis* is a chronic neuromuscular disease that causes gradually increasing muscle weakness.

Preventive Measures

- Perform warm-up exercises before engaging in physical activity.
- Remain active, engaging in walking or exercising every day.
- Receive therapeutic massage to relax stiff muscles.
- Practice relaxation exercises to relieve muscle tension (Chapter 12).
- Use proper lifting techniques.
- Do muscle-strengthening exercises, such as weight lifting.
- Eat adequate amounts of protein.

Age-Related Changes: Muscular System

- Decreased: Muscle mass, tone, and strength
- Increased: Risk of falls

Integumentary

The skin is the largest organ of the body; it accounts for about 15% of total body weight and has a surface area of about 25 square feet in an adult. The skin provides protection from environmental hazards, such as sunrays and bacteria. The nerve endings located in the skin are another protective feature. They respond to touch, heat, cold, pain, and pressure. (See Figure 7–10.) Without this warning system, individuals would not know when to move away from hazards. The skin participates in controlling body temperature through sweating and by widening and narrowing the blood vessels to control the entry and escape of heat. Finally, the skin acts as a waterproofing membrane. Without it, death would occur within minutes from *dehydration* (loss of water).

Fascinating Facts

There are 45 miles of nerves just in the skin of a human being.

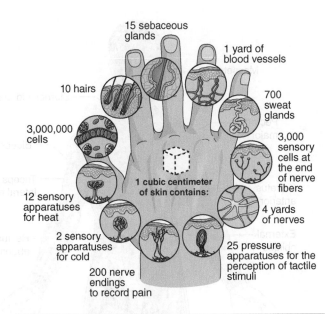

15 sebaceous glands

1 yard of blood vessels

10 hairs

700 sweat glands

3,000,000 cells

3,000 sensory cells at the end of nerve fibers

1 cubic centimeter of skin contains:

12 sensory apparatuses for heat

4 yards of nerves

2 sensory apparatuses for cold

25 pressure apparatuses for the perception of tactile stimuli

200 nerve endings to record pain

FIGURE 7–10 What is in the skin?

The *integumentary system* includes the skin and its appendages. (See Figure 7–11.) The *appendages* include hair, nails, and the sweat and oil glands.

Layers of the skin:

- Epidermis: This outer layer of the skin, consisting of five or six layers, contains no blood supply or nerves. The outermost layer is composed of cells (squamous) that have died from environmental exposure and are shed daily. These lost cells are then replaced with cells produced in the lower layers, a process that continues throughout the lifetime. About 500 million squamous cells are lost every day as we bathe, dry, dress, and move within our environment. Skin pigmentation is determined by the melanocytes that produce the pigment *melanin*. Melanin can be black or brown or have a yellow tint, depending upon racial origin. The amount of melanin (and other skin pigments such as carotene and hemoglobin) produced by the melanocytes determines the various shades of human skin. Patches of melanin are called freckles or, if related to damaged skin areas, "age spots." An albino is a person who has no skin pigmentation.
- Dermis: This is the second layer of skin, which contains involuntary muscles (arrector pili muscles that cause "goose bumps"), blood vessels, nerves, hair follicles, sudoriferous (sweat) glands, and sebaceous (oil) glands.
- Subcutaneous tissue: This is the innermost layer of the skin composed of fatty and connective tissues that fasten the skin to the underlying muscles.

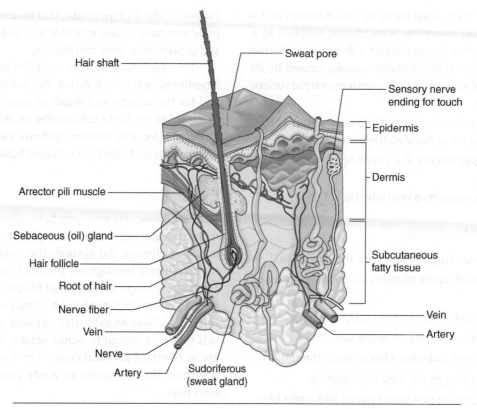

Hair shaft

Sweat pore

Sensory nerve ending for touch

Epidermis

Dermis

Arrector pili muscle

Sebaceous (oil) gland

Hair follicle

Root of hair

Nerve fiber

Subcutaneous fatty tissue

Vein

Vein

Artery

Nerve

Artery

Sudoriferous (sweat gland)

FIGURE 7–11 Structures of the skin.

Fascinating Facts

A fingernail or toenail takes about six months to grow from base to tip. Beards are the fastest-growing hairs on the human body. If never trimmed, a beard could grow to 30 feet in length over the average lifetime.

The appendages:

- Hair: Each hair is encased within a hair follicle and ends in a root where new hair growth occurs. Hair is composed of a fibrous protein called keratin, which is a nonliving cell (a good thing, or haircuts would be very painful).

- Nails: Fingernails and toenails are also composed of keratin. The growth of the nail occurs at the base of the nail under the half-moon-shaped area. The function of the nails is to protect the fingers and toes.

- Sudoriferous (sweat) glands: During perspiration, water mixed with salt and waste products is excreted through the sweat glands. The function of the sweat glands is

to excrete excess water and to assist the cooling of the body by the evaporation of water from the skin.

- Sebaceous (oil) glands: These excrete an oily substance (sebum) to lubricate and protect the skin. Sebum is slightly acidic, so it discourages the growth of bacteria.

Major Diseases and Disorders

- *Acne* is a skin condition that occurs when hair follicles plug with oil and dead skin cells resulting in blackheads and pimples.

- *Athlete's foot* is an infection of the skin caused by a fungus.

- *Boils (furuncles)* are a bacterial infection of the hair follicles or sebaceous glands.

- *Cancer of the skin* has three forms: basal cell, squamous cell, and melanoma. Basal cell is the most common and easiest to treat; squamous cell is more serious; melanoma is the most serious and can be life threatening.

- *Cellulitis* is a bacterial infection of the dermis and subcutaneous layers of the skin.

- *Pressure sores* (bed sores or decubitus ulcers) are areas of skin breakdown that occur over a bony prominence due to excessive and prolonged pressure that prevents adequate circulation to the tissues.

- *Dermatitis* is a general name for inflammation of the skin. *Contact dermatitis* is an allergic reaction to a substance that makes contact with the skin. *Eczema* is a generalized skin irritation usually caused by an irritant that appears as reddened areas on the surface of the skin.
- *Psoriasis* is a chronic, noncontagious, inherited skin disease in which too many epithelial cells are produced.
- *Type 1 herpes simplex* is a viral infection that causes cold sores.
- *Warts* are caused by a viral infection of the skin.

Preventive Measures

- Practice good hygiene and keep the skin clean.
- Do not break open pimples or other growths on the skin.
- Do not scratch insect bites or other irritations.
- Avoid excessive exposure to the sun.
- Use sunscreen and wear a hat when in the sun.
- Have skin changes checked immediately.
- Protect skin from poisonous plants and insect bites.
- Get adequate amounts of vitamins A and C and niacin.

Age-Related Changes: Integumentary System

- Decreased: Elasticity of the skin, subcutaneous fat (insulation), and hair (head, face)
- Increased: Dryness, wrinkles, skin pigmentation, and susceptibility to irritation

SYSTEMS FOR PROVIDING ENERGY AND REMOVING WASTE

These systems work together to provide energy for the body and to remove the products of waste. The circulatory system includes two powerful transportation systems,

Fascinating Facts

Humans shed about 600,000 particles of skin every hour, which is about 1.5 pounds a year. By 70 years of age, the person will have lost 105 pounds of skin.

Humans shed and regrow outer skin cells about every 27 days. That totals almost 1,000 new skins in a lifetime.

cardiovascular and lymphatic, that reach every area of the body and work closely together to maintain fluid balance and prevent infections and disease.

The respiratory system supplies oxygen, and the digestive system turns food into the fuel needed for energy and for the growth and repair of cells. This fuel is then delivered to the body cells via the cardiovascular system. The digestive and urinary systems excrete the waste by-products and help maintain fluid balance.

Circulatory

The cardiovascular and lymphatic systems are the two main transportation (circulatory) systems of the body. In the cardiovascular system, the heart pumps blood that circulates throughout the body and then back to the heart through a network of blood vessels. The lymphatic system does not have a central pumping station, but it does have an extensive network of lymphatic vessels similar in design to blood vessels. The two systems are in constant physical contact and work together to transport fluids, dispose of waste products, and fight infection.

Cardiovascular System

The cardiovascular system transports blood cells and dissolved materials, including nutrients and oxygen, to all areas of the body. The other important function of this system is temperature regulation. Human beings are warm-blooded animals and require a fairly narrow temperature range to maintain homeostasis. This temperature range is maintained by circulating the warmer blood from the center of the body to the surface of the skin where it is cooled. Regulation takes place by the blood vessels dilating to increase heat loss or contracting to reduce heat loss. On hot days the skin is pinker and warmer because the blood vessels are dilated to release heat. The opposite occurs when the outer temperature is cold because the blood flow is restricted. The skin appears pale and feels cool.

The cardiovascular system consists of the heart and blood vessels. The blood vessels that carry blood away from the heart are called *arteries*, and the blood vessels that return blood to the heart are *veins*. Both arteries and veins are like branches on a tree, becoming narrower at each branching. The smallest of the branches are called *capillaries* and their diameter is less than the width of the period at the end of this sentence.

The heart is a strong pump composed of cardiac muscles. Its main function is to pump enough blood at a high enough pressure to supply every part of the body. A fully developed heart is about the size of an adult fist. It is located in the chest cavity, between the lungs, where

Fascinating Facts

Researchers recently discovered a new organ, the *interstitium*. It consists of fluid-filled spaces described as a bubble wrap-like network that is found under that skin and throughout the digestive organs, lungs, blood vessels, and muscles. It was only revealed recently because in previous tissue biopsies and dissections, the fluid dried up and the network became invisible. Research continues to determine the functions of the interstitium.

it is protected by the ribs and sternum. The components of the heart include the following:

- Endocardium: Smooth layer that lines the inside of the heart
- Myocardium: Thick layer of muscle tissue that performs the pumping action
- Pericardium: Sac-like membrane that surrounds the heart
- Four chambers: Two for receiving blood (*atria*) and two for moving it out of the heart (*ventricles*). When blood is pumped out of the chambers, valves snap shut with a "thump-thump" (often referred to as "lub-dub"), which is the sound heard when listening to the heart. The valves prevent backflow of blood.

The blood arriving at the heart from the body takes the following path:

1. Arrives via the *inferior* and *superior vena cavae*
2. Enters the *right atrium* of the heart
3. Passes through a valve to the *right ventricle*
4. Passes through another valve into the right and left *pulmonary arteries*
5. Travels to the *lungs* to pick up fresh oxygen and drop off carbon dioxide
6. Returns to the heart by the *pulmonary veins* to the *left atrium*
7. Passes through another valve to reach the *left ventricle*
8. Leaves the *left ventricle* via the *aorta* to once again circulate throughout the body

Note: The pulmonary artery carries oxygen-poor blood to the lungs. The pulmonary vein carries oxygen-rich blood to the heart. In the rest of the circulatory system, arteries carry oxygen-rich blood to the body. Veins return oxygen-poor blood to the heart. (See Figure 7–12.)

The average adult heart rate is between 60 and 80 beats per minute. The heart rate is higher in children, gradually decreasing from its highest rate at birth until reaching its adult level. Athletes generally have lower rates because their heart muscle is stronger and pumps more blood with each beat. The heart rate varies to accommodate the body's needs. It speeds up during exercise to increase the flow of blood to skeletal muscles, after a meal to send extra blood to the digestive system, and during a fever so more blood flows to the surface of the body to release heat.

The heart has its own blood supply that wraps around its surface to provide it with nourishment and remove wastes. These are called the coronary arteries and veins. It is the blockage of coronary arteries that causes heart attacks. (See Figure 7–13.)

The heart also has its own electrical system that stimulates the cardiac muscle to contract and act as a pump. The electrical impulses, such as the blood, follow their own set path through the heart:

1. An impulse originates at a cluster of nerve cells located in the upper right wall of the right atrium, called the *sinoatrial node (SA node)*. This is the natural pacemaker of the heart, functioning to originate and regulate the heartbeat.
2. The SA node sends the impulse through a network of nerves that reaches all areas of both atria.
3. The right and left atria respond to the impulse by contracting and forcing the blood into the ventricles.
4. The impulse reaches another node, called the *atrioventricular node (AV node)* that is located between the atrium and the ventricle.
5. The AV node sends the impulse through a network of nerve fibers called the *bundle of His* that splits into the *right* and *left bundle fibers* and then terminates in a diffuse network of nerve branches called the *Purkinje fibers*.
6. The right and left ventricles contract.

It is this electrical pattern that is measured during an electrocardiogram (ECG or EKG). The pattern gives information that is helpful in diagnosing heart problems. (See Figure 7–14.)

Blood is carried throughout the body by means of a vast system of vessels, channels that carry fluid. As noted, there are three types of blood vessels: arteries, veins, and capillaries.

- Arteries carry oxygenated blood away from the heart and out to all areas of the body (recall that the pulmonary artery is the only artery that carries oxygen-poor blood, or what is called deoxygenated blood). The aorta, which receives blood pumped from the left ventricle, is the largest artery. On leaving the

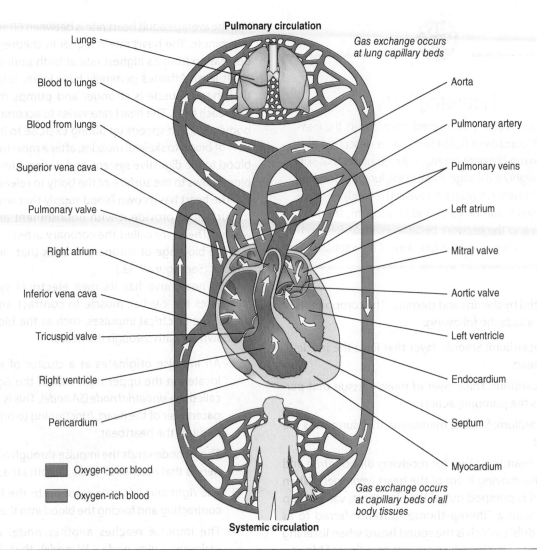

Pulmonary circulation

Lungs

Blood to lungs

Blood from lungs

Superior vena cava

Pulmonary valve

Right atrium

Inferior vena cava

Tricuspid valve

Right ventricle

Pericardium

Gas exchange occurs at lung capillary beds

Aorta

Pulmonary artery

Pulmonary veins

Left atrium

Mitral valve

Aortic valve

Left ventricle

Endocardium

Septum

Myocardium

Oxygen-poor blood

Oxygen-rich blood

Gas exchange occurs at capillary beds of all body tissues

Systemic circulation

FIGURE 7–12 Cardiopulmonary circulation.

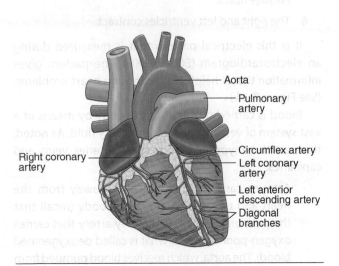

Aorta

Pulmonary artery

Right coronary artery

Circumflex artery

Left coronary artery

Left anterior descending artery

Diagonal branches

FIGURE 7–13 The coronary arteries.

Sinoatrial (SA) node

Atrioventricular (AV) node

AV bundle

Bundle of His

Right and left bundle branches

Purkinje fibers

FIGURE 7–14 The electrical system of the heart.

heart, it immediately begins to branch into smaller and smaller arteries. The smallest arteries are called *arterioles*. Arteries are muscular and elastic in order to handle the force of pumped blood. (See Figure 7–15.)

- Veins carry deoxygenated blood back to the heart from all areas of the body (recall that the pulmonary vein is the only vein that carries oxygenated blood). The farthest veins from the heart, *venules*, are also the smallest. The veins increase in size as they approach the heart. The largest veins are the *inferior* (carrying blood from lower body) and *superior* (carrying blood from upper body) vena cavae. These deliver the blood to the right atrium. Veins have one-way valves that prevent the blood from flowing in a backward direction and are thinner and less muscular than arteries. (See Figure 7–16.)

- Capillaries are the smallest blood vessels. They connect the arterioles with the venules. Their one-cell-thick walls allow substances to exit and enter the bloodstream. Nutrients and oxygen move from the blood into surrounding tissues. Waste materials and carbon dioxide are picked up for transport to the lungs and kidneys for removal from the body. (See Figure 7–17.)

FIGURE 7–15 The major arteries.

Superior sagittal sinus V.
Inferior sagittal sinus V.
Straight sinus V.
Right external jugular V.
Right internal jugular V.
Brachiocephalic V.
Superior vena cava
Right hepatic V.
Inferior vena cava
Superior mesenteric V.
Right renal V.
Right ovarian or testicular V.
Right common iliac V.
Right palmar arch V.
Right great saphenous V.
Right femoral V.
Right small saphenous V.

Left subclavian V.
Left cephalic V.
Great cardiac V.
Left axillary V.
Left basilic V.
Left brachial V.
Left hepatic V.
Hepatic portal V.
Splenic V.
Left renal V.
Left ovarian or testicular V.
Inferior mesenteric V.
Left external iliac V.
Left palmar digitals V.
Left femoral V.
Left great saphenous V.
Left popliteal V.
Left posterior tibial V.
Left anterior tibial V.
Left dorsal venous arch V.

FIGURE 7–16 The major veins.

The blood consists of red blood cells (RBCs), white blood cells (WBCs), platelets, and plasma:

- *Red blood cells* carry oxygen to the body cells. They pick up oxygen in the lungs and bind it to a substance called hemoglobin, then give up the oxygen when they reach the capillaries. An adequate intake of iron in the diet is essential for the production of hemoglobin to carry oxygen. RBCs have no nucleus so they cannot reproduce themselves. They are primarily manufactured in the red bone marrow.

- *White blood cells* fight infections. They pass through the blood vessels to work in the tissues as needed. They function as scavenger cells that engulf and destroy infected cells, a process called *phagocytosis*, and then remove wastes and dead cells. WBCs are manufactured in the bone marrow and the lymphatic system and can be produced on demand as needed by the body.

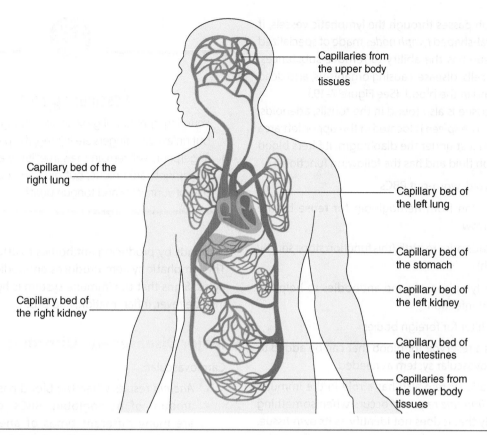

FIGURE 7–17 Examples of capillary beds.

- *Platelets* clump together to form clots when a blood vessel is damaged and aid in preventing loss of blood. Platelets are manufactured in the bone marrow.

- *Plasma* is the liquid part of the blood, consisting mostly of water. Its purpose is to transport the other blood cells along with other nutrients and hormones. It also supplies the fluid needed inside and around the body cells.

Lymphatic System

The second essential transportation system of the body is the *lymphatic system*. (See Figure 7–18.) This network of fluid, called lymph, serves to defend against infection, maintain fluid balance, and remove waste products. Lymph is a straw-colored fluid that consists of water, waste products, digested nutrients, hormones, salts, and lymphocytes (special type of WBC). Lymph travels through vessels that are similar to blood vessels. Lymphatic capillaries combine to form increasingly larger vessels that eventually empty into two *lymphatic ducts*. The ducts, which are walled passageways, then empty into the superior vena cava, and the lymph joins the blood as it enters the right atrium.

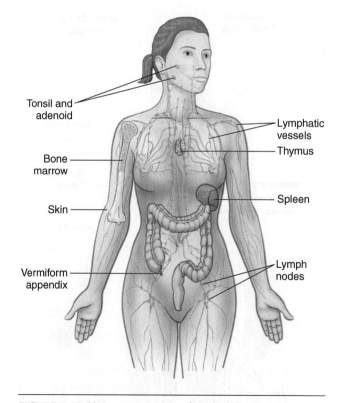

FIGURE 7–18 Major components of the lymphatic system.

As the lymph passes through the lymphatic vessels, it is filtered by oval-shaped *lymph nodes* made of specialized tissue. This tissue has the ability to remove substances, such as cancer cells, disease-causing organisms, and dead blood cells found in the blood. (See Figure 7–19.)

Lymphoid tissue is also found in the tonsils, adenoids, and the spleen. The *spleen* is located in the upper-left area of the abdomen just under the diaphragm. It filters blood instead of lymph fluid and has the following functions:

- Removes old, worn-out RBCs
- Removes iron from hemoglobin for reuse by the bone marrow
- Creates RBCs prior to birth (this function stops shortly after birth)
- Produces lymphocytes and antibodies to help the body fight infection
- Acts as a filter for foreign bodies
- Serves as a reservoir for blood that can be added to the cardiovascular system as needed

The lymphatic system also has a role in the immune response. The *immune response* occurs when something enters the body that it does not identify as its own tissue. Foreign substances are known as *antigens*. Examples include microorganisms, splinters, and poison. The body

Fascinating Facts

Your fingerprints will grow in size during your lifetime, but unless your fingers are injured, the patterns of your fingerprints will remain the same. It is well known that fingerprints are unique, but did you know this is also true of your voice and tongue print?

responds by producing antibodies to attack the antigen. The lymphatic system produces antibodies and lymphocytes. Signs that the immune system is fighting infection include fever, inflammation, and pus.

Major Diseases and Disorders

Cardiovascular:

- *Anemia* results when the blood has an inadequate amount of hemoglobin, RBCs, or both. There are many different types of anemia, including *pernicious anemia* (RBCs not developed due to poor absorption of vitamin B_{12}), *iron-deficiency anemia* (inadequate hemoglobin due to iron shortage), and *aplastic anemia* (bone marrow destroyed by chemicals, radiation, or medications). There are also two genetic forms of anemia, *sickle cell anemia*, most common in people of African origin, and *thalassemia*, most often seen in people of Mediterranean origin.
- *Aneurysm* is a ballooning out of the arterial wall that weakens the wall and disrupts blood flow.
- *Angina pectoris* is heart pain caused by inadequate supply of oxygen to the heart by the coronary arteries. If this condition is severe enough, part of the heart tissue will die, resulting in a *myocardial infarction* (MI; heart attack). A common misconception is that men are more prone to heart disease than women, but it is the number one cause of death in women.
- *Arteriosclerosis* is a hardening or thickening of the arterial walls, resulting in loss of elasticity and contractility.
- *Atherosclerosis* occurs when fatty plaques are deposited on the walls of the arteries, narrowing the lumen (opening). The narrowing decreases or prevents blood flow.
- *Congestive heart failure* is a condition in which the heart fails as a pump.

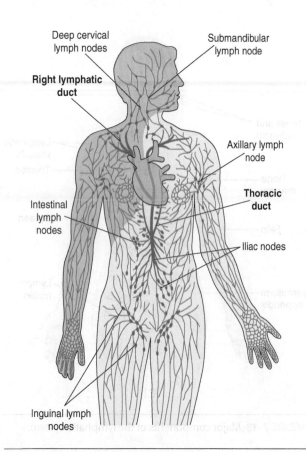

Deep cervical lymph nodes
Submandibular lymph node
Right lymphatic duct
Axillary lymph node
Thoracic duct
Intestinal lymph nodes
Iliac nodes
Inguinal lymph nodes

FIGURE 7–19 The lymphatic system.

- *Hemophilia* is a hereditary condition in which the blood fails to clot normally, resulting in excessive bleeding from even small wounds.

- *Hypertension* is high blood pressure, a condition in which the force of the heart pumping blood is higher than normal. This can result in damage to the heart and blood vessels.

- *Inflammation of the heart* can occur at any of the three layers of the heart: *endocarditis* affects the inner lining of the heart and heart valves; *myocarditis* affects the cardiac muscle; *pericarditis* affects the sac that surrounds the heart.

- *Leukemia* (blood cancer) is an abnormal increase in white blood cells that are immature and less effective than mature cells in fighting infections. These immature cells become so prevalent that they replace the RBCs and cause anemia.

- *Phlebitis* is the inflammation of a vein.

- *Septicemia* (blood poisoning) occurs when an infection enters the blood vessels.

- *Thrombosis* is a blood clot that forms in a blood vessel. If it breaks loose and travels through the body, it is called an *embolus*.

- *Varicose veins* are dilated veins filled with blood. Veins that lose their elasticity allow the blood to pool (stasis), and the result is decreased blood flow.

Lymphatic:

- *Acquired immunodeficiency syndrome* (*AIDS*) is caused by a virus and results in failure of the body's immune system.

- *Autoimmune diseases* occur when the body does not recognize its own tissue and initiates an immune response to destroy the tissue. Examples are *systemic lupus erythematosus*, which affects connective tissue; *Hashimoto's disease*, which destroys the thyroid gland; *rheumatoid arthritis*, which causes inflammation of the lining of the joints; and *celiac disease* in which the ingestion of gluten damages the small intestine.

- *Lymphoma* is cancer of the lymph nodes. There are many types of lymphoma, including *Hodgkin's disease*.

- *Splenomegaly* is an abnormally enlarged spleen which can be caused by many conditions, including infections, liver disease, and some cancers.

- *Tonsillitis* is an infection of the tonsils caused by the large number of microorganisms they are filtering through their lymph tissues.

Preventive Measures

- Practice good nutrition.
- Avoid being overweight.

Fascinating Facts

If the heart beats at the average rate of 70 beats per minute, it will have beat about 2.5 billion times by the age of 70. To appreciate how hard your heart works, try this: let your hand imitate the squeezing action of your heart by fully opening and fully closing your hand at the same rate that your heart beats. Do this for five minutes without stopping. How do the muscles of your hand and forearm feel after five minutes? If your hand got tired, you could always switch to the other hand, but you only have one heart, so take good care of it.

- Get adequate exercise.
- Check blood pressure regularly (hypertension does not have symptoms).
- Treat cuts in the skin promptly to prevent infection.
- Do not smoke.
- Do not cross the legs for long periods.
- Develop coping skills for handling stress (Chapter 12).
- Practice safe sex habits.
- Follow standard precautions and specific techniques and practices to prevent the transmission of diseases. Chapter 10 contains a detailed explanation of standard precautions.

Age-Related Changes

Cardiovascular system:

- Decreased: Arterial elasticity, efficiency of heart valves, cardiac contractility, cardiac output
- Increased: Narrowing of the arteries due to plaque buildup

Lymphatic system:

- Decreased: Inflammatory response, effectiveness of vaccines
- Increased: Susceptibility to viral and bacterial infections

Respiratory

The *respiratory system* consists of the nose, pharynx, larynx, trachea, bronchi (singular form is *bronchus*), and lungs. (See Figure 7–20.) The main function of the system is to deliver air to sites where gas exchange can occur between the air and the circulating blood. The cardiovascular and

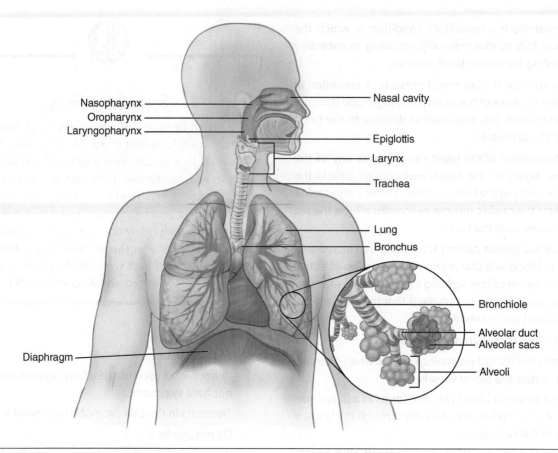

FIGURE 7–20 Structures of the respiratory system.

respiratory systems function together and are sometimes referred to as the *cardiopulmonary system*. The lymphatic system also works closely with the respiratory system to transport excess fluid from the tissues and to destroy any particles that have escaped the filtering systems and traveled deep into the lungs.

- Nose: The sensory organ for smell (olfactory). It is also important in the respiratory system. The nose is the first filter for the incoming air. Hairs and bony ridges in the nasal cavity trap the larger particles, while the nasal cavity has a *mucous* membrane that produces *mucus* to trap smaller particles. (Note that

mucous and mucus sound the same, but are spelled differently.) The nose also humidifies and warms the air as it passes through with moisture from the mucus, sinuses, and tear ducts. *Sinuses* are cavities filled with air that are located around the eyes and nose. Lined with mucous membrane, they also create a resonance to the voice. (The change in the voice during a nasal cold is due to the blockage of sinuses.)

- Pharynx: The throat. Located behind the nasal cavities, it is the passageway for food and liquids, along with air. To prevent swallowed items from entering the passageway to the lungs, there is a flap-like structure called the *epiglottis* that closes off the larynx automatically during swallowing. The soft palate, at the upper rear of the roof of the mouth, blocks food and liquid from entering the nose.

- Larynx: The voice box containing the vocal cords. These are usually relaxed and open. Sounds, such as speech and singing, are produced when the cords are tightened at the same time that air is passed out of the lungs.

- Trachea: The windpipe, which serves as a passageway for air. At its distal end, it splits to form the right and left bronchi.

Fascinating Facts

Laughing lowers levels of stress hormones and strengthens the immune system. Six-year-olds laugh an average of 300 times a day. Adults only laugh 15 to 100 times a day.

- Bronchi: The right and left bronchi continue to branch into smaller and smaller airways until they become the thin-walled *bronchioles*. The bronchioles terminate into tiny, sac-like structures called *alveoli*. It is through the walls of the alveoli that the exchange of oxygen and carbon dioxide takes place.

- Lungs: The right lung has three lobes and the left has two lobes, each containing a branch of the bronchi with its system of airways. The lungs are soft, elastic, spongy, and very light. Each is surrounded with an airtight covering called the pleura. Lungs have no muscles of their own and depend on the muscles around the chest cavity to do their work.

- Diaphragm: A sheet of muscle that separates the chest from the abdomen and stretches from the spine to the front of the rib cage. It provides a movable floor for the lungs. As the diaphragm contracts, it moves downward. This causes the air pressure in the lungs to decrease, which pulls air into the lungs (called inhalation). As the diaphragm relaxes, it moves up, raising air pressure in the lungs and forcing air out (called exhalation). The diaphragm is the major muscle involved in respiration, but there are also some small muscles between the ribs that sometimes help, especially when taking a deep breath.

Important protective structures built into the respiratory system in addition to the mucous membranes are the small, hair-like structures called *cilia*. They sweep mucus upward toward the nose and mouth so that trapped debris can be swallowed, coughed up, and sneezed or blown out. Coughing removes harmful particles that irritate the lining of the throat, trachea, or bronchial passages. Sneezing removes particles from the nasal cavity.

Major Diseases and Disorders

- *Atelectasis* occurs when the alveoli are either partially or totally collapsed. Common causes are blockage in the lung, not breathing deeply due to pain or injury, and inability to cough up secretions.

- *Chronic obstructive pulmonary disease (COPD)* is a general term that refers to chronic diseases that obstruct airflow. For example, *asthma* causes the bronchial tube walls to spasm, which narrows the passageway for airflow. The narrowing prevents an easy exhalation of air and the patient experiences a sense of suffocation. *Chronic bronchitis* is an inflammation of the bronchi and bronchial tubes. *Emphysema* causes the alveoli to become stretched out, which prevents them from efficiently exchanging oxygen and carbon dioxide.

- *Influenza (flu)* is caused by a variety of viruses that infect the nose, throat, and sometimes the lungs. Cases range from mild to so serious that it results in death.

- *Lung cancer* is the growth of tissues in the lung that destroy or block the flow of oxygen to the healthy lung tissue. This results in the entire body being deprived of oxygen. This is the most common fatal cancer, but is largely preventable.

- *Pneumonia* is an inflammation of the lungs that can be caused by bacteria, viruses, or fungi.

- *Pneumothorax* is the collapse of a lung due to air in the chest cavity. The lung can develop an internal leak or air can enter through a hole from the outside, such as a gunshot or stab wound.

- *Sleep apnea* is a disorder in which breathing repeatedly stops and starts during sleep, thus depriving the body of oxygen.

- *Tuberculosis* is a disease that damages the lungs and is caused by the tubercle bacillus (*Mycobacterium tuberculosis*). It is transmitted from person to person through the air.

- *Upper respiratory infection (URI)* is any infection of the upper respiratory structures. For example, *rhinitis* is an inflammation of the nasal mucosa resulting in a runny nose or congestion; *sinusitis* is an inflammation in the sinuses and can cause headache or pressure, congestion, discharge, and change in voice quality; *pharyngitis* (pharynx) causes a sore throat; *laryngitis* (larynx) is inflammation of the vocal cords and can result in hoarseness or loss of voice; *tonsillitis* is a painful inflammation of the lymph nodes. A URI includes the symptoms usually referred to as a common cold.

Preventive Measures

- Do not smoke.
- Use a protective mask when working around dust, toxic fumes, paints, cleaners, and so on.
- Maintain good posture.
- Take deep breaths occasionally.

Age-Related Changes: Respiratory (Pulmonary) System

- Decreased: Lung elasticity, lung expansion, functional alveoli, vital capacity, ciliary action, sense of smell

- Increased: Respiratory rate; diameter of chest (barrel chest), often caused by osteoarthritis in the rib-spine joints; rigidity of lungs

Digestive

The *digestive system* provides energy for the body by processing food. All the body's cells require nutrients to do the work of building, repairing, and controlling body systems. Carbohydrates, proteins, and fats are taken in and converted into glucose, amino acids, and fatty acids that are distributed throughout the body through the capillaries. Minerals and vitamins do not require digestion, but can be absorbed directly by the capillaries. (Chapter 12 contains more information about nutrients.) The body requires an adequate amount of water to maintain and support functions. Undigested food products are eliminated by the digestive system. The entire digestive system consists of a long tube called the *alimentary canal*. This canal is about 30 feet long and extends from the mouth, where food is taken in, to the anus, where waste products are eliminated.

The digestive system uses both mechanical and chemical means to process food. Mechanically the food is chopped, mashed, and mixed. Chemically, food is broken down by digestive enzymes that are produced within the system or added by other organs. Enzymes break down food into absorbable nutrients.

The digestive system is often referred to as the *gastrointestinal system*. The main structures that participate in the digestion of food include the mouth, esophagus, stomach, small intestines, and large intestines. (See Figure 7–21.)

- Mouth: Food enters the mouth, where its taste triggers the saliva glands to produce digestive enzymes that begin the breakdown of carbohydrates. The teeth chop and grind and the tongue mashes the food against the hard palate, mixing it with saliva. The mouth cools or warms the food to body temperature. The tongue moves the food to the back of the throat to be swallowed.

- Esophagus: A strong, muscular tube that connects the pharynx to the stomach. It lies behind the trachea and in front of the spinal column. It is composed of layers of muscle that contract to move the food. This action, called *peristalsis*, is controlled by the autonomic nervous system (processes are not consciously directed). Food passes into the stomach through the *cardiac sphincter*, the muscle that prevents the acidic content of the stomach from backflowing into the esophagus.

- Stomach: A muscular, elastic bag that fits under the diaphragm on the left side of the abdomen and is protected by the lower ribs. Food usually remains in the stomach for two to four hours while its muscles contract to mix it well with digestive juices. The glands in the stomach release hydrochloric acid to kill bacteria, pepsin (an enzyme) to break down protein, and mucus to protect the stomach wall from

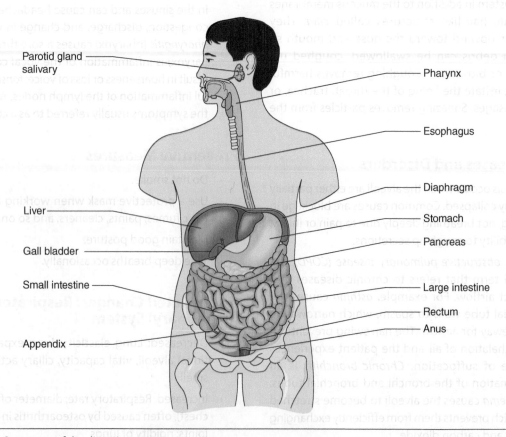

Parotid gland salivary
Pharynx
Esophagus
Diaphragm
Liver
Stomach
Pancreas
Gall bladder
Small intestine
Large intestine
Rectum
Anus
Appendix

FIGURE 7–21 Structures of the digestive system.

the acidic gastric juices. When the partially digested food leaves the stomach, it goes through the *pyloric sphincter* and enters the small intestine.

- Small intestine: Also known as the small bowel, it consists of three parts: *duodenum, jejunum,* and *ileum.* After the food passes into the small intestine, additional intestinal juices are added, including bile from the liver and pancreatic juice from the pancreas. Digestion continues, but the main function of the small intestine is the absorption of nutrients and minerals. This takes place through a network of small, finger-like projections called *villi* that line the small intestine. Each villus contains a network of blood and lymph capillaries; the lymph system absorbs the fatty acids and the blood capillaries absorb the amino acids and simple sugars. Vitamins and minerals pass unchanged from the small intestine into the blood and lymph. The material leaving the small intestine normally consists only of indigestible substances, waste material, and excess water. This passes through the *ileocecal valve* into the large intestine.

- Large intestine: Also known as the large bowel. Nutrients and water not absorbed in the small intestine are absorbed here. The large intestine contains bacteria that work on the undigested substances and synthesize vitamin K (essential for blood clotting), as well as some of the B-complex vitamins (promote various body functions). The *appendix*, located just below the *ileocecal valve* in the lower right quadrant of the abdomen, has no known function. The last portion of the digestive system serves as a storage and elimination structure for indigestible substances.

Accessory organs:

- Liver: Located in the upper right quadrant under the diaphragm; produces thick, green liquid, called bile. Bile breaks down lipids (fat) into fatty acids for absorption. The liver has many other vital functions: maintaining blood sugar levels; filtering out and destroying old RBCs, saving the iron to be used again; storing vitamins; producing prothrombin, necessary for blood clotting; and filtering out harmful toxins (poisons) that have been swallowed, including alcohol and many drugs.

- Gallbladder: Small green organ located on the inferior side of the liver; stores bile made by the liver until it is needed for the digestion of fats.

- Pancreas: Located posterior to the stomach; excretes pancreatic digestive enzymes into the duodenum of the small intestine. These enzymes help digest proteins and fat. The pancreas also functions as an endocrine gland, which will be discussed under the endocrine system presented later in the chapter.

Major Diseases and Disorders

- *Appendicitis* is an inflammation of the appendix from unknown causes. The only treatment is surgical removal (appendectomy).

- *Ascites* is not a disease, but a general term used to describe the abnormal accumulation of fluid in the peritoneal cavity (space between the layers of the membrane that lines the abdominal and pelvic cavities). Cirrhosis, cancer, and advanced congestive heart failure can cause this condition.

- *Cholelithiasis* is the presence of stones in the gallbladder. *Cholecystitis* is an inflammation of the gallbladder.

- *Cirrhosis* is a group of chronic diseases that involve scarring of liver tissue which decreases the liver's ability to perform its functions.

- *Colon cancer* involves an abnormal growth in the large intestines that damages tissue and can cause a blockage of the digestive system.

- *Constipation* is the inability to pass feces, the body's waste that is passed through the anus. The most common causes are lack of dietary fiber, inadequate fluids, certain medications, and lack of exercise. It causes abdominal distension and discomfort.

- *Crohn's disease* is an incurable, chronic inflammatory condition of the gastrointestinal tract. It can be treated with medications and sometimes goes into remission.

- *Diarrhea* is the passage of frequent and watery stools. It can be caused by certain diseases, stress, medications, and diet.

- *Diverticulosis* is the weakening of the colon wall leading to an outpouching in the wall (diverticula). These diverticula can trap digestive material and become infected. *Diverticulitis* is an inflammation of the diverticula.

- *Gastroenteritis* is an inflammation of the mucous membranes that line the stomach and intestines. Causes include food poisoning, infection, and toxins. *Gastritis* is when the lining of the stomach becomes inflamed and can be caused by spicy foods and certain medications.

- *Gastroesophageal reflux disease (GERD, also called heartburn)* occurs when the gastric juices back up through the cardiac sphincter and irritate the lower end of the esophagus, causing a burning sensation in the chest. (The esophagus does not have a protective mucous membrane like the stomach does to protect it against the acidic juices.)

- *Hemorrhoids* are painful, dilated veins in the lower rectum or anus.

- *Hepatitis* is an inflammation of the liver caused by a virus or poison.

- *Pancreatic cancer* has no symptoms in its early stages and therefore is often not detected until it has reached an advanced state. This form of cancer spreads rapidly and has a poor prognosis.

- *Pancreatitis* is an inflammation of the pancreas that can be caused by a variety of factors.

- *Peritonitis* is a condition in which the lining (peritoneum) of the abdominal cavity becomes inflamed.

- An *ulcer* is an open sore in the lining of the digestive system. Pain occurs when the protective lining is damaged and the acidic juices come into contact with the delicate tissues underneath. A *peptic ulcer* can occur in the stomach or duodenum. Stomach ulcers are also called *gastric ulcers*. *Ulcerative colitis* is a severe inflammation of the colon with the formation of ulcers and abscesses (collection of pus in a cavity).

Age-Related Changes: Digestive (Gastrointestinal) System

- Decreased: Peristalsis; control of external sphincter; taste; saliva production; liver size, weight, and efficiency; gastric acid secretion; intestinal movement; appetite

- Increased: gum disease, constipation, indigestion

Preventive Measures

- Eat an adequate amount of fiber.
- Drink plenty of water.
- Avoid excessive alcohol.
- Follow standard precautions (Chapter 10).
- Avoid large amounts of high-fat foods.
- Avoid fad diets and other extreme eating habits.
- Avoid pushing hard during bowel movements (avoid constipation).
- Do not rely on the regular use of laxatives.

Fascinating Facts

A sneeze can exceed the speed of 100 mph.

Every day, the average person produces about a quart of mucus. That comes to a total of over 25,000 quarts in a lifetime (calculated using 70 years), which is enough to fill two swimming pools. What happens to the mucus if it is not coughed out? It is swallowed! Typically, you swallow a quart of mucus every day.

- Make routine dental appointments for examination and cleaning of teeth.

- Have flexible sigmoidoscopy or colonoscopy performed at the age and frequency recommended by your health care provider.

Urinary

The *urinary system* eliminates excess water, salts, and waste products from the body. It consists of the kidneys, ureters, urinary bladder, and urethra. (See Figure 7–22.)

- Kidneys (2): Located behind the peritoneum (lining of the abdominal cavity) and on either side of the spinal column, below the diaphragm. The kidneys clean the blood and regulate the amount of water in the body. The artery that enters the kidney divides into a network of blood vessels that terminate in a grouping of capillaries called a *glomerulus*. Each glomerulus is surrounded by a kidney tubule that forms a capsule called *Bowman's capsule*. This intertwining of the blood capillaries and the kidney tubules is called a *nephron* and is where the real work of the kidney occurs: retaining waste products while returning most of the water, glucose, amino acids, and salts to the body. The nephrons, numbering more than

Fascinating Facts

The kidney is only about 4 inches long, 2 inches wide, and 1 inch thick, but it filters approximately 200 liters (quarts) of blood every day, removing 2 liters (quarts) of toxins, wastes, and water. It accomplishes this with a system of filters and tubes that stretch 140 miles.

FIGURE 7–22 A. Structures of the urinary system. B. Nephron and related structures.

1 million per kidney, are located in the cortex (outer layer) of the kidney. The waste products flow into the *medulla* (inner layer) of the kidney, where water is returned to the body. The average daily fluid output of urine is about 1,500 mL (1-1/2 quarts), but varies with fluid intake.

- Ureters (2): The ureters connect the kidneys with the bladder, forming passageways for the urine.

- Urinary bladder: Stores urine, expanding and contracting its smooth-muscle walls as needed. When the bladder wall is stretched by a large amount of urine, the nerves in the wall send a message to the brain conveying the need to urinate. The opening to the urethra is kept closed by two sphincter muscles, one of which is under voluntary control.

- Urethra: The tube through which urine is passed to the outside of the body. Passage requires relaxation of the voluntary sphincter.

Major Diseases and Disorders

- *Edema* is not a disease but a general term used to describe the abnormal accumulation of fluid in the tissues. Kidney failure, congestive heart failure, and many other conditions can cause edema.

- *Kidney (renal) failure* occurs when the nephrons are unable to filter liquid waste from the blood. The buildup of waste products in the blood is called *uremia*. To sustain life, toxins are removed by regular *dialysis* treatments. Hemodialysis is a procedure in which the blood is passed through a device that functions as an artificial kidney.

- *Kidney (renal) calculi* are kidney stones and are usually composed of uric acid or calcium crystals.

- *Urinary incontinence* is the inability to control urination. *Urinary retention* is the inability to urinate when the urge is felt or the bladder is full. These conditions have many causes.

- *Urinary tract infection (UTI)* is an infection of the lower urinary structures. *Urethritis* is an inflammation of the urethra and *cystitis* is an inflammation of the bladder.

- *Kidney infections* include *nephritis* or *glomerulonephritis*, which refers to an inflammation of the glomerulus (nephrons). *Pyelonephritis* is an inflammation of the kidney tissue and renal pelvis (collecting part of the kidney that narrows into the ureter).

Preventive Measures

- Drink adequate amounts of water (eight glasses per day has been traditionally recommended, but actual amount depends on the individual—some need more, some less).

Fascinating Facts

In a lifetime, each individual spends about six years eating about 700,000 meals, which includes 60 tons of food. And don't forget the fluid—on the average, a person drinks 16,000 gallons of fluids.

- Use proper toilet hygiene to prevent bladder infections.
- If you have hypertension or diabetes, manage it closely because both are primary contributors to renal failure.
- Be aware of and take cautiously any medications that can damage the kidneys. Never take illegal drugs.
- When taking antibiotics, increase your intake of water to prevent crystals from forming in the kidneys.

Age-Related Changes: Urinary System
- Decreased: Glomerular filtration rate, renal blood flow, renal mass, functional nephron units, bladder capacity, sphincter muscle control
- Increased: Frequency and urgency of urination, nocturia (need to urinate during the night)

SYSTEMS FOR SENSING, COORDINATING, AND CONTROLLING

The five senses (seeing, hearing, smelling, tasting, and touching) provide the brain with input from the external environment. The nervous system, in turn, interprets this input into sights, sounds, odors, flavors, or sensations of touch.

Eyes and Ears

The *eye* is often compared to a camera. It receives visual information from light rays through a transparent layer called the *cornea*. The light then enters an opening called the *pupil*, the round, black center of the eye. The *lens* projects the light rays on the *retina*, the innermost layer of the eye. (See Figure 7–23.) An upside-down image is produced, which is then converted to electrical signals and transmitted by the *optic nerve* to the brain, which "sees" it as right side up. A series of muscles attached to the eye coordinate movement so the eyes can focus.

A. Normal vision
Light rays focus on the retina.

B. Hyperopia (farsightedness)
Light rays focus beyond the retina.

C. Myopia (nearsightedness)
Light rays focus in front of the retina.

FIGURE 7–23 Normal vision occurs when the light rays are focused on the retina. An eyeball that is too long or too short prevents the proper focus.

The eye has three layers, the sclera, the choroid, and the retina (Figure 7–24):
- Sclera: The "white of the eye" is tough, fibrous tissue that serves as a protective shield. It contains the *cornea*.
- Choroid: Containing many blood vessels to nourish the eye, it includes the iris, pupil, and lens. The *iris* is the colored part, usually shades of blue, brown, or green and what people refer to when they say you have blue, brown, or hazel eyes. It is a sphincter muscle that controls the size of the pupil opening. In low light the iris relaxes, allowing the pupil to dilate and more light rays to enter for a better image. In bright light it contracts to protect the eye from too much light. Behind the pupil is the *lens* that is attached by ligaments to the *ciliary muscles*, which adjust the

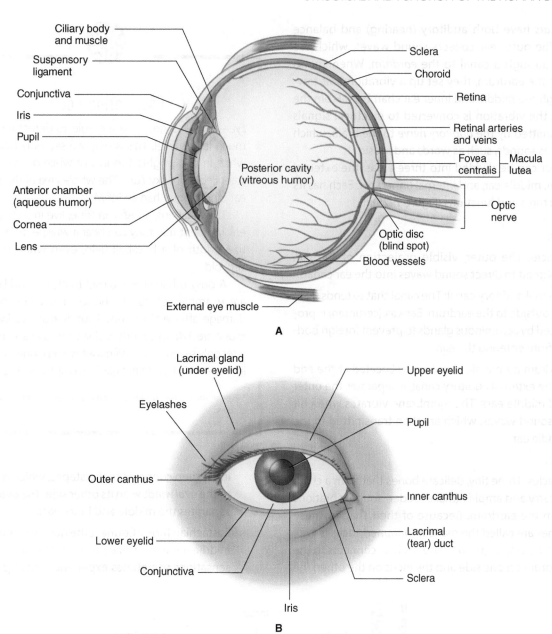

FIGURE 7–24 A. Internal view of the eye. B. External view of the eye.

shape of the lens to ensure that a sharp image is projected on the retina.

- Retina: Thin membrane attached to the back of the eye on which images are projected. It contains two types of light-sensing receptors called *rods* and *cones*. The rods are responsible for seeing in dim light and the cones for seeing colors and in bright light.

A number of structures provide protection for the eye:

- Orbit: Skull bones that form protective cavities for the eye.

- Eyelids, eyelashes, and eyebrows: Eyelids help distribute moisture over the eye and remove small particles that get into the eye. They also automatically close

when an object suddenly comes toward the eye. The eyebrows and eyelashes catch moisture and particles to prevent them from falling into the eye.

- Conjunctiva: Membrane that lines the underside of each eyelid and extends to the cornea on the surface of the eye.

- Lacrimal glands: Produce tears for cleaning and moisturizing the eye.

- Aqueous humor: A clear, watery fluid in the anterior chamber of the eye that bathes the iris, pupil, and lens.

- Vitreous humor: A clear, jelly-like fluid in the posterior chamber that maintains the shape of the eyeball and bends light rays.

The *ears* have both auditory (hearing) and balance organs. The outer ear collects sound waves, which are directed through a canal to the *eardrum*. When sound waves hit the eardrum, they set up a vibration that travels through the middle and inner ear chambers. From the *inner ear*, the vibration is converted to electrical signals and transmitted by the *auditory nerve* to the brain, which "hears" it as sounds, such as words and music.

The ear can be divided into three areas: the external (outer) ear, middle ear, and internal (inner) ear. Each has its own structures and functions (Figure 7–25):

Outer ear:

- Auricle: The outer, visible projection of the ear. Designed to direct sound waves into the ear canal.

- External auditory canal: The canal that extends from the outside to the eardrum. Earwax (cerumen) is produced by ceruminous glands to prevent foreign bodies from entering the ear.

- Eardrum (tympanic membrane): Located at the end of the external auditory canal, it separates the outer and middle ears. The membrane vibrates when hit by sound waves, which are then transmitted to the middle ear.

Middle ear:

- Ossicles: Three tiny, delicate bones that form a chain to carry and amplify (make louder) sound vibrations from the eardrum. Because of their shapes, these bones are called the malleus (*hammer*), incus (*anvil*), and the stapes (*stirrup*). The malleus connects to the eardrum on one side and the incus on the other; the

Fascinating Facts

Eye—Unlike cones, rods are able to detect light at a much lower level. This is why we see only black and white in dimly lighted rooms or while out viewing a star-filled night sky. *Ear*—The whole area of the middle ear is no bigger than an M&M.

The Maabans, an African tribe, live in such a quiet environment that they can hear a whisper from across the length of a baseball field, even when they are very old.

A busy urban street, diesel truck, or food blender are examples of 90 dB* noises and cause hearing damage after eight hours. Thunderclaps or live rock music are 120 dB sounds and start to damage hearing after only seven and a half minutes. Earphones at a high level are 140 dB, and the eardrum ruptures at 150 dB.

*dB is the abbreviation for decibel, a unit used to measure the intensity of sound.

incus then connects to the stapes, which is attached to the *oval window* on its other side. The oval window separates the middle and inner ears.

- Eustachian tubes: Connect the nose and throat to the middle ear to equalize pressure. The uncomfortable sensations sometimes experienced in airplanes and

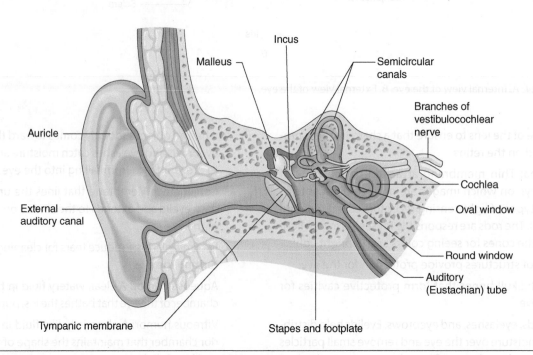

FIGURE 7–25 Structures of the ear.

under water are caused by sudden pressure changes. Chewing gum is recommended in airplanes because it helps open the tubes so that pressure is equalized.

Inner ear:

- Cochlea: A spiral-shaped, bony structure filled with fluid. The vibrations amplified in the middle ear set the fluid in motion. This movement of fluid then starts a wave-like motion in tiny, hair-like receptors, signals that the auditory nerve sends to the brain.

- Semicircular canals: These are the organs of equilibrium (balance). They contain receptor cells that report movements of the head. There are three canals: one is parallel to the ground; a second parallel to the side of the head; and a third is parallel to the face. Dizziness experienced after spinning around rapidly is caused by movement of the fluid in these canals.

Major Diseases and Disorders

Eyes:

- *Cataract* is the condition in which the lens of the eye loses its transparency, preventing light from reaching the inner eye.

- *Conjunctivitis* is an inflammation of the eyelid lining caused by bacteria or irritation from a particle of debris in the eye. It is sometimes referred to as "pink eye."

- *Detached retina* is a serious condition in which the retina pulls away from the layer of blood vessels that provides it with oxygen and nutrients.

- *Glaucoma* occurs when the pressure within the eye increases. This pressure can cause deterioration of the optic nerve.

- *Macular degeneration* is a disorder of the retina that results in dimming and/or distortion of vision.

- *Visual impairments* include a number of very common problems that require corrective lenses. For example, *myopia* (nearsightedness) occurs when the eyeball is longer than normal and cannot focus clearly on faraway objects. *Hyperopia* (farsightedness) occurs when the eyeball is shorter than normal and results in the inability to focus clearly on nearby objects. *Astigmatism* is an imperfect curvature of the cornea that results in blurred vision. *Presbyopia* is farsightedness caused by the loss of lens elasticity that occurs as part of the normal aging process. This is why many people over 40 need to wear "reading" glasses. (See Figure 7–23.)

Ears:

- *Hearing loss* is classified as either conductive or sensory. *Conductive hearing loss* occurs when the sound waves do not reach the inner ear (e.g., wax plug, ruptured eardrum, infection, or obstruction in ear). *Sensory hearing loss* results from damage to the inner ear or auditory nerve. Many cases of hearing loss can be treated with amplification devices (hearing aids), corrective surgery, or cochlear implants (a device that does not restore normal hearing, but allows the individual to hear sounds that can be interpreted for meaning).

- *Labyrinthitis* is an inflammation of the inner ear.

- *Meniere's disease* is a disorder of the inner ear that can cause a spinning sensation (*vertigo*), hearing loss, ear ringing (*tinnitus*), and ear pressure.

- *Otitis externa* is an inflammation of the external auditory canal. For example, *swimmer's ear* occurs in this part of the ear.

- *Otitis media* is an infection of the middle ear.

- *Ruptured eardrum* can occur as a result of infection, a sudden blow to the ear, or a violent change in air pressure such as occurs with an explosion or from an object placed in the ear. Ruptures usually heal without treatment, but massive or repeated injury can cause scar tissue to form and impair hearing.

- *Tinnitus* is not a disease but a medical term for ringing in the ears. It can only be heard by the patient (subjective) and can occur when there is wax buildup in the ear or an ear infection or as a result of an overdose of certain drugs (e.g., quinine or aspirin).

Preventive Measures

Eyes and ears:

- Wear UV-protective sunglasses when in the sun.

- Wear and clean contact lenses only as instructed.

- Get regular eye tests for glaucoma.

- Use eye protective devices around machinery and other hazards.

- Protect the ears from loud noises. Even exposure to one extremely loud noise can damage cells and membranes in the cochlea and cause permanent hearing loss.

- Do not insert objects into the auditory canal.

- Use earplugs when swimming.

Age-Related Changes: Sensory System

Eyes:

- Decreased: Peripheral (side) vision and night vision

- Increased: Difficulty in reading small print and seeing objects at a distance, time to adjust from light to dark, sensitivity to glare, risk for glaucoma and macular degeneration

Ears:

- Decreased: Ability to hear high-frequency sounds (e.g., telephone ringing, doorbell)
- Increased: Difficulty hearing when there is background noise (e.g., music or other people talking)

Nervous

The *nervous system* consists of the brain, spinal cord, and nerves. It detects sensations from all parts of the body and controls all the body's actions. It is also responsible for thoughts, emotions, and memories. A complex network of nerves constantly collects information from both inside and outside the body. This information is then transmitted by electrical stimuli through the spinal cord to the brain for interpretation. The information is stored, and if any response is required, such as pulling the hand away from a hot stove, direction is immediate and usually accomplished by coordinating the activities of other organ systems. In the case of the hot stove, communication would be with the muscles.

As you read this paragraph, your nervous system is performing numerous functions:

1. Directing the eyes to move across the page
2. Recognizing the images as letters and combining them to form words and sentences
3. Storing some of the ideas as memories
4. Recalling previous memories to help in understanding the new information

5. Directing skeletal muscles to maintain a sitting position
6. Causing the eyes to automatically blink to stay moist and clean
7. Controlling the heart rate, blood pressure, and respiration to keep fresh oxygen supplied to the brain to keep it alert
8. Sending sensations of tiredness or hunger after a few hours of studying

These eight examples are just a small fraction of what the nervous system is actually doing at any given moment. It is amazing how complex this system is and how well it works.

The brain makes up only about 2% of the body's weight, but uses 20% of the energy produced. It requires a constant supply of glucose (sugar) and oxygen to function. Low blood sugar causes the brain to partly shut down, resulting in feelings that begin as hunger and irritability and then progress to a weak, faint feeling. The brain is even more sensitive to the lack of oxygen, and brain cells begin to die within five minutes when they are deprived of oxygen.

Central Nervous System

The *central nervous system* (CNS) includes the brain and the spinal cord. The brain consists of the cerebrum, cerebellum, diencephalon, and brain stem. (See Figure 7–26.)

- Cerebrum: Two large hemispheres that control the higher brain functions. Their many folds (*convolutions*) greatly increase the brain's surface

FIGURE 7–26 Cross-section of the brain.

area and thus the storage capacity of the brain. The hemispheres are joined by bands of nerve fibers, including the *corpus callosum* which help the hemispheres communicate. Each hemisphere has a core of white matter surrounded by a layer of gray matter called the *cerebral cortex*. The cerebral cortex controls voluntary actions, including physical action (e.g., running, walking, and chewing), mental activity (e.g., learning, judgment, decision making, and creativity), conscious body sensations (sense of pleasure to what we see or how we are touched), and some emotions. (See Figure 7–27.) It is surprising to note that each hemisphere of the cortex controls the opposite side of the body. That is, the right hemisphere controls the left side of the body and vice versa. For example, a stroke that occurs on the right side of the brain can cause paralysis of the left arm and leg. The left hemisphere is generally responsible for learning and performing tasks that involve speech, reading, writing, math, and logic. The right hemisphere generally affects how an individual learns, performs, and enjoys creative tasks, such as those related to music and art, as well as how a person experiences emotions. When people refer to themselves as either right-brained or left-brained, they are describing their interests and abilities in these areas.

- Cerebellum: Located at the back of the brain between the cerebrum and the brain stem. Working in conjunction with the cerebrum by fine-tuning and coordinating messages for muscular movement, it is also involved in balance, posture, and muscle tone.

- Diencephalon: Contains the *thalamus* and *hypothalamus*. The thalamus relays sensory stimuli to the cerebral cortex. The hypothalamus initiates and controls many involuntary body functions necessary for living, such as water balance and body temperature.

- Brain stem: Consists of the midbrain, pons, and medulla oblongata. It serves as a pathway between the spinal cord and the brain and regulates respiration, blood pressure, and heart rate.

The *spinal cord* carries messages between the brain and other parts of the body. It is attached to the brain and is encased in the spinal column. Thirty-two pairs of nerves branch out from the cord, passing between vertebrae and extending to the various parts of the body. After the nerves branch off from the spinal cord, they are part of the peripheral nervous system.

Besides carrying messages to and from the brain, the spinal cord also serves as a reflex center. Reflexes are automatic responses that do not require any communication with the brain. For example, the jerking that occurs when

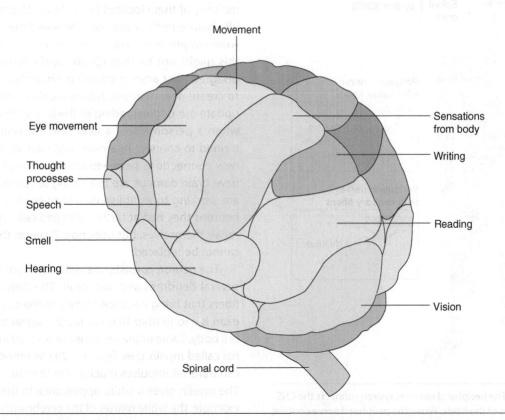

FIGURE 7–27 Functions of the cerebral cortex.

the doctor taps the knee, elbow, or wrist during a physical exam is an automatic reflex action. Also, when a finger touches a hot surface, a reflex occurs to pull it away. The reason pain is not felt until after the finger is removed from the hot surface is that the sensation must travel through the spinal cord to the brain for interpretation as pain.

The brain and the spinal cord are protected not only by bone (skull and vertebrae), but also by membranes and a fluid cushion. Wrapped around the brain and spinal cord are three layers of protective membranes called *meninges*. The two innermost meningeal layers form a space where *cerebrospinal fluid* (*CSF*) flows around the brain and spinal cord.

Peripheral Nervous System

The *peripheral nervous system* consists of the nerves that emerge from the brain (*cranial nerves*) and the spinal cord (*spinal nerves*). These nerves have both a voluntary and an involuntary component. The peripheral nerves contain two types of fibers, one for carrying messages to the central nervous system (sensory fibers) and another for carrying messages from the central nervous system to the skeletal muscles (motor fibers). (See Figure 7–28.)

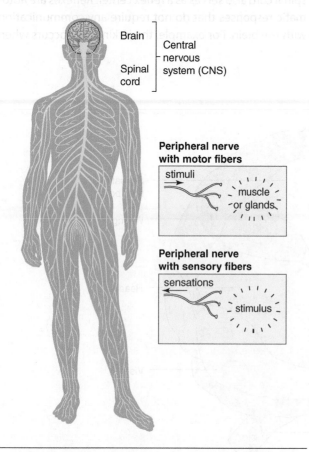

FIGURE 7–28 The peripheral nervous system connects the CNS to the structures of the body. When the peripheral nerve contains both motor and sensory fibers, it is called a mixed nerve.

The *involuntary nerves* of the peripheral nervous system contain fibers leading to and from the internal organs. These nerves belong to the *autonomic nervous system*, which means the individual has no voluntary control over the actions involved. For example, the body cannot be told when and how to digest food, when and how much urine to produce, or where and how much blood to circulate. It is a good thing the body's internal processes are automated or it would be necessary to continually think about taking the next breath or telling the heart to beat.

The autonomic nervous system can be divided into the sympathetic and the parasympathetic systems. The *sympathetic system* is activated in times of stress when the body senses the need to get away from a perceived threat or danger, commonly referred to as the "fight or flight" reaction. The sympathetic nervous system can make the difference between life and death. For example, in a crisis this system has enabled people to perform amazing feats of strength during rescues. But the body cannot tolerate prolonged stress without suffering physical or mental harm. The *parasympathetic system* maintains normal function on a day-to-day basis. (See Table 7–3.)

The autonomic nervous system works closely with the hormones produced by the hypothalamus. This will be discussed in the section on the endocrine system.

Neurons

There are billions of *neurons* (nerve cells) in the body, the majority of them located in the brain. Neurons grow rapidly before birth. It was long believed that new neurons were not produced after birth, but recent research shows this might not be true (Davis, 2018). Although there is disagreement among scientists about the body's ability to create new neurons, future studies will undoubtedly update our understanding of the brain. We do know that when a person learns a new skill, existing neurons are trained to connect in a new way. New ideas come from new connections between neurons. When people who have brain damage are relearning to speak or walk, they are working to establish new connections between the neurons they had at birth. Damaged cells may be able to repair themselves, but until now it seems that dead ones cannot be replaced.

The neuron consists of a *cell body*, from which branch several dendrites and one axon. The *dendrites* are short fibers that bring electrical signals to the cell body, and an *axon* is a long fiber that carries the signal away from the cell body. Some of the neurons are covered in a fatty material called *myelin*. (See Figure 7–29.) Myelin-covered fibers can transmit impulses much faster than uncovered fibers. The myelin gives a white appearance to the neurons. For example, the white matter of the cerebrum is covered with myelin, and the gray matter (cerebral cortex) is not.

Table 7–3 Actions of the Sympathetic and Parasympathetic Nervous Systems

System or Organ	Sympathetic System (to cope with emergencies) "fight or flight"	Parasympathetic System (normal daily functions) "rest and digest"
Heart	Increases rate and force of contraction, which enhances blood flow to skeletal muscles	Decreases rate and force of contraction
Lungs	Dilates airways (bronchioles) to take in more oxygen for body	Constricts the diameter of the air passages (bronchioles) when the need for oxygen has diminished
Arteries	Constricts arteries, thus raising blood pressure	Dilates arteries to lower blood pressure
Gastrointestinal	Diverts blood flow away from the gastrointestinal (GI) tract and skin via vasoconstriction. This results in a slowing of peristalsis and digestive activity to send more blood to the brain and skeletal muscles	Dilates blood vessels leading to the GI tract, increasing blood flow. Speeds peristalsis, increases salivary gland production and digestion to aid in absorption of nutrients
Urinary	Relaxes bladder	Constricts bladder, thus encouraging urination
Eye muscles	Dilates pupils and relaxes the lens, allowing more light to enter the eyes	Constricts pupils and lens
Sweat glands	Increases secretion to prevent overheating of body	Decreases secretion
Hair muscles	Contracts muscles and causes piloerection (goose bumps)	Relaxes muscles, causes hair to lie flat

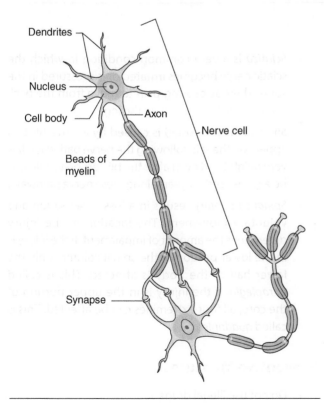

FIGURE 7–29 The neuron.

The neurons do not actually touch each other when impulses are transmitted. When the axon of one cell reaches a dendrite of another cell, they are separated by a gap called a *synapse*. The electric impulse crosses the synapse with the help of chemicals called *neurotransmitters*. For a summary overview of the nervous system, see Figure 7–30.

Major Diseases and Disorders

- *Amyotrophic lateral sclerosis (ALS or Lou Gehrig's disease)* attacks the neurons in the brain and the spinal cord resulting in muscle weakness and eventual paralysis and death from respiratory failure.

- *Cerebral palsy* is caused by abnormal brain development or brain damage and results in a lack of control over the voluntary muscles.

- A *cerebrovascular accident (CVA)* involves the brain and its blood supply and is commonly referred to as a "stroke." A CVA can be caused by a block in the blood flow (e.g., emboli) or result from a ruptured vessel. The disruption of blood flow to the brain can cause tissue damage or even death. The signs and symptoms will depend on what part of the brain has been damaged. Common results are paralysis of one side of the body (*hemiplegia*) and difficulty in or inability to communicate through speech, writing, or signs (*aphasia*). *Transient ischemic attacks (TIAs)*, called "ministrokes," occur when blood flow is only temporarily impaired. TIAs may be warning signs of a future CVA.

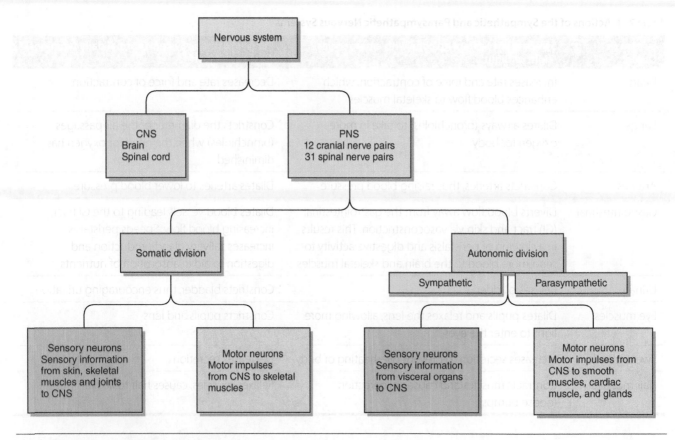

FIGURE 7-30 Divisions of the nervous system.

- *Dementia* is a loss of memory and impairment of intellectual function. *Alzheimer's disease* is only one of several diseases that cause dementia. *Senile dementia* refers to dementia when it occurs in the elderly.

- *Encephalitis* is an infection of the brain.

- *Epilepsy* is a disorder of the brain resulting from abnormal electrical impulses in the neurons. Seizures can range from very mild (petit mal) to generalized severe seizures (grand mal). Anticonvulsant drugs are very effective in controlling epilepsy.

- *Meningitis* is the inflammation of the protective covering (meninges) of the brain and spinal cord.

- *Multiple sclerosis* is a chronic, progressive, disabling condition resulting from a defect in electrical transmission of the neurons, which is caused by degeneration of the myelin sheath.

- *Neuritis* is the inflammation of a nerve. *Neuralgia* is pain, often severe, along the course of a nerve. It can be the result of several conditions, including *shingles* and *diabetes*.

- *Parkinson's disease* is a chronic, progressive condition involving degeneration of brain cells because of a decrease in a neurotransmitter (dopamine). It is characterized by tremors, shuffling walk, muscle rigidity, and loss of facial expression.

- *Sciatica* is a very common condition in which the sciatic nerve becomes irritated or is pressured in the spine, thereby causing pain to move from the back through the hip and down the leg.

- *Shingles (herpes zoster)* is caused by a virus. Blisters appear on the skin following the nerve pathways. It is very painful and even after the blisters heal, pain can be experienced for years along these nerve pathways.

- *Spinal cord injury* results in a loss of sensation and voluntary movement. The location of the injury determines the amount of impairment. If the injury is in the lower portion of the spinal column, only the lower half of the body is affected. This is called *paraplegia*. If the injury is in the upper portion of the cord, all four extremities can be affected. This is called *quadriplegia*.

Preventive Measures

- Do not use illegal drugs.
- Avoid excessive alcohol.
- Continue learning new things throughout life.
- Use protective devices such as helmets and seat belts.
- Get sufficient sleep.

Fascinating Facts

Nerve impulses in your body travel at various speeds. A nerve impulse to signal removing a hand from a hot stove may travel as fast as 330 feet (100 meters) per second. Intellectual pursuit impulses travel much slower, at 70 to 100 feet (20 to 30 meters) per second.

Age-Related Changes: Nervous System

- Decreased: Response and reaction time, number of brain cells, amount of neurotransmitters, ability to sleep, balance and coordination, cerebral blood flow
- Increased: Awakenings during sleep, muscle tremors

Endocrine

The *endocrine system* consists of glands that manufacture hormones. A *hormone* is a chemical substance secreted (produced and released) by a gland in one part of the body that travels via the bloodstream to control the activities of other organ systems and coordinate activities throughout the body. There are many different hormones, and each has its own function.

The nervous and endocrine systems work closely together to coordinate and control the body's functions. For example, recall that the sympathetic nervous system is stimulated in times of crisis. This is caused by a hormone secreted by the adrenal glands, part of the endocrine system.

There are two types of glands: exocrine and endocrine glands. *Exocrine* glands do not produce hormones, but rather produce liquids that flow through a duct (small tube) to reach a body cavity or to the surface of the skin. Examples of exocrine secretions are sweat, saliva, mucus, and digestive juices. The pancreas has the unique characteristic of being both an exocrine (secretes digestive enzyme) and an endocrine gland (produces the hormone insulin).

The hypothalamus is attached to the brain and spinal cord by many nerves. This organ links the autonomic nervous system and endocrine system. It plays an important role in the regulation of most of the involuntary mechanisms of the body and regulates the work of the pituitary gland.

The pituitary gland is often called the "master gland" because it secretes hormones that stimulate other endocrine glands to produce their own hormones. An important feature of the endocrine system is the *feedback mechanism*. This mechanism is similar to the thermostat that controls the temperature in a house. The thermostat measures the internal temperature and then turns heat or air conditioning off or on as needed to maintain the desired temperature. In a similar way, the pituitary determines if there is enough of each hormone circulating in the bloodstream and turns the stimuli to produce hormones on and off. Study Figure 7–31 and Table 7–4 to learn more about each of the endocrine glands, the hormones they produce, and the actions of the hormones. The ovaries and testes are part of the endocrine system, but will be discussed with the female and male reproductive systems.

Major Diseases and Disorders

Adrenal glands:

- *Addison's disease* is caused by inadequate hormone production by the adrenal cortex. It causes excessive skin pigmentation, decreased sugar and salt in the blood, and decreased blood pressure.
- *Cushing's syndrome* is caused by excessive hormone production of the adrenal cortex triggered by oversecretion of adrenocorticotropic hormone (ACTH, from the anterior lobe of pituitary). This results in a redistribution of fat to create a more rounded face (*"moon face"*) and a hump below the back of the neck (*"buffalo hump"*). It also causes increased blood pressure; unusual hair growth called *hirsutism*; and easy bruising.

Pancreas:

- *Diabetes mellitus* is caused by inadequate insulin production. This results in *hyperglycemia* (too much glucose in the blood). The signs and symptoms are *polydipsia* (unusual thirst), *polyuria* (increased urine output), and *polyphagia* (unusual hunger).

Parathyroid glands:

- *Hyperparathyroidism* is caused by excessive parathormone that results in an increased calcium blood level. The excessive calcium levels cause stone formation in the urinary system and elsewhere. The bones are also robbed of their calcium, and this makes them vulnerable to fractures.
- *Hypoparathyroidism* is caused by inadequate parathormone and results in a decreased calcium blood level that interrupts the normal function of nerves. This causes a condition called *tetany*, convulsive muscle twitching, and can lead to death if the respiratory muscles are affected.

Pituitary gland:

- *Acromegaly* is caused by excessive growth hormone (anterior lobe of pituitary) in adults. It causes an enlargement in the bones of the hands, feet, and jaw.

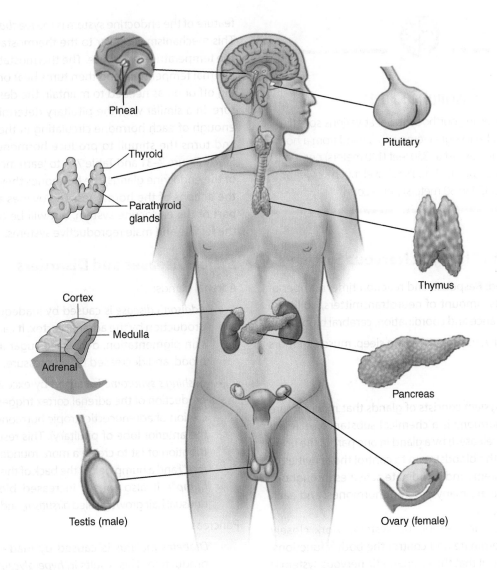

Pineal

Thyroid

Parathyroid
glands

Cortex

Medulla

Adrenal

Testis (male)

Pituitary

Thymus

Pancreas

Ovary (female)

FIGURE 7–31 Locations of the endocrine glands.

Table 7–4 Hormones and Their Actions

Gland and Location	Hormone	Actions
Pituitary (cranium)		
Anterior lobe:	GH—growth hormone	Directs normal growth of body tissues
	ACTH—adrenocorticotropic hormone	Stimulates cortex of adrenal gland
	TSH—thyroid-stimulating hormone	Stimulates thyroid gland
	MSH—melanocyte-stimulating hormone	Stimulates production of melanin, which causes skin pigmentation
	FSH—follicle-stimulating hormone	Promotes egg development in the female and sperm production in the male
	LH—luteinizing hormone	Stimulates ovulation and production of female hormones (estrogen and progesterone)

(continues)

Table 7–4 Hormones and Their Actions *(continued)*

Gland and Location	Hormone	Actions
	ICSH—interstitial cell-stimulating hormone	Stimulates production of male hormone (testosterone)
	LTH—lactogenic hormone or prolactin	Promotes development of breast tissue and production of milk in females
Posterior lobe:	ADH—antidiuretic hormone, or vasopressin	Acts on kidneys to concentrate urine and conserve fluid in the body; also constricts blood vessels
	Oxytocin (pitocin)	Causes contraction of uterus during childbirth; stimulates milk flow
Pineal (cranium)	Melatonin	Controls onset of puberty; affects wake/sleep cycle
Thyroid (neck)	Thyroxine (T_4) and triiodothyronine (T_3)	Controls metabolism and stimulates physical and mental growth
	Calcitonin	Moves calcium from the bloodstream into the bones for storage
Parathyroid (neck)	PTH—parathormone	Promotes absorption of calcium from the intestines, decreases calcium excretion by the kidneys, and moves calcium from the bones to the blood (opposite effect of calcitonin)
Thymus (chest beneath sternum)	Thymosin	Stimulates production of antibodies in early life
Adrenals: (one on top of each kidney)		
Cortex:	Mineralocorticoids (aldosterone)	Regulates the balance of electrolytes (chemicals that, when dissolved in water, can conduct electrical current) by stimulating the kidneys to retain salt (sodium) and excrete potassium
	Glucocorticoids (cortisone)	Aids in metabolism of proteins, fats, and carbohydrates; provides resistance to stress; depresses immune responses (anti-inflammatory)
	Gonadocorticoids (androgens)	Sex hormone, produced by both males and females; function is unclear
Medulla:	Epinephrine (adrenaline) and norepinephrine	Activates sympathetic nervous system in times of stress; increases blood pressure by constricting blood vessels
Pancreas (mid-abdomen under stomach)	Insulin	Regulates the transport of glucose (sugar) from the blood into the body cells
	Glucagon	Increases the amount of glucose in the blood by stimulating the liver to convert glycogen (stored form of glucose) to glucose (type of sugar that is the main source of energy to cells)

- *Diabetes insipidus* is caused by a decrease in antidiuretic hormone (posterior lobe of pituitary). It causes an increase in urine production that can lead to dehydration and electrolyte imbalances.

- *Dwarfism* can be caused by inadequate secretion of growth hormone as a child develops. The body does not develop to an average adult size.

- *Gigantism* is caused by excessive secretion of growth hormone as a child develops. This causes elongation of the long bones and results in excessive height.

Thyroid glands:

- *Hyperthyroidism* is caused by excessive thyroid hormones. It results in nervousness, increased pulse rate, weight loss, irritability, sensitivity to heat, and increased blood sugar. *Grave's disease* is a disorder in which the immune system attacks the thyroid and causes it to produce more thyroid hormone than the body needs.

- *Hypothyroidism* is caused by inadequate thyroid hormones. Hypothyroidism results in edema (excessive fluid in tissues), obesity, lethargy (extreme fatigue), decrease in heart rate, decreased mental function, cold sensitivity, and thinning of the hair.

Preventive Measures

- Maintain healthy weight.
- Avoid excessive refined sugars.
- Take children for checkups to monitor growth and development.
- Avoid the use of steroids unless prescribed (never use for purposes of muscle building during weight training programs).

Age-Related Changes: Endocrine System

- Decreased: Thyroid gland function, basal metabolic rate (energy needed to maintain body functions), adrenal gland function, insulin release, ability to break down glucose to provide energy for the body

- Increased: Incidence of hyperglycemia (increase in blood sugar) with ingestion of sugar

SYSTEMS FOR PRODUCING NEW LIFE

Reproduction is one of the most fundamental functions common to all living organisms. The reproductive system allows the creation of a new human being who is both like and unlike each of the two parents. Reproduction is essential for the continuation of human life on the earth.

Thinking It Through

Mary Steward recently retired after 40 years of teaching high school. Since her retirement, she has noticed that she is increasingly tired, sleeping much more than usual, and seems to feel cold all the time. She loved her job and at first thought that her tiredness was just part of adjusting to retirement and that feeling cold was from lack of exercise. But the symptoms have become more severe, and she made an appointment with her family physician. After an examination and blood work, Mrs. Steward is informed that she has hypothyroidism.

1. What is the function of the thyroid gland?

2. Based on the symptoms, does Mrs. Steward have too much or too little thyroid function?

3. Is the thyroid an exocrine or an endocrine gland? Why?

Female Reproductive

The *female reproductive system* can be divided into the internal and external reproductive organs (Figure 7–32).

Internal reproductive organs:

- Ovaries: There are two ovaries, one on each side of the uterus, which is located in the lower abdomen. They produce the hormones *estrogen* and *progesterone*, which determine the female characteristics (body shape, hair patterns, and breast development) and are necessary for pregnancy and subsequent childbirth to occur. Within each ovary are tiny sacs called *graafian follicles*, each of which contains one *ovum* (egg). The ovum is the female sex cell.

- Fallopian tubes: Arise from the upper portion of the uterus and end in finger-like projections (*fimbriae*) that draw the ovum, released from an ovary, down into the tube. Sperm (male sex cells) travel up into these tubes, which is where fertilization takes place. After being fertilized, the ovum moves down into the uterus.

- Uterus (womb): A muscular, hollow organ located behind the urinary bladder and in front of the rectum. It has three parts: the *fundus* (upper portion where fallopian tubes attach), the *corpus* (body or middle section), and the *cervix* (narrow, bottom area that attaches to the vagina). When the fertilized ovum reaches the uterus, it implants itself into the wall and grows and develops into a fetus. If a

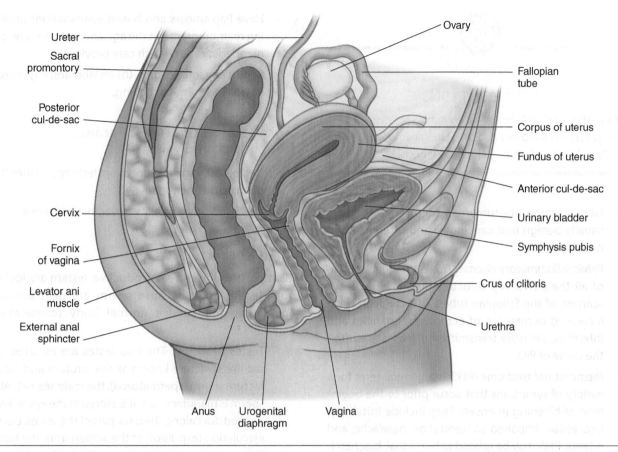

FIGURE 7–32 Cross-section of the female reproductive organs.

fertilized ovum is not implanted, blood and other materials that line the uterus are shed and menstruation occurs.

- Vagina: Opening that connects the outside of the body to the uterus. Made of smooth muscle and lined with a mucous membrane, it is capable of expanding to allow for childbirth and then contracting back to original size.

External reproductive organs (*genitalia*):

- Labia majora: Large fleshy folds of fat tissue that surround and protect the opening of the external female genitalia. They are covered with hair on their outer surfaces.
- Labia minora: Smaller fleshy folds that lay inside the boundaries of the labia majora for further protection.
- Clitoris: Located at the top junction of the labia minora, this is a very sensitive organ composed of erectile tissue similar to that of the male penis.
- Bartholin's glands: Located on each side of the external opening of the vagina, these produce mucus secretions that lubricate the vagina.

The *breasts (mammary glands)* are composed of connective and fatty tissues and contain milk ducts. The female hormones signal when milk production (*lactation*) is needed after childbirth.

Major Diseases and Disorders

- *Menstrual disorders* can result from hormonal imbalances, structural deformities, excessive exercise or stress, and nutritional imbalances. *Amenorrhea* is the absence of menstruation. *Menorrhagia* is excessive bleeding. *Dysmenorrhea* is painful menstrual cramps.
- *Ectopic pregnancy* occurs when the fertilized ovum becomes implanted outside the uterus. The most common site is in the fallopian tube. As the embryo develops, pain is caused by the distension of the tube. The tube will eventually rupture, which creates a life-threatening situation if excessive internal bleeding occurs.
- *Endometriosis* is the growth of endometrial tissue (which lines the uterus) outside the uterus. The tissue can be transferred from the uterus by the fallopian tubes, blood, lymph, or during surgery.

Fascinating Facts

All of the graafian follicles that a woman will ever have are present in the ovary at birth. During ovulation, typically only one will mature and be released.

- *Fibroid tumors* are tumors in the uterus. They are usually benign (not cancerous) and often produce no symptoms.
- *Pelvic inflammatory disease (PID)* is an inflammation of all the pelvic reproductive organs and causes scarring of the fallopian tubes. This can lead to an increased occurrence of ectopic pregnancies and infertility. Sexually transmitted diseases are often the cause of PID.
- *Premenstrual syndrome (PMS)* is a general term for a variety of symptoms that occur prior to the beginning of bleeding (menses). They include irritability, depression, impaired concentration, headache, and edema. PMS may be related to hormonal, biochemical, or nutritional imbalances.
- *Sexually transmitted disease (STD)* or venereal disease is a general term that refers to any disease transmitted through sexual contact. Examples include gonorrhea, syphilis, chlamydia, scabies, pubic lice, genital herpes, genital warts, trichomoniasis, and acquired immune deficiency syndrome (AIDS).
- *Vaginitis* is a nonspecific infection of the vagina.

Preventive Measures

- Practice safe sex if sexually active (see Chapter 12).
- Use good toilet hygiene.
- If menstrual irregularities occur or PMS is severe, have your health care provider perform an evaluation.
- Have early and routine examinations during pregnancy.
- If using contraception, be informed about the effectiveness of the method and any potential complications.
- Do not routinely perform douches.
- Consult a health care provider if sexual intercourse is uncomfortable or painful.
- Do monthly self-examination of the breasts. Report any lumps or irregularities to your health care provider for further evaluation.

- Have Pap smears and breast examinations (including mammograms) at the age and frequency recommended by your health care provider.
- Report any sores or growths on labia and any unusual vaginal discharge or itching.

Age-Related Changes: Female Reproductive System

- Decreased: Vaginal lubrication; fertility and menstruation cease (menopause)
- Increased: Susceptibility to vaginal infections

Male Reproductive

Most parts of the male reproductive system are located outside the body because sperm are heat sensitive and would not survive normal body temperatures (Figure 7–33):

- Testes (testicles): The two testes are encased in a sac-like structure known as the scrotum and manufacture sperm (spermatozoa), the male sex cell. After sperm is manufactured, it is stored in the epididymis, a coiled duct along the back part of the testes. During ejaculation (expulsion of the semen from the body), the sperm travels through a small tube (vas deferens) that enters the lower pelvic area, goes around the urinary bladder, and back down to join the urethra. The testes also produce a male hormone called testosterone, which aids in the maturation of sperm and is responsible for the development of male characteristics (body and facial hair, large muscles, and deep voice).
- Seminal vesicles: These glands join at the final portion of the vas deferens to form the ejaculatory duct. They produce a thick, yellow secretion that nourishes the sperm.
- Prostate gland: Secretes an alkaline fluid into the ejaculatory duct to aid in the movement of sperm (motility) and neutralize the acidity of the vagina. It contracts during ejaculation to propel the semen forward and to close off the urethra to prevent urine from passing at the same time.
- Penis: Composed of erectile tissue that, when aroused, fills with blood and becomes erect. At the distal end of the penis is an enlarged area known as the glans penis that is covered with a prepuce (foreskin). The foreskin is sometimes removed in a surgical procedure called circumcision.
- Urethra: Connects to the urinary bladder, passes through the penis, and exits at the end of the penis through an external opening called a meatus.

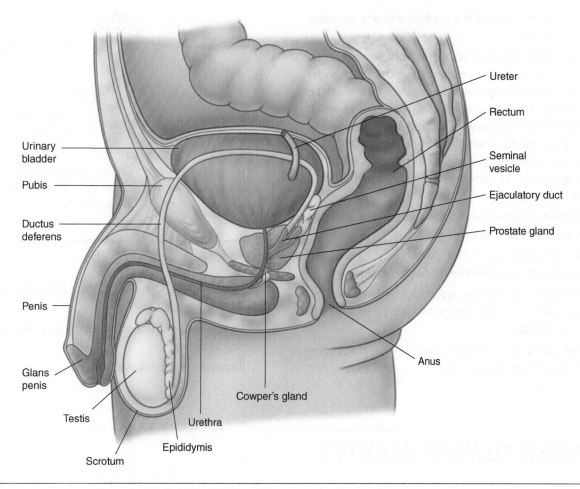

FIGURE 7–33 Cross-section of the male reproductive organs.

It serves as a dual passageway for both urine from the urinary bladder and semen from the reproductive tubes.

- Cowper's (bulbourethral) gland: Produces a thick, white, alkaline secretion to lubricate the urethra and decrease the acidity of urine residue in the urethra.

Major Diseases and Disorders

- *Epididymitis* is an inflammation of the epididymis. It causes intense pain, swelling, and fever.

- *Prostatic hypertrophy* is an enlargement of the prostate that causes symptoms as a result of pressing on the urethra. It can be an age-related condition known as *benign prostatic hypertrophy (BPH)*. It can also be caused by an inflammation, change in hormonal activity, benign (noncancerous) tumor, or malignant (cancerous) tumor.

- *Orchitis* is inflammation of the testes. It causes swelling of the scrotum, pain, and fever. It can lead to atrophy of the testes and cause sterility.

- *Phimosis* refers to a tightness of the foreskin over the end of the penis.

- *Sexually transmitted diseases*—see section under female reproductive diseases and disorders. Some of the diseases listed are asymptomatic (have no symptoms) in males. However, males can be carriers of the disease-causing organism and require treatment to prevent the female from being infected.

- *Testicular cancer* is a form of cancer that mainly affects young men between the ages of 20 and 39.

Preventive Measures

- Practice safe sex if sexually active (more information in Chapter12).

- Use good toilet hygiene.

- Male contraceptive methods are limited to five options (abstinence, condoms, outercourse, vasectomy, and withdrawal). Research may provide other options in the future. As with any contraceptive that may be used, always be informed about the effectiveness of the method and any potential complications.

- If a decrease in libido or ability to obtain an erection develops, discuss this with the health care provider because both physical and emotional factors can be involved. Medications (e.g., antihypertensives, which decrease blood pressure) can also cause this to occur and can be discussed. Do not take medications to increase libido (e.g., Viagra) until there is a thorough examination to detect risk factors and potential complications.

- Consult a health care provider if orgasm or urination is uncomfortable or painful.

- Report any lumps or irregularities of the breasts to your health care provider for further evaluation.

- Have prostate gland examinations performed at the age and frequency recommended by your health care provider.

- Report any discharge from the urethra, and any sores or growths on the genitalia.

Fascinating Facts

The average sperm count is approximately 60 million per milliliter. This number has been decreasing in the past several decades by 1% to 2%. An amount over 20 million is considered normal. Every time a male ejaculates, he releases, on the average, 1 to 6.5 milliliters of semen. An amount of 2 milliliters or more is considered normal.

Age-Related Changes: Male Reproductive System

- Decreased: Production of sperm and seminal fluid, size of testes
- Increased: Size of prostate gland

SUGGESTED LEARNING ACTIVITIES

1. Think of the last time you were ill. Identify the system that was involved (e.g., respiratory for head colds, digestive for stomach flu) and review its anatomy and physiology. Identify the pathophysiological changes that occurred with this illness. What was the etiology of the illness? What were your signs and symptoms? Did you have any diagnostic procedures done? What was the treatment for this illness? What was the prognosis? Are there any preventive measures you can take to avoid a reoccurrence of the problem?

2. Think about the physiological changes you, your parents, or your grandparents have experienced. Can you describe these changes in everyday language?

3. Locate and name as many bones and muscles as you can in your own body by pressing on the surface of your skin.

4. Move your extremities to demonstrate the various positions made possible by your joints.

5. If you have a stethoscope, listen to your heartbeat and identify what is happening in the chambers, with the valves, and in the electrical system of the heart when you hear the "thump-thump" or "lub-dub" sound.

6. Take in a deep breath of fresh air and review the path that will be taken until the oxygen reaches the level of the individual body cell. What physiological actions occur along the way?

7. Next time you have a meal, review the path the solid food and the liquids will take through your body until they are excreted. What physiological actions occur along the way?

8. Change the italicized phrase in the following saying to its correct medical equivalent: "Don't shoot until you see the *whites of their eyes!*"

9. Think of the last time you were very frightened ("fight or flight" reaction) and identify the physiological changes that the sympathetic nervous system would have initiated.

10. Review all the conditions that must be present for pregnancy to occur (remember to include the endocrine system).

WEB ACTIVITIES

Crash Course Lessons

https://www.youtube.com/watch?v=uBGl2BujkPQ

This is a very engaging and entertaining series of illustrated lectures covering all aspects of anatomy and physiology. (Note: Although there is a note about a subscription, it is not necessary to subscribe to view the videos.)

National Geographic Videos

Human Body 101

https://www.youtube.com/watch?v=Ae4MadKPJC0

Brain 101

https://www.youtube.com/watch?v=pRFXSjkpKWA

Quizlet

https://quizlet.com/13696175/anatomy-and-physiology-study-guide-flash-cards/

Review anatomy and physiology with flashcards, games, quizzes, and other activities on this interactive website.

Medline Plus

medlineplus.gov

Click on "Videos & Tools," then on "Health Videos." Choose from among the dozens of very short videos that include topics such as the cardiovascular system, endocrine glands, blood flow, and osteoarthritis.

Human Anatomy Online

www.innerbody.com

View this interactive video, then choose a body system and draw a schematic to detail the structure and function of the system.

The Pathway of Blood Throughout the Heart

https://www.youtube.com/watch?v=rf-rJRs2lLQ
https://www.youtube.com/watch?v=BEWjOCVEN7M

National Human Genome Research Institute

https://www.genome.gov/10001204/specific-genetic-disorders/

Choose one of the disorders listed and write a one-page report on the selected condition.

Human Brain Tour and Alzheimer's Disease

https://alz.org/alzheimers_disease_4719.asp

View an illustrated tour of the healthy brain followed by descriptions of a brain at various stages of Alzheimer's disease. Write a short paper describing the changes that Alzheimer's causes in the brain.

REVIEW QUESTIONS

1. What are the definitions for the terms *anatomy, physiology,* and *pathophysiology*?

2. What is the key difference between wellness and illness?

3. What are the primary anatomical features and physiological actions of the systems for movement and protection of the body?

4. What are the names and actions of the movements made possible by joints?

5. What are the primary anatomical features and physiological actions of the systems for providing energy and for removing waste from the body?

6. What are the primary anatomical features and physiological actions of the systems for sensing and for coordinating and controlling the body?

7. What are the primary anatomical features and physiological actions of the systems for producing new life?

8. What are examples of common diseases or disorders associated with each body system?

9. What are three preventive measures for each body system?

APPLICATION EXERCISES

1. Now that you know the normal anatomy and physiology of the lungs, what signs and symptoms can you anticipate that Mr. Petersen may experience as a result of red cedar disease, discussed in The Case of the Unfamiliar Diagnosis?

2. Kelly Alexico comes into the office and states he was recently diagnosed with diabetes. Wanda Hector, the health care professional, asks him if he is referring to diabetes mellitus or diabetes insipidus. He responds by saying, "I don't know for sure, all I know is that I was peeing a lot."

   a. Is this adequate information to determine if it is diabetes mellitus or diabetes insipidus?

   b. What other questions could the health care professional ask him to determine which type of diabetes is most likely the diagnosis?

   c. If it is diabetes mellitus, what can Wanda tell him about the anatomy and physiology of the related system? What is the pathophysiology of this diagnosis?

   d. If it is diabetes insipidus, what can Wanda tell him about the anatomy and physiology of the related system? What is the pathophysiology of this diagnosis?

PROBLEM-SOLVING PRACTICE

Terrance Pompei is currently taking a class in anatomy and physiology. He enjoys the class and is learning the material easily. Another student in his class is struggling with the material and has asked him to study with her. She states that the instructor speaks too fast and she is unable to grasp the material. Using the five-step problem-solving process, determine what Terrance can do to help his classmate.

CHAPTER 8

Growth and Development

KEY TERMS

chronic illness
cognitive development
deductive reasoning
development
Erikson's stages of psychosocial
    development
Gilligan's stages of the ethics
    of care
growth
Kohlberg's moral stages
life review
physical development
Piaget's cognitive stages
psychosocial development
stages of dying
terminal illness

OBJECTIVES

Studying and applying the material in this chapter will help you to:

1. Explain the differences between *physical, cognitive*, and *psychosocial* as they relate to growth and development.

2. List the nine life stages according to the theory of Erik Erikson and the corresponding age span for each.

3. Describe the physical and cognitive changes that occur at each life stage according to the theory of Erik Erikson.

4. Name the psychosocial stages and describe the changes and developmental tasks to be accomplished according to the theory of Erik Erikson.

5. Describe specific approaches to care at each life stage based on a knowledge of growth and development.

6. Describe the main concepts of the developmental theories of Piaget, Kohlberg, and Gilligan.

7. Identify and describe the five stages of the grieving and dying process.

The Case of the Curious 4-Year-Old

Paul, a 4-year-old child, is brought to the physician's office by his mother for a routine examination. Heathrow Wilson, the medical assistant, directs them to the room and begins to ask the mother routine questions and to take Paul's vital signs (blood pressure, temperature, heart and respiratory rate). Heathrow finds the tasks impossible to accomplish as the child wiggles, tries to pick up or touch everything, and asks continual questions. The mother becomes increasingly frustrated as she repeatedly tells the child to be quiet and sit still.

This may seem like a simple situation that has been observed many times, but there is a deeper dynamic being portrayed. The material in this chapter will help the health care professional to understand that Paul's tremendous curiosity and activity are normal for his age. If Heathrow better understood the stages of growth and development, he could alter his approach and implement a strategy to constructively deal with Paul's behavior. For example, he might encourage the child to participate by giving him something to do to help, asking him questions directly, or first letting Paul listen to his heart with the stethoscope. An age-appropriate response with patients will help prevent frustration and allow them to meet their developmental needs whatever their age.

KNOWING YOUR PATIENT

From before human beings are born until they die, all individuals go through a series of stages in which they develop physically and mentally. Becoming a fully developed person happens over time. The study of growth and development is about these stages in life and what is accomplished in each. Growth refers to the physical changes that take place in the body. Examples of physical changes include:

- Increases in height
- Increases in weight
- Motor sensory adaptation
- Development of the sex organs

Development refers to the increase in mental, emotional, and social capabilities of the individual. Examples include increases in:

- Intellectual (cognitive) ability
- Variety in expression of emotions
- Ability to cope with complex situations
- Social and interpersonal skills

The following terms describe key concepts in human growth and development:

- **Physical development:** Growth of the body, including motor sensory adaptation. Monitoring growth is an important task in health care. The health care professional may be responsible for measuring and recording height, weight, and head circumference for infants and children. The Learning Activities at the end of this chapter cite the address for the government website that publishes the norms for weight, height, body mass, and head circumference according to percentiles. It is important to notify the physician if the measurements fall outside the norms because this may be an indication of a problem that can be addressed before it worsens.
- **Psychosocial development:** Includes both psychological and social development. Psychological refers to the emotions (love, hate, joy, fear, anxiety), attitudes, and other aspects of the mind. Social refers to an individual's interactions and relationships with other members of society.
- **Cognitive development:** Cognitive refers to intellectual processes and includes thought, awareness, and the ability to rationally comprehend the world and determine meaning. Seeking new information and applying it to make judgments and solve problems in positive, productive ways helps develop cognitive ability. An example is using the problem-solving model presented in Chapter 1 to

practice intellectual processing. The information presented in each chapter of this text and the decision-making applications incorporated into the Thinking It Through exercises are designed to develop cognitive ability.

Human needs vary as individuals move through the life span. It is important for health care professionals to understand the developmental milestones of each stage of life, because they may provide care to individuals of all ages. A knowledge of human growth and development, along with individual patient assessment, will guide the health care professional in age-appropriate communication and care. At the same time, it is important to understand that there are always exceptions and that no one individual follows the stages exactly. Generalizations cannot take the place of considering each patient as a unique individual.

LIFE STAGES

The study of growth and development across the life span has traditionally been categorized into time frames. Certain changes and needs characterize each. Although there are a number of variations of these time frames in terms of the months or years that they cover, the age ranges listed in Table 8–1 are commonly used. They start with conception (when an ovum is fertilized) and proceed through infancy, childhood stages, adolescence, and adulthood. A complete study of the life span includes the final stage, that of dying.

In the following sections, the psychosocial aspects of each life stage are based on Erikson's stages of psychosocial development. Erik Erikson, an immigrant from Germany who taught at Yale and Harvard, studied the influence of society and culture on human development. He observed human responses to life's events to gain an understanding of how attitudes and behaviors change throughout the life span. He based his theory, first published in 1950, on the belief that psychosocial development occurs as the result of resolving specific types of conflicts encountered at each stage. Resolving these conflicts, at least in part, allows the individual to advance successfully to the next stage. A unique characteristic of Erikson's life stages is that they include adult development which many developmental theories omit, focusing instead on children. Erikson's developmental tasks are explained in the discussions of each stage later in this chapter.

Although failing to complete a stage can delay the psychosocial growth of the individual, it does not necessarily prevent the successful completion of the stage at a later date. It is also important to understand that transitions are gradual between stages: They do not begin and end abruptly at exact ages. An individual under stress, such as during an illness, may regress (return) to the behaviors characteristic of a previous stage. Some factors

Table 8–1 Life Stages and Erikson's Stages of Psychosocial Development

Life Stage	Age	Erikson Stage
Prenatal	Conception to birth	
Infancy	Birth to 1 year	Trust vs. Mistrust
Toddler	1 to 3 years	Autonomy vs. Shame/Doubt
Preschooler	3 to 6 years	Initiative vs. Guilt
School-Age Child	6 to 12 years	Industry vs. Inferiority
Adolescence	12 to 20 years	Identity vs. Role Confusion
Young Adulthood	20s and 30s	Intimacy vs. Isolation
Middle Adulthood	40 to 65 years	Generativity vs. Stagnation
Later Adulthood:		Ego Integrity vs. Despair
Young–Old	65 to 74 years	
Middle–Old	75 to 84 years	
Old–Old	85 years to death	

can delay normal development. For example, research has found that poverty in childhood may be associated with smaller than normal brain volumes in areas that involve emotion processing and memory (Bidwell, 2013). Erikson did not assign specific beginning and ending ages to each stage, but he emphasized that they occur in the same order for each individual. Researchers and writers have assigned different age ranges to his stages. The ranges chosen for Table 8–1 are representative of the life span of today's adult.

While Erikson's life-stage theory has been used for decades, it is important to note that the world has undergone many changes since his theory was first developed. Some examples of those that are believed to affect human development are the following:

- Television watching by very young children may be linked to delayed language development and kindergarten readiness skills.
- Text messaging on cell phones is changing social interaction skills.
- Distracting very young children with television or electronic games may negatively affect their ability to self-regulate and develop self-discipline.
- Learning electronically may inhibit the development of hands-on skills.

It should also be noted that Erikson's theory does have some limitations. He did not explicitly explain how and why developmental steps take place or how future personality is influenced by the completion of each stage. However, his theory continues to be considered a classic and useful framework for studying human development.

Prenatal

The *prenatal* period begins with conception (fertilization of an ovum by a sperm) and ends with birth. The cell formed when the two reproductive sex cells join is called a *zygote*. The zygote contains all the genetic information from both parents that determines gender and physical characteristics, such as eye color, hair color and texture, and skin pigmentation. Many other areas are not completely determined by genetics. For example, personality, intellect, and other mental characteristics are influenced by many other factors, such as:

- Family relationships
- Cultural customs
- Religion
- Education
- Physical health
- Economic status

Physical growth is affected by factors such as adequate supplies of appropriate food, opportunities for exercise, and access to health care. Individuals are not simply combinations of genetic material, but unique combinations of both genetic and environmental influences.

Human growth and development begin the moment fertilization occurs. The fertilized ovum is implanted into the uterine wall, and rapid cell division and multiplication occur. The period from the second to the eighth week after fertilization is called the *embryo stage*. From 8 weeks until birth, the embryo is called a *fetus*.

Rapid prenatal growth and development make the developing human especially vulnerable to environmental factors. Congenital anomalies (birth defects) can occur if the mother inhales toxins or consumes alcohol, drugs, or nicotine. Therapeutic drugs, beneficial for the mother, can cause harmful side effects in the fetus. Therefore, all over-the-counter (OTC) and prescription medications must be reviewed by the physician to determine whether they are safe to take during pregnancy.

The timeline of prenatal growth is illustrated in Table 8–2.

Table 8–2 Prenatal Development

4 Weeks

By end of 1 month:
- Half the size of a pea
- Heart is beating

8 Weeks

By end of 2 months:
- Approximately 1 inch in length
- Resembles human being
- All body organs have begun forming

12 Weeks

By end of 3 months:
- 2½ to 3 inches long
- Fully formed
- Can swallow and kick (mother cannot usually feel kicks until fourth month)
- External genitalia formed and male or female can be distinguished

24 Weeks

By end of 6 months:
- Weighs 1½ to 2 pounds
- Eyelids can now open and eyes can move up, down, and sideways
- Eyebrows, eyelashes, and taste buds present
- Can hear mother when she talks or sings

40 Weeks

By end of normal term (40 weeks):
- Fetal development is complete
- Weighs 6 to 8 pounds
- Length is 19 to 22 inches

Infancy

During the first month of life, the newborn is often referred to as a *neonate*. In this text, *infant* is used to describe the time frame from birth to 1 year of age.

This is a period of tremendous physical growth. The birth weight triples or quadruples to 21 to 27 pounds by age 1. Length will increase to between 29 and 30 inches. Teeth erupt between ages 8 and 12 months.

The muscular and nervous systems develop rapidly. At first, movements are primarily reflexive rather than being purposefully made by the infant. Over time, infants develop the ability to raise their heads and then move on to turning and rolling over. They increase their ability to focus their eyes. By 1 year many infants crawl, stand alone, and walk with assistance.

Cognitively, vocalization progresses to several words. Infants learn by imitation. During the first few months of life, they learn to manipulate objects, recognize familiar objects and persons, and obey simple commands. It has been proven that infants must receive adequate tactile stimulation (e.g., touching, cuddling, and hugging) to have normal physical and mental development. It has been observed, for example in orphanages, that infants can die from lack of physical affection (Szalavitz, 2010).

Erikson's psychosocial stage for the infant is *trust versus mistrust*. Infants are dependent on others for their physical and emotional survival. Those who receive consistent loving care that satisfies the need for food, warmth, and other physical comforts will develop trust in their caregivers. Inconsistent and inadequate care leads to mistrust of others. (See Figure 8–1.)

Toddler

The *toddler* stage is from 1 to 3 years of age. Physical changes occur as the body grows and proportions change. The characteristic protruding abdomen is still present, but the head no longer looks as oversized for the body as it does in the infant. By 3 years of age, approximately 20 teeth are present, and many toddlers, especially females, have achieved bowel and bladder control.

The motor sensory ability progresses from walking independently to running, jumping, and climbing. This is a very difficult time for the parents, because the activity of the toddler is directed toward continually investigating and searching out new experiences. Keeping the toddler safe and away from hazards requires "child-proofing" the environment and maintaining constant surveillance of the child, as in the following examples:

- Placing breakable items out of their reach
- Locking cabinets
- Using gates to prevent access to swimming pools and other hazards
- Locking away all poisonous substances
- Ensuring that they cannot leave the house by themselves
- Preventing access to any item that can be used for climbing

(See Figure 8–2.)

Cognitive skills develop rapidly as toddlers acquire language skills and begin to speak in sentences. They can understand simple instructions and requests, but their attention span is very short. Toddlers begin to learn ideas, attitudes, and values, but at the same time, they also believe that their point of view is the only one. This belief, combined with an emerging sense of independence, can lead to temper tantrums.

Erikson's psychosocial stage for the toddler is *autonomy versus shame and doubt*. Toddlers will develop confidence in their ability to care for themselves (autonomy) when they receive encouragement to explore their environment

FIGURE 8–1 It is important that the parents bond with the newborn because this will initiate a loving and trusting relationship.

FIGURE 8–2 Toddlers develop motor sensory and cognitive skills as they manipulate and investigate items in their environment.

and learn independent skills such as dressing, feeding, and using the toilet. Parents who are overly protective or have unrealistic expectations, may initiate the development of doubt and shame in their toddler. This can lead to a sense of general inadequacy.

Preschooler

The *preschooler* stage ranges from 3 to 6 years of age. Physically, preschoolers become taller and thinner than toddlers. Self-care skills increase, and they progress to being able to independently dress themselves.

Continuing motor sensory development leads to an improved sense of balance. This allows preschoolers to skip and jump in a coordinated manner and enables them to learn skills such as jumping rope and skating. (See Figure 8–3.)

Cognitively, they can now speak quite well in sentences. They have also developed an awareness of other people who are not in their immediate environment. They still assume that everyone thinks as they do. They have short attention spans but are able to count, recite the alphabet, and recall their address and phone number.

Erikson's psychosocial stage for the preschooler is *initiative versus guilt*. Preschoolers can build on the confidence developed as a toddler to initiate their own learning. They seek out new experiences and knowledge and strive to understand new activities. If their parents severely restrict this initiative, criticize, or scold them for their attempts, a sense of guilt will develop. This feeling of guilt will diminish the preschooler's natural enthusiasm for learning new motor and language skills. As a consequence, they can become hesitant to take on new challenges.

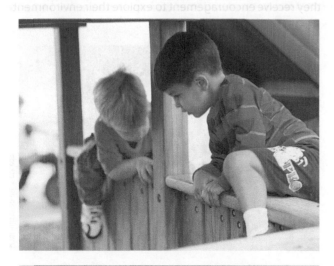

FIGURE 8–3 Preschoolers develop confidence as they succeed at new activities. Socialization skills are also practiced by interacting with their peers in group events.

School-Age Child

The *school-age child* stage ranges from 6 to 12 years of age. The physical growth of the body continues with a more pronounced development between 10 and 12 years with the beginning of puberty (the period in life when boys and girls become functionally capable of reproduction). The permanent teeth also begin to erupt at this stage of growth.

The motor sensory skills become well-coordinated, and the child develops grace and agility. School-age children can assist with household duties and show more responsibility in assigned tasks. They have a desire for both quiet time and intense physical activity. (See Figure 8–4.)

Cognitive development has progressed to logical thinking and the ability to see things from different perspectives. The attention span has increased, and pride is taken in personal accomplishments. Children at this stage reason, problem solve, learn to follow rules, and develop a sense of morality (right and wrong) to guide their behavior.

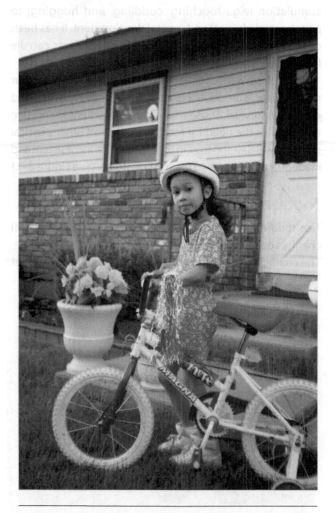

FIGURE 8–4 A school-age child has the motor sensory skills to master activities that require coordination and agility. Protective equipment, such as a helmet, plays an important role in keeping the child safe.

Erikson's psychosocial stage for the school-age child is *industry versus inferiority*. School-age children experience pleasure from the successful completion of projects and anticipate recognition for their accomplishments. They prefer friends to family and are influenced by the approval of their peers. If school-age children are not accepted by peers or cannot meet the expectations of family, a sense of inferiority and lack of self-worth may develop.

Adolescence

Adolescence is the stage ranging from 12 to 20 years of age. There are dramatic physical changes as maturation of the reproductive systems occurs.

The fine motor skills improve, but awkwardness in the gross motor skills is evident. The adolescent may easily become fatigued with activity and requires adequate rest and sleep.

Cognitive abilities greatly increase. Adolescents are able to acquire large quantities of knowledge and are able to use reasoning skills. They have the capacity for introspection and start to develop their philosophy of life and create their future occupational identity. Adolescents are also prone to stress.

Erikson's psychosocial stage for adolescence is *identity versus role confusion*. They are interested in the tremendous changes taking place in their bodies, but are also confused about identities as they move through the transition from child (dependent) to adult (independent). Mood swings are quite common as a result of the hormonal changes. Adolescents may try different roles, including rebellion, in the search for their identity as they work through who they are and who they will become. They may be critical of parents and resent the advice offered or criticism given. Peers continue to exert a significant influence on their behavior, because of strong concerns about how they are perceived. At the same time, they need the help of adults they can trust. If adolescents are unable to determine their identity and direction, they will lack a sense of who they are. This is known as "role confusion." (See Figure 8–5.)

Young Adulthood

Young adulthood includes the 20s and 30s. Physical functioning peaks at about 30 and then starts to slowly diminish as aging continues. For example, after 30 the skin begins to lose moisture, gastrointestinal secretions diminish, and problems with weight gain may begin.

Motor sensory skills also peak during this time and then begin to decline. Muscular strength peaks in the 20s and 30s and then begins to decline after the mid-30s. The visual and auditory senses also start to decline.

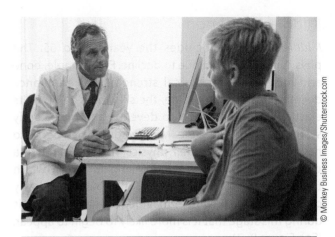

FIGURE 8–5 Adolescents need adults they can easily talk with to share their concerns and to help them understand how their mental and physical health is affected by the decisions they make.

This is a period of maximum potential. Young adults experience optimal cognitive functioning. Their problem-solving skills and creativity are excellent.

Erikson's psychosocial stage for young adulthood is *intimacy versus isolation*. The task of young adults is to complete the transition from dependency to responsibility, to make commitments to others, and to establish themselves in society. The responsibilities during this period can be extensive and may include forming an intimate relationship, having and/or raising children, obtaining advanced education, and/or establishing a career. A fear of making commitments to others may result in isolation and loneliness. (See Figure 8–6.)

FIGURE 8–6 Young adults may experience stress as they try to fill their many roles at this stage. Maintain open communication that allows them to discuss these concerns.

Middle Adulthood

Middle adulthood includes the years 40 to 65. The physical abilities continue to decline. For example, bone and muscle mass, physical strength, and endurance decrease. At the same time, the skin loses some of its elasticity, wrinkles begin to develop, and major body systems begin to decline. Middle adults may begin to have concerns about their physical health. Although a **chronic illness** (health problem of long duration in which the disease or condition shows little change or slowly gets progressively worse) may begin at any time, it is during this stage that it is more likely to begin to appear. (See Figure 8–7.)

The motor sensory skills diminish. The reflexes, muscles, and joints respond more slowly. There is decreased balance and coordination and a more prolonged response to stress. The visual, auditory, and gustatory senses diminish.

Cognitive abilities are still quite strong, although learning may take longer. Problem solving and memory remain consistent until the late middle years. Creativity may increase during this stage.

Erikson's psychosocial stage for middle adulthood is *generativity versus stagnation*. This is a time of shifting concerns from the self to the next generation, as well as toward an increased involvement with friends and community. There is a desire to make a contribution of value. It is a time of self-assessment and evaluation of the accomplishment of goals. There may be many adjustments if children leave home, health issues develop, and concerns arise about retirement. This is the period when many individuals face what is referred to as a "midlife crisis." This may be brought on by the recognition of limitations and unmet goals. If individuals are unable to establish their worth or recognize their contribution to the world, stagnation may occur. This can result in self-absorption and becoming obsessed with health concerns.

Later Adulthood

Later adulthood, as described by Erikson, encompasses age 65 until death. Physical decline continues to occur, with loss of muscle and bone and atrophy of the reproductive organs. The cardiac, renal, and immune systems decline. Decreased peripheral (arms and legs) circulation leads to less tolerance for heat and cold.

The motor sensory abilities also continue their decline. The visual, auditory, gustatory, and olfactory senses diminish. The ability to tolerate pain decreases, physical responses are slower, and some motor skills decline.

Cognitive abilities vary widely among individuals. While many older adults develop dementia, especially after age 80, others retain and even further develop their problem-solving and creative abilities.

Erikson's psychosocial stage for later adulthood is *ego integrity versus despair*. The many challenges are a continuation of changes that began in middle adulthood: retirement, loss of spouse and friends, new family roles (becoming in-laws and grandparents as children marry), and increasing concerns about health. As individuals face their mortality, they review the events of their lives and the related successes and failures. If they experience a sense of satisfaction and pleasure from the events of their lives, a sense of ego integrity will be experienced. In contrast, if the review is interpreted as a series of failures and disappointments, there is a sense of sadness and despair. (See Figure 8–8.)

FIGURE 8–7 Middle adulthood leads to more physical challenges. Keeping active adds to the adult's health, vitality, and longevity.

FIGURE 8–8 Keeping involved and active during later adulthood adds greatly to the enjoyment of life.

Note that in Table 8–1, the later adulthood stage is expanded to identify three subdivisions. Erickson's original stage of later adulthood included ages 65 to death. With the increasing number of individuals living into their 80s, 90s, and even 100s, using only one category is no longer reflective of our society. Our country now commonly sees healthy, active adults age 65 and older who are still making major contributions to society. This is the most rapidly expanding part of the population, which means that the age gap between the health care professional and the patient will increase. It is critical that health care professionals have a respect for and an understanding of the medical, psychological, and cognitive needs of this segment of the population, because this is the primary population seeking medical care today.

Older adults have previously been stereotyped as one group. However, there is a wide difference within the broad category of those who are 65 and older. To compare a person who is 65 years old with someone who is 95 years old would be similar to including a 5-year-old with someone who is 35 years old. The changes that occur in this 30-year period are as significant at the later life span as they are at the younger life span.

The baby boomers are the generation born post–World War II and encompass the 79 million babies born in the United States between 1946 and 1964. This is an average of 4 million babies each year. Prior to this time, an average of 2.5 million babies were born each year. This large group by its sheer mass has impacted every aspect of life as it has moved through society. In 2006, the oldest baby boomers turned 60 years old. In general, the boomers are healthier, more active, better educated, more affluent, and working longer than the generations that preceded them. Many boomers do not silently go into retirement, but still believe that it is possible to make the world a better place. As a result they are making significant contributions by setting up various enterprises to assist others,

getting involved in community projects, or volunteering at nonprofit organizations.

A word of caution to the health care professional: Do not rely on age alone as an indicator of the patient's needs. Assessment of the individual and his or her needs is at the center of good health care. (Information about patient assessment is included in Chapters 15, 16, and 20.) For example, even though the current trend is to break down the 65 and older group into three subdivisions, this does not dictate how to care for them. One 65-year-old may be very frail and suffering from chronic illnesses,

Fascinating Facts

Many young people think that creativity and contributions diminish as one ages. Read the following examples, and evaluate this assumption.

- Sarah Bernhardt (1844–1923) was a famous American actress. She lost a leg in her early 70s but continued acting until her death at age 78.

- Mahatma Gandhi (1869–1948) successfully completed negotiations with Britain to grant India's independence at the age of 77.

- Frank Lloyd Wright (1867–1959), America's most famous architect, designed the Guggenheim Museum in New York City at 91.

- Eleanor Roosevelt (1884–1962), the wife of President Franklin D. Roosevelt, was very active in social causes and chaired the United Nations Commission on Human Rights from ages 62 to 67. She wrote her autobiography, titled *On My Own*, at the age of 74.

- Alfred Hitchcock (1899–1980) directed the movies *Psycho* and *The Birds* in his 60s and *Frenzy* at 73 years of age.

- Nelson Mandela (1918–2013) was inaugurated as president after South Africa's first free election at the age of 75. This was after he had spent 27 years of his life in prison for his political beliefs.

- George Burns (1896–1996), comic and actor, was still appearing in public and telling jokes with perfect timing when he was 100.

- Grandma Moses (1860–1961), the famous American painter whose real name was Anna Mary Robertson, started her art career when she was in her 70s.

Fascinating Facts

Many symptoms experienced by the older persons are thought of as normal for aging, such as falling, weight loss, incontinence, dizziness, or mental impairment. These are not normal aging processes. They are a result of a disease process.

Thinking It Through

Calvin Bell is a dental hygienist in an urban dental clinic. His patients range in age from toddlers to older persons. On one busy day, he saw patients in the following stages: preschooler (3), school age (9), adolescent (15), young adult (26), and later adulthood (83).

1. Explain how his actions might change to be most appropriate with each patient (hint: refer to Table 8–3).

2. What would be the most likely dental health care concerns for each patient?

3. What might be the most effective patient education techniques to use with each?

whereas an 80-year-old may leave you behind on a hiking trail. The health care professional will find a wide variation of mental and physical ability and health status among adults in this age group. The important point to emphasize here is this: *Do not stereotype any person*. Use your assessment skills to help identify the health level of the individual.

CARE CONSIDERATIONS

Each life stage is characterized by its own physical, cognitive, and psychosocial challenges. The advantage of studying general categories is that it assists health care professionals in their understanding of areas to focus on during patient assessment and for determining age-appropriate approaches to care. The danger of using generalizations is that it is possible to make false assumptions about people and lose sight of the unique individual needs of each patient.

All patients at all times need respectful, compassionate, and empathetic care. Families and friends may also be involved in, and affected by, the health of the patient, so the same consideration must be extended to them. A routine question to always ask is if the family members have any concerns, problems, or questions they would like to discuss. When talking with family or friends, the patient's right for confidentiality must always be respected. No information can be shared with anyone else without the consent of the patient. Examples of specific care considerations as they relate to each life stage are presented in Table 8–3. Some considerations apply to most stages, such as involving patients in decisions regarding their care and adapting education and instructions to the patient's level of understanding and preferred way of receiving new information. For example, you might provide written instructions if it appears that the patient is confused by orally

Table 8–3 Care Considerations for the Health Care Professional

Life Stages	Care Considerations
Prenatal (Conception to birth)	• Emphasize care of mother to ensure a normal pregnancy. • Address unhealthy habits such as smoking. • Assist mother in developing strategies to make healthy changes. • Always ask if any over-the-counter medications or products from health food stores are being used. Commonly used medications and products can have harmful effects on unborn babies. • Inquire about mother's nutrition. • Educate the mother about the need for adequate nutrition and fluids.
Infancy (Birth–1 year)	• Involve parents in care. • Provide for safety. • Do not allow the infant to play with objects that have moving or removable parts. • Cuddle and hug infants. • Obtain height, weight, and head circumference measurements to track growth patterns.
Toddler (1–3 years)	• Use a firm, direct approach. • Distract and use a game approach to improve cooperation. • Give only one direction at a time and state it simply. • Involve toddlers in their care by allowing them to make choices when possible. • Prepare them for procedures with simple explanations. • Set limits and maintain safety.

(continues)

Table 8–3 Care Considerations for the Health Care Professional *(continued)*

Life Stages	Care Considerations
Preschooler (3–6 years)	• Explain procedures and unfamiliar objects prior to performing or using them. • Encourage verbalization skills. • Praise good behavior. • To improve acceptance of painful procedures, allow them to make choices when possible (injection site); give a token of bravery, such as a colorful sticker; and use distraction (have them recite alphabet or sing their favorite song).
School-Age Child (6–12 years)	• Explain procedures and equipment using correct terminology, but in words they understand. • Provide for privacy and some personal control. • Define and enforce behavior limits. • Encourage independence. • Educate with clear, simple visual aids.
Adolescence (12–20 years)	• Give explanations along with the rationale. • Encourage questions. • Involve them in the decision-making process. • Determine how they learn best and adapt an approach for their needs, including visual aids and written materials. • Provide privacy. • Do not talk about them where they can overhear the conversation.
Young Adulthood (20s and 30s)	• Involve significant other as appropriate. • Watch body language for clues regarding feelings. • Assess them for stress resulting from the multiple roles and responsibilities of this stage. • Involve them in the decision-making process. • Provide teaching based on how they prefer to receive information.
Middle Adulthood (40–65 years)	• Involve them in the decision-making process. • Encourage self-care. • Explore their concept of illness as it relates to body image and career. • Provide teaching based on how they prefer to receive information. • Encourage lifestyle changes such as quitting smoking, improving nutrition, and increasing exercise to help lessen the effects of natural age-related decline.
Later Adulthood Young–Old (65–74 years)	• If still working, encourage discussion about work plans, activities, and accomplishments. • If retired, encourage social activity with peers (e.g., volunteer, participation in community organizations or clubs). • Encourage active learning, thinking, and use of memory skills. • Assist with adjustment to new roles (e.g., grandparent, widower, balancing independence and dependence).
Middle–Old (75–84 years)	• Explore support systems. • Encourage them to talk about their feelings of loss, grief, and achievements. • Provide support for coping with any impairments. • Provide a safe, comfortable environment. • Be alert to overmedication and sensitivity to medications.
Old–Old (85 years to death)	• Encourage independence by providing physical, mental, and social activities. • Support end-of-life decisions by providing information and resources. • Assist with self-care. • Involve family members in caregiving. • Be sensitive to sensory impairments. • Provide care to maintain skin integrity and regular bowel movements.

presented information. It is also suggested that the health care professional request feedback to check the patient's understanding.

OTHER DEVELOPMENTAL THEORIES

Erickson's stages of psychosocial development offer a classic approach to development that remains the most frequently used theory today. However, other theories have also contributed to the field of life stages and personal development. A few of these are presented in the following sections.

Jean Piaget

Piaget's cognitive stages are concerned with children, rather than people of all ages. According to this psychologist, children progress through four cognitive stages of development. Each stage is marked by how children understand the world. Piaget believed that children are like "little scientists" and they actively try to explore and make sense of the world around them.

Through his observations, Piaget developed a theory of intellectual development that included four distinct stages, as listed in Table 8–4. Piaget considered cognitive development to be a progressive reorganization of mental processes as a result of biological maturation and environmental experiences. Children construct an understanding of the world around them, then experience discrepancies between what they already know and what they discover in their environment.

As with other older theories, there are some who question Piaget's relevancy today. However, many educators still use his ideas to shape curriculum for childhood learning.

Lawrence Kohlberg

Moral development in humans is the focus of Kohlberg's moral stages. He emphasized that human beings develop philosophically and psychologically in a progressive fashion. He identified six stages, preconventional, conventional, and postconventional, each of which is divided into two levels, as seen in Table 8–5. Kohlberg

Table 8–4 Piaget's Cognitive Stages

Cognitive Stage	Age	Comments
Sensorimotor	Birth to 2 years	Infants and toddlers acquire knowledge through sensory experiences and manipulating objects. See Figure 8–9.
Preoperational	2 to 7 years	Children learn through pretend play, but still struggle with logic and being able to take the point of view of other people. See Figure 8–10.
Concrete operational	7 to 12 years	Children begin to think more logically, but their thinking can also be very rigid. They tend to struggle with abstract and hypothetical concepts.
Formal operational	12 years to adulthood	Involves an increase in logic, the ability to use **deductive reasoning** (drawing a logical conclusion from one or more statements), and an understanding of abstract ideas.

Table 8–5 Kohlberg's Moral Stages

Stage/Level	Social Orientation
1. Preconventional	Obedience and Punishment • Generally found at elementary school level • One must behave according to socially acceptable norms as told by some authority figure (parent or teacher) • Obedience is compelled by threat or application of punishment
2. Preconventional	Individualism, Instrumentalism, and exchange • View that right behavior means acting in one's own best interests
3. Conventional	"Good Boy/Girl" • Characterized by an attitude that seeks to do what will gain approval of others
4. Conventional	Law and Order • One is oriented to abiding by the law and responding to obligations of duty
5. Postconventional	Social Contract • Understanding of social mutuality and genuine interest in welfare of others
6. Postconventional	Principled Conscience • Respect for universal principle and demands of individual conscience

FIGURE 8-9 Infants develop their sensorimotor skills by sucking on and manipulating objects.

© Lisa Eastman/Shutterstock.com.

FIGURE 8-10 Children begin to use representational thought through pretend play.

believed that a person could only progress one stage at a time, not "jump" stages, and that most moral development occurs through social interaction. Kohlberg's scale is about how people justify behaviors and his stages are not a

method of ranking how moral someone's behavior is. He also felt that stage 3 was not reached by the majority of adults.

Carol Gilligan

Gilligan worked with Lawrence Kohlberg on his theory of moral development (see previous section), but eventually began to criticize Kohlberg's work. She noted that Kohlberg only studied "privileged, white men and boys," resulting in a biased perspective that overlooked aspects of women's lives. Women's development in terms of their caring effect on human relationships was given less significance than some of the male characteristics of rights and rules. Gilligan observed that as women progress through stages of development, they must learn to address their own interests *and* the interests of others, and that women hesitate to judge because they see the complexities of relationships. Her work outlined features specific to female moral development. **Gilligan's stages of the ethics of care** is divided into three stages of moral development, as seen in Table 8-6.

FUTURE TRENDS

William H. Thomas is a Harvard-educated physician with a special interest in revolutionizing long-term care communities. His book *What Are Old People For? How Elders Will Save the World* (2007) discusses how, with the older population projected to double in the next few years, sweeping changes will be seen. Older people are healthier, more active, and more verbal than ever before in history, and this will change the way aging is experienced in the United States.

Thomas breaks the life span into five groupings, but does not assign specific ages to the groups. He views the aging process as a cycle that begins with a state of "being," transitions through "doing," and ends with "being":

- Infant—the purest example of *being*.

- Adolescent—a time of transition to adulthood. This is not an easy passage and is fraught with complexity

Table 8-6 Gilligan's Stages of the Ethics of Care

Stage	Goal	Orientation
1. Preconventional	Individual survival	Care only for themselves in order to ensure survival (normal in children)
2. Conventional	Self-sacrifice is goodness	More responsibility shown for other people (seen in the roles of mother and wife), but sometimes carries on to ignore needs of self
3. Postconventional	Principle of nonviolence: Do not hurt others or self	Acceptance of care for self and others; transition is from goodness to the truth that she is a person too. Some people never reach this stage

and turbulence. The individual transitions from the joyfulness of play to a clear preference for *doing* over *being*.

- Adult—the focus is on *doing*. The most frequent question asked between two adults is "What do you do?"

- Senescence—a time of transition to elderhood. As in adolescence, this is not an easy passage. Dr. Thomas states, "Sheltered for decades by energy and vitality, adults are utterly convinced of the rightness and goodness of their family and their chosen work. The first sign that you are preparing to grow out of adulthood is the dawning awareness of the heavy toll taken by things that you 'have to do'" (2007). This awareness starts gradually and grows as the individual's insight grows. The senescent person begins to realize that his or her life is not as unique or significantly important as once imagined. Rather, the person begins to understand that his or her family and job are much like those of millions of others who love their families and have contributed significantly in their work. These painful insights lead to the desire to put aside the *have to do* and explore the mysteries of *want to do*. Dr. Thomas states, "It is the beginning of ripening, just as adolescence is the beginning of maturation" (2007).

- Elderhood—this stage completes the cycle and returns the individual back to being. There is a clear preference to put aside the *have to do* for the *want to do*; this is a gift of great value.

Aging is gradual, ongoing, and unstoppable. There are no surprises as we see the process occurring all around us. It does not happen overnight, but it does happen to all of us. An awareness and respect for this process will make you a better and more compassionate health care professional.

DEATH AND DYING

Death is the natural end to life. It is, in a sense, the last stage of human development. Health care professionals may work with patients and their families during this last phase of the life process. To help understand dying, many turn to the classic work of Swiss physician Elisabeth Kübler-Ross. She earned her medical degree at the University of Switzerland in 1957 and her degree in psychiatry from the University of Colorado in 1963. After years of study and research, she published her first book, *On Death and Dying*, in 1969. She was the first person to study and write about death in a way that brought it to public attention. Kübler-Ross conducted extensive interviews with people who knew they were going to die in the foreseeable future

and made notes about the process they followed as they struggled to put their lives in perspective. These studies encouraged general discussion of what had previously been a taboo topic. Her research findings and subsequent books have provided the information that health care professionals and the general public need in order to become more informed about this area.

Based on her research, Kübler-Ross developed a model called the "stages of dying" or "stages of grief." According to the model, people who are dying go through five stages when they learn that they have a **terminal illness** (a condition or disease that, because of its nature, can be expected to cause the patient to die). The five **stages of dying** are summarized as follows:

- Denial: When first learning about a terminal illness, the individual may feel numb and in a state of disbelief. The belief is that this cannot be happening or that a mistake has been made. Common reactions are inability to focus, feeling a sense of it as unreal, hysteria or passivity, or the contemplation of suicide.

- Anger: After the reality of death hits, intense anger may be experienced. It is common for the individual to ask, "Why me?" It seems unfair, and there is envy of those with good health. Acute rage is experienced at the prospect of the upcoming loss. This rage may be directed only toward the illness, but it is also commonly directed toward everyone and everything.

- Bargaining: In this stage the person bargains for the one thing not possible—more time. Dying individuals want time to complete unachieved goals, see their children reach a certain level of maturity, have grandchildren, or travel to unseen parts of the world. The bargaining is often done with whomever they consider to be the higher being who has authority over life and death. They make promises to be better people, to change bad habits, and to live an exemplary life if only given more time.

- Depression: This is a profound sadness felt over the prospect of no longer being alive and not being able to change the course of events. There is a turning inward as they consider all the time that was wasted, the things left undone, and the joys that will not be experienced. Younger individuals feel particularly deprived of a long healthy life and feel they should have had the opportunity to live up to their potential.

- Acceptance: When this stage is reached, there is a dramatic change. Individuals experience a sense of peace with themselves, family, friends, and community. They now accept that they are dying and can focus on tying up any loose ends they perceive need to be resolved in preparation for death. This is referred to as "completing any unfinished business." For example, they may want to talk to certain friends or family to express their feelings or resolve issues or complete any necessary financial arrangements. Another important component of this stage is the need to do a life review. The **life review** involves telling the events of their lives to those close to them (including health care professionals). Part of the process is the desire to put one's life in perspective by performing a self-evaluation. This leads to a sense of closure. During this stage, dying individuals may be very open to talking about their feelings about death. As the time of death approaches, however, withdrawal often occurs. It is as if the external world is no longer important. It is also possible that they do not have the energy to try to communicate with others who do not have the same understanding of life as the dying have now achieved.

During the acceptance stage of dying, it was stated that patients often feel the need to do a life review. This same behavior is also commonly noted in the elderly when no specific terminal illness has been diagnosed. As a health care professional, it is important to take the time to hear (or hear again) these stories because they represent a significant step in the patient's developmental process. You may note that some patients tell their life stories with acceptance of past events, others with bitterness, guilt, or anger. Sometimes the events will be told in a glorified manner. At other times, the telling of stories may be more dispassionate. Another approach is to phrase past events in such a way as to pass on the individual's wisdom or cultural heritage. There is no one right way, and the health care professional can be of most help by showing interest and allowing patients to express themselves in the manner most comfortable to them.

Dying patients do not always go through all these stages, nor do they go through them in an orderly and sequential manner. One of the criticisms of Elisabeth Kübler-Ross's theory is that the stages are too rigid. Theorists who followed her have confirmed these stages, but note that not all people experience all of them, or go through the same sequence, or complete the stages. In addition, tremendous differences are caused by gender, class, and culture.

This model has been presented as it applies to the dying patient, but there is a wider application that will also assist the health care professional. It can be applied to any form of loss. When any loss is perceived, there is

Thinking It Through

Veronica Johnson, age 77, is a home health patient with a terminal illness. She lives in her home and is cared for by her husband. Josephine Mitchell, a hospice nurse, visits Mrs. Johnson on a regular basis to determine if the patient's needs are being met, to educate her husband on how to care for his wife, to offer emotional support, and to help resolve any difficulties that may arise. Mrs. Johnson states, "I am dying. I have known this for some time. I know it will not be much longer now, but I have had a full life and I am not afraid." But she also states, "I want to tell my daughter how much I love her, but I don't know how to do this as there seems to be a distance between us. I'm also afraid I will begin to cry and not be able to stop." Ms. Mitchell speaks with the daughter and determines that the daughter also wishes to talk with her mother to say goodbye, but is reluctant to do so because she is also afraid of starting to cry and not being able to stop.

Mrs. Johnson asks Ms. Mitchell to be present when her daughter arrives to visit her. When the daughter arrives, both mother and daughter repeat their concerns about starting to cry and not being able to stop. Ms. Mitchell then says with humor, "Don't worry about it, I'll start mopping up if it gets too deep." At that point, the daughter rushes to her mother's bedside, and a very loving conversation takes place.

1. What stage of the dying process is Mrs. Johnson in?

2. Mrs. Johnson is in which life stage? According to Erik Erikson's stages of psychosocial development, what is the conflict to be met at this life stage? Does it sound as if she has successfully met this challenge? Why or why not?

3. Should the hospice nurse have been present during the meeting between the mother and the daughter?

4. Was the humor used by the hospice nurse appropriate?

5. What outcome would you anticipate to occur as a result of the daughter and the mother openly sharing their feelings?

suffering and a grieving process is initiated. There are many types of loss:

- Failure to achieve an important goal
- Loss of a job, resulting in a change of social identity
- Divorce
- Death of a pet

- Accident
- Injury
- Upcoming surgery
- Moving away from friends and family
- Grieving about the impending or recent death of a loved one
- Financial setbacks, such as bankruptcy, foreclosure on home, or loss of savings

Helping patients—and others with whom they have contact—handle loss is a valuable skill for health care professionals. Providing caring concern in times of need promotes patient welfare, eases the dying process, and helps others come to terms with their losses. (Chapter 16 contains more information about communicating with terminally ill patients. See Chapter 2 for information about hospice and Chapter 3 for a discussion about the right to die.)

SUGGESTED LEARNING ACTIVITIES

1. Go to the website www.cdc.gov/growthcharts/ to find the growth charts published by the government for the purpose of monitoring normal physical growth. Then answer these questions: What is the normal range in inches and centimeters for the head circumference of a 12-month-old girl? What is the normal weight range in pounds and kilograms for a 15-year-old boy?

2. Observe family members and friends who fit into each of the life stages from infancy to later adulthood and review the information given for each stage. How do your observations with these individuals compare or contrast with the information in the charts? What can you identify in terms of physical, cognitive, or psychosocial behaviors?

3. Which life stage are you currently in? Can you relate your current activities and focus to the life stage?

4. Think of an older person you currently know or have known whom you admire. What did you learn from this person? What was his or her attitude toward life? Where does or did this person's strength of character come from? What are some other reasons you admire this individual?

5. Sit in a relaxed position with no external distractions, close your eyes, take some deep breaths, and clear your mind. Now imagine that you are 85 years old. After you can settle quietly into this process, mentally start to ask yourself questions: Where do you live? What is your health like? Who are your friends? What activities do you enjoy? What is important to you? Are you peaceful about the aging process or frightened by it? When you have completed the activity, open your eyes and discuss the experience with your classmates.

WEB ACTIVITIES

Theories of Human Development
https://www.slideshare.net/peningry/theories-of-human-development

This series of 50 slides contains outlined lectures about the theories of Freud, Erikson, Piaget, Jung, and Maslow. (Note: Maslow is discussed in Chapter 15 of this text.) Write a paper in which you compare and contrast the various theories.

Erik Erikson's Stages of Psychosocial Development
https://www.verywellmind.com/erik-eriksons-stages-of-psychosocial-development-2795740

Use this illustrated article to learn more about Erikson's theory.

Erikson's Psychosocial Theory of Human Development
https://www.businessballs.com/self-management/eriksons-psychosocial-theory-of-human-development-120/#toc-4

A more detailed, but interesting discussion about Erikson: his life, work, and theories.

Stages of Child Development

https://www.slideshare.net/liristhomas/stages-of-child-development

Seventeen illustrated slides that show stages organized a little differently than Erikson's. Compare and contrast with Erikson.

Tufts University Child and Family Web Guide

https://ase.tufts.edu/cfw

Click on "Social Emotional Development" and find a topic of interest to read, then write a report of your findings.

Teen Development

https://medlineplus.gov/teendevelopment.html

This web page contains many links covering various aspects of teen development. Examples include communication and promoting a positive body image. Choose topics to explore and report on.

   Medline Plus also contains sections on "Infant and Newborn Development" and "Toddler Development."

Child Development Theories and Examples: Some Key Ideas

https://www.verywellmind.com/child-development-theories-2795068

This website describes seven of the best-known theories of child development. Read the sections on the theorists not included in this chapter. Is there information you might apply as a health care professional?

What Happens to the Brain as We Age?

https://www.medicalnewstoday.com/articles/319185.php

This article describes how the brain changes over our lifetime. It includes strategies for helping retain healthy brain function. After reading the article, describe how the health care professional can apply this information when working with older patients.

Mayo Clinic

https://www.mayoclinic.org/healthy-lifestyle/healthy-aging/in-depth/aging/art-20046070

Aging: What to Expect Information from the Mayo Clinic about changes that occur with aging and suggestions for seniors to promote their health. Which preventive measures apply to people of any age? How many have you incorporated into your own life?

National Institute on Aging

https://www.nia.nih.gov/

This website contains dozens of topics of interest to the aging adult and those who work with them. Choose a topic to explore in depth and write a paragraph describing what you learn.

Elisabeth Kübler-Ross

www.ekrfoundation.org

Learn more about the woman who researched death and dying to bring to the world an awareness of this process.

American Cancer Society

https://www.cancer.org/treatment/end-of-life-care/grief-and-loss/grieving-process.html

The Grieving Process – Coping with the Loss of a Loved One

   Read this article to learn about the stages of grief experienced by friends and family members who lose a loved one.

REVIEW QUESTIONS

1. What do the terms *physical, cognitive,* and *psychosocial* mean, as they relate to growth and development?

2. What are the nine life stages and the ages represented by each as theorized by Erik Erikson?

3. What are the primary physical and cognitive changes that occur at each of the life stages?

4. What are the psychosocial stages according to Erikson's development theory?

5. What specific considerations can the health care professional use to provide appropriate care to individuals in the various life stages?

6. What are the main theoretical points of Piaget's cognitive stages, Kohlberg's moral stages, and Gilligan's stages of the ethic of care?

7. List the five stages of grief and give an example of behaviors that may be observed during each stage.

APPLICATION EXERCISES

1. Refer to The Case of the Curious Four-Year-Old. What life stage is Paul in, and what are the unique challenges of this stage? What are the possible psychosocial ramifications if his initiative is restricted and he is severely criticized and scolded for his attempts to explore and question his environment? What are the potential positive outcomes if the time is taken to answer his questions and engage him in his care?

2. Ed Klein has been diagnosed with terminal cancer. He has elected to stay at home with his wife, who is his principal caregiver. They also have regular visits from various hospice health care professionals who assist with pain management, bathing, and any problems that arise. The hospice nurse, Sandy Johnson, visits three times a week. She notes that Mr. Klein frequently mentions what he will do as soon as he gets better. Sandy also notices that Mrs. Klein is reluctant to enter the room when she is working with Mr. Klein. On her third visit, Sandy decides to ask Mrs. Klein to come in and assist her with Mr. Klein's care. During the procedure, he acts very angry with his wife and criticizes everything she does to help.

   a. What stage(s) of dying does Mr. Klein demonstrate?

   b. Why do you think the wife was reluctant to enter the room?

   c. Do you think Mr. Klein truly does not know he has a terminal illness?

   d. What type of care assistance do you think this couple needs?

PROBLEM-SOLVING PRACTICE

Your grandmother just arrived at your house to celebrate her 75th birthday. When she drives up, someone in the family comments, "We had better have her stop driving—she is too old to be safe on the road." This idea is upsetting because you know her independence would be greatly curtailed and you are not sure if it is even appropriate. You do some research and discover that crash rates begin to rise at age 70 and continue to rise as age increases. However, older drivers have the lowest crash rate per licensed driver, but the highest fatality rate per vehicle mile driven (older drivers have a high fatality rate because they are more physically fragile than their younger counterparts). Using the five-step problem-solving process, identify what you can do to determine if your grandmother should still be driving or not.

Unit 4 | Personal and Workplace Safety

CHAPTER 9

Body Mechanics

KEY TERMS

body mechanics
carpal tunnel syndrome
ergonomics
exertion injuries
repetitive motion injuries (RMIs)
tendonitis
thoracic outlet syndrome

OBJECTIVES

Studying and applying the material in this chapter will help you to:

1. Explain the importance of practicing good body mechanics and ergonomics at all times to prevent injury.
2. List the risk factors that increase the likelihood of injury.
3. List examples of general health measures that help prevent injuries.
4. Define the terms "body mechanics" and "ergonomics."
5. Explain the meaning of "repetitive motion injuries" and how they occur.
6. Describe the following conditions: carpal tunnel syndrome, thoracic outlet syndrome, and tendonitis.
7. List common symptoms of repetitive motion injuries.
8. Explain how using a computer can result in a repetitive motion injury.
9. List ways to prevent repetitive motion injuries.
10. Describe proper methods of working at the computer to prevent injury.
11. Explain how computer use can cause visual problems.
12. Describe proper methods of sitting when working to prevent injury.
13. Describe proper methods of walking and standing at work to prevent injury.
14. State the causes of exertion injuries.
15. Explain why exertion injuries are increasing in number among health care professionals.
16. Describe the specialized equipment that helps prevent exertion injuries.
17. List actions the health care professionals can take to help prevent exertion injuries.
18. List and describe methods for treating musculoskeletal and nerve injuries.
19. State the arguments for and against the use of back belts.

The Case of Broken Dreams

Rene Alvarez has dreamed of a career in health care for many years. She is thrilled about graduating next month and anticipates that the large medical center where she has been hired will be the fulfillment of her dreams. She has decided to move into a new apartment that is closer to her new employer and only has the weekend to get everything moved, in addition to studying for an important exam. Rene packs quickly and with the help of family and friends

(continues)

starts to load the truck rented for the move. In her haste, Rene forgets to follow proper body mechanics and lifts a box that is very heavy. She feels a tearing sensation in her back, followed by severe pain. She is rushed to the emergency department and is told that she will need to stay in bed for several weeks and surgery may be required if the bed rest provides her no relief.

This chapter will cover the basic principles of good body mechanics and ergonomics that should be followed at all times to prevent personal injury. Health care professionals are particularly at risk for injury because their daily job duties often include lifting equipment, supplies, and patients. Other health care professionals may not lift as much in their jobs but may have long periods of sitting, standing, or working with computers and other tabletop equipment.

THE IMPORTANCE OF PREVENTION

Health care professionals perform a number of mechanical movements with their bodies that can lead to injuries that most frequently involve the musculoskeletal and/or nervous system. In fact, non-fatal injuries and illnesses of health care workers rank among the highest of any industry section (NIOSH, 2017 Healthcare Workers). Activities done every day at work, such as the following examples, can result in injuries:

- Nurses lifting patients
- Insurance coders sitting and working at the computer for long periods
- Surgical technicians standing during long operations
- Medical transcriptionists keyboarding for many hours each day
- Laboratory technicians bending over microscopes for prolonged periods

Following safety guidelines reduces the chance of injury and unnecessary pain and suffering. Many injuries are the result of poor practices over time that involve the repetition of improper movements. In other words, it is not the one-time incident that leads to the greatest number of injuries, but rather the same mistakes repeated over time. As one ages, it is especially important to follow sound practices. As flexibility decreases and recovery time increases, the chance of sustaining injuries is greater.

Certain risk factors increase the likelihood of injury. These include:

- Poor posture
- Poor body mechanics
- Low level of fitness
- Obesity
- Stress, both mechanical and psychological

The best preventive practices are the same as those recommended for good general health:

- Use good posture and proper body mechanics during all activities.
- Stay fit by exercising regularly.
- Use stretching exercises to maintain flexibility.
- Maintain a healthy body weight and good general health by eating correctly.
- Reduce mental stress through good lifestyle habits (see Chapter 12).

Health care professionals should build good habits and safe practices into everyday life. Although the focus of this chapter is on workplace injuries and their prevention, the same principles apply to activities at home, at play, and even at rest.

Body mechanics and ergonomics are two terms used when discussing the prevention of injury. **Body mechanics** refers to the correct positioning of the body for a given task, such as lifting a heavy object or keyboarding. **Ergonomics** is the science of designing and arranging things in the working and living environments for maximum efficiency and maximum health and safety. An ergonomic environment provides the highest possible comfort level and efficiency while limiting possible exposure to discomfort or potential injury. Developing the habit of following proper body mechanics and working in an ergonomically correct workplace are vital to decreasing your chance of injury.

REPETITIVE MOTION INJURIES

Repetitive motion injuries (RMIs) encompass many different injuries, but they are all based on the overuse of one part of the body. Motions that are repeated over time eventually put undue stress on muscles, tendons, nerves, blood vessels, and/or joints and can cause inflammation, swelling, and pain. It is estimated that 50% of all industrial injuries in the United States are attributable to RMIs. Most of these injuries involve the hands, arms, neck, and shoulder area. Common RMIs suffered today include the following:

- **Carpal tunnel syndrome**: compression of the median nerve as it travels through the wrist at the carpel tunnel, the passageway that connects the forearm to the hand

- **Thoracic outlet syndrome**: compression of the nerves, arteries, or veins in the passageway from the lower neck to the armpit

- **Tendonitis**: inflammation of a tendon, the fibrous tissue that attaches a muscle to a bone

RMIs are commonly thought of as work related, but they can occur as a result of academic, leisure-time, or household activities as well. (See Table 9–1.)

The symptoms of RMIs include the following:

- Pain. The pain is typically felt as an aching sensation that gets worse as the affected joint or limb is moved or used.

- Paresthesias. Paresthesia refers to an abnormal sensation or pricking, tingling, or burning in the absence of an external stimulus.

- Numbness, coldness, or loss of sensation

- Clumsiness, weakness, or lack of coordination

- Impaired range of motion or locking of the joint

- Popping, clicking, or crackling sound in the joint

- Swelling or redness in the affected area

Computer Use and Repetitive Motion Injuries

In the past, keying of data was done by a small number of employees and the resulting RMIs were limited to relatively few workers. Today, the prevalence of computers in offices, libraries, schools, and homes for working, communicating with others, making purchases, and conducting research has resulted in a corresponding increase in RMIs. These injuries are the direct result of the repetitive motion of keyboarding or using a mouse as a pointing device. In fact, the extensive use of the mouse as a pointing device when working with a computer has been shown to be a major contributor to RMIs.

Preventing Repetitive Motion Injuries

The following general principles help prevent RMIs:

- Warm up and stretch before and after activities that are repetitive, static (lacking movement), and/or prolonged.

- Avoid static positions for prolonged periods. Muscles fatigue faster when they are held in one position. Take a break and move around every 20 to 30 minutes when it is necessary to maintain a sustained position.

- Change positions or stop whenever activities cause pain.

- Use splints and wrist supports only when recommended by a physician or a therapist. Be sure to follow instructions on the proper use of equipment.

- Sit up straight at your desk or computer station, rather than hunching forward, to maintain the three normal curves of the spine. (See Figure 9–1.)

- Set up computer work stations that fit your physical needs. Figure 9–2 illustrates proper positioning.

- If possible, use an adjustable computer desk or station so you can alternate sitting and standing. (See Figure 9–3.)

- If using a mouse, position it within easy reach so you do not have to stretch to reach it.

- Develop the ability to use the mouse with either hand.

Table 9–1 Most Common RMIs

Condition	Etiology (Cause)	Signs and Symptoms
Carpal tunnel syndrome	Repeated hand motions cause inflammation and swelling that pinch nerves that pass through a tunnel of bones and ligaments in the wrist	• Tingling, numbness, and pain in the hand • Inability to make a fist • Loss of strength in hand
Thoracic outlet syndrome	Repeated motion causes bones or disks to compress nerves in the neck	• Tingling, numbness, and pain in the neck, shoulder, arms, or hands • Poor blood circulation in the hands and fingers • Weakness in arms and hands
Tendonitis	Repeated motion in a joint inflames tendons	• Swelling, tenderness, or weakness in the tendons of the shoulders, elbows, or hands

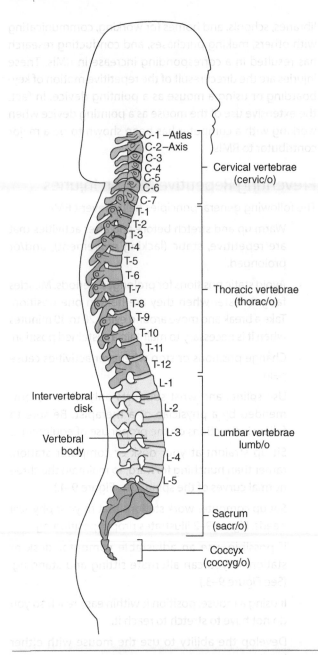

C-1 –Atlas
C-2 –Axis
C-3
C-4
C-5
C-6
C-7

Cervical vertebrae
(cervic/o)

T-1
T-2
T-3
T-4
T-5
T-6
T-7
T-8
T-9
T-10
T-11
T-12

Thoracic vertebrae
(thorac/o)

Intervertebral
disk

L-1
L-2
L-3
L-4
L-5

Lumbar vertebrae
lumb/o

Vertebral
body

Sacrum
(sacr/o)

Coccyx
(coccyg/o)

FIGURE 9–1 Normal curves of the spinal column.

Top of monitor just
below eye level

Back
supported
by chair

Elbow at
90–100°
angle

Wrists
in neutral
position

Feet flat on the floor
or on foot rest

FIGURE 9–2 Proper positioning for seated use of the computer.

FIGURE 9–3 Proper upright standing posture includes a soft bend in the knees or alternating foot on the footplate of the cart, as demonstrated here.

- Learn to use keyboard commands specific to your computer and software to avoid relying on the mouse. Common examples:
  ○ Control/command + s saves a document
  ○ Control/command + p prints a document
  ○ Control/command + w closes a file
- Learn strategies to cope with psychological stress. Tension can be carried in the back, neck, or shoulder muscles, thus reducing blood circulation to the affected tissues.

See Boxes 9–1 and 9–2 for more information about properly sitting, standing, and walking. Box 9–3 contains specific information about properly using the computer. Table 9–2 contains exercises to help prevent computer-use RMIs.

Visual Problems

Visual discomfort is commonly reported as a result of computer work. Eyestrain and headaches are the most common problems. The eyes tire more quickly when looking at a computer screen than when reading printed materials. This is because of the different characteristics of the type. Printed material has dark, dense, consistent lines that are easy to focus on. Computer screens display images with a less consistent density; this results in the eyes having to work much harder to focus. This extra effort can result in eyestrain. See Box 9–4 for guidelines to prevent eyestrain.

People who wear bifocals have an additional challenge to overcome when working on the computer. The lower section of bifocals is used for reading and is adjusted to focus at a closer distance than the typical distance one sits

Box 9-1

While Sitting:

1. Use a chair that supports the normal curves of the back (use a lumbar—lower back—support if needed). Avoid sitting on stools. Don't slouch in chairs or on couches because this causes the natural inward curve of the spine to curve outward.

2. Keep head and shoulders aligned over hips. Avoid bending neck forward for long periods.

3. Avoid pressing the back of the knees against the edge of the chair seat.

4. Minimize twisting and bending motions. Position equipment and work so that the body is directly in front of and close to them.

5. When turning is necessary, pivot entire body in unison or use a swivel chair.

6. Change positions frequently. Get up and move around and stretch at regular intervals.

7. Position your chair so work is at eye level and feet are flat on floor or on a footrest.

8. When using the telephone (even a cell phone) frequently or for extended periods, use a speakerphone or headset.

9. When not using your hands, keep your upper arms close to your body, elbows at a 90- to 100-degree angle, forearms neutral (thumbs toward ceiling), and wrists straight.

Box 9-2

While Standing and Walking:

1. Be aware of your posture. Maintain the three normal curves of the back. (See Figure 9–1.)

2. Keep your neck in a neutral position (avoid jutting the chin forward or slouching).

3. Wear cushioned shoes with good support if work requires a lot of standing or walking.

4. When standing, shift your weight often.

5. If standing in one place for long periods, use a footstool. Alternate placing one foot up on the stool to take the strain off the back.

Box 9-3

While Using the Computer:

1. Position the screen at arm's length to reduce eyestrain and head-forward posture.

2. Position the top of the monitor just below eye level directly in front of the body.

3. Place a document holder next to the screen rather than working from a document placed flat on the desk.

4. Place both feet flat on the floor or on a footrest to reduce back strain.

5. Keep your back in total contact with the back of the chair.

6. Position your abdomen close to the edge of the desk to prevent a forward-leaning posture.

7. Maintain your wrists in a neutral (straight) position when keying or using a pointing device.

8. Position the keyboard so your elbow is at the same height as the keyboard. Slant the keyboard as necessary to maintain your elbows at an angle of 90 to 100 degrees and a neutral wrist position.

9. Rest your eyes and reduce eyestrain by blinking your eyes rapidly, closing them, or focusing on another object away from the computer screen for 10 seconds every 15 minutes.

10. Stretch frequently (shrug shoulders, arch back, nod head, roll feet in circular motion). See Table 9–2 for computer exercises.

11. Use wrist rests during pauses to help maintain neutral position. They are not meant to be used during active keying.

12. Avoid resting wrists against hard surfaces and sharp edges.

13. Try using an ergonomically designed keyboard.

from the computer. Bifocals are also angled downward for reading, so bifocal wearers will typically tilt their heads upward so they can view the screen at this angle. This moves the neck out of the neutral position and can lead to neck problems. One solution is to position the monitor lower than eye level. For the person who does a great deal of computer work, it is preferable to have the ophthalmologist or optometrist prescribe a set of bifocal lenses specifically designed for use at the computer.

Table 9–2 Computer Exercises

Exercise	Description	Benefit
	Make a fist, and then open your hands while spreading fingers apart.	Relaxes muscles of hands, wrists, and forearms
	Interlace the fingers of both hands, then extend your arms at shoulder level, palms facing away from you.	Stretches the muscles of the arms, shoulders, and upper back
	Slowly rotate your head by tilting it to one side, then roll it to a forward position, then to the other side. Repeat.	Stretches the neck muscles and helps relieve tension
	Shrug shoulders up toward the ears, then relax and let them return to their normal position.	Decreases tension in neck and shoulder muscles
	Place your left arm on your right shoulder and turn your head to the left. With your right arm, gently push your left arm for increased stretch. Repeat.	Stretches muscles of upper arm and upper back

Box 9–4

To Prevent Eyestrain:

- Look away from the computer screen and focus on other objects in the environment at frequent intervals.
- Rest the eyes every 20 to 30 minutes.
- Adjust the contrast on the computer screen to a comfortable level.
- Keep the computer screen clean.
- Position the screen to avoid glare from surrounding lights and windows.
- Use a paper holder to prevent having to look down to see text.
- Use a glare screen on the monitor.

EXERTION INJURIES

Injuries caused by lifting, pulling, and pushing occur frequently among health care professionals who work directly with patients or those who move heavy supplies and equipment. These injuries are called exertion injuries and are increasing in number due to the obesity epidemic, shorter hospital stays for patients, and the growing number of elderly patients who need assistance with daily activities. The second two factors have led to an increase in home care services and, as a consequence, more injuries. This is because home environments are not designed for health care: they tend to be more crowded and many beds are not height adjustable. In many homes, there is insufficient room for the nurse, therapist, or aide to maintain a proper posture when lifting or turning a patient. Finally, home health care professionals often work alone without a second trained person to help.

Back injuries alone account for nearly 20% of all injuries and illnesses each year. The most common injuries are sprains and strains. Some exertion injuries can be classified as RMIs; that is, from repeated lifting over time. But they may also occur from a one-time forceful movement. For example, bending forward at the waist and reaching forward to lift or move a patient or heavy object has the spine in its most vulnerable position and can result in an immediate injury. (See Figure 9–4.)

To complicate the problem of exertion injuries, it is reported that certain lifting techniques used to minimize load on the back may increase load on the neck, shoulders, arms, and other joints (Occupational Hazards in Home Healthcare, 2010). (See Box 9–5.)

FIGURE 9–4 When lifting, use the legs rather than bending forward at the waist.

Box 9–5

While Lifting:

1. Move in close to the patient or object to be lifted.

2. Be aware of your posture. Maintain the three normal curves of the back. (See Figure 9–1.)

3. Increase your base of support by positioning your feet 6 to 8 inches apart. Base of support refers to the distance between feet that are both in contact with the ground. A wider base of support improves balance. (See Figure 9–6.)

4. Squat down (bending hips and knees), maintaining normal curves of the back. (See Figure 9–7.) When picking up objects, bend at the knees rather than at the waist.

5. Position your hands underneath the object to be lifted.

6. Take a deep breath and tighten your abdominal muscles prior to lifting. This increases intra-abdominal pressure to increase the support for the spine and back muscles.

7. Lift the load with the legs (not with the back). Use the large muscles of the legs to lift load.

8. Always ask for assistance from other health care professionals when needed.

9. Use two hands to lift rather than one, even with light objects. (See Figure 9–4.)

10. Carry objects close to your body at waist level. (See Figure 9–4.)

11. When turning, move your entire body in unison (avoid twisting). To change directions, use the feet rather than the back: Move and turn the feet instead of twisting the spine while the feet are planted in one position.

12. Avoid reaching overhead with heavy loads (use step stools, ladders, etc.).

13. Push rather than pull heavy objects. The exception to this rule is when on ramps, where you would pull from the higher level.

14. Slide or push objects, when possible, instead of lifting them.

15. Use carts and dollies to carry heavy loads. If possible, break up the load into several trips to avoid lifting heavy loads. Or have someone assist with the lifting of heavy objects.

16. Tilt containers or objects to avoid bending the wrist to pick up objects.

Note: Lifting and moving patients can be a particular challenge for health care professionals who work directly with patients. Many of the principles presented apply to these activities, but additional skills are also required that are beyond the scope of this book. The use of specialized lifting equipment may be available in these settings. Some hospitals have also developed lift teams that can be contacted for assistance in particularly problematic moves involving patients.

Preventing Exertion Injuries

The best way to prevent exertion injuries is to work with a lift team or use specialized equipment. Lift teams consist of at least two physically fit professionals who are trained in proper patient lifting techniques. Some states, including California, require hospitals to have lift teams on staff.

Specialized equipment to prevent injuries include the following:

- Draw sheets: small sheets, made in a variety of materials, placed between the patient and the bottom bed sheet

- Slide boards: very smooth, narrow boards made of strong materials, such as wood or plastic, that provide a "bridge" between transfer points, such as bed and wheelchair

- Rollers: similar to a slide board, this contains rows of hardwood balls to facilitate movement from one transfer point to another

- Transfer belt: specialized, wide belt that is secured around the patient's waist. Contain hand grips for the health care professional

- Hoists: devices in which patient is lifted mechanically in a body sling. Lifting may be done manually or electrically. (See Figure 9–5.)

Regardless of whether any of these devices are available or not, there are a number of actions health care professionals can take to reduce the chance of injury:

- Warm up before and after activities that require lifting, pushing, or pulling.

- Use the largest joints and muscles to do the work (e.g., squat down to lift a box because this uses your leg muscles and not your back).

- When moving a patient, stand close with knees bent, feet apart, and one foot in the direction of the move. (See Figure 9–6.)

FIGURE 9–6 When lifting, maintain proper posture, position feet for a wide base of support, and lift with the leg muscles.

- Avoid bending forward at the waist as you lift an object or to perform a task lower than waist level. (See Figure 9–7.)

- Stretch muscles if they become stiff. Alternately contract and relax muscles to increase blood circulation. (See Box 12–2 in Chapter 12 for muscle relaxation exercises.)

- Change positions as appropriate or stop whenever activities cause pain.

FIGURE 9–5 Using a hoist to lift patients helps prevent back and other exertion injuries.

© Tyler Olson/Shutterstock.com

FIGURE 9–7 Use proper posture when bending at the hips and knees.

- Seek treatment early if problems arise. Do not delay and simply hope the problem will go away.
- As with RMIs, reduce psychological and emotional stress to help prevent injuries.

See Box 9–5 for safe lifting techniques.

TREATMENT OF MUSCULOSKELETAL AND NERVE INJURIES

The treatment of musculoskeletal and nerve injuries varies with the severity of the injury. It may be possible to manage the injury with conservative measures, but surgical intervention is sometimes required. Physical and occupational therapists are an important part of the treatment team, advising about proper use of the injured body part and developing a home exercise program. Psychotherapy may also be appropriate if the injury is related to job dissatisfaction or when an occupation or favorite activity must be given up due to the injury.

After the diagnosis is made, a treatment plan will be developed for the individual. The following are some common conservative treatment measures:

- Resting the affected part; complete rest should last no longer than two to three days as range of motion (the normal full movement of a joint) can be lost
- Applying ice packs or gentle heat

Thinking It Through

Dan McGregor has built model constructions since childhood. His other passion is computer games. Dan admits he spends too much time sedentary as both of these activities require little or no movement. He is very excited about his career path, which is to become a surgical technologist. He realizes this will require him to stand, bend, stoop, or sit for long periods in one location with minimal or no breaks. He will also be expected to manipulate instruments, supplies, and equipment with speed, dexterity, and good eye–hand coordination. Dan feels he is a perfect match for these job skills as they are similar to the activities he prefers and utilizes in his main hobbies.

1. Why might Dan have potential problems with RMIs?
2. Should Dan choose a different career option?
3. What might he do to avoid developing RMIs?

Fascinating Facts

Emotional stress has been shown to influence people's perception of physical pain. Workers who are unhappy in their jobs are more likely to seek treatment for work-related disorders.

- Oral medications (mild pain relievers, anti-inflammatories)
- Corticosteroid injections into joints to reduce inflammation
- Splinting, most commonly used for hand and wrist injuries and can be custom molded by an occupational therapist
- Ergonomic corrections in the home or workplace
- Transcutaneous electrical nerve stimulation (TENS); TENS involves the use of a patient-controlled portable device that sends mild electrical impulses through injured tissues via electrodes placed over the skin. It is reported to relieve pain in 75% to 80% of patients treated for RMIs.
- Acupuncture to reduce pain
- Sports massage, Swedish massage, and shiatsu to encourage improved blood circulation and relaxation of muscles
- Yoga and tai chi, which involve gentle stretching that helps to improve blood circulation and maintain range of motion without tissue damage
- The Alexander technique to emphasize correct posture, particularly the proper position of the head with respect to the spine
- Hydrotherapy (warm whirlpool baths) to improve circulation and relieve pain in injured joints and soft tissue

Musculoskeletal and nerve injuries are treated with surgery only when conservative measures fail to relieve the patient's pain after a trial of 6 to 12 weeks. The most common surgical procedures include the following:

- Nerve decompression: a small portion of bone, under or above the affected nerve, is removed to relieve pressure on the nerve
- Tendon release: tight structures, known as pulleys, are removed when they entrap tendons
- Repair of loose or torn ligaments, the tough connective tissues that connect bones to each other

Fascinating Facts

The Bureau of Labor Statistics reports that 75.2% of all occupational injuries and illnesses occur in service-providing industries.

Rehabilitation programs are tailored to the individual patient and the specific disorder involved.

Recovery from an injury may take only a few days of rest or modified activity, or it may take several months when surgery is required. The prognosis for recovery depends on the specific disorder, the degree of damage, and the patient's compliance with the recommended exercises and activity. Most patients experience adequate pain relief from either conservative measures or surgery. Some, however, will not recover full use of the affected part and must change occupations or give up the activity that produced the original injury. Therefore, taking steps to prevent injury is extremely important for the health care professional.

BACK BELTS

The use of back belts (also known as back supports or abdominal supports) has become a subject of controversy among health care professionals. Back belt advocates state that they are helpful and that back belts increase intra-abdominal pressure, which creates support for the spine and back muscles when performing tasks, such as lifting, that require exertion. They also believe that the belts increase the flexibility of the stomach and back muscles by keeping them warm. Finally, they argue that their presence serves as a reminder to workers to follow proper body mechanics.

Opponents to using back belts argue that the belts increase the worker's blood and pelvic pressures, which can lead to cardiac problems. They also believe that the warmth and sweating created by wearing back belts can cause heat rashes; that belts that don't fit properly can cause abdominal pain and injuries; and that they can give a false sense of

Thinking It Through

Emily Carlson is a nurse who works at Thorsen Rehabilitation Center. One of her patients, John Tucker, is a very obese individual who is recovering from surgery. The physician overseeing Mr. Tucker's care has ordered that the patient be turned every two hours to prevent pressure sores. Mr. Tucker, however, finds being confined to bed uncomfortable and has become irritable, demanding that he be turned every 15 or 30 minutes. One afternoon, when Emily comes to check his vitals, Mr. Tucker demands that he "be turned now!" No other staff or equipment is available to help Emily carry out his request at this time.

1. Should Emily try to turn Mr. Tucker by herself? Why or why not?
2. What might be the reasons for Mr. Tucker's demands?
3. What else, if anything, can Emily do to help Mr. Tucker?

security so that workers may attempt to lift heavier loads than their strength can safely handle. If back belts are used, opponents suggest that they should be tightened only when lifting and left loose the rest of the time.

According to the National Institute for Occupational Safety and Health (NIOSH), there is insufficient scientific evidence to determine the benefits of back belts. Go to www.cdc.gov/niosh/docs/94-127/default.html to view a pamphlet detailing their findings. NIOSH is encouraging more scientific studies to investigate the effectiveness of back belts in the workplace. (Note: back belts may be prescribed for people who have back injuries as part their rehabilitation.)

The current theory is that the most effective way to prevent back injury is to redesign the work environment and work tasks to reduce the hazards of lifting. Training in identifying lifting hazards and using safe lifting techniques and methods should improve program effectiveness.

SUGGESTED LEARNING ACTIVITIES

1. If you have a computer area or office in your home, evaluate your work station. Are there any changes that would improve the ergonomics?
2. Analyze your work, academic, leisure-time, and household activities for actions that may cause overlap of repetitive movements. Did you identify any areas of concern? What can you do now to prevent future problems?

3. Observe health care professionals at work. What measures do they take to avoid workplace injuries?

4. Evaluate your compliance with the guidelines in this chapter. Do you have any "at risk" behaviors? What modifications can you make to decrease the risk of injury?

WEB ACTIVITIES

Ergo Vancouver

http://www.ergovancouver.net/Problems-Fingers.htm

"Finger Problems"

Read the articles on problems caused by computer use. Write a short paper in which you describe potential problems and their causes and then list methods to prevent them.

Computer/Electronic Accommodation Program

http://cap.mil/Documents/CAP_Ergo_Guide.pdf

Workplace Ergonomics Reference Guide 2nd Edition

Read this informative document that describes ergonomic measures for offices and computer workstations. Use the Ergonomic Checklist on page 3 to evaluate your workstation at school, home, and/or work. Then take the quiz on page 16: Ergonomic Economics: Do You Know the Numbers?

U.S. Department of Labor—Occupational Safety and Health Administration (OSHA)

https://www.osha.gov/dsg/hospitals/documents/3.1_Mythbusters_508.pdf

Safe Patient Handling: Busting the Myths

After reading this document, write a paper arguing the benefits of using specialized equipment for lifting and transferring patients.

U.S. Department of Labor—Occupational Safety and Health Administration (OSHA)

https://www.osha.gov/SLTC/healthcarefacilities/safepatienthandling.html

Review this website for links to OSHA websites about safe patient handling for various health care occupations.

U.S. Department of Labor—Occupational Safety and Health Administration (OSHA)

https://www.osha.gov/SLTC/healthcarefacilities/training/index.html

Back Facts – A training workbook to prevent back injuries in nursing homes

Complete the activities. Although the workbook is directed to nursing home workers, the concepts apply to all health care workers who transfer patients.

REVIEW QUESTIONS

1. Why is it important to practice good body mechanics and ergonomics?

2. What are the risk factors that increase the likelihood of injury?

3. What are examples of general health practices that help prevent injuries?

4. What do the following terms mean?

    a. Body mechanics

    b. Ergonomics

5. What are repetitive motion injuries and how are they caused?

6. What are the following RMI conditions?

   a. Carpal tunnel syndrome

   b. Thoracic outlet syndrome

   c. Tendonitis

7. What are the common symptoms of RMIs?

8. How can using a computer result in RMIs?

9. What are practices the health care professional can use to prevent RMIs?

10. What are postures and practices that can help prevent injuries when working at the computer?

11. How can using a computer result in visual problems?

12. How can health care professionals protect themselves from RMIs when sitting?

13. How can health care professionals protect themselves from RMIs when walking and standing?

14. What are the causes of exertion injuries?

15. Why are the number of exertion injuries increasing among health care professionals?

16. What are examples of adaptive devices that can help prevent exertion injuries?

17. What actions can health care professionals take to prevent exertion injuries?

18. What are the treatment options for musculoskeletal and nerve injuries?

19. What are the arguments for and against the use of back belts by health care professionals?

APPLICATION EXERCISES

1. What could Rene, in The Case of Broken Dreams at the beginning of this chapter, have done to decrease her likelihood of sustaining injuries?

2. John Jones, a health care student, has been saving for months to purchase a laptop computer to assist him with his classes. He plans to purchase a computer table and chair as soon as he saves the additional money. In the meantime, he will be using the computer on his lap or at the kitchen table.

   a. What possible injuries is John risking by not having an ergonomically sound setup?

   b. What criteria should he consider when purchasing a computer table and a chair?

   c. What can he do in the meantime to adapt the kitchen to a safe working environment? Include RMI and eyestrain prevention. Describe in detail or prepare a sketch of your suggestions.

PROBLEM-SOLVING PRACTICE

Robert Sherman spends many hours at the computer. He loves to surf the web and play games and now he is also doing a great deal of word processing for his classroom projects. He has heard a lot of talk about carpal tunnel syndrome and wonders if he can prevent this from happening to him. Using the five-step problem-solving process, determine what Robert can do about prevention.

CHAPTER 10

Infection Control

KEY TERMS

aerobic
AIDS
anaerobic
antibiotic
antibodies
antiseptics
asepsis (aseptic technique)
bacteria
bacteriocidal
bacteriostatic
Centers for Disease Control and Prevention (CDC)
chain of infection
communicable disease
contaminated
disinfectants
epidemics
fungi (pl. of fungus)
germ theory
hepatitis B
HIV
HIV positive
hosts
immune response
infection control
infectious disease
medical asepsis (clean technique)
microbes
microorganisms
microscope
neutropenic precautions
normal flora
nosocomial infection
Occupational Safety and Health Administration (OSHA)
opportunistic infection
pandemics

(continues)

OBJECTIVES

Studying and applying the material in this chapter will help you to:

1. Explain the importance of infection control practices in the health care facility to maintain the safety of the health care professional, patients, and others.
2. Explain why infections are a significant problem in health care facilities.
3. Describe the CDC and OSHA and explain their roles in health care safety.
4. Name and describe the five types of microbes and give examples of infectious diseases caused by each type.
5. Give three examples of the body's defense mechanisms.
6. Describe the chain of infection as a model for explaining how infection spreads.
7. Define asepsis and describe the two types.
8. Explain the differences among antiseptics, disinfectants, and sterilization, including the purpose of each.
9. Define sterile field.
10. Explain how to maintain a sterile field.
11. List methods the health care professional can use to break the chain of infection.
12. List the preventive procedures included in the standard precautions.
13. Identify situations for which handwashing is indicated and describe the technique.
14. List the contents of personal protective equipment and state its purpose.
15. Define the meaning of blood-borne pathogens.
16. Explain how the health care professional can avoid sharps injuries.
17. List the three ways that pathogens can be transmitted.
18. Name the three types of transmission-based precautions and when they should be used.
19. Describe the proper method for removing contaminated materials from a patient's room.
20. Describe neutropenic precautions and when they should be used.
21. Describe the effect of influenza on human health and explain what can be done to prevent it.
22. Identify and describe the three major disease risks for health care professionals.
23. Provide the source travelers can access for information about infectious diseases in countries outside the United States.
24. Describe how pathogens become drug resistant and the impact this has on health care.
25. State the purpose of and the policies and procedures that should be included in a facility's exposure control plan.

KEY TERMS *(continued)*

parasite
pathogens
protozoa
rickettsia
spore

standard precautions
sterile fields
sterilization
surgical asepsis
(sterile technique)

transmission-based
precautions
tuberculosis (TB)
virus

The Case of the Traveling Microorganisms

Ralph Romero, a health care professional at a large metropolitan hospital, awakens in the middle of the night with coughing, sneezing, runny nose, and a temperature of 101°F. He is scheduled to work the next day and so takes medications to treat his symptoms and goes back to bed. He awakens still feeling ill and wishes he could stay home, but knows the hospital is always very busy on the weekends and decides to go despite being ill. He works his shift, being careful when he coughs or sneezes to turn his head away from the patient and use some handkerchiefs he brought from home when coughing, sneezing, or blowing his nose. He also makes sure that he washes his hands when entering each patient's room. In this chapter, health care professionals will learn their role in preventing the transmission of microorganisms while performing their duties.

IMPORTANCE OF INFECTION CONTROL IN HEALTH CARE

It is essential that health care professionals have a clear understanding of infections and infection control, the main goal of which is to prevent the spread of infectious diseases. An infectious disease is any disease caused by the growth of pathogens, disease-causing microorganisms (germs), in the body. Until the source of infections was discovered, these diseases were a major cause of death. Because they are easily transmitted among individuals, they sometimes result in epidemics, widespread occurrences of infectious diseases. Even more serious are pandemics in which diseases spread over a vast area, Just over 100 years ago, the 1918 influenza virus infected about one third of the world's population and killed an estimated 50 million people worldwide (https://www.cdc.gov/features/1918-flu-pandemic/index.html). Viruses had not yet been discovered and, therefore, no treatment options existed.

Health care professionals must maintain a safe environment in the health care facility by following specific policies and procedures designed to reduce the risk of transferring infectious diseases. Failure to prevent the spread of an infectious disease can cause unnecessary pain, suffering, and even death. Regulatory standards have been developed to prevent pathogens from being passed from patient to patient, staff to patient, patient to

staff, or staff to staff. Improperly cleaned instruments and equipment are common means of transmitting pathogens. Strict adherence to proper procedures also prevents health care professionals and visitors to facilities from spreading pathogens to the community.

In addition to infectious diseases, such as influenza ("the flu"), an infection may occur in one area of the body, such as an infected wound. It is critical to identify any signs or symptoms of an infection as quickly as possible so an evaluation can be performed and treatment prescribed as indicated. Infections are classified in two ways:

- Generalized (systemic) infections: Affect the whole body with signs and symptoms commonly including headaches, fever, fatigue, vomiting, diarrhea, and an increase in pulse and respiration.
- Localized infections: Affect one area of the body which will be red, swollen, warm to the touch, and painful. There may also be drainage.

Scope of the Problem

It is important to realize that a health care facility by the very nature of its business has a higher concentration of germs than is found in other environments. Combine this with patients who have lowered levels of resistance due to illness and health care personnel who have frequent contact with body fluids, and there exists a potentially deadly situation.

The result is that infections are sometimes acquired through association with health care facilities. The term nosocomial infection (also referred to as health care–associated infection, or HAI) refers to an infection that occurs while a patient is receiving health care. Over the past 25 years, the rate of nosocomial infections per 1,000 patient days has increased by 36%. It is estimated that in U.S. hospitals alone, health care–associated (nosocomial) infections account for an estimated 1.7 million infections and 99,000 associated patient deaths each year (www.cdc.gov/washington/~cdcatWork/pdf/infections.pdf).

The fundamental ethic of health care is that a sick person must receive care. This premise carries an unstated consequence: an occupational risk to health care workers who respond to the needs of contagious patients. When an employee contracts an infectious disease while at work, it is called an industrial illness. There are a number of diseases that the health care professional can be exposed to while caring for infected patients. Examples include the human immunodeficiency virus (HIV), hepatitis B virus (HBV), and hepatitis C virus (HCV). All of them are preventable if the health care professional follows standard precautions (discussed later in the chapter) and other safety practices defined by the health care facility.

Sharps injuries are an important and continuing cause of exposure to serious and fatal diseases among health care professionals. They are defined as a penetrating stab wound from a needle, scalpel, or other sharp object that may result in exposure to blood or other body fluids. The CDC estimates that about 385,000 sharps-related injuries occur annually among health care workers in hospitals (https://www.cdc.gov/niosh/stopsticks/sharpsinjuries.html).

Needlesticks comprise a high number of these injuries; therefore, safer equipment is being made available and more devices are continually being developed by health care manufacturers, such as safety shields for syringes and needleless systems. It is essential that health care professionals learn and apply the means to avoid exposure to infectious agents in the workplace. (Preventing needlesticks is discussed later in this chapter.)

Regulatory Agencies

Two very important regulatory agencies have led the way in the battle against pathogens. They are responsible for developing the guidelines to safeguard health care professionals, their patients, and the public. Understanding the purpose of these agencies and learning the guidelines that pertain to specific occupations is an essential part of health care training.

The Centers for Disease Control and Prevention (CDC) is a government agency that is part of the U.S. Department of Health and Human Services. By studying the causes and distribution of diseases (epidemiology), the CDC is able to formulate safety guidelines to help prevent and control the spread of infectious diseases. Other major tasks include the licensing of clinical laboratories, maintenance of laboratory reference centers for microorganisms, and operation of extensive disease research programs.

The Occupational Safety and Health Administration (OSHA), established in 1970, is a government agency under the Department of Labor. Its two main functions are to establish minimum health and safety standards for the workplace and to enforce those standards. OSHA is the "watchdog" of employee safety and has the authority to conduct onsite inspections to verify compliance with its standards. It is the agency that requires employers to have an exposure control plan and provide hepatitis B vaccines to employees with occupational exposure risk.

MICROORGANISMS

Microorganisms are very small, usually one-celled, living plants or animals. They exist everywhere in the environment but can only be seen with the aid of a microscope (an instrument fitted with a powerful magnifying lens). It is easy to forget their significance because their presence is not obvious. But it is critical to remember that the improper actions of the health care professional can assist destructive microorganisms in their travel, allowing them to infect workers and others.

Not all microorganisms are harmful. Many commonly reside in a particular environment on or in the body and are known as normal flora. The skin, vagina, and intestines are examples of areas that have normal flora. Some microorganisms are even necessary to maintain normal function. For example, the bacterium Escherichia coli aids the digestive process in the colon. In this case, E. coli is a nonpathogen. E. coli can also be a pathogen and create an infection when it invades an area of the body where it is not a part of the normal flora, such as the blood or urine.

Other microorganisms are part of the normal flora, but have no beneficial role. They normally do no harm unless the individual becomes susceptible to an infection due to an alteration in the normal physiological state of the body. This can occur through suppression of the immune response, which is a specific defense used by the body to fight infection and disease by producing antibodies (protective proteins that combat pathogens). Also, long-term antibiotic (medications capable of inhibiting the growth of or destroying microorganisms) therapy suppresses the normal flora and creates an imbalance that can decrease the body's ability to resist pathogens. When an infection occurs due to the weakened physiological state of the body, it is called an opportunistic infection. The ability of the body to resist infection is determined by age, presence of other disease, level of physical health, degree of mental stress, nutritional state, and certain medications.

Microorganisms are either **aerobic** (require oxygen to live) or **anaerobic** (do not require oxygen to live). Many microorganisms prefer a warm, moist, dark environment that provides a source of food. The human body meets these requirements and is thus an ideal environment within which microorganisms can flourish.

Some microorganisms derive nutrients for growth and reproduction from nonliving material and others from living organisms, or **hosts**. If this relationship is beneficial to the host, it is called *symbiosis*. If there is no effect on the host, it is called *neutralism*. But if damage is done to the host, the condition is *parasitic*. An organism that nourishes itself at the expense of other living things and causes them damage is called a **parasite**.

Types of Microbes

Microbes are pathogenic microorganisms. Plant and animal microbes are classified as bacteria, viruses, fungi, rickettsia, and protozoa.

Bacteria

Bacteria are one-celled organisms and can be either pathogenic or nonpathogenic. Many produce *toxins* (poisonous substances). Most bacteria require oxygen and grow best in moderate temperatures. When a group of bacteria grows in one place, it is called a *colony*. Bacteria are categorized

Fascinating Facts

Prior to the **germ theory** (states that bacteria cause specific diseases), it was believed that microorganisms spontaneously arose from decomposing nonliving matter. This theory was based on such observations as noting that maggots (fly larvae) were found in decaying meat and mice would appear when sweat laden shirts were stored with wheat in a dark area.

according to their shapes: round, rod, and spiral. Each type causes certain diseases and conditions. (See Table 10–1.)

Although cocci, round-shaped bacteria, are incapable of movement, some of the rod- and spiral-shaped bacteria have slender whip-like appendages called *flagella* (sing. flagellum) that give them the power of independent locomotion.

Treating Bacterial Infections

Most bacterial infections and diseases can be treated with antibiotics, medicines that destroy bacteria or inhibit their growth. Specific drugs attack specific types of bacteria. (See Table 10–2.) Therefore, diagnosing which bacteria may

Table 10–1 **Major Classifications of Bacteria**

Shape and Configuration	Type/Name	Conditions and Diseases Caused
Cocci – Round or Ovoid Shaped		
Single	Micrococcus	Various skin and wound infections
Pairs	Diplococcus	Gonorrhea, meningitis, some types of pneumonia
Irregular Clusters	Staphylococcus	Pus, some types of pneumonia, abscesses, boils, wound infections, urinary tract infections
Chains	Streptococcus	Rheumatic fever, severe sore throat ("strep" throat)

(continues)

Table 10–1 **Major Classifications of Bacteria** (continued)

Shape and Configuration	Type/Name	Conditions and Diseases Caused
Bacilli – Rod Shaped		
Single	Bacilli	Anthrax, wide variety of infections
Rods are oval shaped	Coccobacilli	
Pairs	Diplobacilli	Tuberculosis, tetanus, pertussis (whooping cough), botulism (severe form of food poisoning), diphtheria, typhoid fever
Chain	Streptobacilli	Rat-bite fever
Spiral		
Curved Rod	Vibrio	Gastrointestinal illness, cholera
Rigid	Spirilla	Bacterial diarrhea Peptic ulcers
Flexible	Spirochete	Syphilis

Table 10–2 **Commonly Prescribed Antibiotics (Generics)**

Antibiotic	Examples of Use
Amoxicillin	Tonsillitis, bronchitis, gonorrhea, ear infections, pneumonia
Doxycycline	Acne, urinary tract, and eye infections, Chlamydia
Cephalexin	Upper respiratory and skin infections
Ciprofloxacin	Exposure to anthrax, certain bacteria such as pseudomonas (this drug may have especially serious side effects)
Clindamycin	Severe middle ear infection, meningitis, some types of pneumonia
Metronidazole	Infections of the vagina, stomach, liver, skin, joints, brain, and respiratory tract
Azithromycin	Many types of infections such as respiratory, ear, and sexually transmitted diseases
Sulfamethoxazole/trimethoprim	Wide variety of infections, including traveler's diarrhea
Amoxicillin and clavulanate	Sinusitis, pneumonia, skin infections
Levofloxacin	Infections of the skin, sinuses, kidneys, bladder, and prostate

Note: Antibiotics are effective against specific types of bacteria. For example, there may be several that can be prescribed for infections of the respiratory tract or pneumonia; the one chosen will depend on the type of bacteria present.

be causing an infection is essential for proper treatment. A laboratory method that is often used to identify the general category of a microorganism is called *Gram staining*. In this method, bacteria are stained with a substance called crystal violet. Bacteria react to staining differently, based on the makeup of their cell walls. This is why their reactions are clues to their identity. There are three categories of reactions:

1. Gram-positive: Retains the stain
2. Gram-negative: Loses the stain
3. Acid-fast: Retains the stain even when treated with acid

This information can be obtained rather quickly and helps determine the class of antibiotic to prescribe.

Another laboratory method usually performed at the same time is to grow the microorganism in various culture media (materials that promote the growth of microorganisms). It can take 24 to 72 hours for colonies to form, but the information obtained can result in the identification of the exact bacteria. Based on this more specific diagnosis, the choice of antibiotics can be reevaluated to determine if a more specific medication should be prescribed. Although most types of bacteria can be destroyed with antibiotics, several types are resistant to antibiotics and are challenging to treat. They create a threat to the health of both patients and health care professionals. Resistant strains of bacteria are discussed later in this chapter.

Some bacteria have the ability to form spores. A **spore** is a thick capsule that the bacterium creates for self-protection. Spores are created when life-supporting conditions are not favorable and are referred to as the "resting stage." Spores are extremely difficult to kill and can lay dormant for months or even years. In this stage, bacteria are still alive but inactive and very resistant to heat, drying, and the action of disinfectants. When supportive conditions return, the bacteria become active again. Extremely high temperatures, such as that reached by steam, must be used for sterilization to ensure that all spores are killed.

Fascinating Facts

It is estimated that the average person carries 39 trillion bacterial cells in and on her body, although this number can vary significantly from person to person. (http://www.microbiomeinstitute.org/blog/2016/1/20/how-many-bacterial-vs-human-cells-are-in-the-body).

Viruses

Viruses are the smallest of the microbes and cannot be seen under the traditional light microscope. A special piece of equipment called an electron microscope is necessary to identify them. (See Figure 10–1.) Viruses are not whole cells and depend on living cells to provide food, nutrients, and a means of reproduction. Because they can only live inside another living organism, they are referred to as *obligate intracellular parasites.*

More than 200 viruses that infect humans have been identified by researchers and three or four more are discovered each year. Viruses are the cause of the common cold, influenza (flu), pneumonia, chickenpox, croup, hepatitis B, acquired immune deficiency syndrome (AIDS), measles, mumps, herpes, warts, and polio.

Viral infections can be extremely difficult to treat because viruses multiply rapidly and are easily transmitted by blood and other body secretions. They are resistant to many disinfectants and are not killed by the antibiotics that kill bacteria. Treatment for viral infections focuses on treating the symptoms until the immune system can fight off the virus. Antiviral drugs have been developed that do not destroy viruses, but rather inhibit their development. There are three FDA-approved antiviral drugs recommended by the CDC for use against influenza viruses:

1. Rapivab (peramivir)
2. Relenza (zanamivir)
3. Tamiflu (oseltamivir phosphate)

Recent research in Australia has identified a protein in the body's immune system that inhibits its ability to destroy viruses. As a result of this discovery, scientists are looking for ways to stop this protein from interfering with the actions of the immune system (Eunice, Ross Vlahos, et al. 2017) .

Courtesy of CDC/Erskine L. Palmer, Ph.D; M.L. Martin

FIGURE 10–1 Electron micrograph of the influenza virus.

Fungi

Fungi are a large group of organisms that are neither plant nor animal. They have unique characteristics that are not shared by other organisms and are thus placed in a kingdom of their own. Two forms of fungi are potential pathogens: yeast and mold. Yeasts are one-celled and molds are multicelled organisms. Both are present everywhere. Fungi cannot produce their own nutrients, so they rely on *organic* (animal and vegetable forms of life) materials. Some use live and others use dead organic materials for nutrients. Fungi thrive in warm, moist, dark conditions.

Many yeasts and molds are nonpathogenic. In fact, penicillin, an important antibiotic, is produced from a mold. But as with other types of microorganisms, fungi can become pathogenic when the right conditions exist. When this happens they create an opportunistic infection. Fungal infections can range from merely annoying to life-threatening.

Some fungi cause chronic, recurrent infections. Superficial, or *cutaneous*, infections are infections of the skin or mucous membranes; these include fungi that cause ringworm, athlete's foot, and infections of the skin, hair follicles, and scalp. The most serious of the fungal infections are the systemic infections, such as *histoplasmosis* (a systemic respiratory disease). Infections that go beyond the cutaneous level are always difficult, if not impossible, to treat or cure. Treatment of systemic infections requires medications that are toxic to humans. Patients, therefore, must be closely monitored.

Rickettsia

Rickettsia are much smaller than bacteria and have rod or spherical shapes. They stain as gram negative and do not move independently. Rickettsia must live inside the cell of another living organism and so are, like the viruses, referred to as *obligate intracellular parasites*.

Rickettsia cause several types of typhus and Rocky Mountain spotted fever. The microorganism is passed through the bite of fleas, lice, ticks, and mites. Historically, epidemic typhus has wiped out entire villages. Although typhus is not common today, there are occasional outbreaks among the homeless populations in cities such as Los Angeles because of unsanitary living conditions.

Protozoa

Protozoa are the only microorganisms that are classified as animals. Consisting of one cell, they are plentiful in the environment and reside in and on the body. Like other microorganisms, they seek locations that provide nutrients, warmth, and moisture. This is why some of the more than 50,000 identified types of protozoa are constantly present in the intestines and on the skin and mucous membranes of the nose and throat.

Protozoa are also found in decayed materials, water **contaminated** (contains infectious material) with sewage waste, food washed in contaminated water or handled by unwashed hands, bird and animal feces, and insect bites. (See Figure 10–2.)

Some of the most common diseases caused by the pathogenic protozoa include the following:

- *Dysentery*, an intestinal infection resulting in abdominal pain, cramping, and diarrhea, is caused by *Giardia lamblia* and is commonly referred to as "traveler's diarrhea." It is the most common intestinal parasite in the United States. It is acquired through contaminated water or food and is diagnosed by examination of the feces.

- *Trichomoniasis* is a sexually transmitted genital infection.

Fascinating Facts

A fungus is an organism that causes food spoilage. Who has not seen fuzzy or dark moldy spots on spoiled bread, fruits, and vegetables? And you are probably familiar with the characteristic "musty" smell of mold. But there are also commercial uses of fungi, such as the use of yeast in making wine from grapes and beer from malt and creating the carbon dioxide necessary for dough to rise. Molds are also responsible for the flavor of Roquefort and Camembert cheeses.

Fascinating Facts

Here is a chilling fact that emphasizes the need to follow strict infection control procedures: Rickettsia get their name from the physician who first identified the causative agent of Rocky Mountain spotted fever, Dr. Howard T. Ricketts, an American pathologist. *He subsequently died from typhus, having been infected through his own research on the disease.*

Electron micrographs courtesy of the Centers for Disease Control and Prevention, Atlanta, GA

FIGURE 10-2 Intestinal protozoan *Entamoeba coli*.

- *Toxoplasmosis* is of particular significance in pregnant women because it can pass to the unborn child and result in death, blindness, or mental retardation. It is found in the feces of birds and animals.

- *Pneumocystis pneumonia* is caused by a protozoan that is normally not pathogenic. But in patients with weakened immune systems, it is very serious and is a common cause of death among AIDS patients.

- *Malaria* is caused by a parasite that attacks the red blood cells and is characterized by periodic (every 48 to 72 hours) chills, fever, and sweats. The parasite is acquired through the bite of a specific kind of mosquito or through a blood transfusion. Malaria is one of the most severe public health problems worldwide. It is a leading cause of death and disease in many developing countries, especially those in sub-Saharan Africa where it accounts for about 15% of deaths of young children (Baylor College of Medicine, n.d.).

DEFENSE MECHANISMS

One of the marvels of the human body is the number of defense mechanisms present to resist infections. If these mechanisms are intact, along with a strong immune system, the individual can often resist the microorganism and not become ill. Examples of the body's natural defense mechanisms include the following:

- Cilia in the respiratory tract that catch and move pathogens out of the body

- Coughing and sneezing to propel pathogens outward

- Tears, which contain chemicals to kill bacteria

- Hydrochloric acid in the stomach, which destroys pathogens

- Mucous membranes of the respiratory, reproductive, and digestive systems, which serve to trap pathogens

- Rise in body temperature (fever) to a level that will kill microorganisms

- Production of additional leukocytes (white blood cells), which have the specific function of destroying pathogens

HOW INFECTIONS SPREAD

The **chain of infection** is a useful model for explaining how infectious diseases occur and are transmitted. It consists of six elements that must be present for an infection to develop. (See Figure 10-3.)

1. Infectious agent: A pathogen must be present.

2. Reservoir host: The pathogen must have a place to live and grow. Examples of reservoir hosts are the human body, contaminated water or food, animals, insects, birds, and dead or decaying organic material. When humans or animals are capable of transmitting the pathogen but have no outward signs of the disease, they are referred to as *carriers*. Individuals who are carriers may not even be aware that they are spreading an infectious disease.

3. Portal of exit: The pathogen must be able to escape from the reservoir host where it has been growing. Examples of portals of exit are blood, urine, feces, breaks in the skin, wound drainage, and body secretions such as saliva, mucus, and reproductive fluids.

4. Route of transmission: When the pathogen leaves the reservoir host through the portal of exit, it must have a way of being transmitted to a new host. Examples are air, food, insects, and direct contact with an infected person.

5. Portal of entry: The pathogen must have a way of entering the new host. Common ports of entry are the mouth, nostrils, and breaks in the skin.

6. Susceptible host: An individual who has a large number of pathogens invading the body or does not have adequate resistance to the invading pathogen will get the infectious disease.

PREVENTING INFECTION

The practice of **asepsis (aseptic technique)** involves methods used to make the patient, the worker, and the environment as pathogen-free as possible. There are two types:

1. **Medical asepsis (clean technique)** includes procedures to decrease the number and spread of pathogens in the environment. Examples include handwashing, good personal hygiene, the cleaning of rooms between patient use, and disposal of

FIGURE 10–3 The chain of infection. Breaking at least one link stops the infectious disease. Examples of health care practices and procedures that impact the cycle are included.

gloves after contact with body fluids or contaminated objects.

2. **Surgical asepsis (sterile technique)**, includes procedures to completely eliminate the presence of pathogens from objects and areas. Examples of surgical asepsis are wearing sterile caps, gowns, masks, and gloves during surgery; sterilizing and using special techniques to handle instruments to be used with patients; maintaining **sterile fields** (areas designated to be free of microorganisms); changing dressings; and disposing of contaminated materials. (Medical asepsis is discussed in more detail later in this chapter.)

Breaking the Chain of Infection

The chain of infection described previously demonstrates how infectious diseases occur and are spread. The most important concept to remember is that *breaking at least one link stops the infectious disease*. The practices and techniques that health care professionals use daily are designed to break the chain.

Recall that the chain of infection consists of six elements. These six elements are often organized into the following three components:

1. Source of infecting microorganisms (elements 1 and 2—infectious agent and reservoir host—both involve the source of infection)

2. Means of transmission for the microorganism (elements 3, 4, and 5—portal of exit, route of transmission, and portal of entry—all affect transmission)

3. Susceptible host (element 6—susceptible host—is unchanged in this organized format)

The best defenses, then, are to decrease the sources of microorganisms, prevent their transmission, and maximize the resistance of the host. Here are actions, discussed in the following sections of this chapter, that health care professionals can take to prevent the spread of infection:

1. How can I decrease the source of microorganisms?

   • Perform proper handwashing. *The Centers for Disease Control and Prevention states that handwashing is the single most important procedure for preventing health care–acquired infections.*

- Decontaminate surfaces and equipment (antiseptics, disinfectants, and sterilization).

- Avoid contact with patients and others when you are harboring infectious microorganisms; for example, the force of a sneeze can propel microorganisms for many feet (the spray travels in the shape of a cone, so as the distance increases from the nose, the spray widens).

2. How can I prevent the transmission of microorganisms?

- Wear personal protective equipment (PPE) when indicated. PPE includes caps, gloves, gowns, masks, booties, and eye protection.

- Follow isolation procedures when indicated. These are additional precautions used when working with patients who have highly contagious diseases.

3. How can I maximize the resistance of the host?

- Provide good hygiene

- Ensure proper nutrition and fluid intake

- Decrease stressors that weaken the immune response

Handwashing

The first line of defense in medical asepsis and the most effective way to help prevent the spread of microorganisms is good handwashing technique. Many microorganisms are normal flora, always present on the body. For example, staphylococci occur naturally on the hands. But when transferred to a wound site, they can cause pus-producing infections. (See Figure 10–4.)

Two types of normal flora are found on the hands. *Transient flora*, whether pathogenic or nonpathogenic, are picked up during our activities of daily living and are easily removed from the hands with frequent and thorough handwashing. *Resident flora* are present at all times, and considerable scrubbing is required to remove these deeply embedded microbes. It is not possible to completely remove all the microorganisms from the hands, but the transient flora can be removed and the resident flora diminished with diligent handwashing. In individuals who do not maintain proper hygiene, it is possible that even the transient flora will become resident flora. This results in the person becoming a carrier of that particular organism.

FIGURE 10–4 Clean hands are caring hands.

Always perform proper handwashing technique as indicated to avoid the transfer of microorganisms to you, your patients, others, or the environment. Examples of appropriate times to do handwashing are as follows:

- When coming on duty
- When taking a break or leaving work
- Between patient contacts
- Before applying and immediately upon removing gloves
- Before and after touching your face in any way (manipulating contact lenses, applying lip balm, blowing your nose, coughing, and sneezing)
- After contact with anything considered contaminated (picking up items from the floor, touching equipment or environmental surfaces that may be contaminated, handling soiled linens)
- Before touching any items considered clean, such as a patient's food or drink
- Before and after eating and/or drinking
- After using the restroom

It is necessary to wash the hands between tasks and procedures on the same patient if there is the possibility of cross-contaminating different body sites. The hands must also be washed and the gloves changed before touching nonintact skin or mucous membranes and after touching nonintact skin, mucous membranes, blood, or any moist body fluid, secretions, or excretions.

Check the Infection Control Program policy in your facility to determine which type of soap to use. It may state to use plain (nonantimicrobial) soap for routine handwashing and an antimicrobial agent for specific circumstances. (See Procedure 10–1, Handwashing and Figures 10–5a–d.)

Related to handwashing is the use of nail polish. It is recommended that health care professionals do not wear nail polish, especially colored polish that can hide dirt under the nails. In addition, research has found that chipped polish can harbor microorganisms that resist removal by handwashing (Cimon and Featherstone, 2017).

Most health care facilities have waterless handwashing foams, gels, or lotions available. The waterless hand-cleaning products contain alcohol as the antiseptic and a moisturizer to prevent drying of the skin. (See Figure 10–6.) A major advantage of this system is availability as they can be placed in multiple locations for easy access. The waterless system can be used between patients when hands are not visibly soiled and when there has been no contact with blood or body fluids. Enough product should be applied to all surfaces of the hands, fingers, nails, and wrists for it to take about

PROCEDURE 10–1

HANDWASHING

Procedure

1. Turn faucet on using a clean, dry paper towel. (See Figure 10–5a.)

2. Run warm water over hands and wrists.

3. Do not lean against the sink, and avoid splashing clothing with water.

4. Keep hands lower than arms during procedure, and keep fingertips pointing downward.

5. Apply liquid soap to hands.

6. Scrub palms in a circular motion while clasping hands together.

7. Scrub wrists 1 to 2 inches above the hands by encircling one wrist with the other hand; then repeat for the other wrist.

8. Scrub the back of each hand with a circular motion by cupping one hand over the other. (See Figure 10–5b.)

Rationale

Faucets are always considered contaminated.

Warm water helps remove superficial dirt and microorganisms.

The sink is always considered contaminated; water splashed from the sink is contaminated, and wet material easily conducts microorganisms.

Prevents contaminated water from running up the arms and dripping on clothes.

Bar soap can carry microorganisms.

Creates lather, and the friction helps to remove microorganisms.

Same as previous.

Same as previous.

(continues)

PROCEDURE

HANDWASHING

10–1

(continued)

Procedure

9. Scrub between the fingers with a back and forth motion by interlacing fingers. (See Figure 10–5c.)

10. Scrub each individual finger and clean under the nails with a cuticle stick, a brush, or a fingernail on the other hand, or by rubbing it against the palm of the other hand.

11. Scrub hands for at least 2 minutes.

12. Rinse each hand thoroughly with running water from the wrists down to the fingertips. (See Figure 10–5d.)

13. Dry thoroughly with a disposable towel(s).

Rationale

Same as previous.

Microorganisms can easily hide under the nails.

Provides thorough cleaning of all surfaces.
Soap residue can cause skin irritation.

Moisture remaining on the skin can cause irritation; reusable towels can harbor microorganisms.

FIGURE 10–5a Use a clean, dry paper towel to turn the faucet on and off.

FIGURE 10–5c Scrub between fingers with back and forth motion by interlacing fingers.

FIGURE 10–5b Keep the fingertips pointed downward. Scrub hands and wrists with a circular motion.

FIGURE 10–5d Rinse each hand thoroughly with running water from the wrists down to fingertips.

14. Use another dry towel to turn off the faucet handle. (See Figure 10–5a.)

15. Clean sink area using dry towels, being careful not to recontaminate hands by touching any surfaces.

16. Use lotion if desired.

Prevents recontamination of hands from microorganisms on the faucet handles; a wet towel would allow microorganisms to travel from the faucet handle back to the hands.

Leaves the area ready for the next person; the faucets and sink are always considered contaminated; wet towels are considered contaminated.

Keeps hands soft and helps prevent chapping and cracking of hands, which are more susceptible to growth of microorganisms.

FIGURE 10–6 If water for handwashing is not easily available, a hand sanitizer may be used.

15 seconds of rubbing for the hands to feel dry. It is important to read the manufacturer's instructions before using any product and to be familiar with the written policies on hand hygiene for the health care facility in which you work.

At the same time, it is important to note that according to the CDC, handwashing is more effective than using a hand sanitizer. Even products with the recommended 60% or higher alcohol content do not kill certain types of microorganisms, such as norovirus (causes vomiting and diarrhea), some parasites, and *Clostridium difficile* (causes severe diarrhea). According to the CDC, proper handwashing is the most effective method of eliminating these microbes (https://www.cdc.gov/handwashing/pdf/hand-sanitizer-factsheet.pdf).

Personal Protective Equipment

Personal protective equipment, commonly referred to as PPE, includes gloves, masks, protective eyewear, gowns, and caps. To be effective, these must be properly used in all situations that have the potential to infect the health care professional.

OSHA requires the use of PPE to reduce employee exposure to infectious hazards in the health care environment.

Employers are required to determine what hazards exist and to implement a PPE program to address these hazards. This program should address the hazards present; the selection, maintenance, and use of PPE; the training of employees; and the monitoring of the program to ensure its ongoing effectiveness.

(See Figure 10–7.)

Gloves

Wear clean, nonsterile gloves when you touch, or have the potential of coming in contact with, blood, body fluids, secretions, excretions, or contaminated items. Put on clean gloves just before touching mucous membranes and nonintact skin. Gloves should be changed between tasks and procedures on the same patient if there is contact with material that may contain a high concentration of microorganisms. Remove gloves promptly after use, before touching noncontaminated items and environmental surfaces, and before going to another patient. After gloves are removed, wash your hands immediately to avoid transferring microorganisms to other patients or environments. (See Procedure 10–2 and Figures 10–8 a–h.)

FIGURE 10–7 Gloves, mask, eye protection, and gown should be worn during procedures and patient-care activities that are likely to generate splashes or sprays of blood, body fluids, secretions, and excretions.

PROCEDURE

10–2

NONSTERILE GLOVES (APPLYING CLEAN GLOVES AND REMOVING CONTAMINATED GLOVES)

Procedure

1. Use proper handwashing technique before applying gloves.

2. Remove appropriate-sized clean gloves from the box and apply. After the hands are washed, no specific technique is necessary for applying gloves, but touch only the gloves you will be using when removing them from the dispenser.

Removing contaminated gloves:

3. Grasp the outside of one glove at the palm with the other gloved hand (see Figure 10–8a); pull the glove down (see Figure 10–8b) and turn it inside out while removing it. (See Figure 10–8c.)

4. Hold the removed glove in the palm of the remaining gloved hand. (See Figures 10–8d and 10–8e.)

Rationale

To remove microorganisms from hands.

Gloves that are too small can split and expose skin, and gloves that are too large are difficult to work with and can expose skin by slipping down; do not contaminate the remaining gloves in the dispenser by touching them.

At no time should the hands touch the outside of the contaminated gloves.

Same as previous.

FIGURE 10–8a Grasp the outside of one glove at palm site with the other gloved hand.

FIGURE 10–8b Begin removing the first glove.

5. Take the ungloved hand and slide it under the cuff of the remaining glove (see Figure 10–8f) and push the glove off. (See Figure 10–8g.) The first glove is now inside the second glove that was removed. (See Figure 10–8h.)

Same as previous.

6. Discard the gloves in an appropriate container according to facility policy.

Isolates the contaminated gloves from contact with other surfaces.

7. Wash hands immediately after removing gloves.

To remove microorganisms from hands.

(continues)

PROCEDURE

NONSTERILE GLOVES (APPLYING CLEAN GLOVES AND REMOVING CONTAMINATED GLOVES)

Procedure

FIGURE 10-8c Turn the glove inside out while removing it. Take care not to touch bare skin with the contaminated glove.

FIGURE 10-8d Inverted glove is completely removed into the contaminated glove.

FIGURE 10-8e Contain the inverted glove completely in the gloved hand.

Rationale

FIGURE 10-8f Take the ungloved hand and slide fingers under the cuff of the remaining contaminated glove.

FIGURE 10-8g Push the glove off while inverting the second glove over the first.

FIGURE 10-8h The first glove is now inside of the second glove that was removed. Dispose of gloves in appropriate container according to facility policy.

Mask, Eye Protection, Face Shield

Wear a mask and eye protection or a face shield to protect the mucous membranes of the eyes, nose, and mouth during procedures and patient care activities that are likely to generate splashes or sprays of blood, body fluids, secretions, or excretions. While the nose and mouth are obvious entry points for infections, the eyes are also portals for microorganisms. In addition to using eye protection equipment, it is important not to touch or rub the eyes when the hands may be contaminated.

Gown

Wear a clean, nonsterile gown to protect the skin and to prevent soiling clothing during procedures and patient care activities that are likely to generate splashes or sprays of blood, body fluids, secretions, or excretions. Select a gown that is appropriate for the activity and amount of fluid likely to be encountered. Remove a soiled gown as promptly as possible and wash your hands to avoid the transfer of microorganisms to other patients or environments.

Application of PPE

When working in contaminated areas, there are guidelines for applying and removing PPE. See Procedure 10–3 and Figures 10–9a–c and 10–10a–c that demonstrate the most commonly used equipment.

Patient-Care Equipment

Handle used patient care equipment that is soiled with blood, body fluids, secretions, and excretions in a manner that prevents skin and mucous membrane exposures, contamination of clothing, and transfer of microorganisms to other patients and environments. Ensure that reusable equipment is not used for the care of another patient until it has been cleaned and reprocessed appropriately. Be sure that single-use items are discarded properly. The correct method will vary, depending on whether the item has been contaminated by a body fluid.

Antiseptics, Disinfectants, and Sterilization

A number of chemical agents and physical methods are used to inhibit the growth of or destroy microorganisms. If the method used only inhibits the growth of the microorganism, the action is described as **bacteriostatic**. If the method results in the microorganisms being killed, the action is **bacteriocidal** or *germicidal*. The methods used can be broken into the following three categories:

- **Antiseptics:** Chemical agents that are antiseptics are only bacteriostatic. They are mild enough to be used on the skin. An example is cleaning with a 70% isopropyl alcohol wipe before giving an injection.

PROCEDURE   10–3

APPLYING AND REMOVING PPE

Procedure

1. Use proper handwashing technique before applying PPE. (See Procedure 10–1.)

2. Put on cap, mask, protective eyewear, and gown.
   No specific sequence of applying these items is required.

3. To apply gown (See Figures 10–9 a–c):
   Put on the gown by placing your hands inside the shoulders.
   Slip your fingers inside the neckband to tie the gown at the neck.
   Overlap the back edges of the gown so your uniform is completely covered before tying the waist ties.

Rationale

To remove microorganisms from hands.

Complete coverage needed to protect against contamination.

Be sure that the cap covers all the hair and ears, the mask fits snugly to the face (press metal clip on mask to fit snugly across bridge of nose), eyewear extends to protect the side of the face, and the gown completely covers the clothing.

(continues)

PROCEDURE

APPLYING AND REMOVING PPE

(continued)

Procedure

4. Apply gloves last. Remove appropriate-sized clean gloves from the box and apply. Touch only the gloves you will be using when removing them from the dispenser.

Rationale

Gloves that are too small can split and expose skin, and gloves that are too large are difficult to work with and can expose skin by slipping down; do not contaminate the remaining gloves in the dispenser by touching them.

FIGURE 10–9a Put on the gown by placing your hands inside the shoulders.

FIGURE 10–9b Slip your fingers inside the neckband to tie the gown at the neck.

5. Pull the cuffs over the sleeves of the gown to create a seal.

Remove PPE prior to leaving the contaminated area, as follows:

6. Untie the waist ties of the gown.

7. Remove contaminated gloves.

8. Wash hands.

9. Remove cap and protective eyewear gently.

   To remove the gown (see Figures 10–10a–c):

   Untie the neck tie of the gown and remove the gown.

   To remove the gown, slip the fingers of one hand under the cuff of the opposite arm and pull the gown down until it covers the hand.

Creates seal against entrance of microorganisms.

The waist ties of the gown are considered contaminated.

See Procedure 10–2.

See Procedure 10–1.

Do gently to prevent dispersion of microorganisms.

The neck ties of the gown are considered clean.

The outside of the gown is considered contaminated and should not be touched.

PROCEDURE

10–3

APPLYING AND REMOVING PPE

Procedure	**Rationale**
Using the gown-covered hand, grasp the outside of the gown on the opposite arm, and pull the gown down until it covers the hand.	The outside of the gown is considered contaminated and should not be touched.

FIGURE 10–9c Overlap the back edges of the gown so your uniform is completely covered before tying the waist ties.

Both hands are now inside the gown and can be used to grasp the outside of the gown. Use your covered hands to grasp the gown at the shoulders and turn the gown inside out (contaminated side on the inside) as you remove it. Roll it up and place in appropriate container according to facility policy.	Keep gown in front of you and away from the body. Avoid excessive motion during procedure because motion causes the spread of organisms.
10. Remove the mask. Hold the mask by the strings to discard it.	The ties of the mask are considered clean. Do not touch any other part of the mask, as it is considered contaminated. The mask is always removed last if the contaminants are airborne.
11. Wash hands. (See Procedure 10–1.)	To remove microorganisms from hands.

FIGURE 10–10a To remove the gown, slip the fingers of one hand under the cuff of the opposite arm and pull the gown down until it covers the hand.

(continues)

PROCEDURE

APPLYING AND REMOVING PPE

(continued)

Procedure | **Rationale**

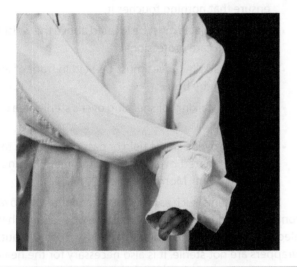

FIGURE 10–10b Using the gown-covered hand, grasp the outside of the gown on the opposite arm, and pull the gown down until it covers the hand.

FIGURE 10–10c Both hands are now inside the gown and can be used to grasp the outside of the gown. Use your covered hands to grasp the gown at the shoulders and turn the gown inside out (contaminated side on the inside) as you remove it. Roll it up and place in appropriate container according to facility policy.

- **Disinfectants:** Agents or methods that destroy most bacteria and viruses. This method of cleaning is used for instruments that do not penetrate the skin and for cleaning the environment (e.g., floors, bathroom, equipment). *Chemical agents* are frequently used as disinfectants. Using a solution comparable to a 10% dilution of common household bleach in water for cleaning the environment (including blood spills) meets OSHA recommendations because it kills hepatitis B, human immunodeficiency virus (HIV), and tuberculosis organisms. Alcohol was mentioned earlier as an example of an antiseptic, but if instruments are soaked for 20 to 30 minutes, it acts as a disinfectant. (See Figure 10–11.) Carefully read and follow the manufacturer's directions when using chemical agents. *Physical disinfectant methods* include boiling instruments in water. This was once commonly used in home health settings, but with the availability of one-time-use equipment, it is rarely used today.

- **Sterilization:** Agents or methods that totally destroy all microorganisms, including viruses and spores. Examples include chemical agents, gas, radiation,

FIGURE 10–11 Chemical agent used as disinfectant. Pour in enough solution to completely cover all instruments.

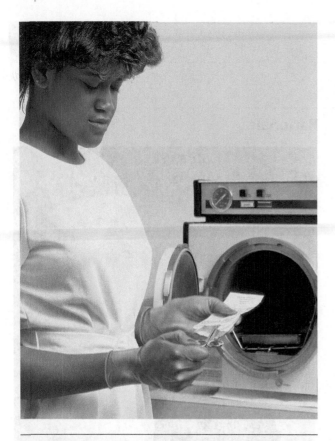

FIGURE 10–12 An autoclave is a pressurized heating system that sterilizes by steam.

and dry or moist heat under pressure. The most common method used is the autoclave, equipment that sterilizes using high-temperature steam created by a pressurized heating system. The size can vary from a small unit for a medical office to a large unit for a hospital. (See Figure 10–12.)

As bacteria mutate, they can become resistant to previously effective methods of inhibiting or destroying them. An example is enterococcus faecium, or E. faecium, that has become resistant to alcohol as an antiseptic or disinfectant. This is especially significant with the wide use of alcohol hand wash in the health care setting as well as the use of alcohol to clean surfaces, equipment, etc. As a result, E. faecium is now a leading bacterial infection in the hospital setting.

Surgical Asepsis

Surgical asepsis (or sterile technique) is a group of principles and related procedures that eliminate the presence of pathogens from objects and areas. To correctly perform these procedures, it is necessary to understand the concept of a sterile field. A sterile field is an area that has been designated as free of microorganisms. An example

is a sterile towel placed on a clean, dry surface. The towel now represents a sterile field. Many health care procedures, such as surgeries, require the use of sterile fields.

The following guidelines protect sterile objects and fields:

- A sterile object may not touch a nonsterile object.
- Sterile objects must not be wet.
- The border between a sterile area and a nonsterile area cannot be less than one inch.
- The sterile area must be constantly observed to ensure that nothing touches it.
- All sterile objects must be located above the waist of the health care professional.
- Hands in sterile gloves must be held in front of and away from the body.
- Coughing, talking, or sneezing over a sterile area can contaminate it.
- Reaching over a sterile field or passing anything that is contaminated over it can contaminate it (Lindh, Tamparo, Dahl, Morris & Correa, 2018).

Sterilized items, such as instruments and surgical gloves, come in sealed packages that must be opened and handled properly to avoid contamination because the outer wrappers are not sterile. It is also necessary for the health care professional to use sterile gloves, applying them in a way that prevents them from being contaminated. (See Procedure 10–4, Figures 10–13a–f.) Always check for expiration dates on the package before using any sterilized items.

Standard Precautions

It is impossible to know which pathogens a patient may carry, so specific procedures have been developed by the CDC. Known as **standard precautions**, it is essential that they be followed at all times and applied to every patient in the health care environment. (See Figure 10–14.)

Standard precautions must be followed to prevent contact with potentially infectious body fluids. Specifically, these fluids include the following:

- Blood
- All body fluids, secretions, and excretions except sweat, regardless of whether or not they contain visible blood
- Nonintact skin
- Mucous membranes
- Any unidentified body fluids

The following sections summarize the specific standard precautions needed by health care professionals.

PROCEDURE

APPLYING STERILE GLOVES

Procedure	Rationale
1. Use proper handwashing technique. (See Procedure 10–1.)	To remove microorganisms from hands.
2. Inspect glove package for tears or stains and do not use if present.	Tears and stains indicate the gloves are no longer sterile and must be discarded or used for nonsterile purposes.
3. Place package of gloves on a clean, dry, flat surface above waist level.	Using a contaminated surface can compromise the sterility of the sterile package.
To apply sterile gloves (see Figures 10–13 a–f):	
Open sterile gloves by pulling back on the tabs without touching the sterile inner border.	Extra caution must be taken to protect the sterility of the gloves.
The gloves should be opened with the cuffs toward you, the palms up, and the thumbs pointing outward. If the gloves are not positioned properly, turn the package around, being careful not to reach over the sterile area or touch the inner surface of the gloves.	Sterile gloves are packaged in this position for ease of application.
Pick up the first glove by grasping the glove on the top edge of the folded-down cuff. Do not drag or dangle the fingers over any nonsterile area.	Picking up the glove by grasping the inner cuff prevents the outer part of the glove from becoming contaminated. Strict adherence to the sterile principles is essential.
Maintain the grasp on the cuff, insert your other hand, and gently pull the glove on by the cuff.	Pull gently to avoid tearing the glove. If contamination occurs, discard the gloves and start again.
Slip the gloved fingers under the cuff of the second glove to lift it from the package and insert the other hand into the glove.	The outside of the second glove is sterile and may be touched only by another sterile surface.
Pull the glove on and adjust the glove into position, being careful not to touch the skin with the gloved hands.	Always be mindful of what is a sterile surface and what is contaminated.
Turn the cuffs up by manipulating only the sterile surface of the gloves (go under the folded cuffs, pull out slightly, and turn cuffs over and up).	Only sterile touches sterile.
Check the gloves for tears, holes, and imperfections.	If any flaws are noted, discard and start again.
4. After gloves are applied, always hold the hands above the waist and away from the body with palms up.	Serves to increase awareness of sterile gloves and prevent inadvertently touching nonsterile areas.

(continues)

PROCEDURE

APPLYING STERILE GLOVES

Procedure

Rationale

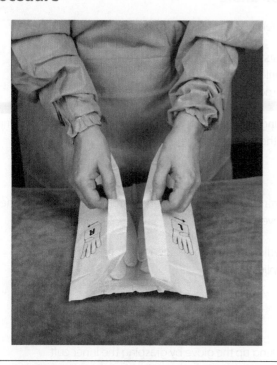

FIGURE 10–13a Open sterile gloves by pulling back on the tabs.

FIGURE 10–13b Pick up the first glove by grasping the glove on the top edge of the folded-down cuff.

FIGURE 10–13c Maintain the grasp on the cuff, insert your other hand, and pull the glove on by the cuff.

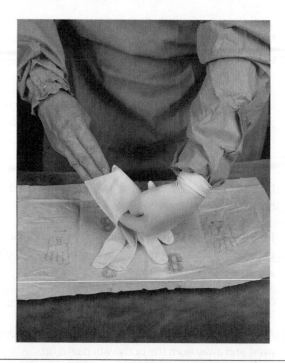

FIGURE 10–13d Slip the gloved fingers under the cuff of the second glove to lift it from the package and insert the other hand into the glove.

(continues)

PROCEDURE

APPLYING STERILE GLOVES

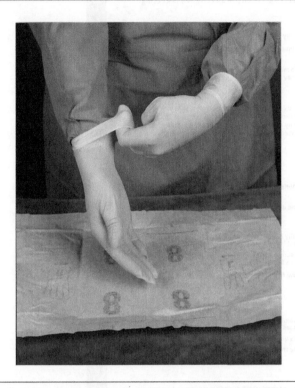

FIGURE 10–13e Pull the glove on and adjust the glove into position, being careful not to touch the skin with the gloved hands.

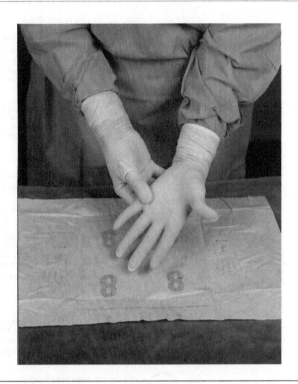

FIGURE 10–13f Check the gloves for tears, holes, and imperfections.

Environmental Control

Procedures must be followed and consistently performed for the routine care, cleaning, and disinfection of environmental surfaces, beds, bed rails, bedside equipment, and other frequently touched surfaces.

Linen

Handle, transport, and process used linen that is soiled with blood, body fluids, secretions, and excretions in a manner that prevents skin and mucous membrane exposures, contamination of your clothing, and transfer of microorganisms to other patients and environments. Some bacteria can survive for days on linen, so it is important that soiled linens be handled carefully and placed in appropriate containers or bags.

Patient Placement

Patients with infections who contaminate the environment or who do not or cannot assist in maintaining appropriate hygiene or environmental control should be placed in a private room. Some hospitals prefer to protect the patient's privacy and post a simple note stating that one must report to the nurse's station prior to entry into the room. If a private room is not available, consult with infection control professionals regarding patient placement or other alternatives.

Blood-Borne Pathogens

The term *blood-borne* is used to identify pathogenic microorganisms that are spread through contact with blood. Blood, however, is not the only route by which they can be transmitted. Infections can also be transmitted through contact with nonintact skin, mucous membranes, secretions, excretions, or any moist body fluid except sweat.

A common way that health care professionals are infected by these pathogens is from injuries sustained when using needles, scalpels, and other sharp instruments or devices; when handling sharp instruments after procedures; when cleaning used instruments; and when disposing of used needles. Place used disposable syringes and needles, scalpel blades, and other sharp items in appropriate puncture-resistant containers. (See Figure 10–15.) These should be located as close as practical to the area in which the items are used. Place reusable syringes and needles in a puncture-resistant container for transport to the reprocessing area.

FIGURE 10–14 Standard precautions.

The following additional precautions must be followed when using needles:

- Never recap used needles. The health care professional needs to be familiar with the facility policies on how to handle contaminated needles because there may be an exception to this rule. Examples include using either a one-handed "scoop" technique or a mechanical device designed for holding the needle sheath.

- Do not remove used needles from disposable syringes by hand and do not bend, break, or otherwise manipulate used needles by hand.

When resuscitation is required, use mouthpieces, resuscitation bags, or other ventilation devices as an alternative to mouth-to-mouth methods. Keep these devices available in areas where the need for resuscitation is predictable.

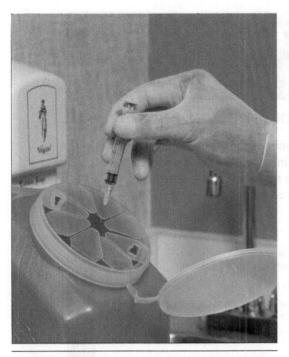

FIGURE 10–15 All needles and sharp objects should be discarded immediately in a puncture-resistant sharp container.

Transmission Precautions

Certain pathogens are especially dangerous because they are easily transmitted and have the potential of causing epidemics. Pathogens can be transmitted in three ways: through the air, in droplets of liquid, or through direct contact with infected persons or contaminated items. (See Table 10–3.)

The CDC recommends the use of transmission-based precautions with patients who are documented or suspected to be infected with these pathogens. There are specific precautions for each type of transmission. They may be combined for diseases that have multiple routes of transmission. *Either alone or in combination, they are to be used in addition to standard precautions.* (See Figures 10–16, 10–17, and 10–18.)

Placing a patient on transmission precautions, however, can present certain disadvantages to the hospital, patients, personnel, and visitors.

- It requires the patient to be in a private room unless it is shared with another patient with the same disease. The rationale for this is to confine the pathogen to the patient's unit.

Table 10-3 Routes of Pathogen Transmission

Type of Transmission	Description	Examples
Airborne	• Airborne droplets or dust particles containing the infectious agent remain suspended in the air for long periods • Can be dispersed widely by air currents within a room or over a long distance • Can be emitted during talking, sneezing, coughing, and whispering	• *Mycobacterium tuberculosis* • Rubeola (measles) • Varicella (chickenpox)
Droplet	• Propelled short distances through the air • Deposited on the host's conjunctiva, nasal mucosa, or mouth • Can be emitted during talking, sneezing, or coughing, and during the performance of certain procedures such as suctioning and bronchoscopy	• Some forms of pneumonia, meningitis, and sepsis • Streptococcal pharyngitis • Mumps • Influenza • Rubella
Contact	• Most important and frequent mode of transmission of nosocomial infections • Divided into two subgroups: direct-contact transmission and indirect-contact transmission • Direct-contact transmission occurs when touching the infectious patient's dry skin—for example, when performing patient care activities such as turning a patient or giving a bath; direct-contact transmission can also occur between two patients, with one serving as the source of the infectious microorganisms and the other as a susceptible host. • Indirect-contact transmission occurs when a contaminated object is touched, such as coming in contact with instruments, needles, dressings, environmental surfaces, or patient care items.	• Some gastrointestinal, respiratory, skin, and wound infections • Herpes simplex virus • Impetigo • Scabies

AIRBORNE PRECAUTIONS
(in addition to Standard Precautions)

VISITORS: Report to nurse before entering.

Use Airborne Precautions as recommended for patients known or suspected to be infected with infectious agents transmitted person-to-person by the airborne route (e.g., M. tuberculosis, measles, chickenpox, disseminated herpes zoster).

Patient placement

Place patients in an **AIIR** (Airborne Infection Isolation Room).
Monitor air pressure daily with visual indicators (e.g., flutter strips).

Keep door closed when not required for entry and exit.

In ambulatory settings instruct patients with a known or suspected airborne infection to wear a surgical mask and observe Respiratory Hygiene/Cough Etiquette. Once in an AIIR, the mask may be removed.

Patient transport

Limit transport and movement of patients to **medically-necessary purposes.**

If transport or movement outside an AIIR is necessary, instruct patients to **wear a surgical mask**, if possible, and observe Respiratory Hygiene/Cough Etiquette.

Hand Hygiene

Hand Hygiene according to Standard Precautions.

Personal Protective Equipment (PPE)

Wear a fit-tested NIOSH-approved **N95** or higher level respirator for respiratory protection when entering the room of a patient when the following diseases are suspected or confirmed: Listed on back.

APR

©2007 Brevis Corporation   www.brevis.com

Reprinted with permission from Brevis Corporation, www.brevis.com

FIGURE 10–16 Airborne precautions.

- It may require specialized equipment and environmental modifications that add to the cost of hospitalization.

- It makes frequent visits by nurses, physicians, and other personnel inconvenient, and may make it more difficult for personnel to give prompt and frequent care that sometimes is required.

- Using a multipatient room for one patient uses valuable space that otherwise might accommodate several patients.

- Forced solitude deprives the patient of normal social relationships and may be psychologically harmful, especially to children and confused patients. As part of the health care team, you must do all you can to decrease these psychological stresses, not only for humanitarian reasons, but also because they compromise the immune system. So, even if it is inconvenient, check on the patient frequently. Remember, you are isolating the pathogen, not the patient. Some hospitals protect the patient's privacy by posting a simple note stating that one must report to the nurse's station before entering the patient's room. (See Figure 10–19.)

DROPLET PRECAUTIONS

(in addition to Standard Precautions)

STOP **VISITORS: Report to nurse before entering.**

Use Droplet Precautions as recommended for patients known or suspected to be infected with pathogens transmitted by respiratory droplets that are generated by a patient who is coughing, sneezing or talking.

Personal Protective Equipment (PPE)

Don a mask upon entry into the patient room or cubicle.

Hand Hygiene

Hand Hygiene according to Standard Precautions.

Patient Placement

Private room, if possible. Cohort or maintain spatial separation of 3 feet from other patients or visitors if private room is not available.

Patient transport

Limit transport and movement of patients to **medically-necessary purposes**.

If transport or movement in any healthcare setting is necessary, instruct patient to **wear a mask** and follow Respiratory Hygiene/Cough Etiquette.

No mask is required for persons transporting patients on Droplet Precautions.

DPR7 ©2007 Brevis Corporation www.brevis.com

FIGURE 10–17 Droplet precautions.

These disadvantages, however, must be weighed against the hospital's mission to prevent the spread of microorganisms that may cause an epidemic.

Disposal of Hazardous Waste

The proper disposal of hazardous waste (contaminated materials) is also essential for maintaining a safe environment. When a patient is in isolation, there will be specially marked hazardous waste containers for trash and for linen located in the room. The only way to remove the contaminated items from the room is by using a *double-bagging* technique. Double-bagging involves taking the contaminated bag from the isolation room (the health care professional has appropriate PPE on) and slipping it into another bag held by a coworker outside the isolation room. Care is taken so that the coworker does not touch the contaminated bag, and the health care professional in the room does not touch the clean bag. The bags are labeled according to the facility policy with hazardous waste or linen markers to alert other personnel to the need for special handling.

CONTACT PRECAUTIONS
(in addition to Standard Precautions)

STOP **VISITORS: Report to nurse before entering.**

Gloves
Don gloves upon entry into the room or cubicle.
Wear gloves whenever touching the patient's intact skin or surfaces and articles in close proximity to the patient.
Remove gloves before leaving patient room.

Hand Hygiene
Hand Hygiene according to Standard Precautions.

Gowns
Don gown upon entry into the room or cubicle.
Remove gown and observe hand hygiene before leaving the patient-care environment.

Patient Transport
Limit transport of patients to medically necessary purposes.
Ensure that infected or colonized areas of the patient's body are contained and covered.
Remove and dispose of contaminated PPE and perform hand hygiene prior to transporting patients on Contact Precautions.
Don clean PPE to handle the patient at the transport destination.

Patient-Care Equipment
Use disposable noncritical patient-care equipment or implement patient-dedicated use of such equipment.

Form No. **CPR7**   BREVIS CORP., 225 West 2855 South, SLC, UT 84115   © 2007 Brevis Corp.

Reprinted with permission from Brevis Corporation, www.brevis.com

FIGURE 10–18 Contact precautions.

In addition to items from isolation rooms, other situations in which blood and body fluids are present require the disposal of hazardous waste. Examples include bloody tissues, culture dishes, and used bandages.

Neutropenic Precautions

Another type of precaution may be ordered for patients who are very susceptible to infections. The procedures followed are meant to protect the patient from infections brought in by people or other sources, rather than protecting the health care professional and visitors from patient infections.

These precautions are called neutropenic precautions, or reverse isolation. This type of precaution will most commonly be seen with an oncology patient who has a repressed immune system secondary to the cancer treatment (i.e., chemotherapy, radiation). A sign similar to Figure 10–19 can be posted on the patient's door. The general guidelines, in addition to standard precautions, are as follows:

- The patient is placed in a private room.

- No one who has an infection should enter the room.

Reprinted with permission of Briggs Corporation

FIGURE 10–19 Report to nurse signage.

- No visitors who have infections or recent exposure to **communicable** (contagious) **diseases** or vaccinations are allowed to enter the room.
- No unwashed fresh fruit or vegetables, raw eggs, or yogurt may be eaten.
- No flowers or plants are allowed in the room.
- Sources of stagnant water (e.g., denture cups, irrigating containers) should be avoided.

THE CHALLENGES

In spite of the great progress made in fighting infectious diseases and infections, there remain infectious diseases that have not been conquered. Viruses are especially problematic because of their ability to quickly mutate and their resistance to drugs. Another problem is that many bacteria, previously controlled by antibiotics, have become resistant to drugs. In the following sections, challenges that will be faced by health care professionals are discussed.

Influenza

Influenza (the flu) is a common infectious disease of the respiratory system that puts a substantial burden on the health of people in the United States. The CDC estimates that influenza has resulted in between 9.2 and 35.6 million illnesses, between 140,000 and 710,000 hospitalizations and between 12,000 and 56,000 deaths annually since 2010 (https://www.cdc.gov/flu/about /disease/burden.htm). It is especially lethal for the very young and the very old.

Common signs and symptoms of the flu include:

- Fever over 100.4 °F (38 °C)
- Aching muscles
- Chills and sweats
- Headache
- Dry, persistent cough
- Fatigue and weakness
- Nasal congestion
- Sore throat

Influenza does not involve the digestion system; that is, stomach upset, vomiting, and diarrhea are not symptoms of this disease.

Each year, vaccines are developed to protect against the flu. However, because of the variety of influenza viruses, scientists must estimate which will be dominant for the short-term future. Also, flu viruses mutate constantly and become resistant to vaccines. In spite of these limitations, the CDC report for 2016–2017 shows that the vaccine prevented the following:

- 5.1 million illnesses
- 2.5 million medical visits
- 71,000 hospitalizations (https://www.cdc.gov/flu /about/burden-averted/2015-16.htm)

Adults between ages 18 and 64 have the lowest rate of vaccination at less than 50% (https://www .cdc.gov/flu/fluvaxview/coverage-1516estimates .htm). If this rate increased, the number of preventions would increase significantly. A common myth is that getting the vaccine may cause an individual to get the flu; however, this is not possible, because the virus used in the vaccines are dead and cannot cause infection.

It is believed that flu virus is spread in droplets when an infected person coughs, sneezes, or talks, with droplets traveling up to six feet. Prevention focuses on being vaccinated each year and taking normal, germ-preventing measures such as frequent handwashing, covering the mouth when coughing, and sanitizing objects that may have flu germs.

Workplace Risks

Certain diseases pose especially serious risks to the health care professional. These include two blood-borne pathogens, hepatitis B virus (HBV) and human immunodeficiency virus (HIV), and an airborne-transmitted disease, tuberculosis (TB). Also of great concern are two drug-resistant infections that create unique challenges.

Hepatitis B

Hepatitis B virus infection (HBV) is the major infectious blood-borne occupational hazard for health care professionals. When an individual becomes infected, the liver, in its attempt to destroy the hepatitis virus, causes an inflammation and subsequent destruction of liver cells (hepat = liver; itis = inflammation of). Symptoms range from very mild to severe jaundice (yellowing of the eyes and skin), dark urine, fatigue, loss of appetite, nausea, abdominal pain, and sometimes joint pain, rash, and fever.

HBV can be spread via several routes:

- Parenteral: Blood transfusion, needle sharing by intravenous (IV) drug users, needlestick, or other sharp instrument
- Mucous membranes: Blood contamination of the eye or mouth
- Sexual contact
- Perinatal: From infected mother to newborn infant

(*Source:* OSHA Online)

Prevention efforts in health care settings are focused on the administration of hepatitis B vaccine, use of PPE, prevention of puncture injuries, and disinfection and sterilization of equipment and surfaces. OSHA mandates that employers provide hepatitis B vaccine for all employees who have an occupational exposure risk. The hepatitis B vaccines are given in three doses over a six-month period. These vaccines, when given according to manufacturer's directions, induce protective antibody levels in 85% to 97% of healthy adults. If there is some doubt about a person's immunity, a blood test can be done to verify presence of the antibody (OSHA Online). An employee has the right to refuse the hepatitis B vaccine, but if declined, the employee must sign a form stating his or her refusal. This releases the facility from responsibility should the health care professional become infected.

Although hepatitis B is the most common and most efficiently transmitted hepatitis virus, there are other hepatitis viruses of which the health care professional must have knowledge. (See Table 10–4.) Note that hepatitis A (HAV) and hepatitis E (HEV) are transmitted by the fecal-oral route. Hepatitis B (HBV), hepatitis C (HCV), and hepatitis D (HDV) are transmitted by blood and body fluids.

Human Immunodeficiency Virus

Human immunodeficiency virus (**HIV**) is the virus that causes acquired immune deficiency syndrome (**AIDS**). The virus destroys cells in the host that are vital to the proper functioning of the immune system. Individuals infected with the virus are said to be **HIV positive**. This is not the same as having AIDS, which means that the immune system has become weakened as a result of the action of the

Thinking It Through

Frank Gello is very excited about his new position as a surgical technologist at the local hospital, although he is somewhat intimidated by the person who is orienting him and is anxious to complete his training and work more independently. As they set up for the next surgery, his preceptor positions himself on the opposite side of the sterile field. As Frank opens the sterile instruments to place them on the sterile field, his preceptor talks him through the procedure and on several occasions he reaches across impatiently to move Frank's placement of the instruments. Frank also knows that he should check all of the packaging on the instruments for integrity to insure sterility has been maintained, but his preceptor abruptly states "I have already done that. Don't waste my time. Keep going as the surgeon is arriving in a few minutes."

1. Does this scenario refer to medical or surgical asepsis? What is the difference between medical and surgical asepsis?

2. Were any of the aseptic principles broken? If so, what are they?

3. Should Frank perform a double-check on the packaging to verify the integrity of the sterility of the instruments even if his preceptor states he has already performed that check?

virus. Until fairly recently, most individuals infected with the virus developed AIDS and died as the result of severe opportunistic infections. These are infections that individuals with normal immune systems rarely experience. The most common opportunistic infection and cause of death of persons with AIDS is *Pneumocystis carinii*.

Today, however, there are medicines called *antiretroviral therapy* (ART) that reduce the amount of HIV in the body. If the infection is diagnosed early and ART taken daily and good medical care received, patients can expect to live as long as people without HIV. Another drug now available can be taken to prevent HIV. Called *pre-exposure prophylaxis (PREP)*, it is taken daily by individuals at high risk for contracting the virus (https://aidsinfo.nih.gov /understanding-hiv-aids/fact-sheets/20/48/the-basics-of-hiv-prevention, 2018).

Carriers of HIV may not have symptoms or even detectable amounts of the virus in the blood during the first six months of infection. It is essential, therefore, that health care professionals understand how the virus is transmitted and follow standard precautions with *all* patients.

Table 10–4 Viral Hepatitis (Liver Diseases)

Type	Infectious Agent	Route of Transmission	Prevention and Recommendations
A	Acute liver disease caused by the hepatitis A virus (HAV), lasting from a few weeks to several months. It does not lead to chronic infection.	Ingestion of fecal matter, even microscopic amounts; from close person-to-person contact; or ingestion of contaminated food or drinks. Once you have had HAV, you cannot get it again.	Hepatitis A vaccination is recommended for all children starting at age 1 year, travelers to certain countries, and others at risk, such as: • Men who have sex with men • Injecting and noninjecting drug users • Persons with clotting-factor disorders (e.g., hemophilia) • Persons with chronic liver disease Short-term protection is obtained when immune globulin is given within 2 weeks of contact with HAV. Always wash hands with soap and water after using the bathroom, changing a diaper, and before preparing and eating food.
B	Liver disease caused by the hepatitis B virus (HBV). It ranges in severity from a mild illness, lasting a few weeks (acute), to a serious long-term (chronic) illness that can lead to liver disease or cancer. An infection occurs when blood or body fluids from an infected person enter the body of a person who is not immune.	Contact with infectious blood, semen, and other body fluids from an infected person, sharing contaminated needles to inject drugs, or from an infected mother to her newborn. Hepatitis B virus can remain active in dried blood for several days, so proper precautions must be followed when cleaning up dried blood.	Hepatitis B vaccination is recommended for all infants, older children, and adolescents who were not vaccinated previously, and adults at risk for HBV infection. Adults at risk include all health care professionals with an occupational risk. Other recommendations: • If having sex with more than one steady partner, use latex condoms correctly and every time you have sex. If allergic to latex, use a condom made of polyurethane or other synthetic material. The efficacy of latex condoms in preventing infection with HBV is unknown, but proper use may reduce transmission. • If pregnant, get a blood test for hepatitis B; infants born to HBV-infected mothers should be given hepatitis B immune globulin (HBIG) and vaccine within 12 hours after birth. • Do not inject drugs; if you do, stop and get into a treatment program; if you cannot stop, never share drugs, needles, syringes, or water; and get vaccinated against HAV and HBV. • Do not share personal care items that might have blood on them (e.g., razors, toothbrushes). • Consider risks if you are thinking about getting a tattoo or body piercing. You might become infected if the tools have someone else's blood on them or if the artist or piercer does not follow good health practices. • If you have or had HBV, do not donate blood, organs, or tissue. • If you are a health care or public safety worker, get vaccinated against HBV and always follow routine standard precautions and safely handle needles and other sharps.

(continues)

Table 10–4 Viral Hepatitis (Liver Diseases) *(continued)*

Type	Infectious Agent	Route of Transmission	Prevention and Recommendations
C	Liver disease caused by hepatitis C virus (HCV). HCV infection sometimes results in an acute illness, but most often becomes a chronic condition that can lead to cirrhosis of the liver and liver cancer.	Contact with the blood of an infected person, primarily through sharing contaminated needles to inject drugs.	There is no vaccine to prevent HCV. • Antiviral drugs are now available that cure 90% of cases. • Do not inject drugs; if you do, stop and get into a treatment program; if you cannot stop, never share needles, syringes, water, or any personal care items and get vaccinated against HAV and HBV. • Do not share personal care items that might have blood on them (e.g., razors, toothbrushes). • If you are a health care or public safety worker, always follow routine standard precautions and safely handle needles and other sharps; get vaccinated against HBV. • Consider risks if you are thinking about getting a tattoo or body piercing. You might become infected if the tools have someone else's blood on them or if the artist or piercer does not follow good health practices. • Can be spread by sex, but this is rare. If you are having sex with more than one steady sex partner, use latex condoms correctly and every time to prevent the spread of sexually transmitted diseases (if allergic to latex, use a condom made of polyurethane or other synthetic material); also get vaccinated against HBV. • If you are HCV positive, do not donate blood, organs, or tissue.
D	Serious liver disease caused by the hepatitis D virus (HDV), which relies on HBV to replicate. It is uncommon in the United States.	Contact with infectious blood, similar to the mechanisms by which HBV is spread.	There is no vaccine to prevent HDV. Recommendations are the same as for HCV.
E	Hepatitis E is a serious liver disease caused by the hepatitis E virus (HEV). It usually results in an acute infection and does not lead to a chronic infection. While rare in the United States, hepatitis E is common in many parts of the world. It is found in the stool (feces) of persons and animals with HEV.	Ingestion of fecal matter, even in microscopic amounts; outbreaks are usually associated with contaminated water supply in countries with poor sanitation. Transmission from person to person occurs less commonly than with HAV.	There is no vaccine to prevent HEV. • Always wash hands with soap and water after using the bathroom, changing a diaper, and before preparing and eating food. • Avoid drinking water (and beverages with ice) of unknown purity and avoid eating uncooked shellfish and uncooked fruits or vegetables that are not peeled or prepared by the traveler.

(continued)

Infection with HIV may be identified through testing the blood for the presence of HIV antibodies. Most people infected with HIV have detectable antibodies within six months of infection, with the majority generating detectable antibodies between six and 12 weeks after exposure. After individuals are HIV positive, they become lifelong carriers and can spread the virus to others.

HIV has been isolated from human blood, semen, breast milk, vaginal secretions, saliva, tears, urine, cerebrospinal fluid, and amniotic fluid; however, only blood, semen, vaginal secretions, and breast milk have been proven to transmit the virus. It is important to understand that *HIV is not transmitted by casual contact*. No evidence exists that HIV is transmitted by shaking hands or talking; by sharing food, eating utensils, plates, drinking glasses, or towels; by sharing the same house or household facilities; or by "personal interactions expected of family members," including hugging and kissing on the cheek or lips. HIV is also not transmitted by mosquitoes or other animals (OSHA Online).

The rate of infection from exposure is in relationship to the amount of infected material introduced into the body. For example, a person receiving a contaminated blood transfusion has a much greater chance of infection than a health care professional injured with a contaminated needle.

Fascinating Facts

Measles killed nearly 90,000 people globally in 2016, according to the World Health Organization. Nine out of the ten people who have not been vaccinated will develop an infection if they are exposed to someone with the virus and can even become infected if they walk into a room where an infected person has been.

Source: Fox (2018).

In fact, only 2.3 health care professionals out of 1,000 will become infected when injured with contaminated needles (https://www.cdc.gov/hiv/workplace/healthcareworkers .html). This is *not* to downplay the impact of acquiring such a devastating disease, but only to put the risk in perspective. Most health care professionals fear being infected by AIDS more than HBV, yet the infection and death rates of HBV far exceed those of AIDS. (See Table 10–5.)

Table 10–5 **HIV/AIDS**

Route of Transmission	Major Symptoms	Treatment	Prevention
AIDS is caused by the blood-borne virus HIV and is transmitted by: • Vaginal, oral, and anal sex • Sharing needles to inject drugs, body piercing, or tattooing • Contaminated blood products (rare) • Infected mother to newborn *Note*: It is *not* transmitted by shaking hands, social kisses, utensils, animals, hugging, swimming pools, toilet seats, food, insects, or coughing.	This disease mimics symptoms of many other infections, such as: • Flu-like illness • Swollen lymph nodes • Persistent fevers • Night sweats • Prolonged diarrhea • Unexplained weight loss • Purple bumps on skin or inside mouth and nose • Chronic fatigue • Recurrent respiratory infections *Note*: These symptoms are not specific for HIV and may have other causes. Most people with HIV have no symptoms at all for several years.	No preventative vaccine or cure is available, although current research is progressing in finding a cure. Early diagnosis and treatment can extend life for years. Keep immune system as strong as possible with medications and life style. Antiviral drugs slow cell processes and can extend life. Prompt treatment of AIDS-related illnesses decreases death due to complications. Medications are available for HIV-infected pregnant women to greatly reduce the chance of passing infection to newborn.	Prevention is similar to that for other blood-borne diseases: • Always use latex condoms/latex barriers during sex (if allergic to latex, use a condom made of polyurethane or other synthetic material). • Do not share needles for drugs, tattooing, or body piercings. • Limit number of sex partners. • Be tested and have potential partners tested for HIV; this can be done by providers, sexually transmitted disease (STD) clinics, and HIV counseling and testing sites. • Notify sex and needle-sharing partners immediately if HIV infected. A health care worker can prevent workplace exposure by following standard precautions and avoiding needlestick injuries.

Tuberculosis

Tuberculosis (TB) is caused by *Mycobacterium tuberculosis*, an airborne pathogen. Working with tuberculosis patients requires the use of special PPE, such as special masks fitted to the individual health care professional, to avoid inhaling the tiny droplets that carry the pathogen through the air. The TB bacteria are put into the air when a person with TB disease of the lungs or throat coughs, sneezes, speaks, or sings. People nearby may breathe in these bacteria and become infected.

TB is *not* spread by:

- Shaking someone's hand
- Sharing food or drink
- Touching bed linens or toilet seats
- Sharing toothbrushes
- Kissing

Once considered to be nearly eliminated from the United States, the number of cases of TB have increased recently. This is due in part to more global travel and the fact that some bacteria have become resistant to drug therapy. The development of resistant strains has occurred because medications must be taken for at least six months. Failure by some patients to complete the full length of treatment has allowed certain strains of the bacterium to develop resistance to the drugs.

Although renewed efforts to control TB have resulted in a slow, but steady decrease in cases, it remains one of the world's deadliest diseases. Depending on the source, it is estimated that between one fourth and one third of the world's population is infected with latent TB. In 2016, 10.4 million people around the world became sick with TB and there were 1.7 million TB-related deaths worldwide (https://www.cdc.gov/tb/statistics/default.htm).

The screening test for TB is a skin test. A positive test result does not necessarily indicate active disease, but does indicate that the person has had an exposure to the pathogen. A chest X-ray and other tests are done to determine if active disease is present. TB primarily affects the lungs, but can affect other parts of the body, such as the kidney, spine, and brain. Patients hospitalized with suspected TB are placed in isolation for two to three weeks during which time antibiotic treatment is given.

Not everyone infected with TB bacteria becomes sick. As a result, two TB-related conditions exist: latent TB infection and active TB disease.

- Latent TB infection: This condition is present when TB bacteria live in the body without making the person sick. In most people who breathe in TB bacteria and become infected, the body is able to fight the bacteria to stop them from growing.
- TB disease: TB bacteria become active if the immune system cannot stop them from growing. After the

Thinking It Through

Monica Stokes is a volunteer at a local extended care facility. Her duties include pushing a cart with books around to the patients' rooms to ask if they would like to borrow a library book. When she enters Mr. Haskin's room, the nurse asks her if she would please take the dirty linens and place them in the linen basket down the hall. She is new and unclear if this is one of her duties, but also desires to be helpful, and surely the nurse would not ask her if it were not appropriate. So she picks up the linens from the floor, carries them close to her, and places them in the linen basket. She notices some stains on her clothes, so she goes to the sink and rinses them off with cold water in the hope there will be no permanent stain. She then returns to her duties of distributing books to patients.

1. Was it appropriate for the nurse to ask the volunteer to assist with the linens?
2. Are all the links present in the chain of infection?
3. What breaks in standard precautions can you identify?

bacteria are active (multiplying in the body), the person will be sick with TB disease and can spread the disease to others. Some people develop TB disease soon after becoming infected (within weeks), before their immune system can fight the TB bacteria. Other people may become sick years later, when their immune system becomes weak for another reason. For persons whose immune systems are weak, especially those with HIV infection, the risk of developing TB disease is much higher than for persons with normal immune systems. (See Table 10–6.)

Fascinating Facts

More than 1.1 million people in the United States are living with HIV infection, and almost 1 in 6 (15.8%) are unaware of their infection. About 1 in 4 HIV infections are among youth ages 13 to 24. Most of them do not know they are infected, are not getting treated, and can unknowingly pass the virus on to others (https://www.hiv.gov/hiv-basics/overview/data-and-trends/statistics).

Table 10–6 Differences between Latent TB Infection and TB Disease

Person with Latent TB Infection	Person with TB Disease
Has no symptoms	Has symptoms that may include: • Bad cough that lasts 3 weeks or longer • Pain in the chest • Coughing up blood or sputum • Weakness or fatigue • Weight loss • No appetite • Chills • Fever • Sweating at night
Does not feel sick	Usually feels sick
Cannot spread TB bacteria to others	May spread TB bacteria to others
Usually has a skin test or blood test result indicating TB infection	Usually has a skin test or blood test result indicating TB infection
Has a normal chest X-ray and a negative sputum smear	May have an abnormal chest X-ray or positive sputum smear or culture
Needs treatment for latent TB infection to prevent active TB disease	Needs treatment to treat active TB disease

Source: CDC Online. www.cdc.gov

Other Infectious Diseases

Over the past several years, other contagious diseases have received a lot of media coverage. These include ebola, bird flu, mad cow disease, and swine flu which currently are not commonly seen in the United States. Today, the diseases that pose the most risks in other countries include yellow fever and zika virus. All these diseases can have a global impact because organisms easily cross borders, usually carried by international travelers. When an outbreak of a disease is first noted in another country, the United States immediately becomes involved in developing a plan of action. The CDC is actively involved in this process, working with partners throughout the nation and the world to monitor health, detect and investigate health problems, conduct research to enhance prevention, develop and advocate sound public health policies, implement prevention strategies, promote healthy behaviors, foster safe and healthful environments, and provide leadership and training. The CDC also lists specific warnings for travelers who plan to visit countries in which these diseases pose a danger on its website Travelers' Health, https://wwwnc.cdc.gov/travel.

In the United States, West Nile virus is the most common pathogen spread by mosquitoes. During the summer, there are cases reported in every state. About 1 in 5 people who are infected develop a fever and other symptoms while about 1 out of the 150 infected people develop a serious, sometimes fatal, illness (https://www.cdc.gov/westnile/index.html).

Drug-Resistant Organisms

The development of drug-resistant organisms is a fairly recent occurrence, the result of antibiotic usage. The CDC reports that this is one of the biggest health challenges of our time. Each year in the United States, at least 2 million people become infected with bacteria that are resistant to antibiotics and at least 23,000 people die each year as a direct result of these infections. Many more people die from other conditions that are complicated by an antibiotic-resistant infection (https://www.cdc.gov/drugresistance/index.html).

Antibiotics and similar drugs, together called antimicrobial agents, have been used for the past 70 years to treat patients who have infectious diseases. Penicillin, the first commercialized antibiotic, was discovered in 1928 by Alexander Fleming. Since the 1940s, these drugs have greatly reduced illness and death from infectious diseases. However, they have been used so widely and for so long that some of the infectious organisms the antibiotics are designed to kill have adapted to them, making the drugs less effective.

Another contributing factor is that antibiotics have routinely been overused by being prescribed for minor conditions. In addition, many patients fail to complete an entire course of antibiotic as prescribed. These two actions create conditions that encourage pathogens to become resistant to antibiotics. It is important to explain to patients why they must take all the medication prescribed for them, because many people have a tendency stop taking the antibiotic when they feel better.

The CDC lists antibiotic-resistant microorganisms by threat level. The 2013 report has 3 microorganisms at the urgent threat level, 21 at the serious threat level, and 3 at the concerning threat level. The CDC is currently working on updating and releasing a threat-level report in the fall of 2019 (https://www.cdc.gov/drugresistance/biggest_threats.html).

Two of these drug-resistant organisms commonly encountered in health care are *methicillin-resistant Staphylococcus aureus (MRSA)* and *vancomycin-resistant Enterococcus (VRE)*. Both are difficult to control and treat and can cause very serious infections. If there is a treatment available, it is usually very expensive and can have severe side effects, such as liver, kidney, and hearing damage. Because these infections occur most frequently in elderly patients who are more susceptible to the side effects and already have weakened resistance, they often result in death. (See Table 10–7.)

Table 10–7 Drug-Resistant Infections

Infectious Agent	Source/Route of Transmission	Major Symptoms	Prevention and Recommendations
MRSA (methicillin-resistant *Staphylococcus aureus*) is most frequently (85%) seen in persons in health care facilities who have weakened immune systems. This is called HA-MRSA (health care-associated or acquired MRSA). MRSA infections occurring outside of the health care setting in otherwise healthy people is known as CA-MRSA (community-associated or acquired MRSA). *Note*: MRSA is a type of staph that is resistant to certain antibiotics, such as methicillin, oxacillin, penicillin, and amoxicillin.	*S. aureus* bacteria are commonly carried on the skin or in the nose of healthy people. Approximately 25% to 30% of the population is colonized (when bacteria are present, but not causing an infection) in the nose with staph bacteria and about 1% are colonized with MRSA.	HA-MRSA symptoms vary with location of infection (skin, surgical wound, bloodstream, urinary tract, pneumonia). CA-MRSA is usually manifested as skin infections, such as pimples and boils and can be red, swollen, painful, or have pus or other drainage.	To prevent HA-MRSA: • See guidelines for VRE that follow. To prevent CA-MRSA: • Keep hands clean by washing thoroughly with soap and water or using an alcohol-based hand sanitizer • Good general hygiene • Keep cuts and scrapes clean and covered with a bandage until healed • Avoid contact with other people's wounds or bandages • Avoid sharing personal items, such as towels or razors Diagnosis of MRSA is frequently done by culture, which can take 2–3 days. If available, Xpert MRSA is a test that provides results in about an hour.
VRE (vancomycin-resistant enterococci) *Note*: Vancomycin is an antibiotic that is often used to treat infections caused by enterococci. When enterococci become resistant to this drug, it is called VRE. Enterococci infections are among the most common type acquired by hospitalized patients, almost always by patients who are already ill.	Enterococci are normally present in the human intestines, in the female genital tract, and are often found in the environment. VRE can also live here without causing disease (called colonization). However, sometimes it can cause infections of the urinary tract, the bloodstream, or of wounds. It is transmitted from person to person by the hands of caregivers or after contact with contaminated surfaces.	Varies with the location of the infection	• Handwashing • Keeping surfaces clean • Wearing gloves • Standard precautions • Follow facility guidelines for contact precautions in caring for patients with VRE

Source: https://medlineplus.gov/mrsa.html and the CDC

Fascinating Facts

Imagine ¼ teaspoon of HBV mixed into a 24,000-gallon swimming pool of water. Someone draws ¼ teaspoon of that water into a syringe and injects you with it. Although the virus is diluted well, you will become HBV positive. Now imagine that 10 people are in a room. Someone takes ¼ teaspoon of HIV and mixes it into a quart of water. Then ¼ teaspoon of this solution is injected into each person. Only one person in the room will become HIV positive. Hepatitis B is thus a much greater threat to health care professionals than HIV (Acello, 2009).

Another organism that the CDC states is an immediate public health threat requiring urgent and aggressive action is *Clostridium difficile*. Infections most often occur in people who have had both recent medical care and antibiotics. *C. difficile* causes life-threatening diarrhea. Although resistance to the antibiotics used to treat *C. difficile* is not yet a problem, the bacteria spread rapidly because they are naturally resistant to many drugs used to treat other infections. In 2011, the latest year reported by the CDC, 500,000 people became infected with 29,000 dying within 30 days of diagnosis (https://www.cdc.gov/HAI/organisms/cdiff/Cdiff_infect.html).

The seriousness of these infections emphasizes the importance of always following standard precautions and

Fascinating Facts

Persons exposed to TB may develop *latent* (inactive) TB infection. Almost 2 billion people (*one* fourth *of the world's population*) have latent TB infection, and about 10% of these infected individuals will develop active disease sometime during their lifetime. In an era marked by increased international travel and a global marketplace, no region of the world is immune from outside influences. International collaboration will be essential to eliminate TB (https://www.hiv.gov/hiv-basics/overview/data-and-trends/statistics).

any additional procedures developed by the health care facility to prevent their spread. Actions on the part of the health care professional can determine whether infections are kept under control or are spread among patients and other workers.

REPORTING ACCIDENTAL EXPOSURE

Any injury or accident involving exposure to blood or body fluids requires immediate washing of the affected area. After a thorough washing of the area, the next action is to report the incident to the supervisor. This must be followed by completion of a written incident or injury report according to facility or agency requirements. Prompt reporting allows for evaluation, appropriate treatment (if indicated), and follow-up of any problems resulting from the exposure. Failure to report an incident can result in negative health consequences for the health care professional and others, as well as the need to take time off from work to recover.

OSHA regulations require every facility to have an exposure control plan, written specifically for that facility. This plan has many components, including the predetermination of employee exposure risk to blood-borne pathogens, description of how employees at risk will be protected, and training and annual retraining and testing requirements for employees. Plans must also include policies and procedures to be followed if exposure does occur. The policies and procedures should include the following:

- Actions to be taken immediately upon exposure, such as washing the exposed area immediately with warm water and soap, or, if the eye or mucous membranes are involved, rinsing with normal saline

- Time frames for reporting

- To whom the incident must be reported

- Form(s) to complete and information that must be included, such as how exposure occurred and the name of the patient

- Recommended procedure for evaluating the risk and outcome of the exposure. For example, a baseline blood test would be run on the health care professional and then repeated at specified intervals, the patient's blood would be drawn to determine HBV and HIV status, and postexposure treatment would begin if indicated. Blood draws and treatments require the consent of the involved individual.

- Plan for counseling and information on safe practices to protect self and others

SUGGESTED LEARNING ACTIVITIES

1. If you have access to a microscope, take samples from various areas, such as your skin or mucous membranes, stagnant pond water, or decaying food, and look for microorganisms.

2. Watch a medical program on television and evaluate the action for breaks in aseptic technique (medical and surgical).

3. Practice handwashing technique in your home environment.

4. Observe the handwashing techniques of others when out in the community.

5. Research additional sources and read about the lives and contributions made by Louis Pasteur, Oliver Wendell Holmes, and Lord Joseph Lister, leaders in the history of infection control.

6. Practice donning and removing PPE using a robe as a gown, any type of gloves you may have, and a mask made with paper and a plastic strap.

7. Identify how your actions at work can affect the health and safety of your family.

WEB ACTIVITIES

Weather.com

50 Striking images of viruses and bacteria

https://weather.com/health/cold-flu/news/2019-01-30-stunning-microscopic-images-viruses-bacteria

Scan the images to view colored images of a variety of microbes.

Centers for Disease Control and Prevention

- Handwashing: Clean Hands Save Lives

https://www.cdc.gov/handwashing/

Read the information on the home page, then explore links of interest. Watch the video on proper handwashing technique. How can you use this information to help educate patients about habits that prevent the spread of germs?

- Antibiotic/Antimicrobial Resistance

https://www.cdc.gov/drugresistance/index.html

Explore the links to learn more about this important topic, then answer the following questions:

1. How serious is antibiotic resistance?

2. How can people protect themselves against infections?

3. What is the CDC doing to combat antibiotic resistance?

- Trends in Tuberculosis – 2016

https://www.cdc.gov/tb/publications/factsheets/statistics/tbtrends.htm

After reading the fact sheet, list 10 key facts about TB in the United States today.

- Standard Precautions in All Patient Care

https://www.cdc.gov/infectioncontrol/basics/standard-precautions.html

Link to information about handwashing, PPE, patient placement, etc. to review the information presented in this chapter.

- Remembering the 1918 Influenza Pandemic

https://www.cdc.gov/features/1918-flu-pandemic/index.html

After reading the web page, answer the following questions:

1. What were the reasons for the severity of the 1918 pandemic?

2. What is being done today to prevent future influenza pandemics?

- Yellow Fever Travel Information

https://wwwnc.cdc.gov/travel/page/yellow-fever-information

1. What causes yellow fever?
2. Where is there a current outbreak?
3. How can travelers protect themselves?

- Zika Travel Information

https://wwwnc.cdc.gov/travel/page/zika-travel-information

1. What is the most serious result of a zika infection?
2. What parts of the world are currently affected by the zika virus?

- Environmental Cleaning and Disinfecting for MRSA

https://www.cdc.gov/mrsa/community/environment/index.html

List 10 actions that can provide protection against MRSA.

Occupational Safety and Health Administration

- OSHA Model Exposure Control Plan

https://www.osha.gov/OshDoc/Directive_pdf/CPL_2-2_69_APPD.pdf

Review the example of a facility exposure plan to learn what health care facilities must do to comply with OSHA standards. When hired, you will be expected to read your facility's policies and procedures and follow them in case of an exposure.

- Infectious Diseases

https://www.osha.gov/SLTC/healthcarefacilities/infectious_diseases.html

Choose one of the links to CDC guidelines and report on your findings.

- Hepatitis B Vaccination Protection

https://www.osha.gov/OshDoc/data_BloodborneFacts/bbfact05.pdf

Read this OSHA notice to learn about how health care workers can be protected against Hepatitis B.

1. Would you choose to receive the vaccination if it is offered by your employer?
2. Why or why not?

- Bloodborne Pathogens Slide Presentation – OSHA

Enter "OSHA bloodborne pathogens slide presentation," then click on the website listed to access the slides.

View the slideshow for a visual review of the information presented in this chapter.

Worldometers

www.worldometers.info

Go to this website, scroll down the page to HEALTH and report on the following worldwide statistics:

1. Number of deaths due to communicable diseases this year
2. Number of HIV/AIDS infected people
3. Deaths caused by HIV/AIDS this year
4. Deaths caused by malaria this year

World Health Organization

Fact Sheets: Infectious Diseases

http://www.who.int/topics/infectious_diseases/factsheets/en/

Choose an infectious disease to read about and write a summary of what you learn.

American Council on Science and Health

Bloom, J., 36 Years Since AIDS hit – Now the possibility of a cure.

https://www.acsh.org/news/2018/03/17/36-years-aids-hit-now-possibility-cure-12700

How does this new discovery act on HIV to prevent AIDS?

REVIEW QUESTIONS

1. Why is it critical for health care professionals to apply infection control practices in the workplace?

2. Why are infections especially prevalent in health care facilities?

3. What are the roles of the CDC and OSHA in protecting the public against infectious diseases?

4. Name and describe the characteristics of each of the five types of infectious microbes. Include examples of diseases caused by each type.

5. What are three examples of defenses used by the body against infection?

6. What are the elements of the chain of infection?

7. What are medical and surgical asepsis?

8. How do antiseptics, disinfectants, and sterilization differ?

9. What is a sterile field?

10. How is a sterile field maintained?

11. How can the health care professional break the chain of infection?

12. What are the requirements of standard precautions?

13. In what situations is handwashing indicated? Describe the proper technique.

14. What is personal protective equipment and what is its purpose?

15. What is a blood-borne pathogen?

16. How can the health care professional avoid injuries with sharp instruments and needles?

17. What are the three ways that pathogens can be transmitted?

18. What are the three types of transmission-based precautions and what actions are performed in each?

19. What is the proper method for removing contaminated items, such as linen, from a patient's room?

20. What are neutropenic precautions and when should they be used?

21. What are the effects of influenza and what measures can be taken to prevent it?

22. Which three infectious diseases are major risks for health care professionals?

23. What is the source of information for travelers about infectious diseases outside the United States?

24. Name two drug-resistant organisms. What has caused the development of this resistance? What are the specific risks caused by these organisms?

25. What is the purpose of an exposure control plan? What are the policies and procedures that should be included?

APPLICATION EXERCISES

1. What are the behaviors demonstrated by Mr. Romero in the Case of the Traveling Microorganisms that jeopardize both him and his patients?

2. Nurse Kristie Rudzinski oversleeps and has barely enough time to dress and get to work on time. She decides to wait until she gets to the hospital to change the adhesive bandage on the finger she cut while fixing dinner last night. When she arrives at work she hears a patient calling for help. No one else is there, so she immediately goes to the patient's room. On entering, Kristie discovers that the patient's IV has become disconnected and blood is running from the patient's vein onto the linens. Without delay, she is at the bedside and solves the problem by reconnecting the tubing. The patient is very

grateful for her prompt assistance. Kristie leaves the room very pleased that she was able to help, especially because this is a patient she has cared for many times. He is an elderly gentleman who is undergoing chemotherapy and has already had more than his share of problems.

a. Evaluate the scenario to determine which elements in the chain of infection were present.

b. What revisions to Kristie's actions would have to occur to follow the principles of medical and surgical asepsis?

c. Which microorganisms would most likely be a threat to Kristie and to the patient?

PROBLEM-SOLVING PRACTICE

Gene Peterson works at Peaceful Retirement, a local skilled nursing facility, as a nursing assistant. He has always enjoyed working with the elderly population. He finds their wisdom, compassion, and humor very comforting. Prior to going to work, Gene has developed a routine of stopping to visit his grandfather and is just leaving for his visit when his mother calls to tell him his grandfather has been admitted to the hospital with tuberculosis. Gene is very concerned because he knew his grandfather had not been feeling well lately, but had no idea he was that ill. Using the five-step problem-solving process, determine what steps Gene should take next.

CHAPTER 11

Environmental Safety

KEY TERMS

bioterrorism
compatibility
emergency preparedness plan
environmental safety
flammable
incident report
inflammable
PASS
RACE
toxic
triage system

The Case of the Bomb Threat

Johanna Welks is a clinical assistant at the community hospital. As she sits at the nursing station, she reflects on how lucky she is to have a job she loves and one that is located only a few blocks from where she lives. When the phone rings, she answers the phone in a cheerful, professional manner: "Hello, this is 4 West, Mrs. Welks speaking, how may I help you?" What she hears next sends chills down her body. The caller states, "Your hospital killed my little girl, and now I will get my revenge. I have placed a bomb in the hospital." Mrs. Welks feels on the verge of hysteria. She thinks of hanging up and leaving or starting to yell for everyone to evacuate the hospital

(continues)

OBJECTIVES

Studying and applying the material in this chapter will help you to:

1. Explain the importance of environmental safety in maintaining the safety of the health care professional, the patients, and others.
2. List seven types of hazards in the health care environment.
3. Describe safety practices that will help prevent injuries and accidents in health care facilities, including moving, dressing, working with patients, and protecting self and others.
4. Give examples of how changes in the physical and mental health of a patient can increase the risk of injuries and accidents.
5. Explain how unsafe conditions in the workplace should be reported.
6. Define workplace violence and discuss preventive measures.
7. Identify the appropriate steps to take in the event of a fire.
8. Explain the meaning of PASS.
9. Identify the different classes of fire extinguishers and the types of fire on which to use each.
10. Explain the meaning of RACE.
11. List ways to prevent electrical hazards.
12. List the general guidelines that apply when handling chemicals.
13. Explain the risks and preventive actions for health care workers who are potentially exposed to radiation.
14. Define infectious waste and explain how to dispose of it.
15. Describe the precautions necessary when oxygen is in use.
16. Define bioterrorism and state how it should be reported.
17. Explain the organization and use of an emergency code system in a health care facility.
18. Explain the purpose and sample contents of an emergency preparedness plan.
19. List the actions that the health care worker must take when an emergency preparedness plan is in place.
20. Define triage system and give an example of how it works.

immediately. But then her head clears, and she thinks about what would be the smartest thing to do in this situation. She tries to keep the caller on the telephone as long as possible in order to determine more specifically where the bomb is located and when it will explode. At the same time she is listening closely to the voice on the phone (to determine the sex, the age, and whether the caller has an accent) and also for any background noise (e.g., car horns, trains, bells, music). This chapter will address the many environmental hazards found in health care facilities and how to keep patients and workers safe. Also discussed are the nature of an emergency preparedness plan, when it is initiated, and the role of the health care professional when the plan is in effect.

IMPORTANCE OF ENVIRONMENTAL SAFETY IN HEALTH CARE

Environmental safety means identifying and correcting potential hazards that can cause accidents and injuries. Workers in the health care and social assistance sectors suffer more injuries than those in any other industry, even construction and manufacturing. In 2010, there were 653,900 injuries and illnesses reported (https://www.osha.gov/SLTC/healthcarefacilities/index.html). These include the injuries and illnesses discussed in Chapters 9 and 10. In this chapter, we will discuss other types of hazards in the workplace, such as the examples listed in Table 11–1.

The health care professional must understand and follow workplace safety policies and procedures that reduce hazards and prevent accidents and know how to handle incidents correctly if they do occur.

The Occupational Safety and Health Administration (OSHA), in addition to the infection-control measures presented in Chapter 10, has many regulatory requirements that apply to other workplace safety issues. The exact policies and procedures may vary among health care facilities, but they must all meet the regulatory requirements of OSHA.

GENERAL SAFETY GUIDELINES

The best approach to safety is to focus on *prevention*. There are many ways that health care professionals can contribute to the prevention of common accidents and injuries that occur in the health care environment. Personal safety practices include ways to move safely within, and dress for, the workplace; work with patients; provide protection for oneself and others; and determine what, when, and how to report any accidents that do occur. The guidelines in this section present specific safety behaviors.

Moving Safely

Movement creates the potential for accidents such as falls. The following practices will limit such occurrences:

- Never run, even in an emergency. You can move swiftly without running if the situation warrants a fast pace.
- Stay to the right in hallways and be cautious when approaching intersections in order to prevent collisions. Pay attention to warning mirrors on corners.
- Remove any loose rugs from floors to prevent tripping or slipping.
- Open doors slowly to avoid injury to someone on the other side.
- Use handrails when climbing or descending stairs.
- Never run up or down the stairs.
- Never carry uncapped syringes or sharp instruments in hallways or between rooms.
- Watch for wet or greasy floors in areas where such spills might take place.

Dressing for Safety

Work in health care requires specific types of clothing and grooming to ensure the safety of both workers and patients:

- Wear long hair tied back or up to prevent contact with contaminated material or the contamination of clean materials; also, so that it cannot be pulled or caught in equipment.
- Do not wear earrings that extend beyond the earlobe so that they cannot be grabbed or caught.
- Wear enclosed shoes with no more than a 1- to 1½-inch heel to prevent injury to the feet.
- Limit jewelry to a smooth wedding band.
- Keep fingernails short. The longer the nail, both natural and artificial, the more likely it is that bacteria reside under its free edge.

Table 11–1 Common Health Care Workplace Hazards

Type of Hazard	Description	Examples
Chemical	May have toxic effects through inhalation, absorption through the skin or mucous membranes, or ingestion. Some irritate the skin on contact	Chemotherapeutic agents, disinfectants, cleaning solutions, alcohol, anesthesia
Environmental	Unsafe conditions in the workplace	Slip, trip, and fall hazards; cramped working space, inefficient equipment, and inadequate equipment maintenance; fire and electrical hazards
Ergonomic (musculoskeletal)	Unsafe workplace design and lack of appropriate client- and material-handling tools and equipment contributing to increased risk of musculoskeletal disorders. Poor lighting, excessive vibration, and noise are also considered ergonomic hazards.	Activities that require lifting heavy loads; twisting, bending, reaching, and holding body parts and other materials for long periods; standing for long periods; pushing, pulling, awkward postures, and repetitive motions; high detail work in dimly lighted area; noisy environment *Note:* Ergonomics is covered in Chapter 9.
Infectious (biological)	May cause infection through inhalation, direct contact with skin or mucosa, skin puncture, or through ingestion (eating or drinking)	Bacteria, viruses, fungi, and other living microorganisms *Note:* This topic is covered in Chapter 10.
Physical	Agents that can cause physical injury and tissue damage	Radiation, noise, explosive objects or substances (e.g., oxygen)
Psychosocial	Stressors in the workplace causing workplace anxiety, emotional fatigue, and burnout	Providing constant emotional support, coping with emergency situations, inadequate staffing, lack of supervisor support, and frequent schedule changes; bioterrorism *Note:* Coping with stressors and avoiding burnout is covered in Chapter 12.
Workplace violence	Any physical assault or verbal abuse that is incurred during the course of performing one's duties at work	Being pushed, hit, or restrained; spoken to in a loud or demeaning manner, cursed at or berated; this type of hazard could also be listed under physical or psychosocial hazards depending on the nature of the violence

Source: Adapted from *Working Safely in Health Care: A Practical Guide,* by Deborah L. Fell-Carlson, 2008, Clifton Park, NY: Delmar Cengage Learning.

Working Safely with Patients

Patient safety is always a primary concern. Focusing on the task at hand and thinking through patient care activities are essential ways to promote safety.

- Do not perform any procedure on patients until you have received adequate training and do not alter the correct procedure (avoid shortcuts).
- Observe and note conditions in patients that might increase their risk of accident and injury. (See Table 11–2.)

- Be absolutely positive you have the correct patient. Always identify your patient by checking his or her wristband against the patient's record. In some health care settings, patients will not have a wristband (e.g., a physician's office). These patients can be identified by asking them to tell you their full name. Do not ask, "Are you Mr. Jones?" because many confused patients will reply affirmatively. Many facilities require two forms of identification, such as having them state their name and their birth date.

Table 11–2 Physical and Mental Changes That Increase the Risk of Injuries and Accidents

Physical or Mental	Change the Risk	Health Care Considerations
Changes in vision	Unable to see unsafe conditions and/or unable to judge distances	Identify yourself when approaching or entering the room. Provide unobstructed walkways. Place items needed by patients within their visual field. Explain the location of items orally.
Changes in hearing	Unable to hear warnings or approaching carts and equipment	Face the patient when speaking. Speak clearly, but do not yell. Notice when patients do not react to warning sounds.
Altered neurological function	Shaking or tremors can affect balance and increase the risk of falls; decreased sensation can prevent normal warning signals (e.g., can step on sharp object and not be aware of injury)	Pay increased attention to physical signs of injury. Give extra assistance, as needed. Do not leave patient alone on treatment table or under any conditions where falls might occur.
Changes in blood vessels	Dizziness when attempting to stand and increased risk of falls	Instruct patients to get up slowly. Assist patients as necessary.
Slowed reflexes (automatic reactions that cause us to pull away from danger)	Unable to move away quickly from danger (e.g., removing hand from hot surface or from under hot water, or unable to stop in time to avoid collision)	Provide patient and family with information about possible unsafe behaviors and ways to safeguard the home.
Changes in mental function	Confusion and forgetfulness can impair good judgment and decrease awareness of common dangers	Provide family with information about medications, home health resources, and safeguarding the home.
Weakness from illness or injury	More prone to falls	Observe patients carefully. Provide extra assistance. Instruct the family about extra precautions needed.
Taking medications	Side effects of some medications cause dizziness, visual disturbances, and other problems that increase the risk of injury	Instruct patient and family to report symptoms immediately. Monitor patients carefully when administering medications and do not leave them alone immediately afterward; watch for possible reactions.

- Always verify that the patient has given consent, because patients have the right to refuse any procedure or medication.
- Observe patients closely and report any changes immediately or assist them as needed. Do not leave patients unattended on treatment tables.
- Leave the bed in a low position, side rails up (if needed), wheels locked, and place the call signal, telephone, and bed controls within the patient's reach.
- Keep the work area clean, dry, and organized for efficient use. Place all supplies and equipment in their proper storage location.

Protecting Yourself and Others

Health care environments contain many potential hazards. It is essential to apply safety practices that consider the well-being of others:

- Follow the standard precautions discussed in Chapter 10.
- Do not open more than one file cabinet drawer at a time to prevent tipping.
- Do not leave cabinet doors open because someone may hit his or her head or trip.
- Do not place food in a refrigerator that contains lab specimens or medications.

FIGURE 11–1 Sweep up broken glass. Wear gloves.

FIGURE 11–2 Clean up spills immediately. When bodily secretions or blood are involved, follow standard precautions.

- Do not wear uniforms in nonwork settings.
- Keep floors clear by immediately picking up dropped objects. Use OSHA standards when cleaning up glass, spilled specimens, and liquids. Never use your hands to pick up broken glass: use a brush or broom and dustpan, or if these are not available, scoop up with pieces of cardboard or heavy paper (Figure 11–1) and place in puncture-resistant wrap or container, prior to placing in a plastic bag. This will prevent cuts on the hands of anyone who handles the bag. When the spill involves bodily secretions or blood, follow standard precautions by using gloves and disposing of waste in special bags designated for biohazardous waste. (See Figure 11–2.)

Reporting for Safety

Properly reporting unsafe conditions and accidents provides a means of making corrections and preventing future problems.

- Report any unsafe conditions immediately, such as burned-out exit sign lights, equipment or flooring in need of repair, frayed electrical cords, and side rails or signal lights that do not work.
- Report any accidents or injuries immediately and complete an incident report. An **incident report** is a

written document completed when any unexpected situation occurs that can cause harm to a patient, an employee, or any other person. It contains only factual information, and most facilities have policies that specify not to include the report in the patient's chart or to refer to the incident or the incident report in any of the patient's health documentation. The following are examples of what might be included in an incident report for a fall:

- Circumstances—how it happened
- Date, time, and location
- Accounts of any witnesses
- Any hazards that contributed to the fall
- Care given to the person who fell

WORKPLACE VIOLENCE

The National Institute for Occupational Safety and Health (NIOSH) defines workplace violence as "violent acts (including physical assaults and threats of assaults) directed toward persons at work or on duty." Health care workers are at more risk for workplace violence than those in other industries. In fact, they are four times more likely to suffer an injury than workers in construction and manufacturing. The highest rate of violence against health care workers occurs in psychiatric and

Thinking It Through

Peta Fry works as a respiratory therapist at a busy medical center. This particular day is busier than usual and it seems no matter how quickly Peta works, she cannot get her assignments done to keep on schedule. It is important for Peta to finish on time because she has a friend picking her up in front of the hospital right after work to go out for dinner. While working with Mrs. Homer, a bottle of water is accidentally tipped over because the patient did not see it due to her poor vision. Peta makes a mental note to call housekeeping when she finishes, so they can clean up the spill. When she finishes with Mrs. Homer, Peta realizes that she is going to be late and is afraid her friend will be upset. In an effort to save time, she decides not to change into the street clothes she brought with her to work and runs as quickly as she can to meet her friend.

1. Identify at least three behaviors of Peta that jeopardize environmental safety. What are the possible consequences of these unsafe behaviors?

2. What health care considerations could Peta have followed when working with the patient with impaired vision that may have prevented the bottle of water from spilling?

substance abuse hospitals (Dressner, 2017). Hospital nurses and nursing assistants who have the most direct contact with patients are also at higher risk. In response to reports that 20% of nurses and nursing students are being physically assaulted annually, the American Nursing Association launched the NurseAbuse Initiative in 2018. The Association wants health care professionals to sign a pledge supporting zero tolerance for violence against nurses and also for nurses to feel empowered to come forward to report abuse.

In addition to physical assaults, workplace prevention programs may include measures to prevent verbal violence, such as verbal abuse, hostility, and harassment that can cause psychological trauma and stress.

Depending on the source, between 80% and 93% of violent incidences in health care settings are caused by client aggression toward caregivers. In other workplaces, such as convenience stores and taxicabs, violence most often relates to robbery. Violence in a health care facility usually results from patients—and occasionally from their family members—who feel frustrated, vulnerable, and powerless. In addition, head injuries, mental health issues, and the effects of anesthesia can cause patients to act out against their caregivers.

Examples of violence are demonstrated in the following actual case reports:

- An elderly patient verbally abused a nurse and pulled her hair when she prevented him from leaving the hospital to go home in the middle of the night.
- An agitated psychotic patient attacked a nurse, broke her arm, and scratched and bruised her.
- A disturbed family member whose father had died in surgery at the community hospital walked into the emergency department and fired a small-caliber handgun, killing a nurse and an emergency medical technician and wounding the emergency physician.

Unfortunately, many incidents go unreported, in some settings up to 30%. Bullying and other forms of verbal abuse among employees are frequently unreported due to the lack of a reporting policy, lack of faith that anything will be done, and a fear of retaliation.

Much rarer, but still a problem, are events involving gang violence in the emergency department and domestic disputes that enter the workplace.

The effects of violence go further than the actual injuries and psychological trauma. Violence may also have negative organizational outcomes, such as low worker morale, increased job stress, increased worker turnover, reduced trust of management and coworkers, and a hostile working environment. These factors can then result in a higher risk of medication errors and patient infections.

Both the employer and the employee have a responsibility to decrease violent occurrences. Review Table 11–3 for some methods of preventing or decreasing workplace violence.

FIRE AND ELECTRICAL HAZARDS

Fires in health care facilities can result from a number of hazards, such as damaged equipment, overloaded circuits, defects in heating systems, spontaneous combustion, improper trash disposal, and smoking. It is important to familiarize yourself with the recommended policies and procedures for the health care facility in which you work. When a fire starts, there is no time to read the policy and procedure manual, and valuable minutes are lost if you hesitate to act promptly and correctly.

It is critical to stay calm during an emergency. A number of decisions must be made, and clear thinking is needed to properly assess the problem. If your safety is at risk, leave the area and sound the alarm. If the fire is small

Table 11–3 **Workplace Violence Preventive Measures**

Employer	Employee
Environmental designs: • Develop emergency signaling, alarms, and monitoring systems. • Install security devices such as metal detectors to prevent armed persons from entering. • Install other security devices, such as cameras and good lighting, in hallways. • Provide security escorts to the parking lots at night. • Design waiting areas to accommodate and assist visitors and patients who may have a delay in service. • Design the triage area and other public areas to minimize the risk of assault (provide staff restrooms and emergency exits, install enclosed nurses' stations, install deep service counters to increase distance from patients or bullet-resistant and shatterproof glass enclosures in reception areas, arrange furniture and other objects to minimize their use as weapons). Administrative controls: • Design staffing patterns to prevent personnel from working alone and to minimize patient waiting time. • Restrict the movement of the public in hospitals by card-controlled access. • Develop a system for alerting security personnel when violence is threatened. Behavior modification: • Provide all workers with training in recognizing and managing assaults, resolving conflicts, and maintaining hazard awareness.	Watch for signals that may be associated with impending violence: • Verbally expressed anger and frustration • Body language such as threatening gestures • Signs of drug or alcohol use • Presence of a weapon Maintain behavior that helps diffuse anger: • Present a calm, caring attitude. • Do not match the threats. • Do not give orders. • Acknowledge the person's feelings (e.g., "I know you are frustrated"). • Avoid any behavior that may be interpreted as aggressive (e.g., moving rapidly, getting too close, touching, or speaking loudly). Be alert: • Evaluate each situation for potential violence when you enter a room or begin to relate to a patient or visitor. • Be vigilant throughout the encounter. • Do not isolate yourself with a potentially violent person. • Always keep an open path for exiting—do not let the potentially violent person stand between you and the door. Take these steps if you cannot defuse the situation quickly: • Remove yourself from the situation. • Call Security for help. • Report any violent incidents to your management.

and contained and your safety and that of others are not at risk, determine which type of extinguisher is appropriate to use and proceed with the proper handling procedure. Remember that your safety and that of others come first.

Fires require three things to start: oxygen or air, an item that will burn to supply fuel (trash, linen, chemicals), and a source of heat (sparks, flames, matches). (See Figure 11–3.) To respond promptly and correctly to a fire, you must be knowledgeable in the following areas:

• The location of fire alarms and extinguishers

• How to use a fire extinguisher—carry the extinguisher upright. To help remember the proper sequence of operation, think **PASS**:

1. **P**ull the pin.
2. **A**im the nozzle at the *base* of the fire.
3. **S**queeze the handle.
4. **S**weep back and forth along the *base* of the fire. (See Figures 11–4 a–c.)

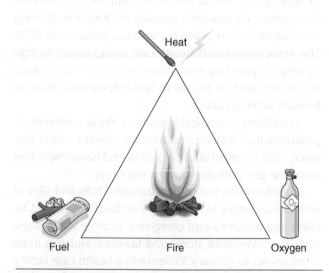

FIGURE 11–3 The fire triangle: elements needed for combustion (burning).

FIGURE 11–4a Verify that the fire extinguisher is the correct class to use.

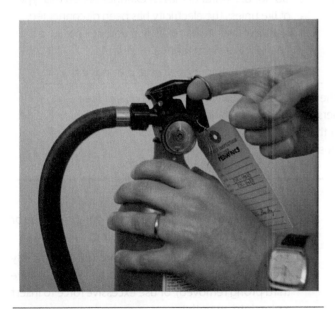

FIGURE 11–4b *Pull* the pin.

- How to respond to each type of fire—fire extinguishers vary for different types of fire. Using the wrong type of fire extinguisher can result in spreading a fire rather than putting it out. (See Table 11–4.)
- The emergency evacuation routes (See Figure 11–5.)
- What procedures to follow—although procedures may vary at individual facilities, there are generally accepted guidelines to use when a fire occurs. These are outlined in Table 11–5. To help you remember the proper sequence, think **RACE**:

FIGURE 11–4c *Aim* the nozzle at the base of the fire and *squeeze* handle. *Sweep* back and forth along the base of the fire.

1. **R**emove patients
2. **A**ctivate alarm
3. **C**ontain the fire
4. **E**xtinguish the fire or **E**vacuate the area (See Figure 11–6.)

- In case of a major fire, follow all instructions carefully. Your duties may include assisting patients into wheelchairs or onto stretchers. Advise ambulatory (able to walk) patients about evacuation routes.
- Many facilities have a policy that no personal electrical equipment can be brought into the hospital because the possibility that it may be defective is a fire risk. Larger facilities will have environmental safety personnel who verify the safety of facility equipment. Check the policy manual to determine if the environmental safety personnel will also check personal equipment. If so, they will attach a tag verifying the completion of the safety check.

Most electrical hazards can be avoided by following a few general safety practices:

- Always be thoroughly familiar with any equipment before attempting to use it independently for the first time. Know and follow all safety precautions.
- Review and follow the manufacturer's operating instructions. The health care professional should not use shortcuts or experiment with unfamiliar equipment.
- If any damage to the equipment is noted, do not attempt to use it, but report it to the proper person for repair. If the health care professional is not trained

Table 11–4 Types of Fires and How to Extinguish

Type of Fire	How to Extinguish	Cautions
Class A Most common type of fires (ordinary combustibles, e.g., paper, cloth, rubber, plastic, wood, trash, or mattress fires)	Use either water, a Class A fire extinguisher, or a Class ABC fire extinguisher. Class A extinguishers are water based and contain pressurized water or aqueous film-forming foam (AFFF). Class ABC extinguishers release a multipurpose dry chemical (monoammonium phosphate) that blankets the burning area and interrupts the chemical chain reaction.	Class A extinguishers—no special precautions; follow the proper sequence of operation (PASS) required with all extinguishers. Class ABC extinguishers—leave a white powdery residue irritating to skin and eyes. Do not stand too close to the fire. Take care when using extinguisher. Wash skin as soon as possible after extinguishing fire. The chemical is corrosive and will damage computers and electrical equipment.
Class B **Flammable** (easily set on fire; same as **inflammable**) and combustible liquids (e.g., gas, oil, paint, solvents, and cooking fat fires)	Use Class B, BC, or ABC fire extinguishers. Class B extinguishers release carbon dioxide (CO_2), which forms a cloud of dry ice or snow. The cloud displaces air and cuts off the fire's oxygen supply, thereby providing a smothering action.	Do not use water or a Class A fire extinguisher on a Class B fire because most burning liquids will float on top of the water, which spreads the fire further. Class B extinguishers—no special precautions; they are noncorrosive and do not damage computers and other electrical equipment, but are heavy and have a shorter discharge range. Class ABC extinguishers—see previous entry.
Class C Electrical fires (e.g., electrical equipment, fuse boxes, wiring, and appliances)	Use Class C, BC, or ABC extinguisher. Same as Class B because carbon dioxide is used, which is nonconducting and provides a smothering action.	Do not use water or Class A extinguisher on this type of fire unless the electricity has been disconnected. Electrical fires are particularly hazardous because the possibility of electrocution is present. Class ABC extinguishers—see previous entry.
Class D Burning metals (not typically seen in the health care environment)	Use Class D extinguisher or smother with dry sand. Class D extinguishers release a sodium chloride powder that when heated forms a crust. The crust excludes air and fire is smothered.	Do not use any of the other types of fire extinguishers on this type of fire.

FIGURE 11–5 All personnel should be familiar with the emergency evacuation plan established by the facility in which they work.

in the repair of a particular piece of equipment, he or she should never attempt to repair it.

- Never use electrical cords that are not completely intact, use plugs that have been altered (i.e., have third prong removed), or use excessive force to insert a plug into an outlet.

- Never handle any electrical equipment around water because electrocution can occur (water conducts electrical currents). Holding electrical equipment with wet hands, standing in water, or removing equipment that has been accidentally dropped in water can be life threatening. Always dry hands, clean up any spilled water, and remove the power source.

- If someone is being shocked (electrically), do not touch the person or pull the plug from the wall because this places you at risk. Instead, turn the main source of power off immediately and be prepared to administer emergency care and call for help.

Table 11–5 What to Do When You Discover a Fire: RACE

Guideline	Rationale
R Remove any patient who is in danger. Ambulatory patients can walk to safety; others may need wheelchairs or can be pushed in beds. Never use elevators during a fire; instead, carry nonambulatory patients in a linen sling, held at each end by a health care professional, while descending steps.	Places patient safety first. Fires can travel through elevator shafts, cables can be damaged, and elevators can get stalled between floors if power fails.
A Activate the fire alarm and notify the facility telephone operator/receptionist.	Pulling the fire alarm sends an alarm call to the fire station. The facility telephone operator(s) are often key to communication, and an exact location of the fire should be given to them.
C Contain the fire by closing all windows and doors. Follow facility procedure for turning off oxygen and electrical equipment.	Decreases the amount of air available to the fire. Drafts (air currents) cause fire to spread more rapidly. Prevents explosions and further fueling of the fire
E Extinguish small fires with an extinguisher. Stand 6 to 10 feet from the nearest edge of the flame and aim at the base of the fire. For large fires, follow or start evacuation procedures.	Allows for immediate extinguishing of fire before it spreads farther. If fire is too large, do not attempt to put out; instead, use that time to initiate further evacuation procedures
Keep exits clear at all times.	Allows patients and workers to leave if necessary
Maintain an exit at all times—never let the fire get between you and the exit.	Prevents the health care professional and patients from being trapped in a confined area
If smoke is present, workers and patients should crawl or move close to the floor toward the exit.	Decreases inhalation of smoke because smoke rises. More oxygen is available closer to the floor. All fires give off toxic gases, which are in the smoke.
A damp towel or similar cloth may be used to cover the mouth and nose for breathing.	Decreases the temperature of inhaled air and filters soot particles from the air
Always check the temperature of a door before opening it. If a door is hot to the touch, do not open it.	Prevents burns caused by a sudden burst of flames escaping the room when the door is opened
If you are trapped in a room and the door is hot to the touch, stay in the room (lie on the floor for more oxygen and less smoke) and place wet towels or blankets under the door.	Wet towels decrease the smoke entering the room.

Remove   Activate alarm   Contain   Extinguish or   Evacuate

FIGURE 11–6 Remember the sequence of critical actions to follow in case of fire.

CHEMICAL HAZARDS

Hundreds of chemicals are used in health care, such as cleaning solutions, anesthesia, and drugs used for chemotherapy. Chemicals can often cause harm if swallowed, inhaled, or absorbed through the skin or mucous membranes. Some also create a fire hazard. Great care must be taken when working with or near these agents. As discussed in Chapter 10, OSHA requires all health care facilities to have an exposure control plan.

OSHA has special requirements for hazardous chemicals in its Hazard Communication Standard. Manufacturers and distributors of specified chemicals must prepare Safety Data Sheets (SDSs, formerly called Material Data Safety Sheets or MSDSs) that include precautions to take when handling the chemical, safety instructions for use, requirements for clean-up and disposal, and first aid measures to take if exposure occurs. SDSs for all chemicals used in a facility must be available to all employees.

There are some general guidelines that apply whenever any type of chemicals are handled:

- If the container is not properly labeled or if it cannot be read clearly, do not use it.

- Recheck labels at least three times. Read the label carefully when you first locate it, and then reread it after removing the solution and again before returning it to its proper location.

- Never mix any two chemicals together without first verifying compatibility (i.e., if they can be combined without unfavorable results).

- Avoid contact with the eyes and skin and do not inhale.

- Take precautions not to splash or spill solutions.

- Wear personal protective equipment (PPE) as indicated.

- Make sure chemicals are used only for their intended purpose.

- Store chemicals as directed on the labels. For example, does the chemical require room temperature storage or refrigeration? Can it be stored on the counter or does it require a dark environment? Never place chemicals in direct sunlight or close to heat.

- Do not pour toxic (poisonous), flammable, foul-smelling, or irritating chemicals down the drain. Instead, place them in the specified container as per the policy and procedure manual.

- If you spill any solutions, clean up immediately according to established procedures and dispose of the debris properly.

- If a chemical does come in contact with the skin, rinse immediately under cool water for at least 5 minutes.

Splashes in the eye should be rinsed for a minimum of 15 minutes, preferably with normal saline. Report any accidents immediately to the supervisor and seek medical assistance for evaluation and follow-up.

RADIATION HAZARDS

Health care professionals in areas where X-rays or radiation therapy are used must practice safety precautions to prevent exposure to radiation waves and particles. Excessive radiation exposure can put the employee at risk for developing tissue damage, contracting cancer, or becoming sterile (unable to have children) or may lead to infants being born with birth defects. OSHA requires that employees at risk for radiation exposure must wear safety monitoring film badges, called dosimeters, that record the amount of exposure. Safety guidelines have been developed that determine the maximum level of radiation exposure allowed per employee. These are checked on a regular schedule to ensure that employees are not receiving too much exposure. Lead aprons and gloves are also worn by anyone who may be exposed to direct X-rays or scattered rays.

In most states, only health care workers who have received special training and are licensed can take radiographs or assist in procedures involving radiation. An act was introduced to the U.S. Congress in 2013, still under consideration, that would require all states to certify all personnel who work with radiation therapy modalities.

There are strict guidelines for the proper disposal of radiological waste. Radioactive waste must be placed in a special container and labeled as "radioactive." It should never be placed in the trash, incinerated, placed in a bag with other waste products, or put down a drain. Only a licensed removal facility can remove these wastes from the health care facility.

INFECTIOUS WASTE

Infectious waste is any item or product that has the potential to transmit disease. Infectious waste, also called hazardous waste, must be handled using standard and transmission-based precautions (discussed in Chapter 10), placed in containers or bags labeled as to type of waste (e.g., linen, sharps, trash), and decontaminated or incinerated on site or removed by a licensed removal facility for decontamination. It is the health care professional's responsibility to follow the facility's policies and procedures in the proper handling, containment, cleanup of spills, and disposal of infectious waste. OSHA requires that any employee who may be exposed to hazardous waste be trained on specific handling and disposing techniques.

This training must be updated annually. Any direct contact with waste that puts the worker at risk of infection must be reported per facility policy.

OXYGEN HAZARDS

When a patient is unable to take in adequate oxygen on his or her own, the physician may order the administration of oxygen: how much oxygen to give, what device to use for oxygen delivery (Figures 11–7a and 11–7b), and how long it is to be administered.

Special precautions are necessary when oxygen is in use:

- Most facilities have signs stating "Oxygen in Use" that are posted as specified in the facility policy.

- Sparks can come from some electrical appliances, equipment, or toys. Before using any of these, always check with the supervisor. Examples include hair dryers, heating pads, space heaters, fans, radios, electric shavers, and handheld computer games.

FIGURE 11–7a Oxygen being delivered by nasal cannula.

FIGURE 11–7b Oxygen being delivered by mask.

- Never use flammable liquids, such as alcohol, oils, adhesive tape remover, nail polish, or nail polish remover.

- An oxygen tank should be secured to prevent it from falling over. Do not place it in the sunlight or near heat. The stem-and-valve assembly on the tank is fragile and if mishandled the cylinder can become a missile as the pressurized gas is suddenly released.

- Smoking is not allowed when oxygen is in use, and smoking materials must be removed from the room. Fortunately, most facilities no longer allow smoking at any time, due to the health risk to the person and others. Always be alert for those who disregard the rules. No lighted matches or open flames should be permitted in the area.

- Use cotton blankets, gowns, or clothing. Wool and synthetics are more apt to create static electricity.

BIOTERRORISM

Bioterrorism refers to microbes or toxins used as weapons. Since the devastating attack on the United States that occurred on September 11, 2001, there has been a tremendous amount of discussion about, and preparation for, a bioterrorist attack. However, bioterrorism is not new to our times. It extends back in history to the earliest of human records. In the 14th century, cadavers were catapulted into enemy camps to create an outbreak of plague or to create such a fear that the enemy would flee and thus be defeated. British forces were suspected of giving Native Americans blankets contaminated with smallpox that led to an epidemic. Over the years, there have been numerous examples of attempts to contaminate food sources and develop weapons for the purpose of dispensing biological organisms.

Although bioterrorist attacks in the United States are very rare, the release of inhalational anthrax in a public place or the release of smallpox virus could affect thousands of people. Therefore, one of the functions of an emergency preparedness plan is the incorporation of a biological exposure readiness plan. The first step in this plan is to become aware of, and report, a suspected bioterrorism-related outbreak. If such an attack is suspected, the Federal Bureau of Investigation (FBI) would be immediately notified. But it may not be possible to wait for definitive evidence to determine if there is a biological threat, so the best approach would be to base the suspicion on epidemiological factors, such as a sudden and rapid increase of disease in a normally healthy population, large numbers of people with the same symptoms, or other atypical or unusual presenting factors.

Table 11-6 Bioterrorism Agents

Disease	Transmitted Person to Person?	Type of Precaution Recommended
Anthrax, cutaneous	Possible	Standard
Anthrax, gastrointestinal	No	Standard
Anthrax, pulmonary	No	Standard
Botulism	No	Standard
Plague, bubonic	No	Standard
Plague, pneumonic	Yes	Droplet
Smallpox	Yes	Airborne/contact

There are numerous agents that can be used for bioterrorism-related diseases, but it is believed that the most likely biological weapon would be anthrax, smallpox, botulism, or plague. In the event of an outbreak, the appropriate type of transmission precautions would be in force. (Chapter 10 covers precautions.) The majority of agents of bioterrorism are not transmitted person to person, so exposure to those agents can be contained by the proper precautions. If exposure to anthrax or smallpox does occur, a regimen of antibiotics for anthrax or a vaccination for smallpox can help lessen or even prevent the development of symptoms. (See Table 11-6.)

EMERGENCY CODE SYSTEM

Many health care facilities use a code system to communicate to the employees in the building when certain emergencies occur. Larger facilities with an overhead paging system will announce by using these codes along with a location (if appropriate). A code system prevents patients and visitors from becoming overly concerned. Code Red (fire) and Code Blue (respiratory or cardiac failure) are commonly known outside of health care, but many of the other codes will not be familiar. See Figure 11-8.

Fascinating Facts

Hospitals, dental offices, veterinary clinics, laboratories, nursing homes, medical offices, and other health care facilities generate more than 3 million tons of hazardous medical waste each year. Much of this waste is dangerous, especially when it is potentially toxic, radioactive, or infectious.

EMERGENCY PREPAREDNESS PLAN

Federal law requires every health care agency to have an emergency preparedness plan and to practice twice each year. Each health care professional should know his or her place in the plan. OSHA requires health care facilities to have an **emergency preparedness plan** for handling large numbers of patients in the event of a catastrophe, such as an earthquake, a flood, a tornado, a hurricane, or a bombing. It is the responsibility of health care professionals to be familiar with the requirements and understand their roles. Procedures will vary based on the type of facility, but some examples of what may be included are as follows:

- Whether you should report to work
- How to protect yourself and your patients
- Your specific duties
- How to get communications and updates

Whatever your role, always remain calm. This will help you think clearly, as well as provide needed stability to those who are confused, injured, and frightened. This is a critical time for the health care team to work efficiently and cooperatively.

The following general guidelines are to be followed when an emergency preparedness plan is in effect:

- Stay calm. There will be a great deal of chaos and confusion in a severe emergency, but panic can escalate the fear and related difficulties. Everyone involved will benefit from an approach by the health care professional that communicates control of the situation, competence, and compassion.
- Know who is in charge and report your availability.
- Report to the person in charge at regular intervals for further directions or changes in assignments.
- If unsure about what to do in a particular situation, ask someone in authority.
- Communicate clearly and be cooperative.
- Use telephones only for official business, not for personal calls.

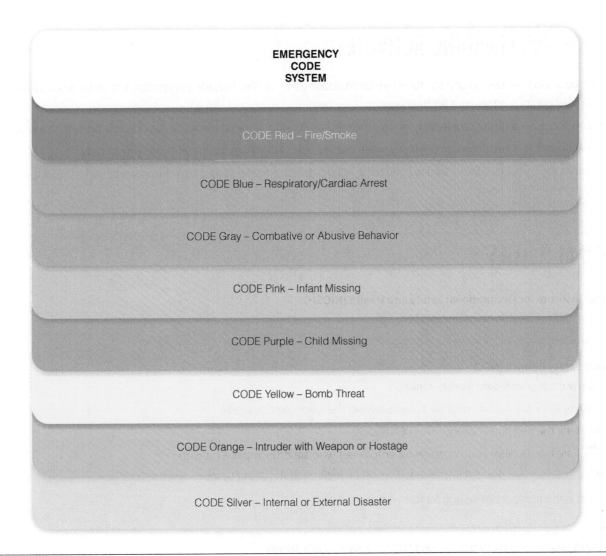

EMERGENCY CODE SYSTEM

CODE Red – Fire/Smoke

CODE Blue – Respiratory/Cardiac Arrest

CODE Gray – Combative or Abusive Behavior

CODE Pink – Infant Missing

CODE Purple – Child Missing

CODE Yellow – Bomb Threat

CODE Orange – Intruder with Weapon or Hostage

CODE Silver – Internal or External Disaster

FIGURE 11–8 Example of an emergency code system. Each page color matches the code name. When the employee opens to any of the colored pages, they will find the criteria to follow upon hearing the code announcement.

Triage

An effectively managed emergency response rests on an established **triage system**. *Triage* is a French word that means "to select." Specially trained personnel follow established triage guidelines to assess patients' conditions and determine where they should be sent and what treatment they should receive.

Triage systems are not just for major natural emergencies but are also used in the emergency department when multiple patients need medical care. An example is a bus accident with multiple passengers or a passenger train that derails sending multiple victims to the emergency department. When there are multiple victims, the available services can be overstrained, so the triage personnel must determine who to treat first, what lab or diagnostic tests receive priority, what procedures to perform immediately, and who to send to surgery. They continually reassess patients who are waiting for services to determine if their condition has changed and if their priority needs to be updated.

A less obvious triage system is in place at all times in the emergency department. For example, there may be a patient waiting to be seen for an earache or another who fell off a bike and may have a possible broken collarbone. Then a third patient arrives with complaints of chest pain and may be having a heart attack. The patient with the potential heart attack will be seen first, because his or her need is more urgent and lack of immediate care could lead to death.

SUGGESTED LEARNING ACTIVITIES

1. Visit your local fire station and ask for information about common fire hazards, prevention, use of fire extinguishers, and availability of training sessions for the public.

2. When you enter a health care facility, look for the fire alarms and an evacuation route plan (usually posted on a wall).

3. Look around your own home and when you are out in public. What potential hazards can you identify?

4. If someone in your family required oxygen to be administered at home, would anything need to be changed to make the situation safe?

WEB ACTIVITIES

National Institute for Occupational Safety and Health (NIOSH)

https://www.cdc.gov/niosh/topics/diseases.html

Choose five items of interest and write a paragraph summarizing each.

National Safety Council (NSC)

https://www.nsc.org/work-safety/safety-topics

After reading the information on this web page, answer the following questions:

1. What are the negative consequences of fatigue?

2. What are the negative consequences for employees who are drug impaired at work?

3. What actions does the NSC advise to help prevent violence in the workplace?

4. What is the number one reason for lost work days?

OSHA

- OSHA Brief – Hazard Communication Standard: Safety Data Sheets

https:www.osha.gov/Publications/OSHA3514.html

Read through the 16 sections required for preparing a Safety Data Sheet. Why do you think the government wants this amount of detailed information about each chemical?

- Caring for Our Caregivers

https://www.osha.gov/dsg/hospitals/understanding_problem.html

Scroll down the page and click on the PDF Download for "How Workers Are Getting Hurt"; you can then download the booklet "Caring for Our Caregivers." As you read the booklet, look for the answers to the following questions:

1. What are five reasons why hospital workers are especially prone to injury?

2. What other health care facilities face similar challenges regarding worker injuries?

3. See Figure 6: What percent of injuries in 2011 were caused by
   - Slips and falls
   - Contact with objects
   - Violence

4. Which hospital workers are at the highest risk for injury?

5. See Figure 19: What are the top two types of injuries in terms of spending on lost-time claims?

6. How do worker injuries negatively affect patients?
   - OSHA Fact Sheet: Protecting Yourself When Handling Contaminated Sharps

https://www.osha.gov/OshDoc/data_BloodborneFacts/bbfact02.pdf

1. What are the responsibilities of employers to prevent sharps injuries?

2. In what types of decisions must non managerial staff be included?

3. Describe a properly designed sharps container.

   - Workplace Violence in Health Care: Understanding the Challenge

https://www.osha.gov/Publications/OSHA3826.pdf

After reading this OSHA publication, answer the following questions:

1. Which health care workers are most likely to experience violence in the workplace?

2. What factors, specific to health care, contribute to underreporting incidences of violence, such as assaults and bullying?

3. List the five elements of an effective workplace violence prevention program.

Managed Care Magazine

Violence Against Nurses: Casualties of Caring

https://www.managedcaremag.com/archives/2018/5/violence-against-nurses-casualties-caring

After reading the article, list methods that various organizations, including the government, are developing to protect nurses from violence in the workplace.

Oregon Health Authority

Radiation Protection: Obtaining and Using Dosimeters

https://www.oregon.gov/oha/PH/HEALTHYENVIRONMENTS/RADIATIONPROTECTION/Pages/dosimetry.aspx

List five things that should not be done with a dosimeter, along with the rationale for each.

Centers for Disease Control and Prevention

Slip, Trip, and Fall Prevention for Healthcare Workers
https://www.cdc.gov/niosh/docs/2011-123/pdfs/2011-123.pdf

1. What are four negative consequences of slip, trip, and fall (STF) injuries?

2. What are the top ten hazards for STFs?

3. Review the checklists starting on page 35. Check your own living environment for the hazards listed.

REVIEW QUESTIONS

1. Why is it important for health care workers to maintain environmental safety in the workplace?

2. What are seven types of hazards in the health care environment?

3. What are actions the health care worker can take to prevent accidents and injuries in the following areas: moving, dressing, working with patients, protecting self and others?

4. What are the physical and mental impairments that make patients more prone to injuries and accidents?

5. What is an incident report, and when should it be completed?

6. What is workplace violence and what are common preventive measures?

7. What are the steps to take in case of a fire?

8. What does PASS mean?

9. What types of portable fire extinguishers are available? How would you decide which one to use? What are the precautions for their use?

10. What does RACE mean?

11. What are the guidelines for preventing electrical hazards?

12. What are the guidelines for safely handling chemicals?

13. What are the risks and safety measures needed for health care workers who work where radiation is used?

14. What is infectious waste and what is the proper method for its disposal?

15. What precautions must be taken when oxygen is being administered and why?

16. What is bioterrorism and how should it be reported?

17. What is an emergency code system? What are examples of the various codes?

18. What is an emergency preparedness plan, and what actions must the health care worker take?

19. What is the meaning of *triage*?

APPLICATION EXERCISES

1. Refer to The Case of the Bomb Threat at the beginning of the chapter and answer these questions:

   a. What would have been the possible consequences if Mrs. Welks had acted on her initial response to flee or yell out for an evacuation?

   b. How could the outcome of this situation be affected by obtaining more information about the location of the bomb and what time it was set to explode?

   c. Why do you think she was trying to listen so carefully to the voice and background noise?

   d. What should Mrs. Welks do when the telephone call is terminated?

   e. Should an emergency preparedness plan be initiated?

2. While at work, Jack Thompson, a health care professional, smells smoke and goes to investigate. He discovers the trash can in the restroom has smoke billowing from it, and he runs to get a fire extinguisher. The fire extinguisher is not where he thought it was, and by the time he returns to the restroom, there is smoke coming out from under the door. Jack opens the door, pulls the pin out of the extinguisher, moves as close as he can to the flames, and aims directly down into the trash can. He then hears someone coughing in one of the bathroom stalls and discovers a patient slumped on the floor. Jack pulls the patient out of the bathroom, but in the process, some of the white powdery residue from the fire extinguisher gets on the patient's skin. Jack is pleased with his actions and thinks to himself, "This patient might have died if I hadn't smelled the smoke and put the fire out."

   a. Evaluate the scenario to determine if Jack followed the recommended procedure. Did he follow RACE and PASS?

   b. What revisions to Jack's actions would have to occur to ensure safety for himself, patients, and coworkers?

   c. Can you determine from the information given, which class of fire extinguisher was used? Was it the correct extinguisher for a trash fire?

   d. Is it of concern that the patient has some of the white powdery residue on his skin?

PROBLEM-SOLVING PRACTICE

After reading the section on workplace violence, Maria Foust finds herself very upset about pursuing a career in health care. She has wanted to work in health care for as long as she can recall. She was raised in a community that was very violent and has finally been able to remove herself from that situation. Now the thought of working in a violent workplace is bringing back a lot of bad memories. Using the five-step problem-solving process, determine what Maria can do about her career choice concerns.

CHAPTER 12

Lifestyle Management

KEY TERMS

- aerobic exercise
- amino acids
- anorexia nervosa
- antioxidants
- assertiveness
- attitude
- binge eating
- body mass index (BMI)
- bulimia
- burnout
- calories
- carbohydrates
- cholesterol
- ChooseMyPlate
- controlled substance
- diet
- fats
- fiber
- free radicals
- legumes
- meditation
- metabolism
- minerals
- muscle relaxation
- nutrients
- nutrition
- obese
- organic
- organic foods
- osteoporosis
- overweight

(continues)

OBJECTIVES

Studying and applying the material in this chapter will help you to:

1. List the four top causes of death in the United States that are influenced by personal health habits.
2. Explain why it is important for health care professionals to practice a healthy lifestyle.
3. List six techniques for developing positive habits.
4. List two ways found effective to help individuals change habits that involve addictive substances.
5. Explain the importance of healthy eating.
6. Give the meaning of the terms "diet" and "nutrition."
7. List the six essential nutrients and the function of each.
8. List four vitamins and four minerals, including their purpose and food sources.
9. Explain the role that fiber plays in the diet.
10. Explain the meaning of a calorie.
11. Describe "good" and "bad" carbohydrates and the effects of each on the body.
12. Explain why added sugars should be limited in the diet.
13. Describe "good" and "bad" fats and the effects of each on the body.
14. Explain the meaning and purpose of cholesterol, including a description of the two types.
15. Explain why trans fats should be avoided.
16. Describe the negative effect of excess sodium in the diet.
17. Describe "processed foods" and give some examples.
18. List the problems associated with highly and ultra-processed foods.
19. Explain why food labels can be confusing for consumers.
20. Explain what makes foods organic, including the three levels of organic foods.
21. List the key recommendations for healthy eating developed by the U.S. Department of Agriculture.
22. Describe the "ChooseMyPlate," including its purpose.
23. List the components of the Mediterranean diet.
24. Give five examples of conditions to which excess body weight contributes.

KEY TERMS *(continued)*

prioritize
processed foods
proteins
refined grains
stress
stressors
trans fat
type 2 diabetes
vitamins
whole grains

25. Give eight examples of factors believed to contribute to the epidemic of overweight and obesity in the United States.
26. State the meaning and purpose of the Body Mass Index, including its limitations.
27. Explain why many weight-loss diets are not healthy.
28. Describe the four types of vegetarian diets.
29. Describe the following conditions: "anorexia nervosa," "bulimia," and "binge eating."
30. Give five examples of the benefits of physical exercise.
31. Define "aerobic exercise."
32. Give three examples of how physical exercise can be incorporated into daily life.
33. Explain the importance of getting adequate sleep.
34. List five suggestions for increasing the length and quality of sleep.
35. List three examples of measures that help prevent health problems from developing or worsening.
36. Define "stress" and list three examples of physical changes that typically accompany it.
37. Define "external stressors" and "internal stressors."
38. Explain why work in health care can be particularly stressful.
39. List methods health care professionals can use to reduce stress.
40. Give five examples of techniques for effectively managing time.
41. Explain the benefits of muscle relaxation.
42. Define meditation and give examples of its long-term benefits.
43. List six methods that have been found to help individuals quit smoking.
44. Define "controlled substance."
45. Explain the reasons for, and potential consequences of, substance abuse among health professionals.
46. Give examples of occupational risks for health care professionals.
47. List five of the most common sexually transmitted diseases.
48. Describe the precautions for avoiding sexually transmitted diseases.
49. Describe burnout and give examples of its causes and symptoms.
50. List ways to help prevent burnout.

The Case of the Cardiac Unit Nurse

Gracie Chin is a nurse working in the cardiac care unit at a large metropolitan hospital. Many of the patients in the unit are recovering from open heart surgery and require continual monitoring and attention. Gracie works three 12-hour shifts each week, and her duties require that she be on her feet during most of that time. She checks each patient frequently and performs such tasks as turning and bathing patients, adjusting the levels of their beds, placing patients on, and removing them from, bedpans, repositioning and maintaining equipment, and reaching to change intravenous fluid bags or to adjust monitoring devices that are located above bed level. In addition to the physical requirements of her job, Gracie must remain mentally alert throughout her shift. Her work requires keen observation skills and good judgment because in patient care, there is no room for error. She must also deal with the stress of working with patients who suffer from serious, often fatal conditions. In this chapter, you will learn about personal habits that enable health care professionals like Gracie to maintain the physical and mental fitness necessary to promote their own and their patients' welfare.

IMPORTANCE OF A HEALTHY LIFESTYLE

The human body consists of systems that are extremely complex and delicately balanced. Cared for properly, the average body is capable, to a great extent, of repairing itself and giving many years of service.

Our state of wellness is largely under our own control. Although the causes of many conditions are still unknown, four of the top five causes of death in the United States today—heart disease, cancer, chronic lower respiratory diseases, and stroke—are often influenced by personal health habits. Unlike previous generations who did not understand the causes of, and ways to prevent, disease, we have the knowledge and power to make healthy choices. To a great extent, individuals today can choose what to eat, how to deal with stress, and how much to exercise each day. Opportunities to raise our level of wellness lie within us, but *each person must accept the responsibility to take advantage of these opportunities.*

Practicing good health habits is especially important for the health care professional. The health professions require adequate physical energy and the ability to handle stress, two results of healthy living practices. In addition, the health care professional can serve as a role model for patients. Patient education is a growing part of the health care professional's duties, because patients are assuming more responsibility for their own health. An effective way to provide this education is to combine being a positive role model with having compassionate conversations with patients that include some wellness advice.

Habits and Health

Maximizing health often requires a change in habits, and this is not always easy. As you read this chapter, you may decide that there are lifestyle habits you would like to change—maybe it's to improve your time management skills, develop an exercise program, or change your eating habits. Being *willing* to change current behavior is the first step. Here are some additional tips for eliminating old habits and developing new ones:

1. Recognize that making changes may not be easy at first. Accepting this fact will help prevent you from becoming discouraged in the beginning.

2. Be patient with yourself. Changes do not occur overnight.

3. Set reasonable goals. Do not try to make so many changes at once that you feel defeated from the start.

4. Focus on the positive. Think about the long-term benefits you will enjoy.

5. Track your progress. Make a chart, maintain a journal or diary, or create some other personal recording system.

6. Plan rewards for your achievements.

Some habits, such as smoking, involve the use of addictive substances. These habits are particularly difficult to change. Many people have found that seeking professional assistance or participating in self-help groups are the most effective ways of dealing with addictive behaviors.

The purpose of attaining good health is more than hoping to prevent disease and extend the length of life. It includes improving the *quality* of living throughout the entire life span. It means waking up refreshed with the energy and well-being necessary to enjoy each day. The following sections of this chapter contain general guidelines and suggestions for achieving maximum wellness. What is appropriate for each individual will vary. Identify your strengths and weaknesses and develop a plan that works for you.

DIET AND NUTRITION

Eating right is one of the cornerstones of good health. What we eat determines, to a great extent, our risk for heart disease, stroke, cancer, and diabetes. Not only does eating a healthy diet help prevent disease, it provides us with the energy and feeling of well-being to live an active, productive life. The importance of diet has been recognized since ancient times. More than 1,600 years ago, Hippocrates said, "Let food be your medicine and medicine be your food."

To many people, the word "diet" means an eating plan designed to help them lose weight. However, the more general meaning of **diet** is the kinds of food a person or people habitually eat. For example, we might say that a typical Japanese diet contains more fish than the diet of most Americans. The word diet is also used to describe various types of eating plans, such as a vegan diet or low-salt diet.

Nutrients

Nutrition means the process of obtaining food necessary for health and growth. **Nutrients** are the various substances the body uses to grow and function properly. There are six classes of nutrients and each is essential to good health:

1. **Proteins:** Food substances containing **amino acids**, which are necessary for both building and maintaining the structural components of the body. Common sources are meat, fish, poultry, eggs, **legumes** (plants with seed pods, such as peas), nuts, seeds, and grains.

2. **Carbohydrates:** Food substances composed of starches and sugars that provide the body with immediate energy. Common sources are fruits, grains, legumes, breads, cereals, and pasta.

3. **Fats:** Food substances consisting of fatty acids that provide the most concentrated forms of energy for the body. In addition to oils and butter, fats are found in meat, fish, nuts, eggs, and certain plants such as olives and avocados.

4. **Vitamins:** Organic (related to, or derived from, living organisms) substances found in foods that are essential, in very small quantities, for growth, health, and life.

5. **Minerals:** Inorganic (not derived from living matter) substances that must be supplied to the body, in very

small quantities, in order for it to function properly. (See Table 12–1 for examples of key vitamins and minerals.)

6. **Water:** Essential for life. Water makes up 55% to 80% of human body weight, depending on age.

Table 12–1 Key Vitamins and Minerals that Contribute to Good Health

Nutrient	Essential for	Examples of Food Sources
Vitamin A	• Growth • Prevention of infection • Good vision and healthy skin	Liver, fish oils, eggs, dark green vegetables
Thiamin (Vitamin B$_1$)	• Production of energy from carbohydrates	Whole or enriched grain products, pork, organ meats
Riboflavin (Vitamin B$_2$)	• **Metabolism** of nutrients into energy	Dairy products, organ meats, enriched and fortified grains
Niacin (Vitamin B$_3$)	• Metabolism of nutrients into energy	Poultry, fish, beef, legumes, enriched or fortified grains
Vitamin B$_6$	• Manufacture of amino acids and red blood cells	Fortified cereals, sweet potatoes, chicken and beef liver
Vitamin B$_{12}$	• Production of red blood cells • Maintenance of central nervous system	Beef, dairy products, shellfish
Vitamin C	• Healing of wounds • Healthy bones and gums	Fruits and vegetables (especially citrus fruits and cabbage)
Vitamin D	• Absorption of calcium • Formation and maintenance of bones and teeth	Vitamin D–fortified milk and cereals, cod liver oil *Note*: The skin produces vitamin D when it is exposed to sunlight.
Vitamin E	• Normal function of muscles • Defense of cells against **free radicals** (particles that can harm cells and tissues)	Vegetable oils, wheat germs, nuts, seeds, leafy greens
Vitamin K	• Blood clotting	Eggs, cereal, leafy greens
Calcium	• Building and maintenance of bones • Maintain muscle and nerve function	Dairy products, leafy greens
Folate	• DNA synthesis in making protein	Fortified cereals, enriched grains, leafy greens, legumes, asparagus
Iron	• Transport of oxygen in red blood cells to body cells	Meats, eggs, dark leafy vegetables
Magnesium	• Energy production • Nerve function	Legumes, nuts, whole grains, green vegetables
Phosphorus	• Growth and repair of supporting tissue • Bone and teeth formation	Milk, meat, poultry, fish, eggs, legumes, nuts
Potassium	• Nerve function • Muscle contraction (including heart muscle)	Fruits, vegetables, meat, poultry, fish, milk
Zinc	• Reproduction of cells • Tissue growth and repair	Meat, eggs, seafood, whole grains

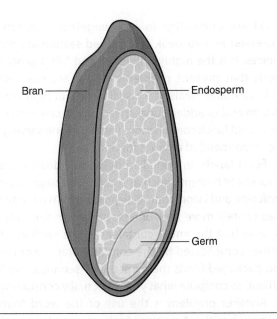

FIGURE 12–1 A grain is considered to be a whole grain as long as all three original parts—the bran, germ, and endosperm—are still present in the same proportions as when the grain was growing in the fields.

In addition to the previously listed nutrients, **fiber** is an important component of the diet. Fibers are food contents, but most cannot be fully digested. Their principal benefits are maintaining a healthy bowel and normalizing bowel movements (preventing constipation). Fiber is found in fruits, vegetables, **whole grains** (contain all their original parts), and legumes. (See Figure 12–1.)

Calories

The body obtains energy from foods in order to function. The potential energy a food can provide the body is measured in **calories**. A gram of carbohydrates has 4 calories, a gram of protein has 4 calories, and a gram of fat has 9 calories. Our bodies "burn" calories and either use them for immediate energy needs or store them as body fat. For years, "diet experts" advocated decreasing the number of calories taken in as a way to lose and control weight. However, it is currently believed that eating a healthy, well-balanced diet (discussed later in this chapter) is more important than counting and restricting calories.

Carbohydrates

Over the years, carbohydrates have been blamed for weight gain and health problems, and many weight-loss diets have been developed that attempt to eliminate them or at least severely decrease the amount permitted. The fact is that carbohydrates exist naturally in many healthy foods, such as fruits, vegetables, and whole grains, and are vital for health:

- They are the body's main fuel source.
- Some evidence suggests that whole grains help decrease the risk of cardiovascular disease.
- Eating fruits, vegetables, and whole grains helps control weight (https://www.mayoclinic.org/healthy-lifestyle/nutrition-and-healthy-eating/in-depth/carbohydrates/art-20045705?p=1).

Foods containing carbohydrates that are high-calorie but low in nutrition are considered to be "bad carbs" and the ones that should be limited. These include **refined grains** (modified so most nutrients are removed) and foods with added sugar, discussed in the next section.

Sugars

Added sugars, according to some nutrition experts, are the worst ingredient in the modern American diet. Many foods, such as fruits, naturally contain sugar. It is the *addition of sugar* in any form (white, brown, honey, etc.) that is the cause of concern. This is because added sugars contain no nutrients while at the same time they add calories, often in high amounts. It is believed that these sugars contribute to overweight and obesity, especially if consuming them replaces more nutritious foods. They also increase the level of triglycerides, a type of fat in the bloodstream, and the likelihood of cavities (https://www.mayoclinic.org/healthy-lifestyle/nutrition-and-healthy-eating/in-depth/added-sugar/art-20045328). The worst offenders of added sugar, according to many sources, are sodas and sugary fruit drinks.

Fats

Fats contain the highest number of calories per gram of all the nutrients. For years it has been recommended that they be avoided in a healthy diet and certainly by people who wish to lose weight. However, research has distinguished between types of fats and some actually help prevent type 2 diabetes and heart disease. "Good fats" are those found in certain types of fish (Omega-3 fats), olive oil, nuts, and seeds. Examples of foods still recommended to be eaten in moderation because of their "bad fat" content are fatty meats, cream, butter, and cheese. Eaten in excess, these can contribute to heart disease and certain types of cancer.

Cholesterol

Our knowledge of what constitutes good nutrition is constantly updated as research continues into the complex ways that foods are processed by our bodies. One example is the effect that the cholesterol in food has on our bodies. **Cholesterol** is a type of fat produced by the liver and also found in foods. It circulates in the blood and, when present in excess quantities, can contribute to plaque that builds up in the arteries, causing atherosclerosis (hardening of the arteries). At the same time, certain amounts of cholesterol are essential for a number of body functions, including making hormones and building cell membranes.

There are two types of cholesterol: low-density lipoprotein (LDL) and high-density lipoprotein (HDL). The LDL is the type that contributes to plaque in the arteries, thus it is referred to as "bad cholesterol." HDL, or "good cholesterol," is believed to carry LDL cholesterol away from the arteries and back to the liver where it is broken down and carried away from the body (https://www.heart.org/en /health-topics/cholesterol/hdl-good-ldl-bad-cholesterol- and-triglycerides). Therefore, if the body is producing too much cholesterol, eating certain foods is recommended to help raise HDL levels. These include the foods recommended in the previous section as "good fats."

Trans Fats

One component of many processed foods that you want to *avoid* rather than include in your diet is trans fat. A trans fat is not natural, but results when hydrogen is added to vegetable oil, which is then identified on food labels as "partially hydrogenated oil." The problem with trans fats is that they raise the level of LDL ("bad cholesterol") while decreasing HDL ("good cholesterol"). The use of trans fats by food manufacturers is not illegal in the United States.

Salt (Sodium)

Salt adds flavor to foods and a certain amount of sodium is necessary for the body to function properly. However, excessive amounts contribute to high blood pressure which in turn can cause a heart attack or stroke. The American Heart Association recommends a maximum of 2,300 milligrams (1 teaspoon) per day, with 1,500 milligrams being the ideal amount for most adults, especially those with high or slightly elevated blood pressure. According to the Harvard School of Public Health, most Americans consume 1.5 teaspoons each day, largely a result of the sodium added to processed foods (https://www.hsph.harvard.edu /nutritionsource/salt-and-sodium/).

Processed Foods

Many Americans include a large number of processed foods in their diet. As defined by the Academy of Nutrition and Dietetics, these are defined as foods that have been "cooked, canned, frozen, packaged or changed in nutritional composition with fortifying, preserving or preparing in different ways" (https://www.eatright .org/food/nutrition/nutrition-facts-and-food-labels /processed-foods-whats-ok-and-what-to-avoid).

Examples of processed foods include prewashed salad greens, frozen vegetables, canned tuna, canned soups, chips, cookies, and microwave meals. Not all processed foods are unhealthy; in fact, vegetables frozen and preserved at their peak and canned salmon are healthy choices. It is the highly processed and "ultra-processed" foods that present problems. These are ready-to-eat and pre-made meals that usually contain high levels of sodium and/or added sugar. In fact, some common highly processed foods contain more sodium in one serving than the recommended amount for one day.

Food labels, intended to help individuals learn the amounts of contents, such as sodium and sugar, are often confusing and incomplete. One problem is that many packages contain more than one serving when the consumer expects that the entire container is one serving. This is further complicated by the common practice of canned and packaged foods that contain 3.5 servings, making it difficult to compute what you are actually consuming.

Another problem is the use of the word "natural" to imply healthy. A popular "natural granola" cereal lists sugar as the second ingredient. One-half cup contains 210 calories, a relatively high number for that amount of cereal. The "all-natural" combination of oats, almonds, brown sugar, and honey results in something more like cookies than a healthy breakfast food.

Organic Foods

Organic foods are growing in popularity. The term organic, when applied to foods, refers to the way they are grown and processed. Table 12–2 lists the major differences between organic and conventional farming methods. The USDA has established an organic certification program that includes standards that need to be met in order for foods to be designated as organic:

- "100% organic": Completely organic
- "Organic": At least 95% organic
- "Made with organic ingredients": Contains at least 70% organic ingredients

Other terms that apply to foods include "all-natural," "free range," and "hormone-free," but these are not the same as organic. They can also be misleading. For example, the term *free range* implies that animals are allowed unlimited movement during their lifetime. However, they may have limited space and be allowed their freedom for only a few hours each day. And all-natural products may have natural ingredients, but they can also have a high sugar content that removes them from a healthy food list.

Studies comparing the nutritional value of traditionally grown foods with organic foods have led to conflicting results: Some researchers have shown that organic produce is far superior in nutritional value while others have found no significant difference for most food products. For example, a Stanford University study concluded there was little difference between organic and conventionally grown

Table 12–2 Conventional versus Organic Farming Methods

Conventional Farming	Organic Farming
Use chemical fertilizers	Use natural fertilizers such as compost and manure
Spray insecticides	Use insects and birds that eat pests
	Disrupt mating of pests. Set traps
Use chemical weed killers	Rotate crops
	Hand weed
	Apply mulch
Give animals antibiotics and other medications, and growth hormones	Give animals organic feed
Food and Drug Administration (FDA) regulations allow rendered animal by-products and waste to be added to the feed	Provide animals with access to the outdoors to prevent spreading disease
	Use various preventive measures to help prevent disease

produce. However, a recent European study concluded that organic produce contains 20–40% higher levels of **antioxidants** (substances that reduce damage in the body due to oxygen). The studies and controversies will surely continue into the future.

People who are concerned about chemical residues on food may prefer to eat organically grown products. (It should be noted that all fruits and vegetables, regardless of whether organic or not, should be thoroughly washed before eating.) In addition, people who are concerned about chemicals in the environment may be interested in organic foods. The major disadvantage of organic foods is that they are more expensive to grow than conventional foods and therefore cost more to purchase.

HEALTHY EATING

Many types of diets are currently advocated for reaching and maintaining optimal health. The most important factors in choosing a diet are to make sure you include a variety of foods that provide the nutrients listed in the previous section, and that you choose a diet you can make part of your daily life. (See Figure 12–2.)

The U.S. Department of Agriculture (USDA) has developed dietary guidelines, which are updated every few years, to help Americans eat for wellness. The key recommendations for a healthy eating pattern include the following:

- A variety of vegetables from all of the subgroups—dark green, red and orange, legumes (beans and peas)
- Fruits, especially whole fruits
- Grains, at least half of which are whole grains
- Fat-free or low-fat dairy, including milk, yogurt, cheese, and/or fortified soy beverages

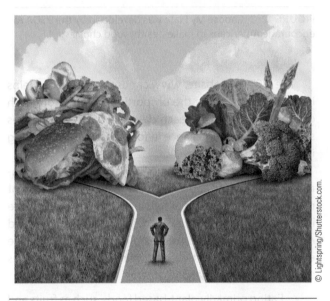

© Lightspring/Shutterstock.com.

FIGURE 12–2 Strive to make healthy food choices for most of your meals.

- A variety of protein foods, including seafood, lean meats and poultry, eggs, legumes (beans and peas), and nuts, seeds, and soy products
- Oils

A visual icon, known as **ChooseMyPlate**, was created by the USDA to help individuals apply the dietary guidelines and make healthy food choices. (See Figure 12–3.) The "plate" is divided into four sections of different sizes to show the recommended proportions of five food groups:

1. Vegetables
2. Grains
3. Protein
4. Fruits
5. Dairy

Courtesy of the U.S. Department of Agriculture.

FIGURE 12–3 Choose My Plate was developed by the USDA to encourage Americans to make healthy food choices.

The USDA's website, www.choosemyplate.gov, helps individuals determine the proportion of food from each group they should eat each day. The USDA emphasizes seeking variety and balance in foods, as well as engaging in adequate physical exercise.

The Mediterranean diet is a way of eating recommended by organizations such as the Mayo Clinic. Recent research also suggests that following this diet may reduce inflammation and the risk of heart disease, stroke, and Alzheimer's. Not a weight-loss diet, it incorporates the everyday cooking, eating, and living styles of countries such as Greece and Italy:

- Eating primarily plant-based foods, such as fruits and vegetables, whole grains, legumes, and nuts
- Replacing butter with healthy fats such as olive oil and canola oil
- Using herbs and spices instead of salt to flavor foods
- Limiting red meat to no more than a few times a month
- Eating fish and poultry at least twice a week
- Enjoying meals with family and friends
- Drinking red wine in moderation (optional)
- Getting plenty of exercise

(https://www.mayoclinic.org/healthy-lifestyle /nutrition-and-healthy-eating/in-depth/mediterranean-diet/art-20047801)

MAINTAINING A HEALTHY WEIGHT

Along with good nutrition, maintaining a healthy weight has repeatedly been shown to contribute to wellness and the prevention of disease. However, it is estimated that at least 71.5% of adults age 20 and over in the United States may be overweight, with 39.8% possibly having obesity (https://www.cdc.gov/nchs/fastats/obesity-overweight. htm). Of particular concern is the increasing number of children and adolescents who may have obesity, as shown by the following percentages reported in 2017:

- Ages 2 to 5 years: 13.9%
- Ages 6 to 11 years: 18.4%
- Ages 12 to 18 years: 20.6% (https://www.cdc.gov /obesity/data/childhood.html)

Young people who are overweight tend to have weight problems as adults.

Many sources call the increasing number of overweight and obese Americans the public health challenge of our time. Thousands of deaths and billions of health care dollars are the direct result of obesity, making it one of the leading causes of preventable deaths in the United States. Excess body weight contributes to a number of uncomfortable conditions and serious diseases, such as the following:

- High blood pressure
- Elevated levels of fats in the blood, including cholesterol
- Type 2 diabetes
- Heart disease
- Stroke
- Gallbladder disease
- Osteoarthritis
- Sleep apnea (condition in which a person stops breathing while sleeping)
- Respiratory problems
- Cancers (endometrial, breast, prostate, and colon)
- Depression

Researchers are investigating why the percentage of overweight and obese Americans continues to grow. It is a complex problem without easy answers and there are many causes:

- Availability and aggressive advertising of inexpensive, calorie-dense foods
- Limited access to markets and stores that sell fresh foods
- The relatively high cost of healthy foods such as fresh vegetables, fruits, fish, and nuts

- Heavy use of the automobile as a means of transportation
- Increased number of hours watching television, using the computer, and playing video games
- Lack of safe places to walk, parks, and economically priced gyms
- Increases in technology and decreases in tasks that require manual labor
- Genes that make some individuals susceptible to weight gain
- Hormone problems, such as an underactive thyroid and Cushing syndrome
- Certain medications, such as some corticosteroids, antidepressants, and seizure medicines
- Stress and emotions such as anger and boredom
- Insufficient sleep

Health care providers, including physicians, are working to find ways to help their patients having realized that simply telling them, "You need to lose weight," is often not an effective solution. Discussing weight issues must be done in a respectful and nonjudgmental way, with the goal of exploring the causes and helping with the issues that are contributing to the patient's condition.

Body Mass Index

Height–weight charts were used for many years to determine if a person was overweight, but the **body mass index (BMI)** is increasingly being used. BMI measures the relationship of weight to height using a mathematical formula. (See Box 12–1.) A BMI of 25.0 to 29.9 is defined as **overweight**. A BMI of 30.0 or higher is considered **obese**.

Although widely used in health care settings, the BMI is not always the best indicator of healthy body weight. For example, muscular individuals may have a number that considers them to be overweight or even obese. This is because muscles weigh more than fat, so this is not a good indication of fitness. Contrarily, a woman may fall within the healthy range for her weight, but has little muscle and too high a percentage of body fat.

Weight-Loss Diets

Dozens of diets and methods have been proposed for losing weight. Many of the most popular diets contradict each other, and it can be difficult to sort fact from fiction. For many people, a diet that provides fewer calories than are burned is likely to result in weight loss. However, weight-loss diets that emphasize one type of food over another or

---

═══ Box 12–1 ═══

Calculating Body Mass Index

1. Multiply weight in pounds by 703.
2. Divide the result by height in inches.
3. Divide the result from step 2 by height in inches.

Example: Calculate the BMI for a man who is 5 feet, 10 inches tall and weighs 236 pounds.

Step 1	$236 \times 703 = 165{,}908$
Step 2	5'10" = 70 inches
	$165{,}908 \div 70 = 2370$
Step 3	$2370 \div 70 = 33.86$
BMI = 33.86	

Fascinating Facts

According to a CDC survey, 1 in 3 Americans eat fast food on a typical day. Nearly half of American men eat fast food for lunch on any given day.

Source: https://www.cdc.gov/nchs/products/databriefs/db322.htm

---

eliminate a whole category of foods that provide essential nutrients can result in a shortage of one or more essential nutrients. Therefore, when planning a weight-loss diet, it is important to include all necessary nutrients rather than focusing only on the restriction of calories.

Vegetarian Diets

Vegetarian diets consist of mainly plant-based foods, such as vegetables, fruits, whole grains, beans, nuts, and seeds. There are at least four types of vegetarian diets:

1. Vegan: Includes only plant-based foods. People who follow this diet do not eat any foods produced by animals such as milk, cheese, and eggs. The meaning of the term *vegan* has expanded beyond food choices and frequently relates to a philosophy that promotes animal rights. Vegans do not use or wear any animal products. When referring to dietary practices, the term *plant-based diet* is a more accurate descriptor than vegan.

Fascinating Facts

Food As Medicine

The Ceres Community Project in Northern California is distributing medically tailored meals each day to low income patients recovering from cancer or suffering from chronic diseases, such as diabetes. To date, individuals who receive the food averaged about $12,000 less a month in medical expenses than those who do not.

Source: California tests food as medicine for chronically ill patients. Bend Bulletin, May 14, 2018. From New York Times News Service.

2. Lacto-vegetarian: Includes milk and milk products along with plant-based foods.

3. Lacto-ovo vegetarian: Includes eggs, milk, and milk products along with plant-based foods.

4. Flexitarian (semi-vegetarian): A mostly plant-based diet, but may occasionally include small amounts of meat, poultry, or fish.

A growing number of scientific studies show that plant-based diets are healthier than meat-based diets. Vegetarian diets may prevent many of the chronic diseases and conditions that have become epidemic in the United States, such as heart disease, cancer, obesity, and diabetes. It is important, however, that plant-based diets be well-planned to include adequate nutrients. A common misconception is that animal products are the only source of protein, but this is not true. Recall that protein is also provided by legumes, seeds, nuts, and grains. A variety of vegetarian eating pyramids have been developed to assist with meal planning.

EATING DISORDERS

Eating disorders, often caused by a fear of obesity and the desire to conform to an unrealistic body image, are a growing problem. Following are the three most common conditions:

1. **Anorexia nervosa**: The distorted belief that one is overweight, even when severely underweight, and the cutting of calories below the number necessary to maintain health. Exact causes are not known, but may be related to social pressures to achieve the unrealistic slimness promoted by the entertainment industry and fashion models. Anorexia can be life threatening, ending in death by starvation. Medical intervention is almost always necessary, and hospitalization is often required.

2. **Bulimia**: A condition characterized by the compulsive eating of huge quantities of food, followed by self-induced vomiting and/or the use of large amounts of laxatives. These actions may be accompanied by feelings of guilt and the fear of being "found out." Stomach acids in vomit may cause the erosion of tooth enamel, development of dental cavities, and eating away of the esophagus.

3. **Binge eating**: The compulsive consumption of large quantities of food, beyond that needed to satisfy hunger. This uncontrolled eating is sometimes used as an escape from boredom, as a means to handle anger, and for other reasons related to handling emotional issues.

Medical assistance, counseling, and support groups offer help with eating disorders.

PHYSICAL ACTIVITY

Like good nutrition, physical activity has been found to have a significant influence on health. It has even been said that if exercise could be put in a tablet form, it would be considered a wonder drug. Exercise has benefits for every body system and can help prevent and treat many illnesses. The many benefits of physical activity include the following:

- Promotes feelings of well-being through the body's production of endorphins, substances that naturally raise the pain threshold and produce sedative effects
- Relieves stress and improves mental outlook
- Improves memory and concentration
- Improves the quality of sleep
- Helps with weight control
- Increases energy level
- Helps prevent lower back pain
- Reduces symptoms of arthritis

Exercise also reduces the risk of developing heart disease. The heart is a muscle and therefore is strengthened by regular exercise that forces it to work by increasing the heartbeat beyond its normal resting rate, within a target range. For a healthy person, the maximum desired heart rate during exercise is 220 minus his or her age. Therefore, the older the person the lower the target heart rate. This type of exercise, known as **aerobic exercise**, increases the heart's strength. In addition to helping prevent heart disease, the number one cause of death in the United States, physical activity decreases the incidence of type 2 diabetes, **osteoporosis**, and certain types of cancer, including breast and colon. Recent studies show that physical fitness may significantly decrease the chance of developing dementia in later life.

It is recommended that adults exercise for at least 30 minutes on five or more days a week. Children and teens need 60 minutes a day. This time may be broken into segments of 10 or 15 minutes and still provide health benefits. In addition to periods of planned exercise, physical activity can be incorporated into daily life. A few alterations can result in a built-in exercise program that does not take too much time in an already busy life. Here are a few ideas:

- Whenever possible, leave the car at home. Walk to the store, library, church, and so on. When using the car, park at the far end of the parking lot.

- Use the stairs instead of elevators.

- Wash the car instead of going to the car wash.

- Do jobs yourself that require physical effort, such as mowing the lawn and washing windows.

- Find a sport or activity you enjoy, such as swimming or dancing. Or shoot baskets with the kids and walk around the neighborhood with a friend. Substitute activity for a few hours of television each week. (See Figure 12–4.)

Fascinating Facts

Studies show that making lifestyle changes, such as in diet and exercise, can reduce the plaque in the arteries. This in turn decreases the risk for a heart attack.

Source: Bend Bulletin, Health Response, June 1, 2018. From the New York Times News Service

FIGURE 12–4 Physical exercise is a key component of good health. Find something you enjoy doing.

© kurhan/Shutterstock.com.

SLEEP

An adequate amount of sleep is necessary because it is during sleep that the body recuperates from the day's activities. Body functions slow down and body temperature drops. It is believed that during the last few hours of sleep before awakening, the time when most dreams occur, mental recuperation takes place. Studies have shown that during sleep the brain is preparing itself for learning and remembering (http://healthysleep.med. harvard.edu/healthy/matters/benefits-of-sleep/learning-memory). This is why it is especially important that students and others who are engaged in learning activities make it a point to get enough sleep. "Enough" varies among individuals but is generally believed to be six to nine hours for adults.

Here are some suggestions for increasing the length and quality of sleep:

- Avoid caffeine—found in coffee, tea, cola drinks, and chocolate—late in the day if it keeps you awake.

- Try to avoid stressful activities or communications just before going to bed.

- Keep a "worry log" to write down things to think about at a set "worry time." Keep the "appointment" and use the time to focus on finding solutions. Knowing that it is possible to get back to worries later can help clear the mind at bedtime.

- Use the time management techniques described later in this chapter to increase personal efficiency and increase the time available for sleep.

- Engage in some form of exercise each day, but avoid very vigorous exercise just before going to bed.

- Develop a routine for getting ready for bed and try to use it every day. This will signal the body to become sleepy.

- Keep the bed for sleeping. Do not do homework and other chores there or the body may program itself to become alert when getting into bed.

- If possible, have a comfortable mattress and pillow.

PREVENTIVE MEASURES

Many health problems can be avoided by practicing preventive measures. These include the following:

- Regular visits to physician or health care practitioner for routine checkups. (See Figure 12–5.)

- Periodic screening for risks associated with your gender and age group.

- Regular visits to the dentist and the practice of proper dental hygiene, including regular flossing. Most gum

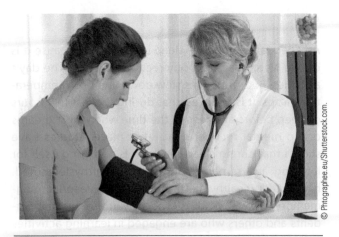

© Phtographee.eu/Shutterstock.com.

FIGURE 12–5 Regular checkups and screening tests are important for maintaining good health.

disease, which can cause the loss of teeth, can be avoided. Untreated tooth decay and abscesses can result in serious infections in other parts of the body, including the heart.

- Treatment of illnesses in their early stages. Positive outcomes are more likely with early treatment.

- Immunizations. Health care employers are required to offer hepatitis B vaccinations for all employees whose work requires them to be exposed to body substances. An annual vaccination against influenza is also highly recommended. This illness may seem like "just the flu," but it causes tens of thousands of death each year. During the 2012–2013 flu season, 56,000 deaths were reported (https://www.cdc.gov/flu/about/disease/us_flu-related_deaths.htm).

Fascinating Facts

The majority of emergency department dental visits were for infections that could have been handled in a dentist's office or prevented with regular dental care. These visits cost $1.9 billion yearly and are not as effectively treated in the ED as in the dental office.

Source: https://www.ahrq.gov/research/findings/nhqrdr/chartbooks/carecoordination/measure2.html

STRESS IN MODERN LIFE

Stress refers to the body's reactions when it responds to danger, either real or imagined. In seeking a state of readiness for action, the body undergoes a series of physical changes that include the following:

- Increased heart rate
- Increased rate of breathing
- Elevated blood pressure
- Raised blood sugar level
- Dilated blood vessels in the muscles to give them the immediate use of sugar
- Dilated pupils of eyes

These reactions, characteristic of the "fight or flight" response explained in Chapter 7, serve individuals well when they must protect themselves, run from a scene, or perform an emergency procedure under pressure. (See Table 7–3.) But the body cannot distinguish between physical danger and fears and worries experienced in the mind or the emotional strain resulting from negative circumstances. For example, worries about losing a job or handling financial problems create the same reaction as being in danger of physical attack. When psychological pressures are continuous or occur frequently, the body can literally wear itself out making preparations to face danger. Responses originally meant to be helpful become sources of harm.

Research studies in recent years have looked for a correlation between stress and various illnesses. Although the evidence is not conclusive, some researchers and physicians believe that the experience of chronic psychological and emotional stress weakens the body's immune system. This reduces the body's ability to defend itself against disease. Stress is also believed by many health professionals to contribute to high blood pressure, heart disease, cancer, and other diseases. In addition to possibly increasing the risk of serious health problems, excessive stress interferes with personal effectiveness, productivity, relationships, and the enjoyment of life.

External and Internal Stressors

Modern life presents many **stressors** (causes of stress). External stressors are those outside one's immediate control. Examples include the fast pace of life, the high cost of living, crowded cities and freeways, and demanding patients. We have limited control over external stressors, although changes can be made in we perceive and deal with them. (See the section on attitude in Chapter 13.)

Internal stressors are self-generated and within the individual's control. Examples include a negative attitude,

Thinking It Through

Mikel Korsov is a recent graduate of a licensed practical nurse program. He has been hired to work in the pediatric ward at Samuelson Hospital. Mikel loves working with children and has a real talent for calming their fears and helping them cope with necessary procedures and medications. He finds, however, that he is physically exhausted at the end of each day. He has little energy left to do much more than drag himself home, eat whatever is available or quick to prepare, and then watch television until bedtime. Mikel weighs about 60 pounds more than the weight suggested for his height and does not participate in much physical exercise beyond that required on the job.

1. What might be the long-term consequences of Mikel's current habits? Consider this from both personal and professional viewpoints.

2. Discuss the possible impact of his health habits on the attitudes of his patients regarding their own health.

3. Suggest five things he can do that can help increase his energy level.

unrealistic goals, poor time management skills, and lack of problem-solving ability. Internal stressors can be controlled by acquiring additional skills, making changes in personal habits, and adjusting one's mental outlook.

Dealing with Stress

There will always be stressors in life. The future may bring achievements and satisfaction, but there is no perfect job or ideal set of conditions that are stress-free. And some degree of stress is actually healthy because it provides the motivation for action. Health care work, by its very nature, can be stressful because workers must be able to do the following:

- Interact with people who are ill or injured
- Remain calm in difficult situations
- Remain constantly attentive
- Apply thinking skills
- Perform tasks accurately
- Work under time constraints
- Respond to changing needs of patients and the facility

Dealing effectively with stress starts with identifying the major stressors in life. Are they internal or external? Which are within your control? Are you adding to your own stress level with ineffective personal habits? Which stressors are outside your control and require adaptive and coping techniques?

Marcos, a respiratory therapy student, is a perfectionist when it comes to his homework assignments. He goes over each one several times, reworking them until he feels satisfied that they are "just right." As a result, Marcos frequently turns in assignments late and never feels caught up. The need for perfection is causing Marcos stress and may be a serious problem when he becomes employed. Workplace tasks, although needing to be performed correctly, must also be completed in a timely way. In this example, knowing when work is satisfactory can alleviate unnecessary stress.

Setting Priorities

Stress can be created when you don't prioritize. To **prioritize** means to rank tasks that need to be done in order of importance. Adult students often experience conflicts between their many responsibilities. School and work are priorities and, at times, choices must be made in order to reduce stress. Ellen, a mother of three, agreed to serve on a parents' committee at her children's school. After enrolling in a dental hygiene program, she found that she did not have the time for the committee meetings, parenting, and studying for her classes. She completed the tasks she had already committed to do, then met with the chairperson to explain her situation and resign from the committee.

Determining which current activities will result in long-term benefits can help you decide what is most important to you. Where can you make compromises now in exchange for future benefits? The time and effort you invest in your studies, for example, will determine your future employment success. And time spent with children is essential to their healthy development. (See Figure 12–6.) The ability to prioritize will continue to be an important skill both on the job and as you balance professional, family, and personal responsibilities.

Time Management

Poor time management is a major cause of stress. Although it is impossible to increase the number of hours in a day, the ones that are available can be used more effectively. Improving the use of time not only can reduce stress, but it can also improve personal performance and increase feelings of personal power.

FIGURE 12-6 Spending time with family and friends supports emotional and physical health and should be a priority.

Start by doing an honest review of your daily habits. It will help to keep a record for a week, listing the amount of time spent on each activity. Are there hours when time is simply "killed" instead of being used effectively or enjoyed? Television, your phone, and the Internet can eat up hours. They may not provide enjoyment in proportion to the time spent. Are there others? Is there adequate time built in for resting and thinking, or is everything too rushed? Are there actions you can take to prevent a future crisis that can be very time-consuming? Try prioritizing activities as a means to identify those that bring the most benefits or enjoyment for the time invested.

Procrastination is a stress producer for many people. This is illustrated by Mohammed, a health information management student. He has assignments that are due throughout the semester. Last semester he was in a continual state of panic and last-minute rushes to complete them. Unexpected delays and interruptions created a sense of emergency. Feelings of desperation mounted and made it difficult to concentrate. Mohammed thought about why he procrastinated and realized that he was afraid to start projects because they seemed overwhelming. He developed the following plan:

1. Break large projects into smaller steps that are more manageable.

2. Set completion dates for each step, starting with the project deadline and moving backward on the calendar.

3. Schedule time to work each day or every other day in order to feel a sense of accomplishment and keep the project moving. (It is important to work even when not in the mood for it.)

4. Seek appropriate help and gather any needed information.

5. Focus on the feelings of accomplishment and control being experienced.

Many time-management techniques can be incorporated into a busy daily schedule:

- Keep a calendar of assignments, tests, field trips, appointments, birthdays, and other "must-remember" activities.

- Write a daily to-do list in the order of most to least important tasks. At the end of each day, cross off completed tasks and carry over undone tasks for the next day.

- When possible, do the hardest things first.

- Keep other lists to help stay organized: shopping, freezer contents, children's chores.

- Organize errands so that several can be accomplished in one trip.

- Keep things in their place so you don't waste time and energy looking for them.

- At work, know the priorities of your supervisor or department.

Time management is a critical work skill. With emphasis on cost containment and efficiency, health care professionals are expected to use time well and accomplish required duties within prescribed time periods. See Chapter 1 for more ideas to help with time management.

Muscle Relaxation Techniques

Muscle Relaxation, as used here, refers to releasing tension in the muscles. This reduces stress, both physical and emotional, by improving blood circulation and allowing the release of blood lactate, a substance that some studies have shown to be associated with anxiety. Using relaxation techniques also produces the sensation of being rested. With practice, it is possible to quickly identify and release muscle tension when it begins to occur. (See Figure 12-7.)

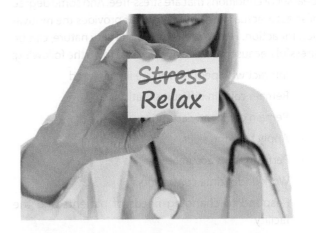

FIGURE 12-7 Relaxation techniques and meditation can help relieve stress.

Box 12–2

Muscle Relaxation Technique

1. Choose a time and place where you can arrange not to be interrupted.

2. Sit in a comfortable position with the spine straight and feet flat on the floor.

3. Starting at the toes, tighten the muscles of each section of the body, experience the feeling of tension, and then relax. Move up as follows:

   a. Toes (flex)

   b. Legs

   c. Hips and abdomen

   d. Chest and upper back

   e. Hands (make a fist) and arms

   f. Shoulders (lift toward ears)

   g. Face, head, and neck (be sure to relax the jaw afterward)

   h. Eyebrows (raise and lower, pull together and release)

4. Tighten the entire body at once, hold as long as possible, then relax as much as possible. (Important note: This step is not recommended for people with hypertension [high blood pressure].)

5. Repeat to yourself: "I am relaxed."

6. Sit for several minutes and experience the lack of tension. If you become aware of any areas of tension, tighten and then release the muscles in that area.

There are several methods for doing muscle relaxation exercises. Although it is outside the scope of this book to provide extensive information, instructions for one popular method can be found in Box 12–2.

Meditation

Meditation is a process for quieting the mind by clearing it of thoughts. It slows the rate of brain waves experienced during normal activity. The regular practice of meditation has been shown to bring about physiological changes that result in both psychological and physiological well-being. An increasing number of health care professionals are recommending meditation as a therapeutic technique because some research suggests that it may help manage the symptoms of the following, among other conditions:

- Anxiety disorders
- Asthma
- Cancer
- Depression
- Digestive disorders
- Heart disease
- High blood pressure

The positive, long-term effects that can be achieved through daily meditation, when it is practiced over an extended period, include the following:

- Positive changes in perception of self, others, and life events
- A freeing of emotions, especially suppressed emotions

- Greater compassion
- Increased capacity for self-love and love for others
- Improved ability to cope with life situations (Milliken & Honeycutt, 2004)

You may have had the experience of finding the solution to a problem when you stopped focusing on it and just "let the mind go." Meditators report similar experiences

Thinking It Through

Janice Nelson, dental assistant for Dr. Grady, is worried about the conversation she had with Dr. Grady this afternoon. He spoke with her privately and expressed concern about her time management practices. He pointed out that Janice had arrived late for work three times in the last two weeks, had left early one day due to child-care problems, and had several times failed to complete assigned work tasks in the designated time. Dr. Grady explained that in a small practice with only a few employees, Janice was having a significant impact on work flow in the office. He warned her that she must improve if she was to continue working there.

1. Discuss the possible impact of Janice's actions on patients, coworkers, and Dr. Grady.

2. Suggest ways that Janice can improve her personal organization and time management.

Box 12–3

A Meditation Method

1. Choose a time and place where you can arrange not to be interrupted.

2. Set a timer. Twenty minutes is best, 10 is the minimum.

3. Sit in a comfortable position in a chair or on the floor. Straighten the spine and place the hands on the thighs.

4. Take a few deep breaths and let your body relax.

5. While breathing naturally, start counting each time you exhale. When you reach four (four breaths), start over.

6. Focus on the counting, not on the breaths.

7. If thoughts enter your mind, let them go by, refocusing on the counting.

---

occurring after completing a meditation session. And meditation has been shown to be very effective in relieving stress.

There are a number of meditation methods. See Box 12–3 for an example.

MINIMIZING HEALTH RISKS

Being aware of commonly encountered health risks enables health care professionals to take preventive measures. These actions provide benefits for workers themselves, as well as for the patients they serve. Armed with knowledge about health risks, workers are better equipped to educate patients about ways to achieve maximum wellness.

Smoking

Most people are familiar with the risks associated with cigarette smoking. It has been linked to many serious health conditions and is estimated to have contributed to approximately 480,000, or one in five, deaths annually. Included in this number are more than 41,000 deaths each year linked to secondhand smoke (https://www.cdc.gov /tobacco/data_statistics/fact_sheets/fast_facts/index .htm). The major causes of these deaths are cancer, stroke, diabetes, and respiratory diseases, such as COPD.

Unfortunately, understanding the dangers does not necessarily make it easy to stop smoking. Nicotine is a physically addictive substance. Although the long-term benefits of quitting are many, the discomfort of withdrawing from the use of tobacco discourages many people who would like to quit. There are methods that some individuals find helpful:

- Groups that meet regularly and offer a structured program that involves quitting gradually. Leaders are usually ex-smokers who offer encouragement. Buddy systems are often organized to provide support between meetings.

- Classes and support groups offered by health care facilities

- Online programs and support groups

- Hypnosis

- Methods that allow the gradual withdrawal from nicotine through the use of skin patches and/or gum

- Medications that reduce the need for nicotine

Withdrawal symptoms vary among individuals. They may include anxiety, inability to concentrate, headaches, irritability, and strong cravings for a cigarette. (These are an

Thinking It Through

Mary Payongayong is stressed out from her job as a radiology technician in a mid-city orthopedic clinic. Her work load has increased as the result of staff reductions, and her current supervisor is demanding. Mary finds it difficult to communicate with him and feels that he is unresponsive to the needs of the staff.

1. What might Mary do to improve her situation at work?

2. What might she do to relieve her stress?

Fascinating Facts

Many sources state that 10 to 20 minutes of meditation are equivalent to a 2-hour nap.

indication of just how strong the effect of nicotine is on the body!) Knowing what to expect and keeping in mind that the symptoms *will disappear* may offer encouragement to stay with the quitting process. Most ex-smokers agree that the temporary discomfort is worth it for them to feel better now and to decrease the risks of illness and premature death.

Substance Abuse

Substance abuse is a growing problem that increases the risk of stress, disease, and injury, accounting for tens of thousands of deaths annually. Paradoxically, it is to *escape* from stress that many individuals turn to alcohol and drugs. However, these habits are likely to create problems and become *additional* sources of stress. Drinking excessive amounts of alcohol in an effort to "relax" after work is an example. At best, alcohol offers only temporary relief. At worst, it can result in poor job performance and dismissal, in addition to health problems, such as liver damage and increased risk of accidents. The Centers for Disease Control and Prevention reports that approximately 88,000 deaths annually in the United States are attributable to excessive alcohol use (https://www.cdc.gov/alcohol/fact-sheets /alcohol-use.htm).

The abuse of drugs, especially prescription drugs that are **controlled substances** (have potential for addiction), has become a serious public health problem. There were 70,237 prescription and over-the-counter overdoses in 2017 (https://www.cdc.gov/drugoverdose/data/statedeaths. html). This problem extends to an increasing number of health care professionals. It is estimated that between 10% and 15% of health care professionals are addicted to drugs or alcohol. There are a number of reasons for drug use among health care professionals:

- Easy access to controlled substance medications
- Stressful job conditions
- Self-medication
- Perceived ability to improve work performance and alertness

Another contributing factor is that some health care professionals are able to call in unauthorized prescriptions for themselves to pharmacies because they know the vocabulary and procedures for ordering.

The dangers of drug abuse, whether with illegal substances or prescription drugs, cannot be overemphasized. Patient care is compromised when health care professionals perform under the influence of either drugs or alcohol because they can cause the following:

- Faulty judgment
- Blackouts
- Memory loss
- Inability to adequately perform tasks requiring physical coordination
- Illegible written documentation

Improper drug use can result in negative physical effects on the health care professional, along with the problems caused by the need to use larger amounts of the substance as the degree of physical tolerance rises. Stealing prescription drugs from a facility is a crime. In addition, patient care can be seriously compromised if health care providers consume the drugs needed by the patients. Even in cases not involving theft, the use of any type of drug or alcohol on the job can result in severe consequences. The fortunate employee may be required to enter a rehabilitation program. The less fortunate one faces imprisonment and a lifetime ban from working in certain health care occupations. Health care students should be aware that a conviction for using illegal drugs can permanently disqualify them from licensure in certain occupations.

There are many effective programs for treating substance abuse, including ones designed especially for health care professionals. The counseling office at most schools is a good source of information about community services. Anyone who believes that he or she may have a problem with drugs or alcohol should seek help immediately. (See also the discussion of opioid abuse in Chapter 2.)

Occupational Hazards

Health care professionals encounter various risks on the job: exposure to infectious disease, to chemicals, and to potentially dangerous equipment. Most risks can be minimized by using proper safety precautions and following facility rules. Occupational safety is discussed throughout this text:

- Avoiding injury through the use of proper body mechanics: Chapter 9
- Protecting oneself against infection and blood-borne pathogens: Chapter 10
- Practicing environmental safety: Chapter 11
- Using the computer safely: Chapter 9

Fascinating Facts

In 2017, 58 opioid prescriptions were written for every 100 Americans.

Source: www.cdc.gov/drugoverdose/data/prescribing.html

Fascinating Facts

In 2016, 10,497 people died in alcohol-impaired driving crashes, accounting for 28% of all traffic-related deaths in the United States.

Source: http://www.cdc.gov/motorvehiclesafety/impaired_driving/impaired-drv_factsheet.html

At each facility where you are employed, carefully read all the safety manuals and instruction books that apply to your work. Never hesitate to ask questions about anything you do not understand. Your safety, and that of patients and coworkers, depends on your knowledge and use of safe practices.

Safe Sex

Sexual practices became a necessary topic of discussion as a result of the global spread of the human immunodeficiency virus (HIV). Although the number of new infections in the United States has declined to 38,000 per year, there are 1.1 million individuals living with the virus (https://www.kff.org/hivaids/fact-sheet/the-hivaids-epidemic-in-the-united-states-the-basics/). It is recommended that everyone between the ages of 13 and 64 be tested at least once as part of a routine health exam, because about one in seven people who have the virus do not know it (https://www.hiv.gov/hiv-basics/hiv-testing/learn-about-hiv-testing/who-should-get-tested).

Although not fatal, genital herpes has reached epidemic proportions in the United States. According to the CDC, one person in six is infected with the virus that causes genital herpes. The number may actually be much higher because many people do not experience symptoms. And herpes may be passed on to an infant during delivery, leading to a potentially deadly infection.

There are a number of other sexually transmitted diseases (STDs) that health care professionals should be aware of. Some of the most common include:

- Human papillomavirus (HPV)
- Chlamydia
- Gonorrhea
- Syphilis
- Trichomoniasis

The only 100% effective means of preventing STDs is abstinence from sexual activity. For individuals who choose to be sexually active, basic precautions can minimize the risk of contracting STDs:

- Discuss risk factors with your potential partner before beginning a sexual relationship. Ask if he or she is aware of having an STD. Herpes is problematic because symptoms can be so mild that many people do not know they are infected.
- With any new partner, mutually agree to be tested for HIV. (*Note:* This is only effective if it has been at least six months since the last sexual contact. It can take that long for the virus to become detectable.)
- Use condoms.
- Get regular screening because some diseases have no signs or symptoms.
- See a physician immediately if symptoms of any STD are experienced. These include sores in the genital area, unusual odors, discharges, and itching.

The American Sexual Health Association (http://www.ashasexualhealth.org/healthcare-providers/) has many resources, including links specifically for health care professionals.

Burnout

Burnout is a form of physical and emotional exhaustion that can be caused by a variety of personal and environmental stressors experienced over an extended period. Burnout occurs in all professions, but health care professionals are particularly susceptible due to the nature of their work. Examples of stressors that can lead to burnout include the following:

- Long hours working under difficult conditions
- Lack of adequate rest
- Inability to deal effectively with frustrating situations
- Inadequate emotional support
- No time for recreational activities
- Emotional involvement with patients who are suffering from terminal diseases
- Poor diet and insufficient exercise

The symptoms of burnout vary among individuals. Commonly noted changes in behavior include the following:

- Negative feelings about work
- Feelings of not being appreciated
- Increased absences due to minor illnesses

- Physical symptoms such as fatigue, gastrointestinal disorders, and headaches
- Irritability
- Making errors and taking longer than previously required to complete tasks

(*Source:* Adapted from *Understanding Human Behavior: A Guide for Health Care Providers* (9th ed.), by M. E. Milliken & A. Honeycutt, 2018, Clifton Park, NY: Cengage Learning.)

The daily practice of good health habits and regular use of stress-prevention techniques are good ways to prevent burnout. Developing good **assertiveness** (expressing feelings freely in a nonthreatening manner) and communication skills (see Chapters 15 and 16) can help resolve workplace issues that might otherwise result in burnout.

Working cooperatively in high-risk situations can help everyone deal with a difficult workload. The nurses in a neonatal unit at a northern California hospital found the stress of caring for heroin-addicted newborns who cried constantly for days at a time to be overwhelming. They agreed to share their assignments so that no one had more than two consecutive shifts working with these babies (P. Bird, personal communication, June 1999). The Cleveland Clinic, rated as one of the best hospitals in the world, has initiated a Code Lavender response team to assist health care professionals in need of emotional support after experiencing troubling or exhaustive times, such as when experiencing the death of a patient (https://consultqd.clevelandclinic.org/code-lavender-offering-emotional-support-holistic-rapid-response/).

HELPING PATIENTS DEVELOP HEALTHY LIFESTYLES

Many health care professionals are required to provide patient education and all the health-promoting techniques described in this chapter can be applied to patients. You may also be expected to give specialized instructions, like the dental hygienist who teaches proper flossing and brushing techniques. Including information about healthy lifestyles is an excellent form of preventive care.

Physical therapy assistants teach exercises as part of their daily work. But other health care professionals, such as medical assistants, also have opportunities to explain the benefits of exercise. The fact is that almost every health care professional has opportunities to share information that will help patients develop healthier lifestyles.

See Chapters 16 and 17 for more information about patient education.

(*Note:* Be sure that your supervisor has approved any information and materials you share with patients.)

See Box 12–4 for a list of websites containing information about the topics in this chapter.

Box 12-4

Useful Websites for Healthy Living

Academy of Nutrition and Dietetics. www.eatright.org

Alcoholics Anonymous. www.aa.org

American Heart Association. www.heart.org

American Sexual Health Association. www.ashasexualhealth.org

Mayo Clinic. www.mayoclinic.org

MedlinePlus. http://medlineplus.gov

Mind Tools (Extensive information on time and stress management). www.mindtools.com

MyPlate. www.choosemyplate.gov

National Council on Alcoholism and Drug Dependence. www.ncadd.org

National Eating Disorders Association. www.nationaleatingdisorders.org

National Institute on Alcohol Abuse and Alcoholism. www.niaaa.nih.gov

Smoke Free. https://smokefree.gov

Substance Abuse and Mental Health Services Administration. http://www.samhsa.gov

U.S. Department of Agriculture, Center for Nutrition Policy and Promotion. www.cnpp.usda.gov

U.S. Department of Health and Human Services (HIV/AIDS information). www.hiv.gov

SUGGESTED LEARNING ACTIVITIES

1. Find articles from credible sources about the benefits of proper nutrition and exercise. What does current research report about best practices?

2. Start a list of articles and information from journals and the Internet about healthy habits.

3. Read packaged food labels. What are the major components of your favorites? Are you surprised by what you discover?

4. Try eating new foods that are high in nutritional value.

5. Start a collection of recipes for healthy dishes.

6. Develop a personal exercise program. Set a reasonable goal, such as three times a week for 20 minutes. Record your progress.

7. Look for examples of stressors in your environment. Which are internal and which are external?

8. Try the relaxation or meditation exercises for two weeks. Do you notice any benefits?

WEB ACTIVITIES

The Atlantic

https://www.theatlantic.com/health/archive/2016/03/less-than-3-percent-of-americans-live-a-healthy-lifestyle/475065/

Less Than 3 Percent of Americans Live a "Healthy Lifestyle"

1. What is defined as a "healthy lifestyle"?

2. Which of the four components seems the most difficult to achieve?

3. Why do you think this is the case?

Vox

https://www.vox.com/2016/8/31/12368246/obesity-america-2018-charts

It's Easy to Become Obese in America: These 7 Charts Explain Why

1. What were the estimated rates of obesity in 2016?

2. What is the percentage growth of obesity rates for men from 1960 to 2014? For women?

3. What components in the food environment contribute to weight gain?

4. Which types of foods are the most expensive? Why is this a problem?

5. How do the following contribute to weight gain: eating in restaurants, common breakfast foods, and ads for snack foods?

6. What are ways the food environment could better support healthful eating?

United States Department of Agriculture

www.choosemyplate.gov

Explore this website to learn more about nutrition and healthy eating.

1. List 10 facts you did not know before researching the site.

2. Write a short report about how you can apply what you learned to your daily eating habits.

Harvard Medical School–Division of Sleep Medicine

http://healthysleep.med.harvard.edu/healthy/matters/benefits-of-sleep/learning-memory

Sleep, Learning, and Memory

1. What are affected by lack of sleep?

2. What are the three functions of learning and memory? When does each take place?

3. What are the three stages of sleep?

4. What type of learning is associated with each sleep stage?

5. In what ways does lack of sleep impact learning and performance?

National Library of Medicine–Medline Plus

http://medlineplus.gov

1. Click on "Health Topics," then on "Health and Wellness." and "Fitness and Exercise."

2. Follow the links to find articles or news reports of interest to read and summarize.

The American Institute of Stress

https://www.stress.org/self-assessment/

1. Take the Stress 360 quiz to determine your stress.

2. Take the Homes–Rahe Stress Inventory to see which life events cause the most stress.

Monster

https://www.monster.com/career-advice/article/stress-management-tips-in-healthcare

Stress-management tips for health care workers

Write a short report describing the suggestions given for combating stress in the health care workplace.

American Institute of Medical Sciences & Education

https://www.aimseducation.edu/blog/10-youtube-videos-boost-productivity/

10 YouTube Videos That Will Boost Your Productivity

The following four videos, presented in different ways, explain reasons behind procrastination and offer suggestions for getting more done and making life easier.

The Science of Productivity

How to Stop Procrastinating

Tips to Structure Your Day

Robin Sharma – How I Beat Procrastination (This video presents the topic in terms of reaching your goals and realizing your dreams for a good life.)

U.S. Department of Justice–Drug Enforcement Administration

https://www.deadiversion.usdoj.gov/pubs/brochures/drug_hc.htm

Drug Addiction in Health Care Professionals

1. What are the health care professional's responsibilities regarding controlled substances (drugs)?

2. What are eight behaviors demonstrated by a drug-impaired individual?

3. How are drug-impaired health care professionals sometimes enabled and not held responsible for their drug problems?

4. What does the DOJ recommend you do if you strongly suspect that a coworker has a drug problem?

REVIEW QUESTIONS

1. Which four of the top causes of death in the United States are influenced by personal health habits?

2. Why is it important for health care professionals to practice a healthy lifestyle?

3. What are six techniques for developing positive habits?

4. What are two ways that have been found effective to help individuals change habits that involve addictive substances?

5. Why is healthy eating important?

6. What is the meaning of the terms diet and nutrition?

7. What are the six essential nutrients? What is the function of each?

8. Choose four examples of vitamins and four of minerals and give their purpose and food sources.

9. What is the role of fiber in the diet?

10. What is a calorie?

11. What are "good" and "bad" carbohydrates and what are the effects of each on the body?

12. Why should added sugars be limited in the diet?

13. What are "good" and "bad" fats and what is the effect of each on the body?

14. What is the meaning and purpose of cholesterol and what are the two types?

15. Why should trans fats be avoided?

16. What is the negative effect of excess sodium in the diet?

17. What are processed foods? What are some examples?

18. What problems are associated with eating processed foods?

19. Why are some food labels confusing for consumers?

20. What makes foods organic? What are the three levels of organic foods?

21. What are the key recommendations for healthy eating developed by the U.S. Department of Agriculture?

22. What is ChooseMyPlate and what is its purpose?

23. What are the components of the Mediterranean diet?

24. What are five conditions to which excess body weight contributes?

25. What are eight factors believed to contribute to the epidemic of overweight and obesity in the United States?

26. What is the meaning and purpose of the Body Mass Index? What are its limitations?

27. Why are many weight-loss diets unhealthy?

28. What are the four types of vegetarian diets?

29. What are the characteristics of the following conditions: anorexia nervosa, bulimia, and binge eating?

30. What are five benefits of physical exercise?

31. What is the definition of aerobic exercise?

32. What are three examples of how physical exercise can be incorporated into daily life?

33. Why is it important to get adequate sleep?

34. What are five suggestions for increasing the length and quality of sleep?

35. What are three measures that help prevent health problems from developing or worsening?

36. What is stress and what are three physical changes that often accompany it?

37. What are external stressors and internal stressors?

38. Why is work in health care particularly stressful?

39. What are some methods health care professionals can use to deal with stress?

40. What are five examples of techniques for effectively managing time?

41. How is muscle relaxation beneficial?

42. What is meditation and what are examples of its long-term benefits?

43. What are six methods found to help individuals quit smoking?

44. What is a controlled substance?

45. What are the reasons that some health care professionals have problems with substance abuse? What are the potential consequences of this abuse?

46. What are some examples of occupational risks for health care professionals?

47. What are five of the most common sexually transmitted diseases?

48. What are the precautions for avoiding sexually transmitted diseases?

49. What is burnout? What are its causes and symptoms?

50. What are some ways to help prevent burnout?

APPLICATION EXERCISES

1. Refer to the Case of the Cardiac Unit Nurse at the beginning of this chapter. Describe the lifestyle habits, based on what you learned in this chapter, that enable Gracie Chin to stay fit for her job as a cardiac nurse.

2. Jorge Chavez is a surgical technologist at a busy ambulatory surgical center. His full-time job requires that he spend many hours on his feet, that he stay mentally alert, and that he quickly and correctly respond to surgeons' requests. Jorge must balance his job with a busy family life. He and his wife have two small children whom he cares for while his wife attends college two evenings a week. Using the information in this chapter, develop a plan that will help Jorge stay healthy, avoid burnout, and remain an effective member of the health care team.

PROBLEM-SOLVING PRACTICE

Sandra is enrolled in a physical therapist assistant program and looking forward to getting her first job. Her father died recently and her elderly mother is making many demands on Sandra's time and energy. She calls Sandra at least once a day to ask questions, complain about how lonely she feels, or ask her daughter to run errands for her.

How can Sandra use the five-step problem-solving process to find ways to help her mother and, at the same time, ensure that she graduates and maintains a job?

CHAPTER 13

Professionalism

KEY TERMS

attitude
compassion
empathy
leadership
professional distance
professionalism

OBJECTIVES

Studying and applying the material in this chapter will help you to:

1. Explain the meaning of professionalism for individuals who work in health care.
2. Define "compassion" and explain why it is important in health care.
3. State the meaning of "attitude."
4. Explain the importance of a positive attitude in health care.
5. State the meaning of "empathy."
6. Explain the importance of empathy in health care.
7. List six ways to demonstrate a professional attitude.
8. List 12 components of professional conduct.
9. Describe the manner in which technical skills must be applied in all work situations.
10. List five ways to develop and maintain your technical skills.
11. Explain what professional appearance communicates to patients.
12. Describe the general requirements for appearance in health care settings.
13. List seven components of a professional appearance.
14. Explain the meaning of "professional distance."
15. Explain how health care professionals can effectively handle difficult situations.
16. Describe how to accept criticism professionally.
17. List behaviors to avoid on social media.
18. Define "leadership" and list the characteristics of a health care leader.

The Case of the Lost Opportunity

Gerald Lenz has worked as an ultrasound technician for just over three years. He performs a variety of duties at a large imaging center. Gerald does what is necessary to complete his work, but believes that his job consists of using his technical skills. He performs them adequately, but makes no effort to "go out of his way" for either his coworkers or patients. Although he is never rude, it is clear to patients that working with them is simply a job Gerald performs in exchange for a salary. Gerald never volunteers to work on extra projects, never contributes new ideas at staff meetings, and never participates in special activities offered outside working hours. Ultrasound technicians are in short supply in Gerald's city, so he remains employed. He was recently passed over for a promotion because his supervisor believed he lacks professionalism. Gerald was disappointed and could not understand why someone who had worked there for just a year and a half got the position instead of him. In this chapter, you will learn about behaviors that make the difference between just getting by on the job and making a positive, professional contribution.

THE MEANING OF PROFESSIONALISM

Professionalism is an essential quality for everyone who works in health care. We often hear someone described as being "very professional" or "acting professionally." Professionalism is difficult to define because it consists of many characteristics and behaviors. Individuals in all health care occupations display professionalism by dedicating themselves to doing their best on the job and providing and maintaining high-quality service. "Caring competence" is one way to express the meaning of **professionalism** in health care. **Compassion**, the sincere concern for others, especially those who are anxious, fearful, and in pain, is the foundation of the caring component of professionalism. It is the basis for developing empathy, discussed in the next section.

The confidence patients have in the care they receive is influenced by each individual they have contact with in the health care system. Health care professionals represent the facilities in which they work. Their attitude and actions are a reflection of all the services and people who work there.

Professional Attitude

Attitude is how a person views a situation—the way she thinks and feels about someone or something. Every situation in life can be viewed in different ways: positively or negatively. For example, problems can be viewed as dreaded difficulties or as challenges that keep life interesting or as opportunities to learn and apply one's skills.

Individuals working in health care who have professional attitudes approach work as positively as possible: upbeat, optimistic, and cheerful. They think in terms of what they can give rather than what they can get. Patient welfare is the primary focus of the employee with a professional attitude, and studies have shown that the attitude of the health care professional has a significant effect on patients. This is true whether the task is preparing accurate billing statements or providing direct patient care. (See Figure 13–1.)

Health care professionals face many situations that can be approached either positively or negatively. Let's look at an example.

Mr. Chang is an 86-year-old resident in an extended care facility. He spent most of his life in Hong Kong, moving to the United States when he was in his 60s. His wife died two years ago, and his children live in other parts of the country. He rarely has visitors. Mr. Chang can be difficult to understand because of his accent, complains a lot about being in the care facility, and is considered generally unpleasant to be around.

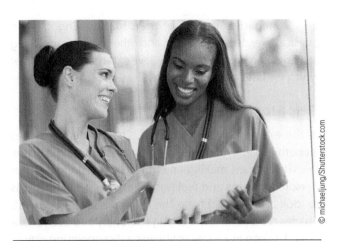

FIGURE 13–1 Approach your work with a positive attitude. Focus on how you and your coworkers can contribute to patient well-being.

Two staff members have contrasting experiences with Mr. Chang:

1. Anne dreads having to enter Mr. Chang's room each morning. He complains and grumbles as she gets him up and dressed. Anne hurries through her tasks and limits her conversation to necessary instructions.

2. Charles works the evening shift and looks forward to working with Mr. Chang. Charles did some research on Chinese culture and learned that for Mr. Chang, living in a care facility away from family is different from how life would have been in Hong Kong where, until recently, families would not consider having senior members live in a facility such as a nursing home. Charles asks Mr. Chang questions and listens carefully. As a result, he has learned a lot about life in another culture and has learned to appreciate the importance of family ties. He has shared stories about his own family with Mr. Chang and offered the elderly resident friendship and relief from loneliness.

When faced with difficult situations, look for ways to turn them into learning experiences or deal with them in ways that create the least amount of stress. Ask yourself:

- Do I fully understand the situation?

- Is my behavior contributing to the problem?

- If so, what can I do differently?

- Are there any positive possibilities, such as those that Charles found, that I have overlooked?

Some situations, in spite of the health care professional's best efforts, do not turn out to be as positive as the example with Charles and Mr. Chang. The best approach in these cases is to perform work in a professional manner, keep emotions under control, and avoid mentally dwelling on the negative aspects of the situation. Engaging in physical exercise, meditation, and other health-promoting activities can help reduce or relieve external stressors over which we have no control.

Empathy

In the example with Mr. Chang, Charles demonstrates empathy, an essential part of professionalism in health care. Empathy means making an effort to understand another person' thoughts and feelings. To experience empathy is to look at the world from the other person's viewpoint. Charles realized that Mr. Chang felt lonely and even abandoned. Living in a care facility was a disappointing way to spend his final years, not what he expected from life.

The old expression, "Walk a mile in my shoes" is a good description of empathy. Put another way, it expresses to patients, "I'm available to walk this road with you" (Tamparo & Lindh, 2008, p. 63). Remember that the roads patients must walk may be painful and scary. Experiencing empathy helps the health care professional understand and more effectively address the needs of each patient.

Empathy includes communicating that you are aware of the other person's feelings. At the same time, it is inappropriate to says, "I know exactly how you feel," because, of course, this is not possible. However, striving to understand patients can help relieve the loneliness and anxiety and encourage them to feel safe about sharing their feelings and discussing their concerns. (See Figure 13–2.)

Demonstrating a Professional Attitude

A professional attitude in health care work can be expressed in many ways:

- Be committed to your work. Believe in the value of what you are doing and your ability to do it.

© Monkey Business Images/Shutterstock.com

FIGURE 13-2 Empathy and compassion provide the foundation of good patient care.

- Keep in mind your impact on patient care and services. Aim to contribute positively to the well-being of patients and their perception of the facility.
- Use an objective approach to situations. This means considering the facts rather than responding emotionally. For example, if a patient you have assisted is rude, think about possible causes. The rudeness may be a reaction to fear or pain and have nothing to do with you personally.
- If you make a mistake or are at fault when working with a patient, take responsibility for correcting the situation.
- View problems as opportunities for positive action. Problems are part of everyday life, and learning to deal with them effectively is essential for achieving work success and satisfaction. (Review the five-step problem-solving process described in Chapter 1.)
- Develop and practice self-discipline. Knowing you can depend on yourself to accomplish what needs to be done results in both competence and self-confidence.

Professional Behaviors

A professional attitude provides the foundation for developing professional behaviors, and these behaviors, in turn, demonstrate "caring competence." The actions of health care professionals directly influence the level of patient satisfaction. Poor outcomes as well as malpractice lawsuits increase when patients are dissatisfied with the service they receive. Patients are health care consumers, and good service increases consumer loyalty. (See Chapter 23.)

The following behaviors are important components of professional conduct:

- Be dependable. Follow through on assignments, meet deadlines, and be on the job and on time as scheduled.
- Perform all duties as assigned and needed. "It's not my job" is rarely heard in today's facilities because employees who say it are not employed for long. (An exception is if a health care professional is asked

Fascinating Facts

When employees in two large-scale studies were asked, "What makes you feel successful at work?" more than half the respondents answered, "Doing a good job."

to do a task that he or she is not trained or legally allowed to perform.) Willingness to always do one's best is the sign of a true professional.

- Be flexible. Health care work is continually changing. Willingness to adapt to these changes is essential.

- Accept differences. Today's patient population is increasingly diverse. (See Chapter 15 for information on cultural diversity.)

- Be aware of how your actions affect others. Treat everyone, patients, coworkers, and supervisors, with courtesy and consideration.

- Practice good communication skills. (See Chapters 15 and 16.)

- Put personal problems aside during work time. Do not discuss them with coworkers or patients. And *never* complain about your work, supervisor, or the facility while you are in the workplace. Patients who hear such complaints may lose confidence in the care they are receiving. Complaining can also negatively affect the morale of coworkers. Keep your conversations focused on creating positive relationships and solving problems rather than creating them. (See Figure 13–1.)

- Be well organized and plan your work. For example, gather all equipment and supplies before beginning a procedure so the patient does not have to wait.

- Behave ethically at all times and set high personal standards. (See Chapter 3.)

- Conduct yourself calmly. This is especially important in emergencies and upsetting situations, when it is necessary to think clearly. Remaining calm also helps patients, who look to health care professionals for reassurance.

- Serve as a role model for good health. As a health care professional, you have an opportunity to encourage good health habits in others. (See Chapter 12.)

- Set professional goals for learning and continual improvement. (See Chapter 14.)

Fascinating Facts

According to Stephen Covey, author of best-selling books on personal effectiveness, the average person spends 80% of his time interacting with others. For most people, then, the majority of their waking hours is spent interacting or communicating with other people—or dealing with the poor results of that interaction.

Technical Skills

Achieving and maintaining a high level of skill is a critical component of professionalism. Tasks must be performed correctly and carefully. Pay attention and think about what you are doing at all times. Nothing can be taken for granted or become routine. Approach each patient as an individual who deserves your best efforts. Here are additional suggestions for developing and maintaining your skill level:

- Develop an in-depth understanding of your work. Learn as much as possible about the theories that support your skills. This will increase the level of your performance and provide a foundation for good decision making and problem solving.

- Observe and listen carefully. Question situations that do not seem right given the circumstances.

- Consult the employee manual at your workplace or ask questions if you are unsure about a policy or procedure.

- Perform all work as neatly and accurately as possible.

- Dedicate time to acquiring new knowledge and skills. (See Chapter 14.)

Professional Appearance

The appearance of those who work in health care occupations is an outward sign of their level of professionalism. It strongly influences the way they are perceived by patients and coworkers. A professional appearance communicates the message, "I take my job and myself seriously. I have self-respect and want patients to have confidence in my abilities."

Professional appearance in health care settings is generally conservative. Some popular fashion trends, such as tattoos and body piercing, were at one time associated with antisocial groups. This is why some patients find them offensive and even frightening. As more people have tattoos and piercings, they are becoming accepted by increasing numbers of employers. In many employment settings, they are not required to be covered *unless* they are frightening (skulls, images suggesting death) or offensive in some other way (racist, gender-biased, etc.). Check with your employer about policies regarding tattoos and body piercings. Keep in mind that it is a sign of respect and consideration for patients to consider their feelings when planning your appearance. (See Figures 13–3 and 13–4.)

Maintaining a professional appearance includes the following:

- Practice personal cleanliness. This includes the hair, hands and fingernails, clothing, and shoes.

- Avoid long and/or painted fingernails. Color on nails can hide dirt that harbors bacteria. Studies have shown that the edges of chipped polish are breeding

FIGURE 13–3 What positive messages are communicated by the appearance of these health care professionals? What effect do you think they have on patients?

FIGURE 13–4 When the job requires regular clothing, it should be neat and conservative.

grounds for bacteria that are hard to remove, even with handwashing.

- Use a deodorant or antiperspirant daily.
- Pay attention to dental hygiene. Flossing and regular dental care help prevent bad breath.
- Avoid the use of perfumes and strong-smelling hair sprays and other personal products. Some people are allergic to fragrances. Many others find them offensive, especially when they are ill. Some fragrances can even trigger asthmatic attacks.
- Avoid extreme styles in dress and grooming, such as unnaturally colored hair and green nail polish.

- Consider personal safety and that of others. Avoid wearing anything that can be grabbed or caught, such as dangling earrings and untied long hair. Wear closed-toed shoes to protect your feet from injury.

Professional Distance

Professional distance refers to a healthy balance in the health professional–patient relationship. It means demonstrating a caring attitude toward patients without the goal of becoming their friend. Although it is appropriate to seek personal satisfaction from work, it is inappropriate to personally depend on the friendship and approval of patients. Working to please, rather than serve appropriately, can be counterproductive. Keep your focus on the patients' health goals and what must be done to achieve them. At the same time, it is appropriate to have empathy and demonstrate a caring attitude toward patients. (See Figure 13–5.)

Handling Difficult Situations Professionally

Health care professionals sometimes deal with challenging and stressful situations. It is natural to react emotionally when faced with an emergency, the death of a child, or an angry patient. Such a response, however, can interfere with your effectiveness. An objective, although not unfeeling, response is necessary for the health care professional to perform professionally and constructively.

Being professional requires that you know yourself well and make an effort to understand the basis of your reactions to workplace problems. Learning to recognize the causes of a behavior can help you change it,

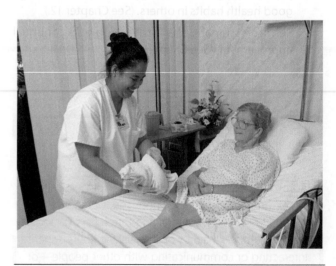

FIGURE 13–5 Professional distance requires focusing on the health care needs of the patient while expressing caring concern.

if necessary. For example, Keith has always had a quick temper. He finds it difficult to be patient and becomes easily irritated by incidents involving disorder, delays, and disorganization. His work as a pharmacy technician in a busy hospital does not always go smoothly, and Keith's impatience is negatively affecting his relationships with coworkers. When he takes time to analyze his behavior and sees that it follows a lifelong pattern, he realizes that he must learn to make adjustments and adapt to workplace conditions.

The problem-solving model described in Chapter 1 provides a constructive way to change negative habits and behaviors. Reviewing and gathering information, as described in the model, helps to separate fact from emotion. Facts provide a basis on which to identify potentially effective resolutions to problems and to make sound decisions.

Professional Acceptance of Criticism

Criticism and correction can be valuable learning resources. These opportunities to learn are often lost because it is hard for people to admit that they might be wrong. It is common to react defensively in these situations and miss the message. Responding gracefully to criticism is a sign of self-confidence and professionalism. Health care professionals who feel secure about themselves are comfortable with suggestions about their work and conduct. They are able to evaluate the information and decide if it applies to them. Being willing to recognize and work on imperfections is a sign of emotional maturity and professionalism. Chapter 23 contains more information about giving and receiving criticism.

Professionalism Outside the Workplace

Working in health care, you represent your profession both on and off the job. Of course, you should enjoy your off time with friends and family, engaging in activities you like. However, inappropriate behaviors should be avoided. Examples include drinking too much at work functions, wearing T-shirts with offensive messages, and exhibiting rude behavior in public.

Social media is a great way to keep in touch with friends and family and express your views and opinions, but it is important to know what to post and what not to post. Many employers now check Facebook and other websites when hiring. Questionable photos, even of what you consider to be harmless fun (overdrinking and acting out at a party, for example), can harm your reputation. Many employers report these kinds of photos as the biggest online mistake, You may have heard news stories about individuals who were fired for posting inappropriate photos or statements that were racist or otherwise

offensive. Professionals in service industries, such as health care and education, cannot afford to damage their reputations online.

Here are other online behaviors to avoid:

- Having a generally negative tone and posting complaints and criticisms (*never* make negative comments about your employer online!)
- Bragging and giving the impression of an inflated ego
- Sharing too much about your personal life
- Using profanity (curse words)
- Sexual content
- Online bullying
- Rude and insensitive comments

Always think before you send: how does this represent me? Remember, what you put online can be viewed by millions and is very difficult, if not impossible, to erase after that send button is pushed.

PROFESSIONAL LEADERSHIP

Leadership involves encouraging people to work together and do their best to achieve common goals. Leaders combine visions of excellence with the ability to inspire

Thinking It Through

An important part of Torst Borgen's work as a physical therapy assistant is working with postoperative patients in their homes. His job is to help them regain strength and range of motion. Exercises prescribed by the supervising physical therapist are often uncomfortable and Torst must encourage as well as instruct patients to perform them. Torst lives alone and enjoys the social aspects of working with patients. He wants them to like him. This sometimes makes it difficult for him to insist that they engage in necessary exercises that are painful.

1. How might Torst's need to be friends with patients interfere with their full recovery?

2. What changes are needed in his view of his role as a physical therapy assistant?

3. What actions in his personal life can he take to achieve the professional distance necessary to best assist patients in their recovery?

Thinking It Through

Certified nursing assistant Barbara Sterndorf has difficulty working independently in her job at Pinehurst Care Home, an extended care facility. Barbara was raised by parents who were quite critical, and she lacks self-confidence. She is afraid of making mistakes and only does exactly what she is directed to do by her supervisor, Carla Thomas. In spite of her self-doubts, Barbara always performs high-quality work and is well liked by the residents. Carla believes her to be well trained and among the most competent CNAs on the staff and tells her this during Barbara's performance evaluation.

1. What might Barbara do to increase her self-confidence at work?

2. How might her self-image and work habits hold her back from advancing in her career?

others. They promote positive changes that benefit their professions and the people they serve. A leader may or may not be a supervisor. It is possible to set an example of excellence and encourage others without having a position of authority.

Effective leaders in health care do the following:

- Demonstrate a high level of competence in their profession

- Commit to providing high-quality service

- Show a willingness to recognize and support the work of others

- Dedicate themselves to meeting high standards

- Believe that necessary changes and improvements can be accomplished

- Show a willingness to serve as an example and complete the tasks necessary to achieve the goals of the group

- Demonstrate an ability to communicate effectively

- Set a good example of professionalism

- Encourage others to be their best

SUGGESTED LEARNING ACTIVITIES

1. Find examples of people you think exhibit professional characteristics. Explain why you chose them.

2. Rate your own level of professionalism in each of the following categories:

   - Attitude

   - Empathy

   - Conduct

   - Appearance

   - Health care skills

Based on your ratings, create a plan to develop and/or improve your professionalism.

3. Interview a health care supervisor about his or her definition of professionalism.

4. Using the material in this chapter as a guide, create your own description of professionalism in your occupational area.

WEB ACTIVITIES

Lockton Affinity

http://locktonmedicalliabilityinsurance.com/positive-attitude-in-healthcare/

A Positive Attitude in Health Care: Make It the Rule, Not the Exception

1. Why is a positive attitude so important in health care?

2. What are three other advantages to having a positive attitude?

3. What are some common causes of a bad attitude?

4. What are ways to deal with job burnout?

5. How can a positive attitude help you succeed in your career?

RN Journal

http://rn-journal.com/journal-of-nursing/attitude-matters-nursing

Although directed to nurses, the information in this article applies to all health care professionals.

1. Do you agree that the set of professional behaviors listed for nurses applies to your future occupation? Why or why not?

2. What are the core values that nurses must have?

3. Do you believe these values apply to you? Do you have these values?

4. What conditions in the health care work environment can cause bad attitudes?

5. Give your impression of this statement: "We all have a choice between self-encouragement and self-pity."

Pomona College

https://www.pomona.edu/administration/pre-health/prepare/characteristics

Characteristics of the Successful Health Care Professional

1. What are the skills and qualities that this school looks for in health care students?

2. What are the core competencies of health care professionals? (Although addressed to medical students, these apply to all.)

Medical GPS

http://blog.medicalgps.com/the-importance-of-empathy-in-healthcare/

The Importance of Empathy in Health Care

    Although directed to physicians, this information applies to all health care professionals.

    According to this article, why is empathy important?

Cleveland Clinic

https://www.youtube.com/watch?v=cDDWvj_q-o8

Watch this powerful video, "The Human Connection to Patient Care." (Note: The previous web activity has a link to this video.)

1. What is your reaction to the video?

2. Do you think you will look at people differently after watching this?

3. How can experiencing empathy make us better people as well as health care professionals?

John Muir Health

https://www.johnmuirhealth.com/get-involved/careers/working-here/professional-appearance.html

See what one employer states about professional appearance for its employees.

Professional Organizations

1. Explore the website of the professional organization(s) for careers of interest to you. (See Appendix 1 for a list of professional organizations and their contact information.)

2. Does the organization contain a definition of professionalism for its members?

3. If you cannot find a section on professionalism, try searching for "professionalism for _____" and insert an occupational area of interest, such as physical therapy.

4. What opportunities does it provide for members to develop professionally?

REVIEW QUESTIONS

1. What is meant by professionalism in health care?

2. What is the meaning of "compassion"? Why is it important in health care?

3. What is the meaning of "attitude"?

4. Why is a positive attitude important in health care?

5. What is the meaning of "empathy"?

6. What is the importance of empathy in health care?

7. What are six ways to demonstrate a professional attitude?

8. What are 12 components of professional conduct?

9. In what way must health care professionals apply their technical skills?

10. What are five ways to develop and maintain your technical skills?

11. What does a professional appearance communicate to patients?

12. What are the general requirements for the health care professional's appearance in the workplace?

13. What are seven components of a professional appearance?

14. What is the meaning of "professional distance"?

15. What are examples of ways that health care professionals can handle difficult situations they encounter in the workplace?

16. What is meant by accepting criticism professionally?

17. Which behaviors should be avoided on social media?

18. What is the definition of "leadership"? What are the characteristics of a health care leader?

APPLICATION EXERCISES

1. What changes does Gerald Lenz, described in the Case of the Lost Opportunity at the beginning of the chapter, need to make in order to increase his level of professionalism as an ultrasound technician?

2. Karin is a dental receptionist for Dr. Sims. She arrives at the office on Monday morning to face the beginning of "one of those days." A long-time patient who has suffered all weekend with a toothache is waiting at the door. The dental hygienist is ill and will not be in, leaving seven patients without appointments. When notified that they will have to reschedule, two patients are very unhappy and express their irritation to Karin. Later in the morning, the office computer freezes up, and the scheduling and billing programs cannot be accessed. In the afternoon, an elderly patient returns to the office after his appointment to say that his car won't start. He asks for help to get it started or to find other transportation home. Discuss how Karin can handle each situation professionally. Include professional attitude as well as actions.

PROBLEM-SOLVING PRACTICE

Max is a licensed practical nurse who has been working in the oncology (cancer) unit of a local hospital for just over a year. He is finding it more and more difficult to remain objective and not become emotionally involved with the patients and their families. It is beginning to disrupt his sleep and he is worried that his feelings might negatively affect his ability to provide the help his patients need. How can Max use the five-step problem-solving process to help maintain a healthy professional distance?

Professional Development and Lifelong Learning

KEY TERMS

- continuing education
- continuing education units (CEUs)
- continuing medical education
- continuing professional education (CPE)
- inservice training
- lifelong learning
- mentor
- professional development
- role model
- self-directed learning

OBJECTIVES

Studying and applying the material in this chapter will help you to:

1. State the meaning of "professional development."
2. List ways the health care professional can grow professionally.
3. State five purposes of professional organizations.
4. List five advantages of participating in one's professional organization.
5. Explain the importance of lifelong learning for the health care professional.
6. Describe the changes and trends in health care and their corresponding learning requirements for health care professionals.
7. Explain the meaning and significance of "expanded scope of practice."
8. Define the following terms: "continuing education units," "continuing professional education," and "continuing medical education."
9. Explain the ways you can earn continuing education units.
10. Provide criteria for choosing quality courses and materials for earning continuing education units.
11. Explain the meaning of "self-directed learning."
12. List ways to incorporate self-directed learning into your daily life.
13. Define the following terms: "role model" and "mentor."
14. List the qualities to look for when choosing a role model.
15. List ways a mentor can help a beginning health care professional.
16. Explain the meaning of "career ladder."
17. Explain how the duties and responsibilities vary with different levels on career ladders.

The Case of Lifetime Success

Mabel Bennett has worked in medical records for many years—so many that she likes to joke and tell people that records were handwritten with feather pens when she started. Mabel enjoys tasks that involve detail and order. She has always received satisfaction from the challenge of maintaining complete and accurate records and has risen to the position of medical records manager at a large suburban rehabilitation hospital. Over the years, Mabel has seen many changes in her field. Her first position was keeping paper records for a country doctor at a time when no one had even thought about desktop computers. Through the years, Mabel has pursued every available opportunity to learn more about her field and has enjoyed her learning experiences. She was one of the first in her profession to realize the potential of computer applications in medical records and became an expert user of computer technology. Mabel credits her long-term career success to her interest in learning all she can and working with the future in mind. In this chapter, you will learn ways in which successful health care professionals like Mabel acquire the knowledge they need to stay current and advance in their fields.

PROFESSIONAL DEVELOPMENT

Professional development means continually striving to improve and be the best at your profession. It also means finding satisfaction in your work and participating in professional activities beyond those required during the normal workday. Obtaining a job is only the first step on the career path. Professional development keeps the journey headed in the right direction. Whether the health care professional spends an entire career at the same job or makes many changes, professional development is necessary for long-term success. All health care occupations are affected by rapidly occurring medical discoveries and technological advances. Continual learning is required to stay current and perform effectively. In many occupations, it is required to maintain a license or certification. Do not view professional education as a burden, but rather as an opportunity to expand your knowledge and opportunities.

There are many ways to grow professionally and maintain a lively interest in work:

- Set goals: Setting attainable goals and periodically reviewing your progress are powerful motivators for growth. Well-planned goals serve as road maps toward a fulfilling future. Here are a few examples of professional goals:

  ○ Increase keyboarding speed to 85 words per minute

  ○ Learn health-related conversational Spanish

  ○ Earn certificate in echocardiography

  ○ Be promoted to supervisory position at hospital within five years

- Join professional organizations: In addition to providing learning opportunities, these organizations are places to share experiences with other health care professionals. Friendship and mutual support increase career satisfaction. Active participation on committees or as an officer is an excellent way to practice teamwork and leadership skills. Professional organizations are also good sources for obtaining necessary continuing education credits. Professional organizations are discussed in the next section.

- Network: Networking is not limited to the initial job search. Maintaining and expanding your networking contacts exposes you to new ideas and opportunities for advancement. Once employed, consider helping others start their careers by giving them information and encouragement. Networking goes in both directions and should be considered a career-long activity.

- Request additional responsibility: This is a way to both show interest and maintain interest in the job. After you have mastered the basic duties and work routine, adding new responsibilities keeps the challenge alive.

- Stay in touch with your mentor: A good mentor keeps you motivated and aiming toward excellence by providing ongoing career advice. Mentors are discussed later in this chapter.

A career in health care involves enormous responsibilities and tremendous rewards. Engaging in professional development activities can help maintain the balance and ensure a long and satisfying career in the service of others.

PROFESSIONAL ORGANIZATIONS

Participating actively in a professional organization can contribute positively to professional development. Most health care occupations have an organization whose purposes include the following:

- Promoting the profession

- Ensuring quality patient care by making certain that professionals have the necessary knowledge and skill sets

- Sponsoring **continuing education** (learning experiences beyond those needed to earn the initial certificate or degree to work in an occupation, discussed later in this chapter). Some organizations, such as the American Association for Respiratory Care, offer leadership courses to help their members advance in their professions.

- Encouraging networking among members

- Supporting legislation on behalf of the profession and health care in general

Serving on committees, volunteering to help with projects, and running for office are excellent ways to become involved. There are many advantages for health care professionals who participate at any level:

- Learning to work in a group to achieve common goals

- Meeting established professionals who can offer career advice and serve as positive role models

- Keeping current in the field

- Developing management skills

- Receiving the support and the encouragement of colleagues

See Appendix 1 for a list of health care professional organizations.

IMPORTANCE OF LIFELONG LEARNING

Lifelong learning refers to all purposeful learning activities, both formal and informal, that take place throughout our lives. Today, lifelong learning is more important than ever because the world is changing faster than at any other time in history. Until the mid-20th century, people could expect to live in much the same way as their parents and grandparents had. Current advancements in technology now produce significant changes during a single lifetime. For example, people who today are in their seventies grew up without television. Those in their fifties began their professional lives without personal computers, handheld calculators, cellular phones, and many other products that are now considered necessities.

Today, most people take change for granted and incorporate it into their lifestyles. They are no longer surprised by the constant stream of new products available, or the speed of the changes in these products that require them to be updated even before they are worn out by use. What new health care professionals may find surprising is *how much learning will be required after graduation* in order to keep up with the many changes that affect the way jobs are performed. For example, many people in the workforce today learned to use a personal computer *after* they had completed their formal education and were already employed. They had to take the time to read manuals, attend workshops, watch videos, or use tutorials to learn to use what has now become an essential tool for work in health care. And the need to learn in the area of computers alone will continue to grow as new applications and updated versions of software and hardware are developed. (See Chapter 18.)

Keeping Up with Changes in Health Care

Changes in the delivery of health care are taking place continually. Knowledge quickly becomes outdated, and within a few years of entering the health care field, an individual who fails to keep up with current information will become incompetent. Your graduation, then, marks the end of formal training and the beginning of lifelong learning.

In addition to technology, the social and demographic changes and trends discussed in Chapter 2 require that health care professionals acquire new knowledge and skills. See Table 14–1 for examples of changes and the corresponding learning requirements for health care professionals. Standard precautions, explained in Chapter 10, are now common knowledge in the workplace. And yet they are actually a relatively recent development, created in 1987 in response to the spread of the human immunodeficiency virus (HIV) and hepatitis B. Health care professionals who work in certain positions must be trained and tested on various standards, including undergoing annual reviews. Health information professionals must continue to update their knowledge of contract management, patient eligibility, and billing procedures. And the shift in patient demographics has meant that a large percentage of those who provide direct patient care will spend much of their time working with older adults. (See Figure 14–1.)

Many health care occupations have expanded their scope of practice in an effort to increase the efficiency of patient care delivery. Professionals who previously performed a limited set of tasks are now being cross-trained and becoming multiskilled. Examples of additional duties

Table 14–1 Changes That Affect Health Care

Changes	Corresponding Learning Needs of Health Care Professionals
People living longer	Developmental stages and needs of older adults
	Patient care skills for long-term care
	Care of patients with chronic conditions
Increasing numbers of patients diagnosed with Alzheimer's disease and other forms of dementia	Care of dementia patients
Hospital stays that are much shorter than in the past	Home health patient practices and techniques
	Patient education delivery techniques
Increased ethnic and cultural diversity of U.S. population	Diverse customs and health habits
	Languages other than English
Growing patient interest in complementary health care practices, such as acupuncture and holistic medicine	Knowledge of complementary and alternative medicine
	Understanding of how the use of complementary and alternative health care practices is affecting Western medical practices

(continues)

Table 14–1 Changes That Affect Health Care (continued)

Changes	Corresponding Learning Needs of Health Care Professionals
Increase in third-party payers	Coding and billing practices
	Contract administration, obtaining preauthorizations for treatment, and permission for referral to specialists
Emphasis on wellness and patients' responsibility for their own health	Prevention practices to ward off diseases and disorders
	Patient education on wellness and prevention techniques
Increased computerization	Computer applications in health care: administration, diagnostics, treatment, and education
	Computer operation skills and knowledge of software programs
Increased use of electronic health records, along with the use of more specific diagnostic and treatment codes	Knowledge of electronic health records and new codes
Spread of hepatitis viruses, return of communicable diseases, such as measles, and threat of viruses due to globalization	Use of standard precautions
	Symptoms, treatment, and prevention of specific diseases
Increase in drug-resistant bacteria	Ability to educate patients about proper use of antibiotics, including when they are not necessary
Expansion of roles for health care professionals	Increased skill base
	Flexibility and willingness to perform a variety of tasks
Increased specialization and use of teams to provide patient care	Teamwork skills
	Intraprofessional and interprofessional communication skills
Development of increasingly sophisticated equipment	Operation of equipment and interpretation of results
New information about how the human body functions	New discoveries that affect the professional's occupational area
New diagnostic procedures and treatments	Information and skills that apply to the professional's occupational area
Implementation of the Patient Protection and Affordable Care Act; followed by repeal of some sections and other changes	Education of new patients in how to use the health care system and keep up with changes government has made that can be confusing

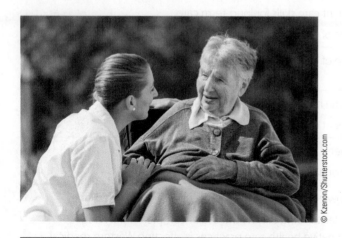

© Kzenon/Shutterstock.com

FIGURE 14–1 Health care professionals must continue to learn about the needs of older patients in order to provide appropriate care for this growing segment of the population.

some facilities are assigning to medical assistants include the following: serving as health coaches and navigators, visiting homes of patients to perform risk assessments, working as pharmacy technicians, and performing the duties of a limited license radiological technician. (Note that some of these duties require additional formal training.)

CONTINUING EDUCATION UNITS

Continuing education units (CEUs) are the credits granted for certain types of learning that take place after the completion of formal education. This type of education is also referred to as **continuing professional education (CPE)** and **continuing medical education (CME)**. Most forms of professional approval, such as licensure, certification, and registration, require that a specific number of CEUs be earned in order to be renewed. Health care professionals should find out the requirements for their occupations well in advance of licensure and certification renewal dates to allow adequate time to meet them. Most professional organizations and licensing boards have sites on the Internet that explain their continuing education requirements. In addition, some states have specific course requirements. For example, at least one state now requires registered nurses to earn seven hours of pain management-related continuing education in response to the current opioid crisis.

The amount of time, as well as the activities involved, vary for earning CEUs. Some credits are granted for assignments completed or tests passed; others require class or workshop attendance. Many schools and organizations offer classes and activities that award CEUs. However, the organizations that grant licenses, certifications, and registrations decide which CEUs they will accept. Not all courses and activities are accepted by all organizations. Before engaging in any activity for the purpose of earning CEUs, be sure that it has been approved by the necessary professional or regulatory organization.

If you participate in workshops or other activities, be *sure* to sign in. Some organizations now have badges that are scanned electronically to record your attendance. Also, ask for a certificate verifying attendance or completion of work. These will be needed as proof that units were earned. Keep certificates in a safe place. Some approval agencies require that they be kept for at least four years. Inquire whether your professional organization maintains a tracking system for CEUs earned by members. Some make a practice of sending out regular "statements" of units earned. These may be kept online and available for you to review. This is a good way for health care professionals to avoid getting caught short at renewal time.

Ways to Earn CEUs

There are many ways to earn CEUs. Health care professional organizations offer a variety of convenient ways to help their members stay current in their field. They can provide you with information about how many CEUs are needed, which subject areas they must be in, and how they can be earned. In addition to traditional classes and workshops, there are other ways to obtain CEUs:

- Special sessions and workshops offered at annual meetings, conferences, and conventions sponsored by professional health care organizations; may require taking a quiz, completing an assignment, or demonstrating in some other way that you have met the objectives

Example CEUs can be earned at the national convention of the American Physical Therapy Association.

- Home study materials published in professional journals

Example Members can read designated articles published in *CMA Today* (published by the American Association of Medical Assistants [AAMA]) and earn units by passing online quizzes about the articles' content. The AAMA articles are available both in the print form of the journal and online.

- Online study courses sponsored by professional organizations

Examples The American Association for Respiratory Care has online courses, some of them free, in various formats, including live webcasts; the National Association for Practical Nurse Education and Service offers a variety of courses online at its Online Learning Center.

- Home study courses offered by approved educational providers

Examples Tech Lectures (www.techlectures.com) is a company that offers a series of printed lectures and exams that enable pharmacy technicians to earn CEUs that are accepted by the Pharmacy Technician Certification Board and the Institute for the Certification of Pharmacy Technicians. Speedy CEUs offers courses for nurses that are approved by the California Board of Registered Nurses and accepted by all states except Delaware.

- Distance education courses offered by colleges and universities—many courses are now available over the Internet; a growing number of institutions provide for-credit classes that include interaction with the instructor and other students

Example University of Phoenix, based in Phoenix, Arizona, was one of the first to develop and offer distance education courses for credit. Its web address is www.phoenix.edu. Today, dozens of colleges and universities offer online courses.

Fascinating Facts

It is estimated that the doubling time of medical knowledge in 1950 was 50 years; in 1980, 7 years, and in 2010, 3.5 years. In 2020 it is projected to be 0.2 years—just 73 days.

Source: http://www.nlm.nih.gov/pubs/factsheets/mesh.html

Thinking It Through

Jan Summers loves her work as an occupational therapy assistant. One of the reasons that Jan wanted to be an occupational therapy assistant was because she likes to interact with other people. Her outgoing personality helps her develop good relationships with patients, and her cheerful disposition makes her a popular assistant. Jan looks forward to the annual occupational therapy conferences, held in different cities around the country. They provide opportunities to see friends she has made in the profession and catch up on all the news. What Jan does not enjoy is attending the informational meetings and workshops. She finds them "boring." She has talked some of her friends into signing her name on the attendance rosters and, so far, has not been caught. In this way she manages to accumulate the credits needed to renew her certification to practice.

1. Even if Jan is not caught, what are the possible future consequences of her failure to attend the meetings and workshops?

2. Is Jan maintaining professional ethical standards? Why or why not?

3. What is the possible impact on her patients?

4. What is the possible impact on her future career?

Not all providers of learning opportunities are high quality, and not all courses are beneficial simply because they grant CEUs. Consider the following criteria for choosing courses and materials that offer maximum value for the time and money invested:

- Recommendations from your professional and/or certification organization
- Skill and knowledge requirements of your current job
- Future career goals
- Credibility and reputation of the educational provider
- Areas of personal and professional weakness that need improvement
- Personal and professional interests
- Accreditation by the International Association for Continuing Education and Training at https://www.iacet.org/resources/accredited-providers-list/

Although it may or may not award continuing education units, **inservice training** may be provided by your employer. This is usually mandatory and consists of training and communication necessary for some aspect of your work.

SELF-DIRECTED LEARNING

Self-directed learning refers to all activities that you plan and participate in to increase your knowledge and skills. It goes beyond learning to earn CEUs—it adds to your value as a professional and gives you fresh perspectives. There are many ways to incorporate learning into your daily life:

- Observe others: Watch how successful, experienced professionals perform their duties. (See Figure 14–2.)

- Ask questions: Learn from the expertise of others. Most people are happy to share what they know. Be sure to choose an appropriate time to ask questions. For example, do not ask questions about patients in their presence or when the other professional is very busy and cannot stop to talk.

- Read books and journal articles: Plan a regular time to keep up on publications related to your occupational area. Most professional organizations publish a newsletter or journal, online or in print. In addition, there are hundreds of specialized journals that cover medical and health care topics. Many large health care facilities have libraries for employees. Some have libraries open to patients and the public. Many universities and colleges allow the public to use their libraries. Some offer checkout privileges for an annual fee. Libraries have become highly computerized. Do not hesitate to ask the librarian for assistance if you have trouble locating materials.

FIGURE 14–2 Health care professionals can learn a lot by observing others at work.

- Study in a small group: Organize a study group with other employees at work. Or, if you belonged to a study group at school, consider encouraging the members to meet regularly after you graduate. You can learn by sharing workplace experiences and working on selected topics to keep current in your field. (See Figure 14–3.) Important note: Remember that sharing personal or identifiable information about your patients is a breach of confidentiality.

- Attend professional conferences and meetings: These often include lectures, workshops, and discussions of current topics.

- Learning channels, public television stations, and those managed by local universities often feature programs of interest to the health care professional.

- Explore the Internet: Information is available on all kinds of topics and in a variety of formats, including webcasts, podcasts, and videos. Youtube.com has dozens of videos on health care topics. Ted Talks addresses current topics, including those related to health care (https://www.ted.com/talks). Here are a few reliable health care websites to get you started:

  - Centers for Disease Control and Prevention

    www.cdc.gov

  - Mayo Clinic

    www.mayoclinic.com

  - National Center for Health Statistics

    www.cdc.gov/nchs

  - National Library of Medicine

    www.medlineplus.gov

  - National Institute of Mental Health

    www.nimh.nih.gov

  - National Institutes of Health

    http://health.nih.gov

See Chapter 18 for tips on evaluating Internet sources.

Planning your own study activities allows you to learn in ways you prefer. Look for activities that make learning enjoyable and incorporate them into your daily life. Think of the world as a giant classroom that offers endless opportunities for learning. Keeping up with changes and adding to your knowledge and skill base should be part of your work routine. You will have the satisfaction of knowing that you are staying current and competent.

In addition to developing health care skills, you can advance your career and personal life by improving nontechnical skills. Oral and written communication, interpersonal relations, computer applications, and time management are examples of important skills that will help you get ahead.

Learn from Role Models and Mentors

A **role model** is a person who serves as a positive example. Role models demonstrate high levels of professionalism and competence. They strive to be their best and provide inspiration through their abilities, courage, and dedication. Following the example of appropriate role models is an excellent way for the new health care professional to continue the education received during formal training.

What are the qualities to look for when choosing role models?

- Dedication to their profession
- Good technical skills
- Respectful of others
- High standards
- Confidence gained through experience
- High level of integrity
- Ability to work well with people
- Understanding of the health care field

A **mentor** is a combination coach and advisor. A mentor should also have the qualities of a role model. Having a good mentor is a tremendous career advantage. However, it does not happen automatically. Look for someone with professional experience, expertise, an interest in helping others, and time to spend with you. This person might work in the same department or facility or be someone you meet at a professional meeting or through networking activities pursued during the job search.

© Rido/Shutterstock.com

FIGURE 14–3 Studying in a small group allows the exchange of ideas and can be a productive way to learn.

314 | CHAPTER 14

Nursing career path in research at the NIH clinical center

Nurse practitioner

Registered nurse

Licensed practical/vocational nurse

Certified nursing assistant

Patient care assistant

Home health aide

FIGURE 14–4 Example of a nursing career ladder, each step requiring more education, training, and certification.

The following are a few of the ways that a mentor can help the beginning health care professional:

- Suggest learning resources
- Offer suggestions and advice about career strategies
- Provide introductions to people in the field
- Pass on information about job openings
- Encourage you to be your best

CAREER LADDERS

Recall from Chapter 1 that occupational areas have positions at different levels, with the levels compared to rungs on a ladder. (See Figure 14–4.) Although many health care professionals obtain career satisfaction and success by remaining at one level, others are interested in "climbing

the ladder" by obtaining additional education and experience. It is important to know that the work at various levels, while in the same field such as physical therapy, may vary. Some examples include:

- The amount of time spent working directly with patients
- The paperwork and reports required
- Working closely with a supervisor or independently
- Working environment
- Additional responsibilities and accountability

It is recommended that anyone considering "moving up the ladder" learn everything possible about the educational requirements, duties performed, and employment prospects of the new level. The tables and suggested resources in Chapter 1 provide a good starting point.

SUGGESTED LEARNING ACTIVITIES

1. Explore the continuing education units required for your occupation of interest.

2. Create a personal plan for self-directed learning.

3. Develop the habit of scanning health care articles and resources on the Internet.

4. Visit your local public or university library. Review periodicals and books on health care. Are there helpful resources in your subject area? Many journals can now be accessed on the Internet.

5. Request a continuing education catalog from a local college or university. What types of courses are offered? Do you see any that might help you develop your personal or professional skills?

6. Choose a health topic you find interesting and conduct an Internet search. Record your findings and develop a webliography (a list of sites with name, Web address, and brief description of contents) of useful sites.

7. Explore the websites mentioned in this chapter.

WEB ACTIVITIES

Professional Organizations

1. Explore the website of the professional organization(s) for your career. (See Appendix 1.)

2. What information does it contain about CEUs?

3. Are there minimum requirements for your certification/licensure/registration (if applicable for your career)?

4. What are various ways you can earn CEUs?

Various Websites

1. Search for "continuing education requirements for …" inserting the occupation in which you are interested.

2. What information is available?

National Library of Medicine—Medline Plus

www.medlineplus.gov

1. Explore the sections on this website, such as Health Videos and Games.

2. Choose three and report on what you learn.

America's Biopharmaceutical Companies

www.innovation.org

1. Choose at least one topic to explore.

2. Write a short report describing what you learn about the role of pharmaceutical products in health care today.

REVIEW QUESTIONS

1. What is the meaning of "professional development"?

2. What are ways the health care professional can grow professionally?

3. What are five purposes of professional organizations?

4. What are five advantages of participating in a professional organization?

5. Why is lifelong learning important for health care professionals?

6. What are some of the changes and trends in health care? What are the learning requirements for the health care professional that correspond to each?

7. What is the meaning and significance of "expanded scope of practice"?

8. What is the meaning of the following terms: "continuing education units," continuing professional education," and "continuing medical education"?

9. What are the ways you can earn continuing education units?

10. What are the criteria for choosing quality courses and materials for earning continuing education units?

11. What is the meaning of "self-directed learning"?

12. What are ways you can incorporate self-directed learning into your daily life?

13. What are the meanings of "role model" and "mentor"?

14. What are the guidelines to look for when choosing a role model?

15. What are ways a mentor can help a beginning health care professional?

16. What is the meaning of "career ladder"?

17. What are ways the duties and responsibilities vary with various levels on a career ladder?

APPLICATION EXERCISES

1. Describe the methods for keeping up to date that Mabel Bennett, described in the Case of Lifetime Success, may have used throughout her career.

2. Debbie Yano is a practical (licensed) vocational nurse working for Dr. Cerutti in a single-physician office in a small town. Dr. Cerutti is a general practitioner and, because of the limited number of health care facilities in the area, many long-time patients rely on this caring physician for the majority of their health care needs. Debbie enjoys the variety of experiences encountered in her work with Dr. Cerutti: patients of all ages with all types of health issues. An important professional goal is to keep her skills up-to-date and to continue to acquire new ones. Learning opportunities are limited by her busy work schedule and family responsibilities and by living in a small town. Develop a comprehensive, long-term plan for Debbie to achieve her goal.

PROBLEM-SOLVING PRACTICE

Laura is pleased to have passed her exam and earned her certification as an occupational therapy assistant. How can she use the five-step problem-solving process to be sure she both stays up to date in her field and maintains her certification?

CHAPTER 15

The Patient as an Individual

KEY TERMS

bias
culture
defense mechanisms
dominant culture
implicit bias
personal space
philosophy of individual worth
physiological needs
prejudice
self-actualization
self-esteem

OBJECTIVES

Studying and applying the material in this chapter will help you to:

1. Explain why it is important for the health care professional to consider each patient as an individual.
2. Explain the meaning of the philosophy of individual worth and how it applies to work in health care.
3. List five conditions that can make it difficult to provide appropriate care to patients.
4. Define empathy.
5. Explain the meaning of prejudice (bias) and explain how it detracts from providing positive and appropriate patient care.
6. Explain the meaning of "implicit bias."
7. List six strategies to overcome prejudice and implicit bias.
8. Define *culture* and describe how it influences all aspects of human beliefs and behavior.
9. Explain the meaning of "dominant culture."
10. Explain why it is difficult for some individuals to adapt to a dominant culture.
11. List the nine diverse groups identified in the text that are components of the U.S. population.
12. List five reasons for gathering information about the ethnic groups you might encounter in your work.
13. Give examples of cultural differences in personal space and touching that can affect health care interactions.
14. Give examples of differences that might be found among cultures and individuals in the following: time orientation, personal space, communication, and family structure.
15. Describe the components of traditional Western medicine.
16. Explain how religious beliefs can influence health care practices and give three examples.
17. Describe the concept of harmony and how it relates to health care, including mind–body–spirit and the four humors.
18. Describe the role of herb and plant medicines in some cultures.
19. Give three examples of different cultural approaches to health care for each of the following categories:
    - Definition of health
    - Sources of good health
    - Causes of illness
    - Methods of treatment

20. What is Maslow's hierarchy of needs?

21. List and describe the five categories of needs proposed by Maslow.

22. List three ways that health care professionals can help patients meet the needs of each category.

23. Explain why Maslow's long-accepted hierarchy of needs is being challenged today.

24. Define "self-esteem" and "self-actualization."

25. Define "defense mechanisms" and explain why people use them.

26. List and describe the 11 defense mechanisms presented in the text.

27. Give five examples of how health care professionals can help reduce the level of anxiety experienced by patients who are demonstrating defense mechanisms.

28. Explain how the health care professional can help patients deal with the experience of loss.

29. List the five recommendations from Britain's National Health Service for knowing patients as individuals.

30. Describe five actions that health care professionals can take to learn about their patients as individuals.

31. Give five examples of questions to ask patients to learn about their needs.

The Case of the Polite Patient

Shortly after graduation from a medical assistant program, Carley Ford moved from her small town to a large city 50 miles away. She has always wanted to experience city life and is excited when she is hired to work in a large downtown clinic. During her first week at the clinic, she meets with Mr. Alvarez, who was recently diagnosed with diabetes. His physician, Dr. Washington, believes that if Mr. Alvarez follows a diabetic diet and a regular plan of exercise, he may avoid having to take insulin injections. Carley spends about 10 minutes carefully explaining the eating plan recommended by Dr. Washington. She speaks slowly and clearly because she has noted that Mr. Alvarez does not speak English fluently. From time to time Carley asks Mr. Alvarez if he understands, and he nods to indicate that he does. She gives him a set of written instructions, including an eating plan, advising him to follow it carefully.

When Mr. Alvarez arrives for his follow-up appointment six months later, Dr. Washington is surprised that his condition has worsened. When he questions Mr. Alvarez—in Spanish—he learns that the elderly widower did not understand much of what Carley had explained to him. The written instructions were not helpful because Mr. Alvarez reads very little Spanish and no English at all. He has not cooked for himself since his wife died. Mr. Alvarez did not say anything to Carley about not understanding because "she was so nice and took her time" so he "didn't want to hurt her feelings." He also did not want to inconvenience the neighbors and family members who supply his meals by asking them to cook in a different way than they do for their families. This chapter discusses how to learn about individual patients in order to best help them meet their health care needs.

PATIENTS AS INDIVIDUALS

The well-being of patients depends on more than the technical competence of health care professionals. It is also very much influenced by the attitude and concern expressed by everyone who works with them in the health care setting. A popular, true saying is: "People don't care how much you know, until they know how much you care." Each patient is a complex individual who represents a combination of cultural influences, personal experiences, and basic human needs. Working effectively with patients, as well as with coworkers, requires understanding and appreciating the differences that make each person unique. The wide variety of people who make up the population of the United States today has been compared with a garden filled with flowers of every color and shape. Although each one is different, they all contribute to the overall beauty of the

FIGURE 15–1 Every patient is worthy of your full attention and respect.

garden. The lesson for health care professionals is that learning to work with a variety of patients can enrich their experience of giving service to fellow human beings, as well as improving the care they provide. (See Figure 15–1.)

Philosophy of Individual Worth

The **philosophy of individual worth** is based on the belief that every human being, "regardless of personal circumstances or personal qualities, has worth and is entitled to respect as a human being" (Milliken & Honeycutt, 2018, p. 14). Health care professionals have the obligation to strive to provide appropriate care to every patient, regardless of race, cultural background, economic status, behavior, physical condition, age, or sexual orientation. This is not always easy, for a number of reasons:

- The health professional's own values and beliefs may conflict with those of the patient.

- The health professional may not understand the cultural beliefs and practices of the patient.

- The patient may be of a different socioeconomic group or have a different level of education not familiar to the health care professional.

- The patient may be challenging, rude, and/or uncooperative.

- The professional's work environment may be challenging, with much work to accomplish in a limited amount of time.

It is natural to find it difficult to work with people you don't understand, who resist your efforts to help them, or who are unpleasant and make your work more difficult. But it is at precisely these times that the philosophy of individual worth should serve as a reminder and

motivator for health care professionals to do their best for every patient. Providing equal care to all, even under demanding circumstances, demonstrates the highest level of professionalism.

Understanding Patients

Empathy provides a foundation for understanding others. Recall from Chapter 13 that empathy means trying your best to understand the thoughts, feelings, and motivation of others. Expressed another way, it means seeing the world from their point of view. As previously stated, each individual is unique, a compilation of his or her culture, race, experiences, genetic make-up, environment, physical characteristics, and more. All will contribute to his or her current experience which is likely to differ significantly from that of the health care professional.

Dealing with Prejudice

Prejudice (also known as **bias**) means having certain beliefs and feelings, usually negative, about a person because he or she belongs to a specific group or has certain characteristics. It can result in judging an individual based on assumptions about the group they belong to. Prejudice also refers to having unfavorable opinions about individuals because of characteristics such as obesity, poverty, and sexual preference. Prejudice prevents people from being considered as unique individuals.

Almost everyone has prejudices of some type. They are not always easy to recognize in ourselves because they become incorporated into our belief systems. They are taken for granted and become part of our reality, making it difficult to understand and accept that there are other acceptable ways of living and viewing the world. **Implicit bias** means bias that is unconscious and outside our immediate intentional control, therefore difficult to identify and overcome. Although more research is recommended, studies to date show that implicit bias exists extensively in health care and is significantly related to how patients and providers interact, treatment decisions, treatment adherence, and overall patient outcomes (http://www.ihi.org/communities/blogs/how-to-reduce-implicit-bias). Becoming aware of our implicit biases takes effort, but health care professionals must make an effort to recognize their own by examining honestly how they regard others. Strategies recommended by psychologists to help overcome both recognized prejudice and implicit bias include the following:

- Examine your responses to others to help you recognize if they are based on stereotypes; then consciously adjust your responses.

- Try imagining the individual as the opposite of the stereotype.

- Strive to see the person as an individual rather than a stereotype (e.g., learn about their personal history and the context that brought them to the health facility).

- Practice empathy: Put yourself in the other person's shoes.

- Increase your contact with individuals from different groups by expanding your network of friends and colleagues and/or attend events where people of other racial and ethnic groups, gender identities, sexual orientation, and other groups may be present.

- Reframe interactions with patients as one between collaborating equals, rather than between high-status persons and low-status persons.

(Adapted from Devine et al. (2012), https://www.ncbi.nlm.nih .gov/pmc/articles/PMC3603687/)

At the same time, it is not necessary to agree with all the beliefs and actions of others. In fact, some behaviors may be harmful to the health of the patient, and it is the duty of health care professionals to encourage positive changes. In order to do this, however, they must understand their patients' beliefs and motivations. And this understanding can only come by listening carefully and resisting the temptation to judge what is heard. When hearing information we believe to be "incorrect," a common reaction is to stop listening. This prevents gathering the very information needed to begin to understand other people's points of view and the reasons for their beliefs.

THE MEANING OF CULTURE

The term **culture** refers to a wide range of factors that include values, shared beliefs and attitudes, social organization, family and personal relationships, language, everyday activities, religious practices, and concepts of time and space. Culture provides a framework for viewing the world and every individual's thinking and actions are influenced to some degree by his or her cultural background. Belief systems and customs are developed over time to help people make sense of their world. Accepted customs provide guidelines for conduct so that daily life can proceed without constant decision-making. They give life predictability and stability and provide the means for people to live together in relative harmony. (See Figure 15-2.)

A broader view of culture includes individuals not by their ethnicity, but by factors such as their socioeconomic status. The United States is considered to be a wealthy nation, but as of 2016, almost 13% (40.6 million people) lived in poverty (https://povertyusa.org/facts). Habits, such as hygiene, can be affected by economic status.

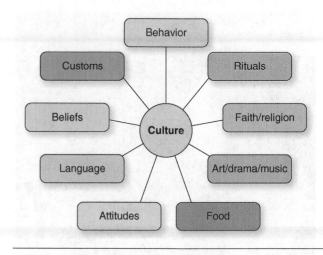

FIGURE 15–2 Cultures are composed of many factors.

Fascinating Facts

Perhaps the greatest example of the application of the philosophy of individual worth was demonstrated by the life of Mother Teresa, who dedicated her life to working with, in her words, "the poorest of the poor." From 1948 until her death in 1997, Mother Teresa worked in Calcutta, India, caring for desperately poor people who were ill, abandoned, and dying. She founded the House for the Dying in 1952 to provide a place for people to die in peace and dignity. Over the years she created other sites that offered medical care and shelter to the needy all over the world. Mother Teresa put into action her belief that *every* human being is worthy of respect and loving care.

For example, an individual who lives in deep poverty may lack the means to bathe regularly, use deodorant, and have regular dental care. And he or she is likely unable to afford the fresh foods that contribute to good health. (See "Improving Social Conditions" in Chapter 2.)

It is natural to take our own beliefs, economic status, and way of life for granted—we seldom question them. This is a common source of miscommunication because behaviors that are considered positive in one culture may be a sign of disrespect in another. Or people, such as the homeless, may not have the means to practice habits considered to be correct or desirable and this could cause these people to be labeled negatively rather than understood.

Dominant Culture

The term **dominant culture** refers to what commonly are considered to be the foundational beliefs and ideal behaviors of a society or country. These beliefs are generally considered to be necessary in order to be successful. This text, for instance, contains examples of attitudes that belong to the dominant culture of the United States:

- The importance of "being on time" and "using one's time effectively": Not all cultures believe that time is something to be controlled—or even that it *can* be controlled. Nor is punctuality an important concern. In some cultures, the belief is that everything will happen in its "own time" with or without the intervention of humans.

- The need to work efficiently: Interactions with people, even if a medical appointment or work assignment takes longer as a result, are given high priority by some cultures. If a health care professional moves quickly, even though competently, through a procedure and fails to inquire about the patient's family and engage in personal conversation, this may be viewed as indicating a lack of interest in and respect for the patient.

- The need to shake hands firmly when meeting new people: Recommended and even rehearsed for important occasions such as job interviews, this behavior is not universally practiced. In some cultures, only men are expected to shake hands and the handshake should be light, not firm. In others, handshakes are not common among persons of either sex. Other forms of greeting, such as a bow, may be used.

Individuals and Culture

The United States is home to an increasingly diverse number of people from a variety of cultural backgrounds. Significant portions of the population are made up of people once considered to be members of "minority groups." Table 15–1 contains statistics that demonstrate the current diversity of the United States population. (See also Figure 15–3.)

Immigrants come to the United States for a variety of reasons. Many have fled wars and unstable political conditions in their own countries. These immigrants are the most likely to live in close-knit communities. Older members tend to retain their native language and many customs.

There also exist other subcultures whose members, although born in the United States, have not fully integrated. The Chinese community in San Francisco is an

Table 15–1 Diversity of the U.S. Population

Group	Percentage
White, non-Hispanic	60.7%
Hispanic	18.1%
African American	13.4%
Asian	5.8%
American Indian and Alaska Native	1.3%
Foreign born persons	13.4%
Language other than English spoken at home	21.3%
Persons under age 65 with a disability	8.7%
Persons living in poverty	12.3%
Source: https://www.census.gov/quickfacts/fact/table/US/PST045217	
Individuals who are obese	39.8%
Source: https://www.cdc.gov/obesity/data/adult.html	
Persons who report as being gay, lesbian, bisexual, or transgender	4.5%
Source: https://www.nbcnews.com/feature/nbc-out/ record-4-5-percent-u-s-adults-identify-lgbt-gallup-n877486	

FIGURE 15-3 America's population is made up of dozens of ethnic groups.

© Rawpixel/Shutterstock.com.

example of a group that has retained the language and customs of the original culture over many generations. (Note: This may be largely due to previous governmental bias against Chinese immigrants, including the Chinese Exclusion Act, federal legislation passed in 1882 that prohibited Chinese labor immigration for ten years. In 1892, another law extended the ban for another ten years.) This does not mean that most members of ethnic groups, including recent immigrants and those who choose to retain traditional beliefs and customs, fail to learn the customs necessary to be successful in the United States. Many customs are quickly learned and integrated into daily life. Some behaviors retained from the culture of origin, however, are based on deeply held beliefs about what is important in life. Making the required changes to life in the United States may involve adopting new behaviors that are considered inappropriate in the original culture. Attitudes are much more difficult to recognize and change when they are based on important values.

While health care professionals must recognize that differences among people are sometimes based on cultural background, they must take care to identify which cultural characteristics each individual patient or coworker may have chosen to identify with and integrate into his or her lifestyle. Making assumptions about individuals based on the group to which they are believed to "belong" is disrespectful because it *takes away from their worth as individuals*. Assumptions also lead to mistakes in communication and misunderstandings. It is essential that health care professionals learn to observe, ask meaningful questions, and listen carefully to the responses. Using these skills, described later in this chapter, they can better meet the needs of all patients.

There is value in learning about the beliefs and practices of the cultural groups that health care professionals might encounter in their work. Gathering cultural information enables them to do the following:

- Realize and appreciate that there are many valid approaches to life. There is never an "only way" or even a "best way"
- Enrich and improve their own lives by increasing their knowledge of other cultures and discovering new ideas they might want to incorporate
- Avoid making the assumption that everything health care professionals do and say will be understood and appreciated
- Understand that certain beliefs *might* be held and certain customs *might* be practiced because of an individual's background
- Ask appropriate and useful questions (more about this later in the chapter)

Cultural Differences

Health care professionals who have close interactions with patients and coworkers daily, should understand customs regarding personal space and personal contact. **Personal space** refers to the distance at which people feel most comfortable when carrying on a conversation. In the dominant culture of the United States, a distance of about 18 inches is considered appropriate for people who know each other very well, such as family members and close friends. Two feet is considered appropriate for acquaintances and friends. In other cultures, people stand very close together when talking. It is appropriate that each speaker feels the breath of the other. On the other hand, some groups tend to maintain more distance than 18 inches when engaged in conversation.

The issue of touch is also relevant in health care. Some medical procedures involve parts of the body considered private by all cultural groups. It is important to be aware that the degree to which any type of physical contact is tolerated varies. For example, some cultures consider the examination of a female by a male physician to be unacceptable.

Harmless touching in one culture may be improper in another. In the United States, lightly patting a child on the head is a sign of acknowledgment or affection. But it can cause extreme distress for some members of Asian cultures, because they believe that the spirits of their ancestors reside there. People who believe in reincarnation (rebirth of the soul in another body following death) may consider the issue of touch to be important even after death. For example, the Hmongs, a group from Asia who immigrated to the United States as a result of the Vietnam

Thinking It Through

Many nurses from the Philippines emigrate to work in the United States. Their educational training is similar and they can speak English. One thing that surprises them when they start work here is that part of their job is to provide personal care to patients. In the Philippines, it is family members who feed and help with hygiene tasks. One nurse reported that in the Filipino hospital where she worked, she had never seen a patient alone.

1. How do you think this might shape Filipino nurses' impressions of typical families in the United States?

2. How would you explain to them why, in this country, personal care is typically performed by the nursing staff, such as nursing assistants?

In one U.S. health care facility, a Filipino nurse was reported to spend a lot of time on her phone during her shift. It was assumed that she was talking with her family and friends. It turned out that she was speaking with Filipino nurses in other parts of the hospital who considered her an expert and were calling her for advice.

1. Why do you think the nurses were calling a colleague in a different department, rather than asking for help from their supervisors or the other nurses on their shift?

Source of examples: Vestal, V., and Kautz, D. D. (2009). International perspectives: Responding to the similarities and differences between Filipino and American nurses. Journal of Nursing Administration, 39, 8–10. DOI: 10.1097/NNA.0b013e31818fe726.

War, oppose autopsies because the disfigurement of the body may prevent reincarnation of the soul (https://www.ncbi.nlm.nih.gov/pmc/articles/PMC5010786/).

The most important point is that often there are no "correct" customs. Exceptions—that is, "incorrect customs"—would be those that are harmful or dangerous to oneself or others. The most important consideration for health care professionals is to establish an environment that is comfortable and reassuring for patients and that promotes their welfare. See Box 15–1 for information about the variety of approaches to life you may encounter with patients and coworkers.

Finally, it is important to note that even individuals who "belong" to the dominant culture can have a variety of beliefs and behaviors that are not considered to be "the norm." Much depends on the personality, health status, childhood environment, and other influencing factors.

Box 15–1

Values, Beliefs, and Behaviors

Time Orientation

Past-oriented

Present is more important than the future

Future-focused and goal-oriented

Punctuality is very important

Being late is acceptable

Time is commodity: can be saved, spent, wasted

Not ruled by precise calendars and schedules

Life follows the cycle of the seasons

Personal Space

Standing close is appropriate

Hugging, touching (arm or shoulder, for example) is acceptable

Touching others not normally done during conversation

Shaking hands is polite, respectful greeting

Bowing is appropriate greeting

Good eye contact shows interest and sincerity

Eye contact shows lack of respect

Communication

May use slang particular to their region, age, etc.

Silence is valued

Criticism and disagreement are avoided

Direct confrontation is disrespectful

Politeness extremely important

English may be limited—this does *not* indicate level of intelligence or education

Body language and gestures important part of communication

Family Structure

Large, extended families

Basic unit is nuclear family: parents and children

Welfare of family as a whole may be valued above individual members

Ancestors are honored

Older members are highly respected

One member may make decisions for all

HEALTH CARE BELIEFS

Health care beliefs and practices vary widely among cultural groups. Traditional Western medicine, defined here as that which is practiced by most physicians in the United States, mainly focuses on the physical aspects of the body and employs scientific methods of diagnosis and treatment. The effect of the mind and spirit tend to be considered less important, except in the case of holistic practitioners, as discussed in Chapter 2. (An exception for traditional Western practitioners is stress, which is recognized as having an impact on health.) Illness is generally attributed to factors that can be measured and explained, such as infection, environmental conditions, and physical changes in the body's structure. Treatment methods, such as medications, must be proven to be both effective and safe through carefully controlled clinical trials. There is emphasis on formal training and official verification of the competence of health care practitioners through licensing and certification.

Traditional Western medicine is beginning to acknowledge the effects of the mind on the functions and health of the body. Some cultures have always believed that there is a strong connection. They have traditionally emphasized the relationship among the mind, body, and spirit,

believing that illness can result when the harmony among these three human components is disrupted.

Religious Beliefs and Health

Religious and spiritual beliefs influence the health practices of many cultural groups and individuals. For example, the traditional healers in some Native American communities have religious status. They use diagnostic and healing methods that have been employed for centuries. These include the widespread use of herbs and special healing ceremonies. At the same time, modern medical science may be combined with traditional methods.

Faith healing is practiced by some Christians. They believe they can be cured from illness and disabilities through prayer and strong religious faith. In fact, 80% of Americans surveyed use prayer to assist their healing (not necessarily cure) from injury and illness (https://www.cbsnews.com/news/many-americans-turn-to-prayer-for-healing/). Some Christians believe that certain members of the clergy have the power to assist with healing. Christian Scientists believe that illness and health are controlled by God and that the patient's Christian faith is the main means to recovery.

Islam is a religion that is predominant in many parts of the world, including North Africa, the Middle East, and Indonesia. Many Muslims believe that what happens in life, including illness, is due to the "will of Allah" (God's will). Illness is a test and a means of having sins forgiven. Therefore, illness may be avoided by religious means which include the use of prayers and reciting verses from the Koran (the sacred text of Islam).

The people of some cultures believe in the effects of evil spirits and the "evil eye," a stare from someone believed to have the power to cause harm. Wearing charms and carrying special objects, such as engraved stones, are practiced to ward off evil spirits. This is not unlike athletes who have lucky objects, such as a special pair of shoes, that they believe they need to have to perform well. Some Latin American peoples have special customs to avoid encountering the evil eye. They are especially protective of young children.

The Catholic religion plays a major role in the life of many people and is the predominant religion in Spanish-speaking countries. Illness is considered by some Catholics to be a form of punishment for sins. Prayers are believed to be helpful, especially when the person calls upon specific saints for help and purchases and lights votive candles.

Harmony and Health

The concept of harmony—the balance of mind, body, and spirit—as necessary for good health is common to

Thinking It Through

Kelly O'Connor handles the billing for Dr. Sinclair's busy orthopedic practice. Patients are sent to Kelly to give her information about their insurance coverage, make payment arrangements, and pay their portion of office calls. One day she is collecting a payment from an elderly patient who came to Dr. Sinclair for treatment of arthritis. He had moved to the United States from a small island in the South Pacific a few years ago. The patient is visibly upset. Kelly asks if Mr. Juarez is all right. He says, "Everything here is so rush-rush. The doctor has no time."

1. How can Kelly appropriately respond to the patient?

2. Are there questions she might ask him to learn more about his feelings?

3. How should she follow up?

4. Should she share this encounter with anyone else in the office? Why?

many cultures. The phrase "mind–body connection" is being heard more often in the United States as people are discovering the benefits of a more holistic approach to medicine. (See the section in Chapter 2 on Complementary, Alternative, and Integrative Health.)

The Chinese civilization is thousands of years old and has developed many time-honored health care practices. Chinese medicine is based in part on the belief that the body has two energy forces, known as *yin* and *yang*. Illness occurs when these forces are out of balance. Diseases and treatments are classified by their relationship to these forces. Activities and treatments believed to promote the integration of the mind and body and enhance the flow of the life force (*qi*) are widely practiced. An example is *t'ai chi*, an ancient form of martial arts, in which slow, relaxed movements are carried out while focusing the mind. T'ai chi is now becoming a popular method in the United States for promoting relaxation, balance, flexibility, and healthy joints.

Traditional beliefs among some Hispanic groups include the theory that the body is controlled by four basic body fluids, known as *humors*. These humors are classified as follows: hot and wet, hot and dry, cold and wet, and cold and dry. Illness results when the humors are out of balance. Disorders and corresponding treatments are organized according to the hot–cold principle: cold illnesses should be treated with hot remedies and hot illnesses with cold ones. For example, a headache is classified as a cold condition and appropriate hot foods include cereals, eggs, beef, and spicy foods; appropriate medical remedies include aspirin, cinnamon, and garlic. See Box 15–2 for more examples.

In addition to beliefs about hot and cold remedies, members of some cultural groups, such as the Chinese, prescribe specific foods as treatments for various conditions.

Herbs and Plant Medicines

Plants and herbs have been used for thousands of years to treat various ailments. Asian cultures have developed thousands of herbal remedies that are widely used today in the practice of Chinese medicine. There has been growing interest in the use of medicinal herbs in the United States by people who believe that, because they are natural, they have fewer dangerous side effects than pharmaceutical drugs. It is important that health care professionals be aware that "natural" treatments are not necessarily safe. Many plants and herbs *can* have harmful side effects. Also, some herbs interact negatively with traditional prescribed medications. Herbal remedies and food supplements are not regulated by the government as are pharmaceutical products.

Box 15–2

Hot and Cold Conditions and Treatments

Hot Conditions	Cold Conditions
Constipation	Cancer
Fever	Colds
Infections	Headache
Sore throat	Pneumonia
Ulcers	Tuberculosis

Cold Food Remedies	Hot Food Remedies
Dairy products	Cereals
Milk	Eggs
Lima beans	Beef
Vegetables	Oils
Honey	Spicy foods
Chicken	Wine
Raisins	

Cold Medical Remedies	Hot Medical Remedies
Bicarbonate of soda	Aspirin
Milk of magnesia	Cinnamon
Orange flower water	Cod liver oil
Sage	Garlic
	Penicillin

Fascinating Facts

There are 62 schools in the United States accredited by the National Association for Acupuncture and Oriental Medicine. These schools offer certificates through doctoral degrees.

Some older members of African-American communities are recognized for their ability to provide effective home remedies, including the preparation of medications from herbs and roots. In many cases, this was likely in response to limited access to medical care and/or discrimination by the health care system. As with other cultural groups, popular remedies may be handed down from one generation to the next.

See Boxes 15–3 through 15–6 for examples of culturally influenced approaches to health.

Box 15-3

Definitions of Health

Absence of disease

Balance of body energy (yin and yang)

Balance of hot/cold and wet/dry forces in the body

Harmony with nature

Integration of body, mind, and spirit

Box 15-4

Sources of Good Health

Nutritious food, rest, and practice of good hygiene

Gift from ancestors

Good self-care practices, such as exercise and not smoking

Reward from God

Will of God

Good luck

Box 15-5

Causes of Illness

Blockage or imbalance of body energy

Disharmony between self and environment

Disharmony caused by demons or spirits

Punishment for sins

Receiving the evil eye or a bad fright

Scientifically explained phenomena, such as microbes

Supernatural forces

Violation of taboo (prohibited activity)

Will of God

Box 15-6

Methods of Treatment

Acupressure

Acupuncture

Consultation with traditional healers

Exercise and changes in eating habits

Fasting (giving up eating all or certain foods for a specific period of time)

Herbs

Meditation

Pharmaceutical drugs

Prayer

Restoration of balance of energy or other bodily forces

Restoration of mind–body–spirit harmony

Rituals and ceremonies

Roots from plants

Surgery

HUMAN NEEDS

Cultural backgrounds form the frameworks for the physical, psychological, and spiritual development of human beings. Within these frameworks, however, each individual develops a unique combination of characteristics and behaviors.

There are many approaches to describing and explaining the complexities of human behavior. One useful approach for the health care professional is based on understanding human needs. A model that has been used by health care professionals for many years to better understand their patients was developed by American psychologist Abraham Maslow. According to Maslow, human behavior is motivated by each individual's efforts to fulfill certain requirements for complete physical, mental, and emotional well-being. He originally developed five categories of human needs, which he then ranked in order of importance for human fulfillment. (As he continued to study human behavior, he added three more categories of needs: knowledge, beauty, and transcendence [the need to help others achieve self-actualization].) As Maslow listed and then ranked the original five needs, he proposed that certain needs had to be fulfilled before an individual would or could fulfill the next higher one. This is known as "Maslow's hierarchy of needs" (a hierarchy being an arrangement in order of rank or grade). The five original categories are listed below:

- **Physiological needs**: Must be satisfied in order to maintain life. These include necessities such as oxygen, water, and food.

- Safety and security: Physical and psychological security, such as living free from the fear of physical harm.

- Love and affection: Need for maintaining satisfying relationships with other people. This need can be met by enjoying friendships and attaining intimacy with another. (See Figure 15–4.)

- Esteem: Need for self-respect and the approval of others as well as respect for oneself.

- **Self-actualization**: Maslow defined this as the achievement of one's greatest potential.

An individual's behavior at any given time to meet the needs described by Maslow are determined by his or her personality, the current situation, and the opportunities available. For example, securing food for survival can be achieved in several ways: earning money, farming, trading, begging, or stealing. The method selected will be influenced by such factors as parental training, educational level, economic status, job availability, physical condition, level of self-esteem, and moral beliefs. In summary, human beings tend to be motivated by their needs, but the urgency, priority, and means of fulfilling these vary among individuals.

FIGURE 15–4 Celebrating with friends helps fulfill the need for love and affection.

In recent years, other researchers have questioned Maslow's assumptions. For example, they believe that there is insufficient scientific evidence to support the notion that each level must be satisfied before an individual can move on to the next. They point out that many high achieving people, such as great artists, writers, and composers, did not have their basic needs fulfilled before completing their masterpieces. In fact, some suffered extreme poverty and isolation. Miguel de Cervantes began writing "Don Quixote," considered a literary masterpiece, while imprisoned in the late 1500s. According to some, Maslow studied mostly high-achieving white males who only represented a small sample of society. More recent studies of human behavior propose that although some needs are universal, such as for food and water, not all individuals have the same needs. In fact, needs may be determined by culture. Reportedly, Maslow was influenced by Blackfoot traditions of ranking needs, although the ones developed by the First Nations' people were listed in the opposite order as presented by Maslow, with self-actualization as the foundation.

Implications for Health Care Professionals

In spite of the challenges to Maslow's theory, health care professionals may find it useful for considering human behavior in general terms. Illness and injury can alter the nature of human needs and the means available to satisfy them. When patients enter the health care world, they may have to develop new strategies for adjusting and coping. It is important for health care professionals to understand how human needs affect patient behavior and recovery. They should also recognize the significant role they can play in helping patients meet their current needs.

Fascinating Facts

Many people throughout history have achieved their greatest potential, labeled by Maslow as self-actualization, in spite of personal difficulties that may have prevented them from fulfilling lower needs on the hierarchy.

Helen Keller: Graduated from college and became an author, political activist, and lecturer in spite of being deaf and blind.

Franklin D. Roosevelt: Served four terms as president of the United States although severely disabled as a result of polio.

Ludwig van Beethoven: Wrote some of the world's most beautiful music after losing his hearing.

Stephen Hawking: Considered one of the most brilliant minds of the 20th century, he became a theoretical physicist and cosmologist despite early-onset amyotrophic lateral sclerosis (ALS), diagnosed when he was 21 years old.

We will use the example of a patient named Carlos to illustrate changing needs throughout the recovery process. Carlos is a 29-year-old welder. His wife cares for their two children and maintains their home. Carlos is involved in a motorcycle accident in which he suffers a spinal cord injury that results in paraplegia, paralysis from the waist down. His injuries will make it impossible for him to ever walk again. (See Figure 15–5.)

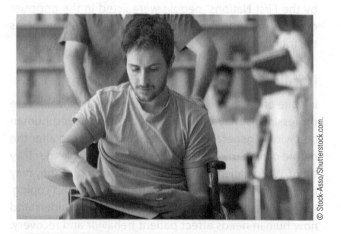

© Stock-Asso/Shutterstock.com.

FIGURE 15–5 Carlos's life and needs changed dramatically following his accident.

Carlos's needs changed significantly as a result of the accident. His progress through the long recovery process begins with meeting the most basic physiological need, which is to survive the physical trauma of the accident. His progress, described in the following sections, will not necessarily be smooth and steady and may not take place in an orderly way.

Physiological Needs

Carlos's survival depends on whether his physiological needs can be met to deal with his injuries. He is now dependent on the health care team to meet his physical needs. His needs, like those of other patients in similar situations, include the following:

- Reassurance
- Knowledge that he is receiving competent care
- Information about where he is and what has happened

After receiving the basic care necessary to save his life, Carlos will remain dependent on the health facility for some time to attend to his physical needs. These include the food and shelter that he used to provide for himself and others.

Safety and Security Needs

Being confined to a health care facility can threaten a patient's feelings of safety and security. Carlos feels uncomfortable in this strange environment, separated from the familiar surroundings of his home and the presence of family members. The feeling of security is increased for patients when they know the following:

- The names of the staff providing their care
- How to contact staff when they need assistance
- The routine for their care, including when to expect meals, personal care, and treatments
- Pain or discomfort they are likely to experience
- Availability of pain medication

Carlos faces a future full of unknowns, and this is causing him considerable anxiety. He often expresses concern about how he will be able to pay for his medical expenses and continue to support his family. Do not try to trivialize his worries, even if well intentioned. Saying, "Now, you shouldn't worry about that—just concentrate on getting well," does not show respect for Carlos nor does it help him find solutions for his problems.

As Carlos learns to trust the members of the health care team, his feelings of security will increase. Team members can encourage the development of trust by demonstrating acceptance of and respect for the patient. They can accomplish this by listening attentively, withholding judgment, and providing answers to questions. Questions from patients that the health care professional is not qualified to answer should be referred promptly to his or her supervisor.

Love and Affection Needs

Paraplegia brings a set of serious challenges, and one of the most difficult areas is how it affects the need for friendship, love, and affection. Before the accident, Carlos's social life centered on active pursuits with his friends. He knows that he will no longer join in on Saturday soccer games and that his days of riding motorcycles on his own are over. Many of the guys have visited him in the hospital, but he wonders how long they will keep spending time with someone who is confined to a wheelchair. Worse yet are his fears about how his wife is adjusting to having a disabled husband. Does she still love him? Will they be able to have sex?

All aspects of Carlos's previous social life seem altered, and the future looks very lonely. He is experiencing intense frustration and fear, and these emotions lead to occasional angry verbal attacks on the health care professionals who provide his care. Although it is a natural response to avoid prolonged contact and communication with an angry patient, it is often at this time that human contact is most needed. If Carlos fears rejection and loneliness, avoidance will only reinforce his belief that he is unlikable and unlovable.

Ways to help patients meet their need for love and affection include the following:

- Expressing sincere interest in them and their well-being
- Behaving in a compassionate way when they exhibit difficult behavior
- Listening attentively
- Touching them on the hand or shoulder as a form of greeting or reassurance
- Allowing them to express themselves even if the topic is difficult or unpleasant
- Helping family and friends feel welcome and comfortable during visits
- Encouraging family and friends to come and celebrate holidays or special events with patients

The health care professional can also alert the supervisor or other appropriate members of the health care team about Carlos's current behavior and possible needs. For example, occupational therapists help patients like Carlos rebuild their lives and achieve the highest level of activity possible, including sexual function. (Remember, however, that legal considerations of confidentiality restrict any discussions about patients to *only* those health care practitioners who work with them.)

Esteem Needs

Esteem refers to the opinions that others have of us, such as respect and admiration, as well as the attention they give us. The feelings and opinions that individuals have about *themselves* at a given time and their opinions of their value as people are known as self-esteem. Self-esteem can fluctuate depending on the person's experiences and perceptions at the moment. Injuries and illnesses that disfigure and cause loss of function often result in a decrease in self-esteem that can last for extended periods. Most people place importance on what others think of them and base their self-esteem, to a great extent, on the opinions of others. Before the accident, Carlos defined himself in terms of his roles as husband, father, son, friend, and worker. In other words, he based his personal value on *what* rather than *who* he was. He took pride in his skills as a welder and was confident of his ability to provide for his family.

In the weeks following the accident, Carlos's self-esteem has plummeted. Before his accident, he was a physically fit, active man. Now he must depend on others to take care of even his most basic physical needs. He doesn't know how he will provide for the financial security of himself or his family. And he has doubts about how he will be treated by friends and family during his long rehabilitation and future life as a paraplegic.

Health care professionals can help reinforce Carlos's self-esteem by sending the message that "You are worth my time. Your disability does not detract from your value as a person." Ways to express this idea to patients include the following:

- Taking the time to listen
- Showing interest by referring back to something the patient said in the past or remembering an occasion or event that is important to the patient
- Giving patients the opportunity to express their needs
- Asking for and respecting their preferences as much as possible
- Protecting their privacy
- Treating them with respect and dignity
- Asking for their permission before giving care
- Asking for patients' opinions of what works best for them *if* there are options

Self-Actualization Needs

Although the means available for Carlos to reach his highest potential have been altered by his accident, it is still possible for him to achieve self-actualization. Some people who have suffered serious health problems see their circumstances as an opportunity to make positive life changes. They even find that in some ways, their quality of life improves, because they realize the value of each day and more fully appreciate what they have. Common life changes include the following:

- Finding work that is more meaningful
- Making time for things they have always wanted to do, such as painting or working with children
- Sharing their recovery experiences with others who are experiencing similar injuries or illnesses
- Becoming involved in health care fund-raising activities to pay for research into and treatment of their condition

Actor Christopher Reeve, star of the Superman movies, was paralyzed from the neck down when he was thrown from his horse in 1995. He returned to films as a director and worked vigorously to promote research focused on developing new treatments for spinal cord injuries until his death in 2004. He remains an example of responding in a self-actualized manner to a catastrophic event. Another example is popular television and movie actor Michael J. Fox, who was diagnosed at age 30 with early-onset Parkinson's disease. He continued his acting career for some years following his diagnosis (including a sit-com about a newsman who is diagnosed with Parkinson's), and currently works to raise public awareness of the disease and funds for research to find a cure. In the case of Carlos, many factors will influence to what extent he succeeds in achieving self-actualization. The way he is treated as an individual in the various health facilities during his recovery is important.

DEFENSE MECHANISMS

Defense mechanisms are a special category of responses that humans employ to deal with conflict, problems, and threats to self-esteem. They help provide relief from the mental discomfort and anxiety caused by internal conflict and are usually performed unconsciously. For example, a student may believe that his inability to arrive on time to class is due to sleep patterns inherited from his father, when in reality it is due to his habit of partying late at night. In this case, he is using *rationalization* to justify his behavior. Although defense mechanisms provide temporary relief, they do not resolve the underlying, anxiety-producing problems that need to be addressed. For example, Mrs. Azordegan discovers a small lump in her left breast. She is afraid that it might be cancer and refuses to take any action. She puts off calling her physician or telling anyone in the family about the lump. Her *denial* is a defense mechanism whose purpose is to avoid facing a potentially unpleasant truth. By the time she seeks medical attention, she learns that she does have cancer and that delaying treatment has allowed it to metastasize (spread to other parts of

the body). The use of a defense mechanism has worsened the very problem that Mrs. Azordegan feared most and hoped to avoid. Even if the lump had not been cancerous, Mrs. Azordegan experienced prolonged and unnecessary stress caused by the delayed diagnosis. In either case, ignoring the situation only caused additional problems.

Defense mechanisms are commonly used at times of stress and anxiety, such as those experienced during illness or injury. Table 15–2 describes some of the defense mechanisms that patients may exhibit. Recognizing defense mechanisms aids health care professionals in understanding patient behavior so they can help reduce the level of threat experienced by patients. Here are examples of ways the health care professional can do this:

- Demonstrate acceptance
- Show sincere interest in patients' well-being
- Provide education and instructions to increase patients' control over their own health issues (see Figure 15–6)
- Allow them to discuss what is really bothering them, if they wish to do so
- Respect their need to use defense mechanisms, which may be needed to get through a very difficult situation

DEALING WITH LOSS

Having to deal with loss can significantly influence patient behavior. Suffering an illness or injury or even undergoing the normal aging process can result in many types of loss. These include loss of independence, a body part or function, control over one's life, appearance and self-image, privacy, financial security, familiar surroundings, and a significant other. The patient who must remain in a health care facility for a long time is likely to suffer multiple losses. Even the removal of a tooth in the dentist's office represents a loss. It can be traumatic for the middle-aged patient who thinks of the loss of a tooth as the beginning of the aging process and only the first of future physical problems and losses. Any health care encounter can represent loss of control for patients.

Just as the methods used to fulfill needs vary among individuals, so will their reactions to loss. Some common examples of ways of dealing with loss include the following:

- Seeking support from family and friends
- Finding comfort in religion
- Drawing on self-esteem
- Employing problem-solving techniques
- Using defense mechanisms
- Becoming angry
- Experiencing depression

Table 15–2 **Examples of Common Defense Mechanisms**

Defense Mechanism	Definition	Example
Acting out	Expressing difficult to communicate feelings by performing an extreme behavior	Husband kicking the wall when angry over wife's criticism of him
Compensation	Attempting to meet a need by substituting something that does not actually satisfy the need	Recently divorced woman overeating to deal with loneliness
Control	Trying to exert excessive control over others to make up for a loss of control elsewhere	Hospitalized patient insisting on being given an exact time schedule for care
Denial	Pretending that something is not true, especially something unpleasant	Business executive refusing to acknowledge testing positive for human immunodeficiency virus (HIV)
Displacement	Transferring feelings that one has about one person to a different person	Nurse becoming angry with her children after working with a demanding patient
Malingering	Pretending to be ill when one is not	Student faking symptoms to avoid taking a test at school
Projection	Failing to see one's own weaknesses or problems while seeing them in others	Overweight mother criticizing her overweight daughter's poor eating habits
Rationalization	Explaining behavior by using a socially acceptable reason	Graduate nurse delaying taking a licensing exam because she is "too busy" when in reality she is afraid she will fail
Regression	Behaving in ways that are more appropriate for a younger person	A 10-year-old boy returning to thumb-sucking after being hospitalized
Repression	Keeping unpleasant thoughts or memories in the subconscious and out of awareness	Young woman lacking conscious memory of having been sexually assaulted as a child
Withdrawal	Refusing to communicate with others or participate in social activities	Teenage boy refusing to take calls from friends or attending social activities after being diagnosed with leukemia

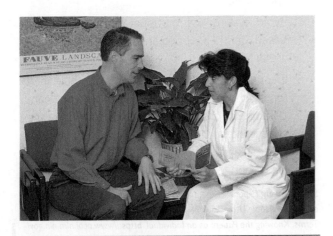

FIGURE 15–6 Educating patients about self-care techniques can reduce anxiety by increasing their control over personal health issues.

Health care professionals can help patients deal with loss by realizing its significance to patients, understanding their reactions to loss and their need to grieve, and being willing to talk with patients who wish to discuss their loss. This gives patients the opportunity to share their feelings, if they wish to do so, and to explore ways to grieve and deal with their loss. (See Figure 15–7.) Death and dying are discussed in Chapter 8.

TREATING PATIENTS AS INDIVIDUALS

As emphasized throughout this chapter, treating each patient as an individual is an essential component of good care. It is important to help patients retain their dignity, and strive to understand and acknowledge their experiences

FIGURE 15–7 Listening and expressing concern can help patients deal with loss.

and needs during the stressful period of illness or injury. (See Box 15–7 for a useful summary of treating patients as individuals developed by Britain's National Health Service.)

The effectiveness of the health care professional's interactions and communication with patients depends to a great degree on understanding and respecting individual differences. Although it is not suggested that the practice of modern health care be compromised to accommodate all the traditional beliefs and individual needs of patients, knowing something about the content and basis of their beliefs and behaviors can help provide a foundation on which to build effective helping relationships. Being sensitive to the variety of perceptions that patients bring to the health care setting enables health care professionals to better meet patient needs. There are a number of ways to learn about patients as individuals:

1. Observe the patient's behavior and ways of interacting with others.
   - Eye contact
   - Degree of formality in conversation and body movements
   - Outward signs of possible emotions such as nervousness, fear, or suspicion
   - Presence of family members
   - Interactions with family members
   - Reaction to touch and close personal contact

Box 15–7

Knowing the Patient as an Individual

Recommendations from the National Health Service in the United Kingdom

1. Develop an understanding of the patient as an individual, including how the condition affects the person, and how the person's circumstances and experiences affect their condition and treatment.

2. Ensure that factors such as physical or learning disabilities, sight, speech or hearing problems and difficulties with reading, understanding, or speaking English are addressed so that the patient is able to participate as fully as possible in consultations and care.

3. Ask the patient about and take into account any factors, such as their domestic, social, and work situation and their previous experience of health care, that may:
   - impact on their health condition and/or
   - affect their ability or willingness to engage with health care services and/or
   - affect their ability to manage their own care and make decisions about self-management and lifestyle choices.

4. Listen to and address any health beliefs, concerns, and preferences that the patient has, and be aware that these affect how and whether they engage with treatment. Respect their views and offer support if needed to help them engage effectively with health care services and participate in self-management as appropriate.

5. Avoid making assumptions about the patient based on their appearance or other personal characteristics.

6. If appropriate, discuss with the patient their need for psychological, social, spiritual, and/or financial support. Offer support and information to the patient and/or direct them to sources of support and information. Review their circumstances and need for support regularly.

Source: Patient Experience in Adult NHS Services: Improving the Experience of Care for People Using Adult NHS Services: Patient Experience in Generic Terms. Knowing the Patient as an Individual. https://www.ncbi.nlm.nih.gov/books/NBK115223/

2. Determine whether language barriers are present.

- Ask patient in what language he or she is most comfortable communicating
- Ask about language preferences for written information and instructions
- Ask if patient needs an interpreter when discussing health care information and treatments

3. Ask questions to determine individual preferences.

a. Health beliefs and practices

- What do you do to help you stay healthy?
- What do you usually do when you are sick or not feeling well?
- Who do you go to first when seeking help with health problems?
- Who in your family is primarily responsible for making health care decisions for members of the family?
- Who will help you at home if you need assistance with health problems?
- In coping with this illness/injury, what are your expectations of the health care team and of yourself?
- What do you think will be the most important factor in your recovery?

- Are you aware of any medical procedures or practices that contradict your spiritual beliefs?

b. Communication styles

- What are the ways you show respect and disrespect?
- Do you have preferences or restrictions related to touching, personal space, making eye contact, or social behaviors that you would like to tell me?

c. General

- Is there anything you would like to tell me that might help us understand your needs?

4. Listen carefully to the patient's responses.

5. Explain what you are doing and why when performing procedures or asking questions that may be difficult for the individual based on what you have learned.

(Source: Estes, M. E. Z. (2011). Health assessment and physical examination (5th ed.). Clifton Park, NY: Cengage Learning.)

In addition to being aware of cultural and individual differences, understanding human motivation and the need to preserve self-esteem will help you communicate effectively and provide appropriate care. The next chapter presents communication techniques such as listening, observing body language, and creating clear messages.

SUGGESTED LEARNING ACTIVITIES

1. Brainstorm ideas on how you can apply the philosophy of individual worth, described in this chapter, in your personal and future work life.

2. Learn more about the various cultural groups in your area. Attend local cultural events, such as diversity fairs and informational workshops.

3. Research two cultural groups that are different from your own. Choose five aspects to compare and contrast between the two groups and with your own.

4. Use illustrations from magazines or images copied from the Internet to create a poster that represents the cultural groups represented in the United States today.

5. Watch for examples of possible defense mechanisms used by people around you: friends, family members, and classmates. If observed, why do you think these mechanisms were employed?

6. Think about your own behaviors and reactions to events in your life. Are you using any defense mechanisms?

WEB ACTIVITIES

Institute for Health Care Improvement

How to Reduce Implicit Bias

http://www.ihi.org/communities/blogs/how-to-reduce-implicit-bias

1. An opening quote in this article states, "the uncomfortable truth is that we live in a society in which stereotypes about groups of people are ubiquitous, and it follows that almost everyone has some implicit bias" ("ubiquitous" means found everywhere).

    a. What does this mean?

    b. Do you agree? Why or why not?

2. What is the difference between "intentional bias" and "ubiquitous bias"?

3. How does race sometimes influence the type of health care provided?

Exactly What Is . . . Time

Time in Different Cultures

http://www.exactlywhatistime.com/OTHER-ASPECTS-OF-TIME/TIME-IN-DIFFERENT-CULTURES/

1. How have our concepts of time changed over the last 100 years?

2. Compare and contrast past-oriented and future-oriented cultures.

3. How are concepts of time of pre-industrial cultures different from post-industrial cultures? Give examples of groups today that remain pre-industrial.

4. Give the meaning of the following terms, including countries in which the dominant culture practices them: monochronic, polychronic, and variably monochronic.

5. How can understanding different orientation to time help you as a health care professional?

99% Invisible

It's Chinatown

https://99percentinvisible.org/episode/its-chinatown/

1. Read the article (To learn even more, you can also listen to the 39-minute audio portion).

2. When San Francisco's Chinatown was rebuilt after the 1906 earthquake, why did it look foreign to Chinese immigrants?

3. Why do tourists like Chinatown?

4. How was Chinese cooking adapted to American tastes? What are examples of "Chinese food" that isn't Chinese at all?

5. Explain how San Francisco's Chinatown is an example of combining two very different cultures.

6. Do you think that Chinatown gives a false impression of what modern China is like? Explain your answer.

Ethnomed

Clinical Pearls

https://ethnomed.org/clinical/clinical%20pearls

1. Choose three pearls (short articles) to read or videos to watch.

2. Report on what you learned about the effects of culture on health care.

3. What can health care professionals do to help patients from other cultures?

Psych Central

https://psychcentral.com/lib/15-common-defense-mechanisms/

1. Did you learn anything new about the various defense mechanisms?

2. Write a brief description of the mechanisms described in the article that are not included in this chapter.

Simply Psychology

Psychology Perspectives

https://www.simplypsychology.org/perspective.html

1. Read about different approaches to psychology and human behavior.

2. Choose a perspective that interests you and explain why.

3. How can having a basic understanding of psychology help you work more effectively with patients?

REVIEW QUESTIONS

1. Why is it important for the health care professional to consider each patient as an individual?

2. What is the meaning of the "philosophy of individual worth" and how does it apply to work in health care?

3. What are five conditions that can make it difficult to give appropriate care to patients?

4. What is the meaning of "empathy"?

5. What is the meaning of "prejudice" (also known as "bias")? How does it detract from providing positive and appropriate patient care?

6. What is the meaning of "implicit bias"?

7. What are six strategies to overcome prejudice and implicit bias?

8. What is the definition of "culture"? How does it influence human beliefs and behavior?

9. What is the meaning of "dominant culture"?

10. Why is it difficult for some individuals to adapt to a dominant culture?

11. What are the nine diverse groups identified in this text that are components of the U.S. population?

12. What are five reasons for to gathering information about ethnic groups you might encounter in your work?

13. What are some examples of cultural differences in perceptions of personal space and touching?

14. What are some examples of different cultural approaches to the following: time orientation, personal space, communication, and family structure?

15. What are the components of traditional Western medicine?

16. How can religious beliefs influence health care practices? Give three examples.

17. What is the concept of harmony as it applies to health, including the mind–body–spirit connection and the four humors?

18. What is the role of herb and plant medicines in some cultures?

19. What are three examples of different cultural approaches to health care for each of the following categories:
    - Definition of health
    - Sources of good health
    - Causes of illness
    - Methods of treatment

20. What is Maslow's hierarchy of needs?

21. What are the five categories of needs proposed by Maslow?

22. What are three ways the health care professional can help patients meet their needs in the following categories: physiological, safety and security, love and affection, self-esteem, and self-actualization.

23. Why is Maslow's hierarchy of needs being challenged today?

24. What are the definitions of "self-esteem" and "self-actualization"?

25. What is a defense mechanism? Why do people use them?

26. What are the 11 defense mechanisms listed in the text? Briefly explain each one.

27. What are five examples of how health care professionals can help reduce the level of anxiety experienced by patients who are demonstrating defense mechanisms?

28. What are three examples of ways the health care professional can help patients deal with loss?

29. What are the five recommendations from Britain's National Health Service for knowing patients as individuals?

30. What are five actions that health care professionals can take to learn about their patients as individuals?

31. What are five examples of questions to ask to learn about a patient's needs?

APPLICATION EXERCISES

1. Refer back to the Case of the Polite Patient at the beginning of the chapter. What assumptions did Carley make? How could she have learned more about Mr. Alvarez? After she learned about his situation, what could she have done to better help him understand and carry out the diet and exercise program prescribed by Dr. Washington?

2. You are working as a medical assistant in the private medical office of an oncologist (cancer specialist). Mrs. Ramirez, an elderly woman who lived in Guatemala until she was 56, comes to the office accompanied by her granddaughter. Mrs. Ramirez speaks very little English, but her granddaughter is bilingual. This visit was at the granddaughter's insistence after her grandmother admitted finding a small lump in her breast. Mrs. Ramirez is very anxious about the visit. Describe how you would work with this patient, including a review of cultural factors and individual needs.

PROBLEM-SOLVING PRACTICE

Katelin works as a nurse in a public school. Many of the children with whom she works are from homes with parents who are immigrants from a variety of countries. Katelin often finds herself unable to communicate with these parents. How might she apply the problem-solving process to improve her ability to work with families from different cultural backgrounds?

CHAPTER 16

The Communication Process

KEY TERMS

active listening
asking questions
barriers
clinical depression
closed-ended questions
communication
feedback
health literacy
leading questions
learning objectives
nonverbal communication
open-ended questions
pantomime
paraphrasing
probing questions
receiver
reflecting
requesting examples
sender
teach back
therapeutic communication

OBJECTIVES

Studying and applying the material in this chapter will help you to:

1. Define communication.
2. Explain the meaning of "successful communication."
3. Explain the importance of effective communication in health care.
4. List four factors that have increased the need for competent communication in health care.
5. State the foundation for good communication in health care.
6. Explain how health care professionals can use communication to help patients deal with stress, anxiety, and loneliness.
7. Define "health literacy."
8. List five reasons why patients do not follow medical advice.
9. List four ways that messages can be exchanged.
10. List the six steps in the communication process.
11. Explain the meaning of "teach back."
12. List three goals that should be included in every interaction with a patient.
13. List four factors that should be considered about patients when creating communication goals.
14. Explain why medical terminology should not be used when communicating with most patients.
15. List eight strategies for organizing long messages.
16. Define and explain when to use the four types of questions.
17. Explain how humor can be used in health care situations.
18. Describe appropriate ways to address older patients.
19. Explain the meaning and importance of nonverbal communication.
20. List eight examples of positive body language.
21. Define "pantomime" and explain its use in health care communication.
22. Describe the appropriate use of touch when working with patients.
23. List five environmental factors that affect communication.
24. Explain the meaning of "active listening."
25. Explain the purpose of feedback and describe the four types.
26. Explain how to evaluate a completed communication.
27. Describe the considerations when communicating with children, adolescents, adults, and older adults.
28. List techniques for communicating with patients who are:
    a. Terminally ill
    b. In pain, medicated, confused, or disoriented
    c. Suffering from dementia

d. Depressed

e. Anxious

f. Hearing impaired

g. Visually impaired

h. Speech impaired

i. Angry

j. Unable to speak or understand English

29. List eight professional telephone techniques and explain their importance.

30. Explain the importance of patient education.

31. List and describe the six-step process for delivering patient education.

32. List seven strategies for preparing and giving presentations to groups.

33. Describe three ways to discourage and avoid gossip.

34. Explain why it is unacceptable to discuss a patient with anyone who is not involved in the patient's care.

The Case of the Coder Who Lacked Confidence

Jenny McAbee has worked as a medical insurance coder and biller for Appleton Medical Clinic for three years. She enjoys working with detailed information and performing tasks on the computer. Her coding is accurate and very few claims she submits to insurance companies are denied. Jenny chose this career partly because she is shy and enjoys working by herself. Dr. Morton, the director of the clinic, has noted that many patients are confused about their insurance coverage, which payments are their responsibility, how to fill out and submit the proper paperwork, and other insurance details. He believes it would be helpful if Jenny could spend less time on paperwork and more time interacting with patients, answering their questions, and explaining their insurance plans. Therefore, he provides her with an assistant so she will have time to spend with the clinic's patients. Although Jenny has a thorough understanding of medical insurance and a desire to help the clinic's patients, she does not feel confident about her communication skills. Many of the clinic's patients have hearing impairments. Others speak very little English. She wonders how she can best help them. This chapter covers the communication process and techniques for becoming an effective communicator.

IMPORTANCE OF COMMUNICATION IN HEALTH CARE

Communication is the process in which messages are exchanged between a sender and a receiver. The **sender**, also referred to as the *speaker*, is the person who creates and delivers a message. The **receiver**, also called the *listener*, is the person to whom the sender directs the message. Communication is successful when the receiver interprets and understands the sender's message as it was intended.

Good communication is essential for the delivery of safe, effective health care. Modern health care systems rely on the efficient and accurate delivery of large amounts of information. Diagnoses and treatments are usually based on a variety of data that must be shared among many health care providers. There are vast networks of primary care providers, specialists, therapists, testing centers, medical facilities, and insurance companies that work together to provide and coordinate patient care. Chances of miscommunication increase as systems become larger and more complex.

Good face-to-face communication is also essential. It is reported that the root cause of nearly 66% of medical errors is the result of poor team communication (https://healthcarecomm.org/about-us/impact-of-communication-in-healthcare). Health care professional dissatisfaction and turnover also increase when there is poor communication among staff. (See Figure 16–1.)

Communication with Patients

The ability to communicate well can be as important to the professional success of the phlebotomist as her ability to safely draw blood. The well-being of patients depends on more than technical competence. For example, if a nurse is

FIGURE 16–1 Good communication between members of the health care team is essential for providing good patient care.

instructing a patient about how to change the dressing on a wound, the patient's understanding of these instructions is critical for successfully carrying out self-care practices at home. Studies have shown that health and treatment outcomes are significantly influenced by the quality of communication between patients and health care providers.

Several factors have increased the need for competent communication:

- Increasingly complex coverage of health care costs: Costs covered by private insurance, Medicare, Medicaid, and other insurance plans can be difficult to identify and understand. Patients need clear communication to determine which treatments and drugs they qualify for.

- Significant decrease in the length of time patients spend in hospitals and other health care facilities: Patients are now more responsible for their own follow-up care and need clear instructions to correctly carry out necessary self-care procedures.

- Shift in major causes of death from infectious diseases to cancer, heart disease, chronic obstructive pulmonary disease (COPD), and stroke: There has been an increase in chronic illness because people are living longer. An important part of the health care professional's responsibilities is providing patient education about factors that promote wellness.

- New medications: Many patients take a large number of medications and this makes it more difficult for them to organize and take them properly.

The attitudes of health care professionals influence their ability to communicate effectively with patients. Therefore, the first step in achieving excellent communication skills

is to develop respect for, and an understanding of, individual patients and their needs, as discussed in Chapter 15. Effective communication involves more than applying a set of techniques. It must be based on sincere compassion and concern for patients and their welfare. (See Figure 16–2.)

The health care world can be intimidating for patients. They may be anxious about receiving negative test results and learning that they have serious medical conditions. Or they may fear experiencing pain and discomfort during treatments. Still others are worried about losing control over portions of their lives as a result of their physical conditions. These concerns, combined with the physical stress caused by illness or injury, can negatively affect patient recovery. Health care professionals can help relieve patient stress by showing compassion, providing appropriate information, and answering questions. *Good communication has been shown to increase the speed of patient recovery.*

Loneliness and depression are commonly experienced by patients during their stay in health care facilities. This is especially common among older patients in facilities such as nursing homes. Health care professionals may be their principal contact with the outside world. Being willing to talk and, even more important, to *listen* to patients can lift their spirits.

Situations do not have to involve a direct threat to health to be stressful experiences for patients. As discussed in Chapter 15, any health care encounter can represent a loss for the patient and be a source of anxiety. Well-chosen words and a willingness to listen can help relieve anxiety. Patients' satisfaction is determined, to a great extent, by the quality of their communication with health care staff. As stated in Chapter 3, poor communication between

FIGURE 16–2 Good communication skills, combined with sincere caring about others, are essential for effective patient care.

patients and their providers is a major cause of medical malpractice lawsuits.

Another factor that affects communication with patients is **health literacy**. This is defined as "the ability to obtain, process, and understand basic health information and services needed to make appropriate health decisions" (https://www.cdc.gov/healthliteracy/training/page572.html). A significant percentage of Americans read at a grade-school level and do not understand instructions on prescription bottles, appointment reminders, and other written materials. They also report not understanding what their health providers tell them orally, but are too embarrassed to admit they miss what is said. The American Medical Association Foundation has produced an excellent video featuring real patients who explain their difficulties in understanding what health care professionals tell them. It is available at www.youtube.com/watch?v=cGtTZ_vxjyA.

There are other reasons, related to communication, that patients do not follow medical advice:

- 39% disagreed with the recommended treatment
- 27% were concerned about cost
- 25% found the instructions for self-care too difficult to follow
- 20% felt it was against their personal beliefs
- 7% stated they didn't understand what they were supposed to do

Source: https://healthcarecomm.org/about-us/impact-of-communication-in-healthcare

When patients are not comfortable expressing these concerns to their health care providers, there is no opportunity to address them. Good communication skills, discussed in this chapter, can assist health care professionals to better help their patients discuss their concerns.

THE COMMUNICATION PROCESS

Messages can be exchanged in at least four ways:

1. Orally (this chapter)
2. Nonverbally (this chapter)
3. In written form (Chapter 17)
4. Electronically (Chapter 18)

It is commonly believed that oral communication consists of simply talking and listening, activities that most people have been doing all their lives. We carry on dozens of conversations daily with family members, friends, classmates, and coworkers. Effective communication in health care, often referred to as **therapeutic communication**, is specifically aimed at meeting the needs of patients. It involves the application of a set of skills that can be acquired through practice.

In this text, communication is organized into a six-step process. This process provides a structured approach for studying and learning the skills that make up effective communication. Like other health care skills, communication cannot be taken for granted or performed in a routine manner. Each communication encounter presents its own set of circumstances and requires the health care professional's full attention. Good communication involves applying the thinking skills presented in Chapter 1.

The Six Steps of the Communication Process

1. Set communication goals: Determine what is to be accomplished. This requires considering the receiver's needs, current circumstances, and the duties assigned to the health care professional.
2. Create the message: Select and organize appropriate content based on the communication goals and characteristics of the receiver.
3. Deliver the message: Choose the delivery method best suited for ensuring that the receiver will understand the intent of the message.
4. Listen to the response: Employ listening and observational techniques to determine whether the message was received as intended.
5. Offer feedback and seek clarification: Rephrase what you hear and/or ask questions or use **teach back** (asking receivers to explain what you have said in their own words) to check the receiver's understanding.
6. Evaluate the encounter and revise the message, if necessary: Determine whether the goal was met. If not, why not? What other options are available? What should be the next step?

(See Figure 16–3.)

Step One: Set Communication Goals

Much of our everyday communication is spontaneous and superficial and requires little or no planning. This includes everyday greetings ("Hi, how are you?"), which are said automatically and from which little real information is usually expected. Interactions in health care settings are more purposeful. Suppose a nurse has a goal of learning about the current health status of a patient. Instead of asking the patient "How are you?" which may result in a programmed response of "Fine," she needs to ask more specific questions. These will be based on communication goals. Examples of specific questions include the following:

- On a scale of 1 to 10, what is your pain level?
- Do you have any questions about your care?
- Are you feeling nervous about the procedure?

FIGURE 16–3 The six steps in the communication process.

Here are some examples of health care goals:

- Gather objective and subjective information about a patient's condition.
- Instruct individuals on postsurgical home care procedures so family members can understand and follow them correctly.
- Inform a patient about the benefits of the recommended treatment.
- Report patient care information to a coworker who is taking over the care of the patient.

In addition to goals that are specific to the situation, there are three more that should be included in every interaction with a patient:

1. Demonstrate sincere concern for the patient's welfare.
   - Have a warm smile.
   - Use a gentle manner.
   - Do not act hurried.
   - Listen carefully.
2. Establish trust.
   - Establish eye contact as culturally appropriate.
   - Explain why a procedure, treatment, or test is necessary.
   - Explain in advance everything you are going to do.
   - Follow through with anything you say you will do (return in five minutes, call patient at home to check on progress, and so on).
3. Enhance the patient's self-esteem.
   - Involve the patient in decision-making whenever possible.
   - Clarify the patient's communication if you're unsure of meaning.
   - Address the patient properly and respectfully.
   - Provide for privacy.
   - Ask the patient for input on how he or she wants things done, when appropriate.

These goals are based on the philosophy of individual worth, discussed in Chapter 15. It may seem unrealistic to try to achieve these goals in the brief time the health care professional spends with patients. There are other tasks to accomplish, such as taking a blood sample or performing a breathing treatment. Good communication, however, depends more on quality than quantity. A warm smile and informative reassurance are not time-consuming and can be included in any encounter. Patients today receive much of their care from strangers who are in a hurry. It is for this very reason that an effort should be made to personalize interactions as much as possible.

Collect Information

To set appropriate goals, it is important to collect and review information that might affect communication. This includes the cultural and behavioral factors discussed in Chapter 15 as well as circumstances specific to the situation. The following factors should be considered:

- Patient's level of understanding
  - Is the patient very young?
  - Does the patient speak English?
  - If so, is English the second language?
  - Does the patient have a learning disability that affects his or her ability to understand?
  - Does the patient appear to be confused or disoriented?
  - What is the patient's ability to retain information? Is there short-term memory loss?
  - What is the appropriate terminology to use?
- Emotional factors
  - Does the patient's behavior indicate fear or anxiety?
  - Are there signs that the patient is using a defense mechanism? (See Chapter 15.)
  - Is the patient ready to accept the information that is to be offered?

- Physical factors
  - Is the patient in pain?
  - Is the patient on medication that causes drowsiness or affects the ability to concentrate?
  - Does the patient have a hearing, visual, or speech impairment that affects the communication process?
- Urgency of the communication
  - Must the communication take place now?
  - Is this the appropriate setting for the communication?
  - What are the consequences if it does not take place or if it is unsuccessful?

Learning to make these determinations quickly is an important health care skill that is developed over time. One technique for new health care professionals is to use mental checklists to help them prepare for communication encounters.

Step Two: Create the Message

Creating an appropriate message requires the selection of content and use of language that is based on the answers to the questions listed earlier. (Creating a message is also called *encoding*.) Health care communication usually takes place at a deeper level than everyday conversation and must be clear and accurate. It may involve sharing very personal information, such as a patient's fears.

Information must be presented in a manner that the receiver understands. For example, although the use of medical terminology helps ensure accuracy in communications with other health care professionals, it can confuse and intimidate patients. Even everyday language may have to be simplified into common terms for some patients, depending on their age and language skills. For example, "number two" might be substituted for "bowel movement." At the same time, take care not to talk down to patients.

Organize long messages to make them easier to follow. Here are some examples of organizational strategies:

- Explain what you plan to do and what the patient should expect to hear, feel, and so on.
- Rank information in order of importance.
- List a sequence of steps for the patient to follow.
- State facts, following each with an explanation.
- Present an overview of a procedure before detailing the individual steps.
- Give instructions along with a description of possible consequences if they are not followed.

- Break information into sections, if possible, so the patient can grasp each part or set of facts before moving on to the next.
- Use teach back: Have patients demonstrate understanding by explaining the information *in their own words* or by performing the task or exercise being taught.

Asking Questions

Some messages are phrased as questions. There are several types of questions:

1. **Closed-ended questions** can be answered with a single word or a response of "yes" or "no." This type of question is used to gather factual information. For example, the health care professional may ask closed-ended questions when obtaining background information about a patient. Closed-ended questions are not recommended when checking for understanding. Many patients will answer "Yes" to the question "Do you understand?" even if they do not. They are afraid of appearing dumb or do not want to "bother you" by having the information repeated.

2. **Open-ended questions** cannot be answered with a simple "yes" or "no." They require a more complete response and are used to encourage patients to provide more detailed information or explanations. These questions can be used to learn about the patient's symptoms, to encourage them to share feelings and opinions, or to check understanding of the message.

3. **Probing questions** are requests for additional information or clarification. For example, they can be used to lead patients to more fully discuss their symptoms. If a patient states, "My stomach hurts," appropriate probing questions would inquire about the exact location and type of pain, when it first occurred, and when it is experienced. It is important not to confuse the purposeful use of probing questions with digging for unnecessary personal details, which patients may find offensive.

4. **Leading questions** are those in which all or part of the answer is included in the wording of the question. Leading questions should be avoided when they encourage the receiver to give the answer believed to be correct or what the health care professional wants to hear. However, leading questions can be useful when used with patients who have difficulty speaking or who do not understand English well enough to phrase a complete answer. In these situations, take extra care to check for understanding to ensure that the patient is not simply agreeing with you. See Table 16–1 for examples of each type of question.

Table 16–1 Common Types of Questions

Question Type	Examples
Closed-ended	What is your date of birth?
	Are you taking any medications?
Open-ended	How did you fall?
	Why do you think you are feeling sad?
Probing	You said that you've been experiencing pain in your chest. Where, exactly, in your chest do you feel the pain?
	When is it the most severe?
	Can you tell me more about when you get these headaches?
Leading	Would you describe the pain as sharp, dull, throbbing, or aching?
	Do you feel more nauseated in the morning, afternoon, evening, or during the night?

After asking a question, it is important to pause and give the receiver sufficient time to respond. Some people need more time than others to formulate answers. Do not interrupt or finish sentences for patients. If it is obvious that they do not understand the question or are unable to reply, reword the question and provide another opportunity for a response. Consider the state of each patient and his or her ability to answer questions. For example, Mrs. Feinstein is an elderly patient who has difficulty remembering. Hospitalized for severe back pain, she cannot accurately respond to questions about how she is feeling today compared to yesterday. A more effective way to get the needed information is to ask her to rate her pain level on a scale of 0 to 10, with 0 being no pain and 10 being the highest level she can imagine. (See Chapter 20 for more information about assessing pain.)

Using Humor

Messages need not always be serious. The careful use of humor can offer relief from the difficult situations faced by patients and their families. It can help relieve tension and promote the open discussion of sensitive issues. Humor, however, should *never* be at the expense of anyone, even in the person's absence.

Patients will sometimes joke about their condition as a cover-up for fear or embarrassment, but the health care professional should never initiate this type of humor. Listen carefully in these situations, because these jokes may indicate the patient's need for help in dealing with a difficult condition. It is appropriate to let patients know that if they wish, they can discuss fears they have or request information they need.

Step Three: Deliver the Message

It is important to first determine to whom the message should be delivered. This is not always obvious. For example, if the patient is a child, elderly person, or disabled,

Thinking It Through

Robin Winters is starting her career as a dental hygienist for Dr. Castro at an urban dental clinic. Robin has noted that many of the patients appear to have poor dental care habits: Their teeth have accumulations of plaque and a high number of caries (cavities), and the patients suffer from gingivitis (inflammation of the gums). When she asks patients if they take care of their teeth at home, most respond, "Yes."

1. How can Robin use questions more effectively to learn about her patient's dental care habits?

2. Give examples of questions that she might ask.

should communication be directed to the patient or to a family member? Patients who are able to understand any or all of the message should be addressed directly. Detailed information or instructions can also be given to a family member later. For example, a medical assistant who greets 87-year-old Mrs. Hernandez by asking her daughter, "How is your mother doing today?" is failing to show respect for the patient. Older patients often face the biases of a youth-oriented society. Using titles, such as Mrs., Ms., and Mr., demonstrates respect for patients. It is inappropriate to address older persons as "dearie" or "hon." Although this may be considered a sign of affection, it is offensive to some patients. A common guideline for health care professionals is to address patients older than themselves more formally than those who are the same age or younger. If in doubt, it is best to ask patients how they wish to be addressed.

Some cultural groups designate a family member, often the oldest or a male, to make decisions on behalf of the patient. Although it is important for the health care professional to understand the dynamics of the patient's family, this does not suggest that the laws governing confidentiality can be broken in order to accommodate cultural preferences. Well-meaning family members, friends, and others who appear to have a valid right to know *cannot* be given information unless the patient has signed a release. It is essential to recognize which messages have a restricted audience and exactly who that audience is.

Advance directives and a health care power of attorney, discussed in Chapter 3, serve as the links between health care professionals and patients who have lost their ability to communicate. It is essential to know what medical treatments patients desire to be performed and who may receive information and speak on their behalf.

It is believed that many patients who cannot speak or respond can hear and experience touch. Under these circumstances, health care professionals can provide comfort by maintaining communication. They should speak reassuringly and consider making appropriate physical contact, such as touching the patient's hand or shoulder when speaking.

Nonverbal Communication

How a message is delivered can either reinforce or change the intended meaning. For example, an otherwise friendly remark, stated in a sarcastic voice, distorts the intended message. The words "that's a nice thing to say" can be delivered in a way that indicates the sender's pleasure. The same words, delivered in a mocking tone with stress on the word "that's," convey the opposite meaning. It sends the message that what was said was hurtful.

Nonverbal communication includes tone of voice, body language, gestures, facial expressions, touch, and physical appearance. Up to 70% of the meaning of messages are expressed nonverbally. Nonverbal communication is usually the most accurate expression of what the sender truly feels and believes. This is because it comes from within and is conveyed without the awareness of the sender. It takes place subconsciously.

Health care professionals must be aware of the nonverbal communication of both themselves and others. The nonverbal communication of patients should always be observed. For example, if a patient reports feeling "fine" but appears very tense and nervous, the verbal and nonverbal messages do not match. In such cases, the health care professional needs to observe carefully, ask questions, and provide opportunities for the patient to share what he or she is really experiencing.

The appearance of the health professional is a form of nonverbal communication. It can influence the patient's confidence in the worker's competence, which in turn can affect how messages are perceived. (See Chapter 13 for a discussion of professional appearance.)

Body Language

Body posture and movements convey messages. Some body language can have a negative impact on the receiver. Examples include crossing the arms, shrugging the shoulders, tapping the fingers or feet, clenching the fists, and rolling the eyes. These can communicate disagreement, lack of interest, disbelief, and impatience.

Positive body language conveys interest, caring, and the willingness to listen to the sender's message, even if there is disagreement. It encourages sharing information and promotes exchanging honest messages. Positive body language includes the following:

- Looking at the other person
- Directing the body toward the other person
- Leaning slightly toward the person being addressed
- Holding the body in a relaxed position
- Nodding or verbalizing ("uh huh," "yes," "tell me more") occasionally to indicate acknowledgment
- Having open and warm facial expressions
- Approaching the patient, if standing at a distance
- Stopping the performance of tasks to give your full attention

Positive body posture communicates "I am focused on, and paying attention to, you and what you are saying." (See Figure 16–4.) Actions must match words. For example, if a patient wants to discuss a sensitive matter and the health care professional listens while facing toward the door, the message to the patient may be "I'm really in a hurry to leave." In another example, a health care professional

FIGURE 16–4 What positive body language is this health care professional demonstrating?

wants to reassure a patient, but looks away nervously while speaking. The message will seem false and the patient will sense that important information, possibly negative, is being left unsaid. Establishing trust, an essential ingredient in effective communication, requires that spoken and nonverbal communications match.

The use of pantomime, body movements that convey ideas or actions, can communicate when speaking is not possible or when the patient does not understand English. For example, acting out the movements a patient must make when performing an exercise can demonstrate exactly what needs to be done.

Gestures are helpful when patients cannot be attended to immediately. Acknowledging their presence conveys respect and creates good will. For example, if the medical receptionist is speaking on the telephone when a patient arrives for an appointment, the patient should be greeted with a smile, nod of the head, and quick hand gesture to indicate that he or she will be attended to shortly.

Facial Expressions

Facial expressions are an important form of nonverbal communication. The health care professional's expressions can be a source of reassurance or anxiety for patients, so it is important to learn to be aware of, and control, them. This can be difficult when dealing with situations that are challenging, unpleasant, or offensive. For example, you may feel very frustrated with the behavior of an angry patient. Efforts at calming the patient will be less effective if your face reflects signs of impatience and annoyance. The health care professional's face should reflect warmth, confidence, and interest in the welfare of the patient.

Use of Touch

The use of touch has become a difficult issue in health care today. Although a friendly pat or squeeze of the hand has been a traditional way of communicating care and interest, any touching that a patient considers to be inappropriate can lead to legal problems. It is essential that health care professionals always practice good judgment and use common sense. It is also important that they be aware that patients may have cultural preferences regarding touch, as discussed in Chapter 15. Many health care activities require entering personal space that is normally reserved for only the closest and most trusted people in the patient's life. It is important that patients be told what is to take place and why. Explain what they should expect to see, hear, and feel. For example, when administering an injection, the health care professional should inform the patient of its purpose, where it will be given, and what sensations might be experienced.

The health care professional should avoid touching areas that are considered sexual (buttocks, breasts, genital area) unless it is necessary when performing a procedure. Any unnecessary roughness, even done in a playful manner, can be interpreted as abusive and must be avoided.

Gestures and body movements that are either positive or neutral to one person may be unacceptable to others. As discussed in Chapter 15, health care professionals should be sensitive to the possibility of such differences, willing to learn about various cultural practices, and observant of patient reactions. If a patient seems uncomfortable with any contact that was intended to be a sign of caring or reassurance, seek clarification by stating your intention and asking if the gesture was unacceptable.

Physical Environment

The physical environment and how the health care professional is positioned in relation to the patient can affect the delivery of the message. Sitting behind a desk or standing over the other person projects a sign of authority or dominance. Other factors to consider include the following:

- Light sources: Can the patient see you clearly? Is there a glare on anything the patient is expected to see? Is light shining in the patient's eyes?

- Sounds: Can the patient hear you clearly? Are there unnecessary noises that are distracting? Should the television or radio be turned off?

- Privacy: Are there other people in the area who can hear the communication? If privacy is necessary, how can it be arranged? Are you speaking directly to the patient and only as loudly as necessary?

- Activity: Do you appear to be more focused on taking notes or entering data into a computer than on the patient?

- Comfort: Is the patient exposed or in an awkward position? Can communication wait?

Step Four: Listen to the Response

Listening is not passive, but an active process that requires the following:

- Concentration
- Attention
- Observation

Hearing and taking in words take place at a rate that is several times faster than the rate of speech. This is helpful when taking notes, but it also allows time for the mind to wander. Active listening is characterized by focusing fully on what the speaker is saying. (Listening and trying to understand a message is also called "decoding.")

Effective listening can be hindered by receivers' reactions to what the sender is saying. For example, if the receiver strongly disagrees with the message, his or her

mind may become occupied formulating mental arguments instead of listening carefully. Another common interference to listening is thinking about how one is going to respond when the speaker stops talking. The mind becomes engaged in self-talk and stops listening.

Good listening also requires that receivers do not interrupt senders or complete messages for them. Allow enough time for senders to complete their messages. Encouraging remarks and gestures may be used as prompts: "I see," "Go on," or a nod of the head. Interrupting, however, can convey a lack of respect and impatience. It can also distort the sender's intended message, preventing important information from being conveyed.

Effective listening skills can be developed. This is worth the effort because patients report that being listened to is a major determinant in their opinions of health care providers (Anderson, Barbara, & Feldman, 2007). Start by becoming aware of lapses in your attention. When you realize you are losing focus, bring your mind back to the speaker. With practice, you can decrease internal interference and poor attention. See Box 16–1 for a summary of good listening skills.

Periods of silence can be a meaningful component of communication. The purpose of health care encounters is not to maintain a steady stream of conversation, but to help patients solve their health problems. Silence allows time for thought and reflection. It also provides a chance to observe the nonverbal communication that takes place during silence. Some cultures have a high respect for the value of silence. Allowing periods of silence may feel awkward at first, but they can be a valuable tool in promoting good communication.

Step Five: Ask for Feedback

Feedback is a method used to check understanding of what is said. Did the message come across as the sender intended? All of us have had the experience of believing we understood a message perfectly, only to discover later that we had misinterpreted it. Obtaining feedback helps avoid misunderstandings.

Here are four ways to obtain feedback:

1. **Paraphrasing** The receiver rewords the sender's message in the receiver's own words and then asks the sender for confirmation.

   Example "I understood you to say that you have experienced these headaches every day for the past two weeks. Is that correct?"

2. **Reflecting** This is similar to paraphrasing, but prompts the receiver to either complete or add more detail to the original message.

   Example "You say that it's difficult for you to do the exercises the therapist has recommended because _____." (Pause and allow time for response.)

3. **Asking questions** Request clarification and additional information. Many words, such as "difficult," "painful," and "a lot," have different meanings for people. In health care, the use of questions can help patients describe their conditions more clearly. Accurate diagnoses and appropriate treatments depend, in part, on the clarity and completeness of information supplied by the patient.

   Example "What symptoms are you experiencing when you say you are feeling terrible?"

   Questions can be used to check the receiver's understanding of important information. Instead of asking if the receiver understands, ask a question whose answer will demonstrate understanding.

   Example "Can you list for me the three steps you'll take when giving your son his medication?" This is an example of teach back.

   Open-ended questions, discussed earlier, can be used to encourage patients to talk about their values and beliefs. Although it is not the role of the health care professional to make value judgments about patients, what is learned can help you better understand the behavior and motivations of patients and find ways to meet their needs.

   Example "Why do you say that you deserved to have the accident?"

   This question may help in understanding why a patient is making no effort to perform the exercises that will assist in recovering from injuries.

4. **Requesting examples** Examples can help to more clearly explain and fill in meaning.

   Example "Tell me about the kind of situations in which you feel lightheaded."

Box 16-1

Summary of Good Listening Skills

Clear your mind of distractions

Face the sender

Focus your full attention on the sender

Maintain eye contact as appropriate for the culture

Turn off "self-talk"

Do not make value judgments about what you hear

Mentally note anything that needs clarification

Do not interrupt

Establishing clear channels of communication by using feedback also helps maintain good relationships with coworkers and supervisors. Developing competence as a health care professional requires monitoring personal progress and learning from mistakes. Feedback can be an important tool for fostering professional growth. For example, Rosie's supervisor informs her that a report she has prepared is "unacceptable." Rosie can request more specific feedback by asking questions such as "What did I do or not do that made my performance on this task unacceptable?" and "Can you tell me exactly what it is that makes the report unacceptable?" These questions will encourage the supervisor to be specific and provide details from which Rosie can learn.

Step Six: Evaluate the Encounter

The purpose of evaluation is to determine whether the communication goals have been met, demonstrated by the response or behavior of the receiver. If the goal is not met, the following questions can help identify the difficulty:

- Did I clearly state my messages?
- Did I present them at a level appropriate for the receiver?
- Did I listen actively?
- Which part of the message was misunderstood?

The evaluation process actually continues throughout every communication encounter. A good communicator constantly checks for understanding by listening, observing, and asking for feedback as needed. That way, adjustments can be made as needed.

Some communication goals are achieved over time, and the evaluation must be delayed. For example, if cardiac patient Heinrich Mueller is instructed about improving his eating habits, it may be weeks before the dietician finds out if he understood and was motivated to follow the low-fat eating plan. Another example of a long-term communication goal is making an effort over time to improve a relationship with a coworker.

COMMUNICATION THROUGH THE LIFE SPAN

Chapter 8 gave an overview of the human life span and discussed the various stages of human growth and development. Each stage has certain characteristics and needs which should be considered when communicating with individuals in each group.

When communicating with young children, it is important to help them understand what is happening to them and how you are helping them. They may be fearful and need help reducing their anxiety. At the same time, children should be included as much as possible in decision-making and allowed to help with their care when appropriate. As with patients of any age, it is important to listen actively to children and answer their questions using age-appropriate language. (See Figure 16–5.)

Adolescents must be treated with respect and dignity. Show an interest in them as individuals by learning about what is important to them. They may be struggling to establish their identity as they move from childhood to adulthood. Do not talk down to them, but fully explain what you are doing and why.

Adulthood is a busy time of life with many responsibilities, such as career and family. Illness and injury at this time can be extremely stressful and it is important for the health care professional to listen to patients' concerns. Do not assume that adults understand medical vocabulary, detailed instructions, and preventive measures they should take now to avoid health problems as they age. Use teach back to check understanding.

Fascinating Facts

- Between 70% and 80% of our waking hours are spent in some form of communication: approximately 30% speaking and 45% listening.

- The average person speaks at 125 to 175 words per minute and can understand 400 words per minute.

- After listening to a 10-minute presentation, the average person retains 50% of what was said. After 48 hours, retention drops to 25%.

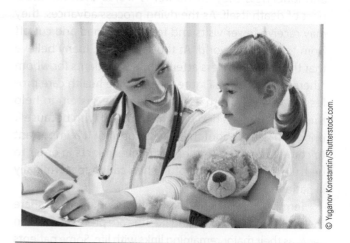

FIGURE 16–5 Your communication must be adjusted to the age and other characteristics of the receiver.

© Yuganov Konstantin/Shutterstock.com.

Older adults may have the most variation among individuals, from those who are active and mentally sharp into their nineties to individuals suffering from dementia. (Communicating with dementia patients is covered in a later section.) A goal for the health care professional is to help patients remain independent as long as possible by providing them with the information they need to maintain their health. They need honest conversations about any chronic conditions as well as help in making end-of-life decisions. Strive for an approach that is respectful but not overprotective.

(Information in this section adapted from Tamparo and Lindh (2017).)

OVERCOMING COMMUNICATION BARRIERS

Obstacles known as **barriers** sometimes block communication. Barriers include the following:

- Language differences
- Cultural influences
- Defense mechanisms (see Chapter 15)
- Physical distractions
- Sensory impairments
- Medication effects
- Pain

Identifying and overcoming barriers requires the use of empathy, observation, questions, and feedback. Specific techniques can be employed and extra time allowed to promote effective communication.

Patients Who Are Terminally Ill

Patients who are dying have reported that the isolation and loneliness they encounter is worse than the prospect of death itself. As the dying process advances, they may receive fewer visits and feel abandoned and cut off from the outside world. At the same time, many believe that they are given less attention than patients for whom "there is hope." (See Figure 16–6.) Some health care professionals view death as a failure of the system to help the patient. Others find it difficult to deal with because it brings up issues about their own mortality. It is important to come to terms with these difficult subjects in order to be truly effective and helpful when caring for terminally ill patients.

Terminally ill patients may have strong needs to share their fears and concerns, and health care professionals can serve as their major remaining links with life. Some patients want to talk about death and their desire to complete

FIGURE 16–6 Dying patients often suffer from loneliness and feelings of isolation.

Thinking It Through

Craig Segal is a recently graduated licensed vocational nurse (LVN) who has been hired at an oncology clinic in his home town. Craig works with patients who are dealing with a potentially fatal disease. This is difficult because he has known many of them and their families for many years. He finds himself wondering how he can best communicate with patients and their families. Craig wants them to know that he cares and wants to be of assistance, but he is not sure how to approach what he believes to be emotional topics and finds himself keeping conversation to a minimum.

1. How can Craig use the steps of the communication process to help him feel more confident about communicating with patients?

2. Which techniques do you think he might find most effective?

unfinished life tasks. The health care professional can improve the quality of this final phase by seeking, rather than avoiding, opportunities for communication. Be willing to listen and show that you care. Patients who cannot speak or respond may still be able to hear, so maintain oral communication. For example, greet the patient and explain what you are doing. Do not speak as if the patient is not in the room. (Home Care Institute, 2009). (See Chapter 8 for a discussion of death and dying.)

Patients Who Are in Pain, Medicated, Confused, or Disoriented

Patients who are in pain, medicated, confused, or disoriented may have difficulty communicating. Health care professionals can assist them by taking extra time and following these guidelines:

- Identify yourself and say the patient's name.
- Maintain eye contact.
- Speak slowly and clearly in a moderate pitch of voice.
- Use simple language. Avoid slang and expressions that do not mean exactly what they say.
- Keep each message short and to the point. For example, do not give a series of instructions or ask more than one question at a time.
- Give the patient time to respond.
- Use touch if the patient is comfortable with it.
- Try to schedule interactions when patients are in the least amount of pain.
- Repeat the message as needed, without changing the content or words.
- Review the content with the patient to assess retention of the message.
- When appropriate, give the patient written information that can be referred to later.

Source: Adapted from Nursing Assistant: A Nursing Process Approach *(11th ed.), by B. Acello & B. Hegner, 2016, Boston: Cengage Learning.*

Patients with Dementia

Alzheimer's disease causes up to 80% of cases of dementia, but there are other conditions, such as vascular dementia that can follow a stroke. In addition to memory loss, dementia decreases the ability to communicate, both in understanding others and expressing oneself orally. Patients may forget the meaning of words and phrases, have difficulty finding the right words, and invent words to express themselves, such as calling a watch an "arm clock." As verbal skills decline, they may rely more on gestures (http://contemporaryclinic.pharmacytimes.com/chronic-care/how-to-communicate-effectively-with-dementia-patients).

Patients may also exhibit difficult behavior, such as shouting, name-calling, hitting, and pushing. Health care professionals must be compassionate and patient, stay calm, and not take this behavior personally. It is also important to continue to communicate with dementia patients in spite of the barriers. The following suggestions may be helpful for maintaining and improving communication:

- Limit distractions and noise.
- Approach patients from the front and introduce yourself.
- Get the patient's attention: establish eye contact and call them by name.
- Do not assume that the patient cannot understand or does not want to communicate.
- Maintain a friendly expression.
- Use simple language and short sentences.
- Be patient: allow long pauses for patients to formulate a response.
- Agree or distract with a different subject when what the patient says does not make sense or is repetitive.
- Respond to the patient's feelings rather than the words.
- Do not confront, argue, or try to reason with the patient.
- If the patient does not understand what you say, rephrase rather than repeating.
- Offer suggestions instead of corrections. For example, if a patient mistakes her brother for someone else, say, "I think this is your brother, Gordon."
- If the patient is unable to communicate orally, observe their body language to learn what they want or need.

Patients Who Are Depressed

It is not uncommon for patients with serious conditions, such as cancer, to be depressed. This is usually a temporary condition, as opposed to **clinical depression** (a mood disorder that causes persistent feelings of sadness and loss of interest), but it can result in feelings of distress and interfere with the patient's functioning and ability to communicate. Let depressed patients know: "I am here for you." "I'm glad to listen." At the same time, realize that these patients may respond negatively to whatever you say. Specific suggestions for communication include the following:

- Invite, but do not force patients to talk about their fears, concerns, and how they are feeling.
- Listen carefully without judging.
- Offer hope, but do not advise them to "Cheer up" or "Be positive."
- Allow for silence.

Source: Adapted from American Cancer Society. Caring for the patient with cancer at home. Depression. (From American Cancer Society, Depression. https://www.cancer.org/treatment/treatments-and-side-effects/physical-side-effects/changes-in-mood-or-thinking/depression.html)

Patients Who Are Anxious

In addition to depression, anxiety is a common experience for patients. Even a visit to the dentist can bring on anxiety for patients who fear needles, pain, or embarrassment about the condition of their teeth. Anxious patients may have difficulty focusing and responding, so exercise patience. Be empathetic and reassuring. At the same time, do not trivialize the patients' feelings by telling them, "It's silly to be anxious" or "There's nothing to be afraid of." Clearly, for the patient, the situation is fearful. Instead, try the following suggestions:

- Approach the patient calmly and with a smile.
- Ask the patient to express his or her concerns.
- Let the patient talk and *listen* carefully.
- Keep your messages simple and to the point.
- Stick to one topic to make it easier for the patient to follow.
- Use feedback to check the patient's understanding of your message.

Patients Who Have Hearing Impairments

Hearing loss affects a significant number of Americans, as illustrated by the following statistics:

- Approximately 15% (37.5 million) Americans aged 18 and over have some trouble hearing.
- Who has disabling hearing loss?
  - 2% of adults 45 to 54 years old
  - 8.5% of adults 55 to 64 years old
  - 25% of adults 65 to 74 years old
  - 50% of adults age 75 or older
- About 2 to 3 out of every 1,000 children in the United States are born with a detectable level of hearing loss.

Source: https://www.nidcd.nih.gov/health/statistics/quick-statistics-hearing

When initiating conversation, especially with older adults, carefully observe the receiver and use appropriate feedback to check for understanding. It is important not to assume that people can hear just because they are not wearing a hearing aid or do not ask you to speak up. In fact, it is reported that only 30% of adults over age 70 who could benefit from using hearing aids actually wear them. Also, many people who experience hearing loss are unaware of it because it can happen gradually over the years or they are embarrassed to admit it. Following are signs that a person may have difficulty hearing:

- Leaning forward and turning the head
- Asking you to repeat information
- Failing to hear when not facing the speaker
- Not responding to you when you ask a question or finish speaking

American Sign Language (ASL) provides a means of communication for people with significant or complete hearing loss. It consists of hand movements and shapes, facial expressions, and corresponding body postures to convey meaning. (See Figure 16–7.) Partly due to the difficulty experienced in trying to communicate with people who have normal hearing, many hearing-impaired individuals consider themselves to be members of a unique cultural group they refer to as "deaf culture."

The following suggestions can improve communication with the hearing impaired:

- Position yourself close to the receiver and speak face-to-face.
- Remove or turn off sources of noise.
- Have the light source directed to your face.
- Make sure your mouth is visible to the receiver.
- Keep your hands away from your face.
- Say the person's name before beginning the conversation.
- Determine if the person hears better in one ear than the other.
- Introduce the general topic of the conversation.
- Speak distinctly and do not mumble.

HURT, PAIN, ACHED, SORE NO HELLO, HI! GOOD MORNING

FIGURE 16–7 Sign language is a means of communication for many people who are hearing impaired.

- Speak slowly, but naturally.
- Do not shout or exaggerate words. This can make it even more difficult for the person to understand.
- Maintain a low to moderate pitch of voice.
- Use short sentences.
- Watch for signs of comprehension.
- Do not change the subject without warning.

Source: Alexander Graham Bell Association, 1996; University of California San Francisco Medical Center, n.d. Communicating with People with Hearing Loss. https://www.ucsfhealth.org/education/communicating_with_people_with_hearing_loss/

When necessary, video remote services with ASL interpreters are available for communication with deaf patients when on-site interpreters are not available.

Patients Who Have Visual Impairments

Patients who have visual limitations need special consideration, too. They do not have visual clues with which to orient themselves physically. With up to 70% of the meaning of communication being conveyed nonverbally, it is understandable that the visually impaired person experiences special communication challenges. Here are some ways to assist visually impaired patients:

- Start all communication by announcing your presence and identifying yourself.
- Before starting a procedure, describe any equipment to be used and its position in relation to the patient.
- As you proceed, explain what will be done and where you will be touching the patient.
- Explain what noises the patient will hear.
- Give clear and complete directions. For example, say, "Raise your left arm directly in front of you to a 45-degree angle," not "Raise your arm like this," or "Lift your arm."
- Let the patient know when you are leaving the area.
- If the patient is to leave unaccompanied, give specific instructions about doorways and other landmarks and obstacles, such as uneven surfaces, that the patient will encounter.
- Give extra verbal information to describe anything that would usually be expressed through facial expressions, gestures, head nods, and other movements.

Source: Adapted from Nursing Assistant: A Nursing Process Approach (11th ed.), by B. Acello & B. Hegner, 2016, Boston: Cengage Learning.

Patients Who Have Speech Impairments

Patients may be unable to speak because of an injury, stroke, or other neurological condition. The condition may be temporary, such as when on a ventilator or using an artificial airway. Patients who are unable to express themselves can become anxious, frustrated, and even panicked. Communication can be aided by the use of pantomime, pictures and drawings, writing, and specially designed communication boards that have the most common patient requests to which they can point.

Aphasia is a condition in which individuals have trouble saying (and/or writing) words correctly. Problems vary from having difficulty finding the correct word to saying whole sentences that do not make sense. The main cause of aphasia is stroke. It may also be the result of loss of brain function, as happens with Alzheimer's disease. Here are some ways to improve communication for people with aphasia:

- Remove noise and distractions.
- Use adult language. Do not treat patients as if they were children.
- Ask yes and no questions.
- Give clear choices for possible answers.
- Use visual cues. (See Figure 16–8.)
- Encourage the patient to communicate with you through gestures and drawings.
- Check for understanding.

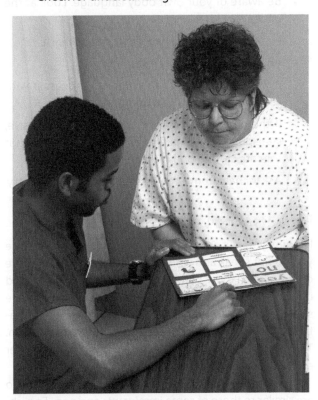

FIGURE 16–8 Picture cards help enable communication with patients who cannot speak or who do not speak English.

Patients Who Are Angry

Anger is the emotional response of displeasure or extreme annoyance to a perceived wrong. The loss of personal control experienced due to illness or injury, worries about the expense of health care, and the inconvenience of having to wait for service can all result in patient anger. Anger can also be caused by problems unrelated to health care, such as family difficulties or the loss of a job.

When dealing with an angry patient, try to determine the cause. In most cases, the anger is not the fault of the health care professional. Recall the defense mechanisms discussed in Chapter 15. Anger may be a form of displacement in which the patient is unable to direct anger at the real cause. However, if you discover that you have done something to upset the patient, apologize sincerely and try to establish good communication aimed at meeting the patient's needs. The following guidelines are helpful when dealing with angry patients:

- Do not respond in anger or argue with the patient.
- Remain calm and courteous.
- Listen attentively to the patient's concerns.
- Offer a sincere apology, if necessary.
- Do not raise your voice.
- Be aware of your own body language. Look at the patient.
- Express concern and interest, not annoyance.
- Answer the patient's questions.
- If you cannot resolve the problem, discuss it with your supervisor or other appropriate person.
- If the patient is cursing or being verbally abusive, state politely that you are willing to listen but will not tolerate cursing or threatening language.
- Ask for help from a coworker or security, if necessary.

Patients Who Do Not Speak English

Imagine yourself as a tourist in a country whose language you do not speak and where the health care practices are different from those of the United States. You are involved in an accident and taken to a hospital where no one speaks English. You cannot explain your needs, the location of your pain, or ask questions about your condition. The treatments are different from anything you have ever experienced.

The fear and confusion experienced in this scenario are similar to those of some immigrants and non–English-speaking patients in the United States. Health care

professionals can demonstrate compassion and care for these patients by learning at least a few common phrases of the major languages spoken in their community. In addition, the following ideas are helpful when working with non–English-speaking patients:

- A smile is a universal sign of good will.
- Determine if the patient speaks or understands any English at all.
- Find out if an English-speaking family member or friend is available to help. (Be sure that the patient agrees to have the other person involved so that confidentiality is not violated.)
- Speak slowly and clearly.
- Do not raise your voice. It will not help the other person understand.
- Use simple words and sentences.
- Do not use slang or expressions that may be misunderstood.
- Try repeating your message in different words.
- Use gestures and pantomime to demonstrate what you need the patient to do.
- Write the message.
- Use pictures, if available.
- Request the services of an interpreter, if necessary. In addition to on-site, face-to-face interpreting, there are services that enable health care providers to communicate with patients who speak other languages.

Hispanics, at 58.9 million, make up the largest population in the United States who may speak a language other than English (https://www.census.gov/newsroom/facts-for-features/2018/hispanic-heritage-month.html). Although 62% of Hispanics speak English, 38% mainly use Spanish (https://ucanr.edu/blogs/blogcore/postdetail.cfm?postnum=25033). If a patient speaks a little English, take care not to assume that health care communication will be understood. Health care professionals who are likely to work with Spanish-speaking patients can better help patients by learning a few words and phrases. See Appendix 2 for a list of conversational and health-related phrases.

SPECIAL APPLICATIONS OF COMMUNICATION SKILLS

There are a variety of special applications of communication skills in health care work. Each application requires the use of specific techniques.

Telephone Communication

The telephone is often the first means of contact between patients and health care facilities. The impression that patients, other professionals, and the general public receive at this time influences their perception of the facility and helps set the tone for all future communication. Businesses, including health care facilities, lose customers and patients when employees cannot communicate effectively. It is essential that caring, interest, and competence be projected to callers.

The quality of the voice is an important factor in all types of oral communication, but it is especially significant when speaking on the telephone. The receiver has no visual clues and must depend on words and voice to understand the message. The following guidelines can help create a telephone manner that is both welcoming and professional:

- Identify yourself.
- If necessary, ask permission to place the caller on hold.
- Speak clearly and pronounce words correctly and distinctly.
- Speak at a moderate rate of speed. When giving instructions or directions, speak more slowly.
- Strive for a pleasant tone, not too high-pitched.
- Project warmth, friendliness, and caring.
- Smile as you speak unless it is inappropriate in the situation, as in a call for emergency help.
- Put expression in your voice. Avoid speaking in a monotone.
- Allow appropriate periods of silence to give the other person an opportunity to speak.
- Never chew gum or eat when speaking on the telephone.

The Health Insurance Portability and Accountability Act (HIPAA) guidelines regarding patient confidentiality apply to telephone messages. Protected information, such as test results, cannot be given to anyone except the patient to whom the information applies. It is important, therefore, to determine the identity of the person with whom you are speaking. While it is acceptable to leave reminders of appointments or requests to call on answering machines, do not leave messages that contain confidential information unless the patient has given written permission to do so.

Patient Education

Patients who have knowledge about their health condition and understand the reasons for self-care techniques are more likely to follow their provider's recommendations.

With shorter hospital stays, patients and their families must take more responsibility for their own care. It has been shown that good health education can positively influence healing and recovery.

In the physician's office, patients receive information such as prevention strategies, chronic illness management, and medications, One study reported that patients only recalled 40% of the information they were given and almost half of what they remembered was incorrect (https://medicalreview.columbia.edu/article/communication-healthcare/). Obviously, there is a growing need for good patient education that includes teach back to check patient understanding. (See Table 16–2 for examples of patient education topics.)

The steps in the communication process described in this chapter can be adapted to provide a process for delivering patient education:

1. Set educational goals

    Educators call these **learning objectives** and create them to describe what students will be able to do as a result of the instruction. What does the patient need to know? Examples of goals for patients include the following:

    - Self-administer insulin injection following correct procedure

Table 16–2 Examples of Patient Education Subject Categories

Category	Examples
Promote wellness	Hygiene
	Nutrition
	Exercise
Prevent illness	First aid
	Safety
	Immunizations
	Management of risk factors
Restore health	Orientation to treatment
	Introduction to staff
	Information about the illness
	Self-care practices
Improve coping skills	Stress management
	Grief counseling
	Community resources

Source: Adapted from Fundamentals of Nursing: The Art and Science of Nursing Care (6th ed.), by C. Taylor, C. Lillis, & P. LeMone, 2006, Philadelphia, PA: Lippincott-Raven Publishers.

- Take blood pressure medicine as prescribed
- Identify medication side effects that require calling the physician

2. Create the instructional message

When creating effective instruction, determine additional facts about the patient:

- Level of knowledge: What does the patient already know about the topic?
- Patient preference: How is information best presented?
- Motivation: How important does the patient believe the information to be?
- Ability to learn: Is the patient able to acquire and retain new information at this time?

Use nontechnical language and divide information into sections and relate it to something the patient already knows. To avoid overwhelming the patient, do not give too much information at one time.

3. Deliver the instruction. Methods include:

- Instruction works best using a mixed media approach
- Oral explanations
- Audiovisual materials such as videos, diagrams, and charts
- Written materials such as instructional sheets, lists, informational reports, pamphlets, reprints of journal articles (See Chapter 17 for information about creating written documents.)
- Discussion groups
- Demonstrations of procedures, exercises, self-care techniques
- Computerized instruction such as CDs, DVDs, interactive software programs, and information available on the Internet, such as YouTube videos (See Chapter 18 about computer uses in education.)

4. Listen

Encourage patients to ask questions

5. Check for understanding

Use teach back, described previously, by asking patients to state what they learned using their own words. If appropriate, have them demonstrate what they learned.

6. Evaluate

- Were the instructional goals met?
- Is the patient able to re-state information correctly and/or satisfactorily demonstrate the skills?

Presentations to Groups

You may not need to give formal speeches as a health care professional, but there can be occasions when it is necessary to talk to a group. Examples include explaining home care procedures to a patient's family members, giving a report at a professional meeting, and demonstrating a new procedure to coworkers.

It is important to plan in advance what you are going to say, even when the audience is a small, informal group. Patient health may depend on the clarity of the presentation. The following strategies can help improve its effectiveness:

- Be clear about the purpose and most important points.
- Determine the needs and level of understanding of the audience.
- Organize material so it is easy for the audience to follow.
- Avoid jumping from topic to topic or adding unnecessary information that can be confusing.
- Speak at a moderate rate.
- Prepare notes or a checklist to prevent forgetting important points.
- Look at the audience while you are speaking.

Gossip and Patient Privacy

Gossip is unnecessary conversation, often negative, about people who are not present. It serves no constructive purpose and should always be avoided. Gossip about one's coworkers can disrupt the harmony of the health care team and compromise the quality of the patient care delivered. If it involves inappropriately sharing patient information, it can result in a lawsuit. (See information on patient confidentiality in Chapter 3.) Any type of gossip is a time-waster and cannot be justified in the busy schedules maintained by health care facilities. If a coworker tries to engage you in gossip, the following techniques may be helpful:

- Explain that you believe such conversation is unfair to the subject of the gossip. ("I don't think we know enough about the situation to discuss it," or "I don't think it's fair to talk about people behind their back.")
- State that you believe it is inappropriate for discussion. ("You know, I really don't feel comfortable talking about that.")
- Change the subject. ("What I really need to talk to you about is . . .")

Thinking It Through

Robin Winters, the dental hygienist with Dr. Castro, wants to create a patient education program to teach effective dental home care and nutritional practices. Her patients range from toddlers to the elderly. They come from a variety of cultural backgrounds. Some speak English as a second language.

1. What should Robin take into consideration when planning a patient education program?
2. What types of methods would you suggest she use?
3. How can she check for patient understanding?
4. How can she evaluate the effectiveness of her program?

Take care that private patient information is not included in social conversations with coworkers. Avoid making comments in public areas that might be overheard by the patient's friends or family members. Even sympathetic remarks such as, "I feel so bad. My favorite patient, Mr. Phillips, was just diagnosed with lung cancer," can be damaging if overheard. Patient names, along with personal information, should not be used during telephone conversations that can be heard by others. For example, when transferring a telephone call from the front desk, say "A patient is calling to follow up as you requested," *not* "Mr. Sanders is calling to get the results of his HIV test." If patient information is shared with another health professional in the patient's presence, it is best to include the patient in the conversation. Being "talked about," even by health care professionals discussing the patient's condition will be considered inappropriate and disrespectful. Patients want to be acknowledged as individuals and not made to feel like "cases."

SUGGESTED LEARNING ACTIVITIES

1. Make a poster that illustrates the six steps in the communication process.

2. Observe people as they communicate. What communication techniques are they using? Do they appear to be effective? Why or why not?

3. Apply what you have learned in this chapter to your everyday life. Use the listening techniques when communicating with your instructors, friends, and family members.

4. Practice asking different types of questions and using feedback in your everyday encounters.

5. Create a list or chart of various forms of nonverbal communication.

6. Look for examples of nonverbal communication in your daily life. List the instances when the nonverbal message does not seem to match the verbal message.

7. Mentally monitor your telephone conversations over the next week. Note the conversations you find most pleasant and those that are most unpleasant. Explain why in each case.

8. Create a teaching situation with a friend or family member. Apply the education process presented in the chapter and describe the results.

WEB ACTIVITIES

American Medical Association Foundation

www.youtube.com/watch?v=cGtTZ_vxjyA

Health Literacy and Patient Safety: Help Patients Understand

This is an excellent and very informative video, well worth the 23 minutes it takes to watch it. Although created for physicians, this video has excellent information about communicating with the many patients who have difficulty understanding the information they receive from their health care providers.

1. After watching the video, write a summary that explains the reasons why patients have trouble understanding health information.

2. Why don't patients tell their health care providers that they don't understand what they've been told?

3. What are some of the most serious consequences of patients not understanding their health care providers?

4. List suggestions for health care professionals to improve their communication with patients.

American Academy of Family Physicians

https://www.aafp.org/news/blogs/leadervoices/entry/20180518lv-hearpatient.html

Our Patients Want—and Need—to Be Heard

1. What is the writer's new meaning of "Where is the patient"?

2. How has data interfered with treating patients as individuals?

3. What is the difference between an encounter and a visit with a patient?

The Focusing Institute

http://www.focusing.org/klagsbrun.html

Listening and Focusing: Holistic Health Care Tools for Nurses

This is an excellent article that includes examples of exchanges between nurses and patients. Although addressed to nurses, it is applicable to all health care professionals who work with patients.

1. What is the meaning of "holistic communication"?

2. How does the author define "active listening"?

3. How can you apply active listening to your future occupation?

4. What is the process of focusing?

5. How might focusing be helpful for patients?

Effective Communication—Student's Choice

1. Using the term "effective communication techniques," conduct an Internet search.

2. Review at least three articles and choose one you think contains helpful methods for the health care professional.

3. Write a summary of this article and try out at least two of the methods in your daily communications.

Health Literacy Consulting

https://healthliteracy.com/2003/07/01/humor/

1. Do you agree that humor can be an effective communication tool when working with patients? Explain why or why not.

2. What are the four ways the author suggests for using humor in communications with patients?

Teach Back

http://www.teachbacktraining.org/assets/files/PDFS/Teach%20Back%20-%2010%20Elements%20of%20Competence.pdf

10 Elements of Competence for Using Teach Back Effectively

1. Practice explaining something you have learned in class to a friend or family member, then use teach back to check their understanding.

2. Copy the list of elements and review from time to time.

Health Literacy Consulting

https://healthliteracy.com/2001/08/01/anxious-angry-patients/

Know When to Speak and When to Listen: Communicating with Patients Who Are Angry or Anxious

1. Have you had an experience that made you anxious? In health care? If so, did you get help? If so, what was it that helped you?

2. How can you "put yourself in the patients' shoes" to better understand how they are feeling?

3. Why is it important not to use judgmental language when communicating with an angry patient?

REVIEW QUESTIONS

1. What is the definition of "communication"?

2. What is the meaning of "successful communication"?

3. Why is effective communication important in health care delivery?

4. What are four factors that have increased the need for competent communication in health care?

5. What is the foundation for good communication in health care?

6. How can health care professionals use communication to help patients deal with stress, anxiety, and loneliness?

7. What is the definition of "health literacy"?

8. What are five reasons why patients do not follow medical advice?

9. What are four ways that messages can be exchanged?

10. What are the six steps of the communication process?

11. What is the meaning of "teach back"?

12. What are the three goals that should be included in every interaction with a patient?

13. What are four factors that should be considered about patients when creating communication goals?

14. Why should medical terminology not be used when speaking with most patients?

15. What are eight strategies for organizing long messages?

16. What is the definition and use of the four types of questions?

17. How can humor be used in health care situations?

18. What are appropriate ways to address older patients?

19. What is the meaning and importance of nonverbal communication?

20. What are eight examples of positive body language?

21. What is "pantomime" and how can it be used in health care communication?

22. What is the appropriate use of touch when working with patients?

23. What are five environmental factors that affect communication?

24. What is the meaning of "active listening"?

25. What is the purpose of feedback and what are the four types?

26. How do you evaluate a completed communication?

27. What are considerations to take when communicating with children, adolescents, adults, and older adults?

28. List techniques for communicating with patients who are:

    a. Terminally ill

    b. In pain, medicated, confused, or disoriented

    c. Suffering from dementia

    d. Depressed

    e. Anxious

    f. Hearing impaired

    g. Visually impaired

    h. Speech impaired

    i. Angry

    j. Unable to speak or understand English

29. What are eight ways to project a professional impression when speaking on the telephone?

30. Why is patient education important?

31. What are the six steps for developing and delivering effective patient education?

32. What are seven strategies for preparing and giving presentations to groups?

33. What are three ways to discourage and avoid gossip?

34. Why is it unacceptable to discuss a patient with anyone who is not involved in the patient's care?

APPLICATION EXERCISES

1. Refer to the Case of the Coder Who Lacked Confidence at the beginning of the chapter. What would you recommend that Jenny do in order to increase her communication skills?

2. Compare and contrast how you would initiate communication with each of the following patients. Include your communication goal, what information you would need to gather about the patient, and important factors to consider in preparing your message.

   a. You are a medical assistant. The patient has a severe hearing impairment. She is seeing the physician for a routine physical examination.

   b. You are a dental hygienist. The patient is 5 years old and terrified of the dentist's office.

   c. You are a physical therapist assistant. The patient is a well-to-do man in his 50s. He is furious about having had to wait for 20 minutes while you finished working with your previous patient.

PROBLEM-SOLVING PRACTICE

Josie has a new job at an imaging center conveniently located near her home. She loves working with the patients and applying what she learned in her radiology classes. But the manager of the center has poor supervisory skills and the staff constantly complains and gossips about the woman and sometimes about each other. Everyone seems to be taking sides. How can Josie use the five-step problem-solving process to help her improve her work situation?

CHAPTER 17

Written Communication

KEY TERMS

agenda
block letter
consonant
contraction
cross-training
etiquette
grammar
independent clauses
justified
modified block letter
quotation
salutation
semi-block letter
suffix
syllable
vowel
word processing

OBJECTIVES

Studying and applying the material in this chapter will help you to:

1. Explain why the ability to write clearly and correctly is an important skill for the health care professional.
2. Describe four steps to follow when planning and organizing written documents.
3. Describe the following ways to organize content when starting to write: formal outline, informal outline, and mind map.
4. Explain why it is important to use correct spelling in all written communication.
5. List six resources that can help the health care professional with spelling.
6. List nine major spelling rules.
7. List four ways to master words that are difficult to spell in English.
8. Explain the instances in which words should be capitalized.
9. Give the rules for using the following punctuation marks: period, comma, semicolon, colon, apostrophe, and quotation marks.
10. Explain the rules for placement when using more than one punctuation mark.
11. Give the rules for writing numbers correctly.
12. Give the rules for writing titles correctly.
13. Explain how the content of an effective business letter should be organized.
14. Explain how to write, format, and send effective business letters.
15. Describe the following types of letter formats: block, modified block, and semi-block.
16. Explain the purpose and characteristics of a good memo.
17. List what should be included in meeting agendas and minutes.
18. List five techniques for creating effective written patient education materials.
19. Discuss the proper handling of written documents to protect patient confidentiality.
20. List ways to improve proofreading skills.

The Case of the Surprised Therapist

Al Trent was recently hired by Cathy Barnes, a physical therapist in private practice. When Al started work, he imagined that his tasks would consist mainly of working with patients. He was surprised when Cathy asked him to help her with several special projects that required good writing skills. She is active at both the local and state level of two professional organizations. Believing that professional organizations are important for the promotion of physical therapy, she has encouraged Al to become active and has requested his help in preparing agendas and reports for the meetings. Cathy has also asked him to prepare written instruction sheets for patients to use when doing exercises at home. Although there is an administrative assistant who does the billing, bookkeeping, and other clerical tasks, Cathy believes that Al's physical therapy education better qualifies him for writing materials that are directly related to physical therapy. This chapter covers the basics of effective written communication that may be required of today's health care professionals.

WRITTEN COMMUNICATION: A VITAL LINK IN HEALTH CARE

The quality of modern health care delivery depends heavily on the completeness and accuracy of written communications prepared by health care professionals. Many kinds of documents are created daily. They range from notes made in a patient's medical record to technical reports to formal business letters. The type of writing done by each health care professional depends on his or her specific occupation and employment circumstances. However, even those who spend most of their time providing hands-on patient care may prepare written documentation and may be required to write an occasional letter or patient instruction sheet. Writing skills are also used when preparing résumés, cover letters, and letters inquiring about employment opportunities. Health care professionals who decide to pursue additional education may find themselves assigned research papers and other writing assignments. The ability to write clearly and correctly is a mark of professionalism and increases the health care professional's value and promotional opportunities.

Written documents provide important links among the many professionals and facilities that make up the web of care for today's patients. However, while the growth in specialty services raises the level of care, it also increases the chances for miscommunication and lost information. Consider the communication trail created during the routine annual exam of Mrs. Kardinski, a 55-year-old patient of Dr. Landau:

1. Dr. Landau's administrative medical assistant, Denise Carter, sends Mrs. Kardinski a *reminder letter* to encourage her to make an appointment for her annual physical exam.

2. On the day of the appointment, Denise locates the patient's *file*, for the clinical medical assistant, Lachelle Hayes. (In many offices today, the file will be digitally stored on a computer which the medical assistant and physician will use as they work with the patient.)

3. Lachelle updates the *medical record* with Mrs. Kardinski's weight, blood pressure, and other vital signs.

4. Lachelle adds further notes to the *medical record* at the direction of Dr. Landau during the exam.

5. Dr. Landau signs *request forms* for routine tests to be performed at other facilities.

6. Mrs. Kardinski visits an off-site lab to have blood drawn for routine tests, and the lab sends the results in a *report* to Dr. Landau's office.

7. Mrs. Kardinski then visits an imaging center for a mammogram, and the center sends a *report* to Dr. Landau's office.

8. The cytology lab that examines the Pap specimen sends a *report* to Dr. Landau's office.

9. All reports are normal, so Denise sends a *letter* to Mrs. Kardinski, notifying her of the results.

10. Denise sends a *statement* to Mrs. Kardinski's insurance company.

Mrs. Kardinski's routine visit involves at least 10 written documents that contain essential information for ensuring that she receives consistent and appropriate care. A lot of the information in these examples may be sent electronically, but the words and sentences still must be correct. This need for accuracy includes the spelling of medical terms which, if incorrect, can result in errors and misunderstandings. Appropriate care depends on the smooth flow of clearly and accurately prepared written communications among health care providers and between them and their patients.

THE COMPONENTS OF GOOD WRITING

Good writing is characterized by logical organization and attention to detail, including spelling, grammar, and format. In addition to helping ensure good patient care, complete and accurate written documents are viewed by many as the sign of a competent professional. Writing that contains errors and is poorly presented reflects negatively on the quality of the individual as well as on the facility. Patients may question the competence of the facility to deliver quality health care if they receive a letter or hand-out that is sloppily prepared, contains spelling errors, or is difficult to understand.

Organizing Content

All types of written communication, whether they consist of one paragraph or several pages, must be organized in a way that is easy for the reader to follow and understand. Unlike oral communication, in which the speaker can request feedback and make necessary adjustments, written communication must stand on its own. Writers cannot use non-verbal language to enhance and emphasize their messages.

The steps for organizing written content described in this section are designed as a guide for creating all types of written communication. The specific techniques used and the time spent on each are determined by the type of document being prepared. For example, a short memo might take 10 minutes to plan and write, whereas a research report could take more than a month and require attention to each step in the process. Whatever the length of a document, good writing requires that consideration be given to planning and organizing.

Preparing to Write

1. Determine the purpose for writing.
   - Inform
   - Persuade
   - Gather information
   - Encourage action

   It is possible to have more than one purpose. A patient information sheet about physical exercise, for example, may be designed to provide information about the health benefits of exercise *and* encourage patients to participate in regular physical activity.

2. Generate ideas for content based on the purpose of the document.
   - List as many ideas as come to mind. Write down everything you already know about the topic.
   - Gather facts. Sources include professional journals, books, publications from professional organizations, and credible websites. (See Chapter 18 for information on evaluating the quality of websites.)
   - Talk with others. Get content information from experts. Ask potential readers what they want to know.

3. Consider the readers:
   - Knowledge of the subject matter
   - Reading level (age, native language, level of education)
   - Interest in the subject
   - Reason for needing the information

   It is appropriate to use medical terminology and abbreviations in writing that is directed to health care professionals because, as the "language of medicine," your message will be more clear and specific. This is why mastering medical terminology is important for health care professionals. At the same time, this language can confuse patients who do not have a background in health care. It is also important to know that some abbreviations are unacceptable because they can confuse even health care professionals. (See Chapter 4.)

   The tone, which is the writer's attitude toward the topic, must be appropriate for the situation. Tone is expressed through the writer's choice of words. The following two sentences basically say the same thing, but notice the difference in tone:
   - You must be here on time.
   - We would appreciate it if you could be here on time.

   The tone should be adapted to the circumstances. Take the example of collection letters for late payment. A long-time patient who always pays medical bills promptly but is currently experiencing financial difficulties might receive a different letter than the one directed to a patient with a history of late payments.

   Many professional writers suggest getting words down as quickly as possible when starting to write a long document. Content, rather than grammar and spelling, should be emphasized at this time. Creativity can be lost when the focus on details is too great. On the first draft, it can be intimidating that the writing becomes overwhelmed. The first draft, however, does not have to be perfect; that can be done later.

Thinking It Through

For each of the documents involved in Mrs. Kardinski's routine visit, discuss the possible consequences for the patient and health care providers if it were:

1. Written inaccurately
2. Sent to the wrong facility or person

4. Organize the content.

The material should flow in a way that makes sense to the reader. The traditional structure of a written document includes three parts:

- Introduction—State the topic and purpose. Interesting facts and questions can be used to attract the reader's attention.

- Body—Fully develop the topic or message. Provide supporting facts and information. Ways to present information include:
  - Examples and illustrations
  - Description, using specific details
  - List of steps in a process
  - List of reasons
  - Grouping of items into categories

- Conclusion—Summarize the information contained in the body. Effective endings include restating the purpose or pointing out how the facts given support the purpose.

Starting to Write

The task of writing can be simplified by using one of the following organizing techniques. Even short documents can be improved by making a few notes before preparing the "real thing."

- Create a formal outline. Use letters and numbers to create a detailed outline, which is fleshed out when you begin to write. (See Figure 17–1 for an example.)

- Create an informal outline. Omit letters and numbers. Simply list major ideas and indent supporting ideas.

- Draw a diagram, also known as a mind map, using circles and lines to connect major and supporting ideas. You may also want to use colors to clarify the relationships of ideas. Figure 17–2 shows how the information contained in the formal outline in Figure 17–1 looks in mind map form.

Many professional writers suggest writing the first draft as quickly as possible when starting to write a long document. Content, rather than grammar and spelling, should be emphasized at this time. Creativity can be lost when the focus is on detail. Trying for perfection on the first draft can be so intimidating that the writer becomes overwhelmed. The final draft, however, should have perfect spelling and grammar.

Spell Your Way to Success

Spelling errors in medical documents can have serious consequences. Apart from giving the impression of carelessness, misspelled words can cause confusion that

---

Using an Outline to Organize Content
Subject: Hepatitis B

I. Introduction
   A. Threat to health
   B. Vaccine available
II. Symptoms
   A. Loss of appetite
   B. Fatigue
   C. Nausea
   D. Headache
   E. Fever
   F. Jaundice
III. Transmission
   A. Contact with virus
      1. Sexual contact
      2. Blood
      3. Body fluids
         a. Vaginal secretions
         b. Semen
         c. Fluids from body cavities
         d. Sputum
IV. Treatment
   A. Dietary measures
      1. Decrease dietary fat
      2. Low protein
      3. Small, frequent high-calorie meals (if nausea present)
      4. Decrease fluids (if retaining)
   B. Bed rest
V. Prevention
   A. Hepatitis B vaccine for employees at risk for exposure
   B. Standard precautions
      1. Handwashing
      2. Gloves
      3. Personal protective equipment
      4. Proper handling of needles
      5. Proper disposal of hazardous waste

FIGURE 17–1 Sample of formal outline to organize content for writing.

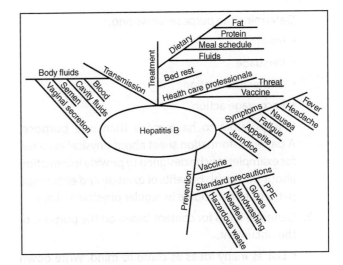

FIGURE 17–2 Some students find mind maps to be a helpful way to organize content.

negatively affects patient care. As discussed in Chapter 4, many medical terms can present difficulties because they were borrowed from Latin and Greek, are long, have silent letters, or have spelling that is similar to other words with different meanings. A medical dictionary, either printed or computerized, is a good tool for the medical professional. Online medical spell checkers are also available and can be located by entering the search term "online medical spell checker" into a search engine, such as Google or Bing. There are also a number of online medical dictionaries, including one at medlineplus.gov, a service of the National Library of Medicine.

If you are ever in doubt about the spelling of any word, take the time to check it. Not doing so is negligent. There are many tools available to assist with proper spelling:

- General English dictionary. If English is your second language, you may also need a bilingual dictionary.

- Medical dictionaries, available in print, online, and as apps

- Word books for health care specialties

- Online dictionaries

- Spell-checkers on **word processing** software (programs for creating written documents on a computer). These are available for general English and medical vocabulary. Do not depend on spell-checkers to catch all errors, because the computer cannot identify words that are spelled correctly but used incorrectly. For example, "to" is spelled correctly, but is incorrect if you meant to write "too" or "toe."

- Pharmaceutical reference guides, such as the *Prescriber's Digital Reference* (PDR), available online at www.pdr.net/browse-by-drug-name

Spelling Tips

Everyday English, as well as medical spelling, can be challenging, but it is well worth the time and effort necessary to achieve mastery. Here are a few suggestions for improving spelling:

1. Learn the major spelling rules listed in Table 17–1. Each rule governs the spelling of many words and prevents having to learn to spell each word individually.

2. Memorize words that are look-alikes, exceptions to the rules, or ones you usually misspell. Here are some suggestions for mastering this vocabulary:

   - Write each word several times.
   - Spell each word out loud several times.
   - Make flashcards for practice and self-quizzes.
   - List words on a wall chart and place it where you will see it often.

- Create rhymes or associations. For example, the sentence "He was vain about owning a big van" might help distinguish between "vain" and "vein."

- Create a personal dictionary of words with which you have trouble. This can be handwritten or stored electronically. Review the list regularly.

3. Review troublesome words regularly for mastery. See Table 17–2 for a list of frequently misspelled words that are commonly used in health care.

4. Set weekly goals. Challenge yourself to learn a certain number of new words. Create self-quizzes and give yourself small rewards for perfect scores.

Grammar at a Glance

Every language has a set of rules that determines proper word order, sentence construction, punctuation, and capitalization. Collectively these are referred to as **grammar**. The use of correct grammar is a sign of a good education, competence, and professionalism. As representatives of the facilities in which they work, health care professionals need to achieve a level of grammar that gives a favorable impression of both them and their employers.

The following sections are designed to provide a quick review of English grammar. If you are unsure about your knowledge of grammar, plan to take an English class, purchase educational software, or locate a workbook with review exercises. Time spent now can make a significant difference in your professional life. A good grammar reference book will be useful now and on the job. Most word processing software programs have grammar-checkers. It is the authors' experience, however, that more than half the suggestions made by the grammar-checker in one popular word processing program are incorrect.

Capitalization Rules

Capitalizing correctly is an important mark of good written English. The following conditions require capitalization:

- First word in a sentence

- Proper names of people, countries, organizations, companies, products, holidays, and so on

- Names of months and days of the week

- Medical acronyms: AIDS, ECG

- Titles used with a person's name: Dr. Castanedo, Mrs. Cranston

- First word of a **quotation** (words written exactly as spoken): The patient asked, "Why do I need this surgery?"

Table 17–1 Major Spelling Rules

Rule	Examples
Place *i* before *e* except after *c* or in words in which the *ei* sounds like ay. *Exceptions:* seize either weird height foreign leisure	relieve receive weight
Drop the final silent *e* before adding a **suffix** (word ending) that begins with a **vowel** (the letters *a, e, i, o, u*). Keep the *e* if the suffix begins with a **consonant** (all letters except *a, e, i, o, u*).	care ⟶ caring care ⟶ careful achieve ⟶ achievable achieve ⟶ achievement
Change the final *y* to *ie* when adding *s* or *d* when the *y* is preceded by a consonant.	laboratory ⟶ laboratories dry ⟶ dried
Double the final consonant when adding a suffix if all the following conditions are met: 1. The final consonant is preceded by a vowel. 2. The suffix begins with a vowel. 3. The word is only one **syllable** (part of a word that has a single spoken sound) or the final syllable is stressed.	sit ⟶ sitting commit ⟶ committed
Add *k* to words ending in *c* before adding suffixes that begin with *e, i*.	panic ⟶ panicking, panicked
Add *s* to make most words plural.	patient ⟶ patients X-ray ⟶ X-rays
Add *es* to make the plural form of words that end in *s, sh, ch, x*.	abscess ⟶ abscesses dish ⟶ dishes crutch ⟶ crutches suffix ⟶ suffixes
Add *s* to make the plural form of words that end in *o* if it is preceded by a vowel. Add *es* if *o* is preceded by a consonant.	ratio ⟶ ratios tomato ⟶ tomatoes
Some words that were borrowed from other languages, mainly Latin and Greek, keep their original plural forms, which do not use the letter *s*.	diverticulum (singular) ⟶ diverticula (plural) (pouch in mucous membrane lining) curriculum (singular) ⟶ curricula (plural)

Punctuation Rules

Punctuation marks help the reader understand written messages. Incorrect or missing punctuation can lead to confusion and distorted meanings. Here are guidelines for the most common uses of punctuation marks:

1. The *period* is used at the end of a sentence and after some abbreviations.

    Examples Respiratory therapists must have good technical skills.

    Dr. Hansen is a noted thoracic surgeon.

Table 17–2 Commonly Misspelled Words

abscess	eligible	maneuver	rhythm
absence	eliminate	miscellaneous	schedule
accidentally	embarrass	necessary	scissors
accommodate	emphasize	negligence	secretary
accumulate	encourage	negligible	seize
address	enthusiastic	neighbor	seizure
aggravate	environment	noticeable	separate
analyze	equipped	occasionally	severely
appropriate	equivalent	occur	significance
assistant	especially	occurrence	similar
association	exaggerate	often	strategy
behavior	exercise	pamphlet	strictly
belief	exhausted	parallel	substantial
beneficial	experience	particular	succeed
business	extremely	patience	success
cafeteria	fatigue	persistent	surprise
caffeine	February	physically	sympathy
calendar	fluctuation	physician	technique
cancel, canceled	foreign	pneumonia	temperature
column	forty	possession	thorough
commitment	fourth	practical	though
communicate	fragile	precede	tongue
comparative	friend	prejudice	transferred
cooperate	government	privilege	typical
correspond	harass, harassment	proceed	urgent
criticism	height	prominent	vacuum
criticize	intelligence	psychiatry	vague
decision	judgment	psychology	vegetable
deficiency	knowledge	qualified	Wednesday
definitely	knowledgeable	quantity	weight
describe	label	questionnaire	writing
disease	laboratory	recommend	
efficiency	license	reference	
eighth	maintenance	resuscitate	

Source: Adapted from Delmar's Comprehensive Medical Assisting: Administrative and Clinical Competencies, by W. Lindh, M. Pooler, C. Tamparo, & J. Cerrato, 1998, Clifton Park, NY: Delmar Cengage Learning.

2. The *comma* is used:

a. To join two independent clauses (parts of a sentence that can stand on their own as complete sentences) joined by *and, but, or, nor, for, so, yet*

Example Brushing the teeth after each meal is important, but flossing is also necessary.

b. To separate three or more words or phrases that appear in a series

Example The three energy nutrients are carbohydrates, fats, and proteins.

c. At the end of an introductory group of words

Examples When the patient arrived at the office, he was having trouble breathing.

Efficient and well organized, Dr. Bancini's office staff rarely got behind schedule.

Buried under piles of papers, Mrs. North's medical chart was nowhere to be seen.

d. Around inessential phrases that describe or add information

Examples The patient, who lives in my neighborhood, came to the clinic on Monday. (*Phrase adds interesting but unnecessary information.*)

The physician, who specializes in pulmonary disorders, agreed to see the patient this afternoon. (Phrase adds important information about the physician.)

e. To set off transitional expressions: *however, therefore, for example, in other words, as a matter of fact*

Examples Practicing sterile technique, for example, is an important skill for surgical technologists.

Giving medical advice, however, can be done only by the physician.

f. With dates and addresses

Examples The clinic first opened on June 2, 1985, in Omaha, Nebraska.

The nearest hospital is located at 417 Santa Clara Road, San Diego, California.

3. The *semicolon* is used:

a. Between independent clauses that are *not* joined with connecting words such as *and, but, or, nor, for, so, yet*

Example The physician referred Mr. Denton to a physical therapist; his leg requires special exercises to regain strength and range of motion.

b. Between independent clauses joined by transitional expressions such as *also, besides, finally, furthermore, for example, in conclusion, on the contrary*

Example Good health is influenced by proper nutrition; also, exercise plays an important role.

4. The *colon* is used:

a. At the end of an independent clause that introduces a list or a quotation

Example The major functions of the integumentary system include the following: provide protection from the external environment, control body temperature, and maintain homeostasis.

b. Between independent clauses when the second clause explains, illustrates, or expands on the first

Example The clinic director called a staff meeting: he wanted to discuss the new guidelines for reporting accidents in the lab.

c. After the salutation (greeting) in a business letter

Example Dear Dr. Phillips:

5. The *apostrophe* is used:

a. To create the possessive form of a noun

Example The nurse's stethoscope lay on the counter.

b. To indicate the contraction (combining) of two words

Example It's a busy day at the clinic. (It's = It is)

6. Quotation marks are used:

a. To enclose direct quotes (exact words of a speaker)

Example "I need you to help me turn Mrs. Sands," said Nurse Ames to the CNA.

b. Around titles of magazine and newspaper articles, chapters in books, stories, songs, and poems. (Note: titles of books, plays, movies, and names of magazines and newspapers are put in italics—*like this*—or underlined.)

Using More than One Punctuation Mark

- Always place periods and commas inside quotation marks.

  Example This month's journal had an interesting article titled "Postoperative Pain in Knee-Replacement Patients."

- Place exclamation and question marks inside quotation marks unless they apply to the entire sentence.

  Examples When Dr. Pedersen told Mr. Watson that his cholesterol was lower as a result of the new medication, the patient exclaimed, "That's great news!"

Box 17–1

How Punctuation Affects Meaning: The Result Can Be Quite Humorous!

We're going to learn to cut and paste kids!

We're going to learn to cut and paste, kids!

Let's eat grandpa.

Let's eat, grandpa.

A woman: without her, man is nothing.

A woman, without her man, is nothing.

Eat your dinner.

Eat! You're dinner.

Twenty five-dollar bills. ($100)

Twenty-five dollar bills. ($25)

I want to thank my parents, Joan and God.

I want to thank my parents, Joan, and God.

I'm sorry I love you.

I'm sorry; I love you.

I really enjoy cooking my family and my dog.

I really enjoy cooking, my family, and my dog.

Have you read Chapter 10, "Infection Control"?

See Box 17–1 for examples of how punctuation can change the meaning of a sentence, sometimes with a humorous result.

Writing Numbers Correctly

The general rule when using numbers in sentences is to write them out as words when:

- They consist of only one or two words (Note: Hyphenate compound numbers from twenty-one to ninety-nine.)
- They are the first word in a sentence

Otherwise, they are written as figures. See the following examples:

- There were five patients waiting to see the doctor.
- There were 25,000 cases reported last year in the United States.
- Twenty-five thousand new cases were reported last year in the United States.

In technical writing, such as that used in health care, using figures rather than writing out words for numbers is sometimes preferred. Check the preferences for your specific profession and facility. The American Psychological Association (APA) and the American Medical Association (AMA), for example, publish style manuals. They have their own rules for writing numbers as figures or words. Figures are also used in the following situations:

- When expressing time with a.m. or p.m. (am and pm are also correct)

  Example Your next appointment is scheduled for 3:15 p.m. on Monday, January 12, 2015.

  Otherwise, write the numbers out in words.

  Example Mr. Hashimoto's surgery is scheduled to begin at eight o'clock in the morning.

- Percentages

  Example The range of normal hematocrit (volume percentage of red blood cells in whole blood) values for newborns is 45% to 60%. (The word *percent* may also be spelled out.)

- Temperature

  Example His temperature was below normal at 97.6 degrees.

- Fractions and decimals

  Examples A quart is equal to 1/4 gallon.

  The specific gravity (weight compared to equal volume of water) of normal urine ranges from 1.003 to 1.035.

Writing Titles Correctly

Use standard abbreviations if the title appears immediately before or after names (never in both places).

Dr. Joanna Carter	or	Joanna Carter, MD (Doctor of Medicine)
Dr. Esteban Alvarez	or	Esteban Alvarez, Ph.D. (Doctor of Philosophy)
Dr. Mary O'Leary	or	Mary O'Leary, D.D.S. (Doctor of Dental Surgery)

Periods have traditionally followed abbreviations for titles. However, usage varies and periods are often omitted, except for the abbreviation Dr. Use the form preferred by your employer or professional organization.

BUSINESS LETTERS

A trend in health care employment today is **cross-training** employees. This means that they learn to perform tasks in addition to those traditionally performed by individuals with their job titles. For example, more administrative tasks are being required of health care professionals who provide direct patient care. Even in our digital age, the ability to write business letters correctly is a necessary skill for an increasing number of occupations.

Business letters create an important link between health care providers and their patients and colleagues. The following types of letters are commonly used in health care:

- Appointment: Reminds a patient of the date and time of the next appointment

- Recall: Requests a patient to call and make an appointment

- Collection: Requests a patient to pay a bill

- Follow-up: Summarizes reports regarding test results, outlines further treatment needs

- Consultation: Requests another professional to examine a patient

- Explanation: Provides an excuse from work or school, explains special needs for patient accommodation

- Inquiry: Requests information about products or processes

- Special occasion: Accepts an invitation or sends regrets, offers congratulations

- Announcement: States new office hours or other policies, announces new associate or retirement of staff member

Thinking It Through

Karin McFarland is the office manager for Drs. Kern, Wilkes, and Ruiz. She recently hired a new medical receptionist, Wanda Belini, whom patients like for her warm, friendly personality. Wanda has excellent telephone skills and good judgment about handling calls appropriately. Karin is concerned, however, about Wanda's writing skills. The short documents such as memos and meeting announcements that she has prepared have contained spelling and punctuation errors. Karin believes that Wanda is a valuable asset to the office and wants to help her improve.

1. Why is it important for memos and meeting announcements to be written properly if they are only seen by people who work in the office?

2. What might Wanda do to improve her writing skills?

3. What impact might Wanda's poor writing skills have on her future career if she does not improve them?

Using Form Letters

Many letters and email messages are sent out repeatedly with the same information. Creating form letters can save time. With today's word processing software, it is possible to personalize form letters and print them without the telltale signs of repeated passes through the copy machine. The patient's name and address can be entered, and personal notes included within the text. Form letters should be personally signed whenever possible.

Writing Effective Letters

Effective business letters are courteous, clear, and direct. Getting to the point, without being abrupt, is a sign of respect for the reader's time. Although they should be businesslike, letters to patients should never be so formal as to seem uncaring. The message of a letter is organized in the same way as for other types of writing:

1. State the purpose in the introduction.

2. Develop ideas in the body. Provide necessary information and explanations. Use an appropriate tone. For example, a collection letter might be written using a firm tone.

3. Summarize, and state what you want the reader to do.

Carefully proofread all letters for content, grammar, and spelling. A letter that contains even a single error is not considered mailable.

Business Letter Formats

Certain traditions govern the appearance of business letters. Like dressing appropriately for a business occasion, the correct use of a prescribed letter format is a sign of proper business etiquette (manners). Remember that the quality and appearance of correspondence represent the level of professionalism of the sender.

The three most commonly used letter formats are block, modified block, and semi-block. The main difference between the formats is how the lines of text are justified (lined up with the margins).

- **Block letter:** All lines are flush (lined up evenly) with the left margin. This is the most efficient format to use because it eliminates the need for extra keystrokes to indent the lines. (See Figure 17–3.)

- **Modified block letter:** All lines are flush with the left margin except the date, closing, and signature. These begin just to the right of the center of the page. (See Figure 17–4.)

- **Semi-block letter:** The same as block, except that the first line of each paragraph is indented five spaces and the subject line begins just to the right of the center of the page. This format is considered the least formal of the three and is the least used. (See Figure 17–5.)

WINSTON LEWIS, MD
2501 CENTER STREET
NORTHBOROUGH, OH 12345

NORTHBOROUGH
FAMILY MEDICAL GROUP

Date Line

January 12, 20___ (approximately 15th line)

Inside Address

Jeremy Brown, MD (approximately 20th line)
111 S Main
Blossom, UT 10283-1120
　　　　(double-space)

Salutation

Dear Dr. Brown:
　　　　(double-space)

Subject Line

Blossom Medical Society Meeting
　　　　(double-space)
Thank you for inviting me to speak at the Blossom Medical Society
Meeting on June 15, 20___. As requested, my topic will describe
using MRI scans to make more accurate diagnoses without resorting to
invasive procedures. I will send you the exact title of my speech
by next Friday.
　　　　(double-space)
Please have your office manager send me information about the
number of participants expected, the time of the meeting, location,
and any other details that will assist me in preparing my speech.

I will write or call if I have any additional questions.
　　　　(double-space)

Complimentary
Closing

Yours truly,

Winston Lewis, MD (4–5 line spaces)

Keyed Signature

Winston Lewis, MD
　　　　(double-space)

Reference Initials

WL:jg (Who dictated the letter: who prepared the letter)
　　　　(double-space)

Enclosure Notation

Enclosure: Handout on MRI

FIGURE 17–3 Block style letter format. The contents of a standard business letter are labeled.

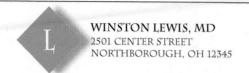

WINSTON LEWIS, MD
2501 CENTER STREET
NORTHBOROUGH, OH 12345

NORTHBOROUGH
FAMILY MEDICAL GROUP

January 12, 20___ (approximately 15th line)

Jeremy Brown, MD (approximately 20th line)
111 S Main
Blossom, UT 10283-1120

Dear Dr. Brown:

Blossom Medical Society Meeting

Thank you for inviting me to speak at the Blossom Medical Society
Meeting on June 15, 20___. As requested, my topic will describe using
MRI scans to make more accurate diagnoses without resorting to invasive
procedures. I will send you the exact title of my speech will by
next Friday.

Please have your office manager send me information regarding the number of
participants expected, the time of the meeting, location, and any other details
that will assist me in preparing my speech.

I will write or call if I have any additional questions.

Yours truly,

Winston Lewis, MD

Winston Lewis, MD

WL:jg (Who dictated the letter: who prepared the letter)

Enclosure: Handout on MRI

FIGURE 17-4 Modified block style business letter format.

NORTHBOROUGH
FAMILY MEDICAL GROUP

WINSTON LEWIS, MD
2501 CENTER STREET
NORTHBOROUGH, OH 12345

January 12, 20____ (approximately 15th line)

Jeremy Brown, MD (approximately 20th line)
111 S Main
Blossom, UT 10283-1120

Dear Dr. Brown:

Blossom Medical Society Meeting

    Thank you for inviting me to speak at the Blossom Medical Society
Meeting on June 15, 20____. As requested, my topic will describe using
MRI scans to make more accurate diagnoses without resorting to invasive
procedures. I will send you the exact title of my speech will by
next Friday.

    Please have your office manager send me information regarding the number of
participants expected, the time of the meeting, location, and any other details
that will assist me in preparing my speech.

    I will write or call if I have any additional questions.

               Yours truly,

               Winston Lewis, MD

               Winston Lewis, MD

WL:jg (Who dictated the letter: who prepared the letter)

Enclosure: Handout on MRI

FIGURE 17–5 Semi-block style business letter format.

Winston Lewis, MD
2501 Center Street
Northborough, OH 12345

JEREMY BROWN MD
111 S MAIN
BLOSSOM UT 10283-1120

FIGURE 17–6 Correctly addressed envelope.

Preparing Letters for Mailing

When a letter requires more than one sheet, use a piece of plain matching paper (without the information about the sender and receiver) for the second page. Proper delivery is ensured if the envelope is addressed according to the following guidelines:

- Write the address in all uppercase (capital) letters.
- Do not use punctuation in the address.
- Use the zip code. Add the additional zip + 4 code when possible.
- Do not write in the lower-right corner.
- Include a complete return address in the upper-left corner.

(See Figure 17–6.)

MEMOS

Memos are written to share information within an organization. Examples of typical memo topics include policy changes, staff schedules, explanations of procedures, announcements about new staff or equipment, and safety reminders.

Memos should be written clearly, concisely, and to the point. It is important that they can be read and understood quickly and easily. The message should be useful to the recipient. Employees who receive too many memos begin to ignore them. All suggestions regarding memos pertain to both paper and electronically sent memos (emails).

Prepare memos with the same care given to outgoing letters. The quality of memos can set the tone for work standards at a facility. Poorly prepared memos and other internal documents can send the message that quality paperwork and attention to detail are not valued. See Figure 17–7 for a sample memo format.

MEETING AGENDAS

Whether for a meeting at work or for a professional organization, the health care professional may be called upon to prepare a meeting agenda. An agenda lists what is to take place at a meeting. Agendas promote efficiency by helping attendees prepare in advance and by keeping meetings focused on what needs to be discussed and accomplished. A good agenda should include the following:

1. Date of the meeting
2. Start and end times
3. Exact location
4. Topics to be discussed
5. What attendees should bring, if applicable
6. Guest speaker(s), if applicable

MINUTES OF MEETINGS

Minutes provide written documentation of what happens at meetings. They serve several purposes:

- Inform those who did not attend about important decisions and announcements that took place.

Wilsonville Orthopedic Clinic

MEMO

To: Person(s) to whom the memo is being sent
From: Person sending the memo
CC: Names of other individuals to whom a copy of the memo is being sent
Date: Date memo is written and/or sent
Re: Subject of the memo. Helps recipient prioritize and organize memos if they are saved

Body of message here

FIGURE 17–7 Sample memo format.

Thinking It Through

Kendra Washington is the administrative assistant for Dr. Benson, the director of an inner-city community clinic. The clinic depends on charitable contributions for a significant portion of its operating funds. Dr. Benson has asked Kendra to draft a letter to past and potential contributors in anticipation of the clinic's annual fundraising drive. The purpose of the letter is to explain the progress of the clinic over the last year and how it contributes to the community. The most important part is to ask the recipient to make a donation. Kendra knows that the organization and wording of the letter are important in order for it to be effective.

1. What must Kendra consider when deciding how to write this letter?

2. What steps should she take to plan its content?

3. What tone do you think would be most appropriate? Explain.

4. If she decides to use a form letter, how could it be personalized for the recipients?

- Create a record of facility business. Document, for regulatory and accrediting purposes, that specific items were discussed.

- Serve as a guide for the next meeting's agenda.

- Provide a resource for future reference and a reminder of decisions made.

- The following items are commonly included in minutes:

  1. Date and time the meeting is called to order

  2. Members present and absent

  3. Acceptance of previous minutes, including any corrections or additions

  4. Announcements

  5. Short write-up of discussions, decisions made, and conclusions agreed on

  6. Date and time of next meeting

  7. Time of adjournment

  8. Signature of the person preparing the minutes and of the chairperson

PATIENT EDUCATION MATERIALS

High-quality written materials are an important part of effective patient education, as introduced in Chapter 16. Written materials are appropriate for providing information on many topics:

- Diets
- Exercises
- Medications
- Postoperative instructions
- Preparing for a diagnostic test
- Self-exams
- Tips for quitting smoking
- Wound care

Whether the content is original information or material borrowed from other sources, it should be verified for accuracy. Organize the material in an easy-to-follow format. Bulleted or numbered lists may be easier for patients to follow than solid text. Create a logical order. For example, when listing possible postoperative complications, start with the most serious. Clearly indicate which ones require notifying the physician. When explaining the steps of a procedure, list them in the order in which they are performed.

Write at a reading level that is appropriate for patients. Avoid technical language that may be confusing or misunderstood. Use diagrams to illustrate important points or procedures. Use a larger-than-standard font size for patients with poor eyesight. Keep clear master copies so that repeated copying does not result in poor-quality print. An even more effective way is to maintain computerized patient information and education files. Doing so makes it easier to keep materials up to date with medical advances and facility policies. The materials can even be edited to meet the individual needs of patients. Good sources for patient education information include the National Library of Medicine (Medline Plus) at http://medlineplus.gov and the Mayo Clinic at www.mayoclinic.org.

CONFIDENTIALITY OF WRITTEN MATERIALS

All written materials containing patient information must be secure from the sight or possession of any unauthorized person. As discussed in Chapters 3 and 19, patient confidentiality must be respected at all times. Seemingly innocent documents, such as appointment reminder letters, are considered confidential if patients' names are visible. These, along with similar written materials, should never be left out where they can be seen by other patients, vendors, or other office visitors.

PROOFREADING WRITTEN WORK

All written work should be proofread for content, grammar, punctuation, spelling, and appearance. It is easy to overlook errors, because most people read more than one word at a time. The brain, reading for content, fills in missing letters and even whole words. Here are some tips for proofreading effectively:

- Reread the document to verify content. Check all facts for accuracy.
- Check the organization of the material. Does it make sense? Does it flow well?
- Read aloud. Listen for odd-sounding phrases and words.
- Check spelling by reading backward, word by word. This way, you concentrate on the appearance and spelling of words rather than on the meaning.
- Use the spell-checker feature on the computer. (However, as cautioned previously, do not depend on the spell-checker to catch all errors.)
- Print out documents created on the computer if you find it easier to read material on paper than on the screen. It is worth using extra paper and printer ink to ensure that documents are well written and accurate.

Box 17–2

Written Communication Checklist

_____ Appearance: margins, formatting, print quality

_____ Completeness: all information filled in

_____ Accuracy: numbers, dates, facts verified

_____ Grammar

_____ Punctuation

_____ Capitalization

_____ Corrections done properly

_____ Confidentiality protected

- If you are unsure about any aspect of a document, ask a qualified person for help.
- Have your written work checked as required by your facility.

See Box 17–2 for a list of items to check when reviewing written work.

Fascinating Facts

The following examples show why it is sometimes difficult to catch spelling errors. Our brains, as Live Science explains, are "code-cracking machines."

> For emaxlpe, it deson't mttaer in waht oredr the ltteers in a wrod aepapr, the olny iprmoatnt tihng is taht the frist and lsat ltteer are in the rghit pcale. The rset can be a toatl mses and you can sitll raed it wouthit a pobelrm.
>
> S1M1L4RLY, Y0UR M1ND 15 R34D1NG 7H15 4U70M471C4LLY W17H0U7 3V3N 7H1NK1NG 4B0U7 17.

Source: Breaking the Code: Why Yuor Barin Can Raed Tihs, by N. Wolchover, 2012, Live Science, http://www.livescience.com/18392-reading-jumbled-words.html.

SUGGESTED LEARNING ACTIVITIES

1. Quiz yourself on the spelling of the words in the list of frequently misspelled words.
2. Start your own personal dictionary for words you misspell. Dedicate time each week to studying and mastering these words.

3. Collect samples from health care facilities of nonconfidential written documents, such as instruction sheets, form letters, and office policies. Compare their quality and look for examples that illustrate good written communication.

4. Pay attention to writing styles as you read your textbooks, magazine and newspaper articles, and novels. Identify characteristics you believe make writing effective. Start a scrapbook of good examples.

WEB ACTIVITIES

How Stuff Works

https://people.howstuffworks.com/why-spellcheck-is-so-good-and-grammar-check-is-so-bad.htm

Why Spellcheck Is So Good and Grammar Check Is So Bad

    Why is it difficult for a computer program to identify correct English grammar?

Purdue University's Online Writing Lab

http://owl.english.purdue.edu

1. Click on *Online Writing Lab*.

2. Click on *General Writing* at the top of the list on the left side of the screen. Choose one or more of the following sections: Mechanics, Grammar, and/or Punctuation.

3. Review at least five topics.

4. Under the *Suggested Resources* listed on the left side of the web pages, click on *OWL Exercises* and complete any you believe might be helpful.

Study Guides and Strategies

www.studygs.net

Scroll down the page to "Guides: Writing and Vocabulary." Explore the topics to find 10 ideas you think might help you improve your writing.

Guide to Grammar and Writing

http://guidetogrammar.org/grammar/index.htm

Explore the many topics available and report on what you learn.

REVIEW QUESTIONS

1. Why is the ability to write clearly and correctly important for every health care professional?

2. What are the four steps to take when starting to write?

3. What are the characteristics of the following ways to organize content: formal outline, informal outline, and mind map?

4. Why is it important that the health care professional use correct spelling in all written documents?

5. What are six resources health professionals can use to check their spelling?

6. What are the nine major spelling rules?

7. What are four ways to master spelling?

8. When should words be capitalized?

9. What are the rules for using the following punctuation marks: period, comma, semicolon, colon, apostrophe, and quotation marks?

10. What are the rules for placing punctuation marks when there is more than one?

11. What are the rules for correctly writing numbers?

12. What are the rules for writing titles correctly?

13. How should the content of an effective business letter be organized?

14. How are effective written letters written, formatted, and sent?

15. Compare and contrast the three major business letter formats.

16. What are the purpose and characteristics of a good memo?

17. What items should be included when preparing meeting agendas and minutes?

18. What are five strategies for preparing effective written materials for patient education?

19. How can patient confidentiality be protected when handling written documents?

20. What are five good proofreading techniques?

APPLICATION EXERCISES

1. Refer to The Case of the Surprised Therapist at the beginning of the chapter. Explain what AI can do to ensure that the agendas, reports, and instruction sheets are written effectively and correctly.

2. Dental assistant Tanya Lucas is the chair of the program planning committee for her local professional organization. She has written the letter in Figure 17–8 to Dr. Samantha Speares, a local dentist, inviting her to speak to the group.

   a. Should Tanya send her letter as written to Dr. Speares?

   b. If not, explain what she should do to make it "mailable." Apply what you learned in this chapter about spelling, capitalization, punctuation, and letter formats.

```
                                          Tanya Lucas, RDA
                                          943 Castro Lane
                                          Oakland, CA 94662




January 14, 2020




Dr. Samantha Speares, D.D. S.
Speares Pediatric Dentistry
7920 Glenwood Circle
Oakland, Ca 94662

Dear Dr. Speares,
On behalf of the Oakland Dental Assistants Society, I would like to invite you to speak
to our group about pediatric dentistry. Many of our members are interested in working
with children, they are thinking about working in pediatric dentistry and would
like to know more about it. It would definately be a priviledge to have you as our
speaker.

The meeting will be held on Febuary 18, 2016, at seven o'clock P.M. at the Town and
Country hotel located at 2275 Scenic Road Oakland. I sincerely hope you can attend.
Please call me or our secretary, Diana LaMer at (510) 123-4567.

Sincerely,



Tanya Lucas
Program Committee Chair
```

FIGURE 17–8 Letter Tanya has written to Dr. Speares.

PROBLEM-SOLVING PRACTICE

Teresa is in an associate's degree program studying to be a respiratory therapist. She is having difficulty with her English composition class. Teresa spends a lot of time writing her papers, but is disappointed when the instructor returns them marked up with many grammar and spelling errors. How can Teresa use the five-step problem-solving process to improve her writing skills?

CHAPTER 18

Computers and Technology in Health Care

KEY TERMS

artificial intelligence
bioinformatics
cloud storage
computer literate
computer viruses
database
electronic mail
electronic spreadsheet
fiber optics
fields
file
Internet
lasers
networks
plagiarism
point-of-care charting
RAM
record
search engine
site licenses
telemedicine
virtual communities

OBJECTIVES

Studying and applying the material in this chapter will help you to:

1. Explain why it is important for today's health care professional to be computer literate.
2. List at least two ways that computers and technology are applied in the following areas of health care:
   a. Information management
   b. Creation of documents
   c. Numerical calculations
   d. Diagnostics
   e. Treatment
   f. Rehabilitation
   g. Patient monitoring
   h. Research
   i. Education
   j. Communication
3. List six guidelines for evaluating websites.
4. Provide eight guidelines for writing professional emails.
5. Explain what should be avoided when posting on social media.
6. Define telemedicine and list five ways it is helpful in the practice of medicine.
7. State four obstacles to the use of telemedicine.
8. List six guidelines for using computers effectively.
9. Describe precautions that the health care professional can take to ensure the security of computerized records.
10. Explain how to maintain the human touch when using computers while working with patients.
11. List three ways that health care professionals can acquire and/or improve their computer skills.

The Case of the Therapist Who Wants to Add to Her Computer System

Carol Lindstrom has maintained a physical therapy practice in a small community for more than 30 years. Her interpersonal communication skills are excellent, and she is known for her ability to motivate her patients to reach their highest physical potential following accidents and surgeries. Carol recognizes the worth of computers to her practice and has a system capable of word processing, bookkeeping, and accessing the Internet. Her assistant, Graciela, uses the computer mainly for correspondence and billing. Carol is aware that she and Graciela could be using computer technology in additional ways, both to make the practice more efficient and to better help patients. Carol discusses this with Graciela and assigns her the task of investigating additional computer applications. This chapter includes a discussion of the many ways that computers are being used to provide enhanced services to patients.

COMPUTERS IN HEALTH CARE

Computers and their applications have influenced every aspect of modern health care. From patient check-in procedures to diagnostics and research, technology is changing the way that health care is delivered. All health care professionals now function as information managers, and the ability to use computers has become an essential part of health care competency.

Computers perform three major types of operations:

1. Store huge amounts of data

2. Calculate, manipulate, organize, and retrieve data quickly and accurately

3. Enable high-speed communication

We can see more clearly the impact of computers on health care by following one patient, Mr. Johnson. Mr. Johnson was mowing his lawn on a Saturday afternoon when he experienced chest pains and nausea. His wife took him to the emergency department at nearby Ames General Hospital. Here are some of the many ways that computer technology was used during his stay at Ames:

1. Mr. Johnson was seen by a physician immediately, because of the possibility that he was suffering a myocardial infarction (heart attack). Mrs. Johnson gave information about Mr. Johnson and their health insurance coverage to the admitting clerk, who entered it on the hospital's *computerized patient record system*.

2. An electrocardiogram (ECG, a diagnostic method used to measure the heart's electrical activity) was performed on Mr. Johnson. The results were interpreted by a *computer*.

3. Dr. Sanchez, the cardiologist on duty, examined Mr. Johnson and decided to admit him to the hospital for observation. He dictated his observations, using *voice recognition software*, into the medical record.

4. A room was scheduled for Mr. Johnson using the hospital's *computerized scheduling program*.

5. Orders for medications prescribed by Dr. Sanchez were sent via a *computer network* to the hospital pharmacy.

6. A hospital pharmacy technician used a *pharmaceutical software program* to compare the new medications with those that Mr. Johnson was already taking to check for possible drug interactions.

7. All supplies used for Mr. Johnson's hospitalization were tracked on a *computerized inventory system*. This information was used for reordering supplies and preparing billing statements.

8. Mr. Johnson's blood pressure and pulse were intermittently monitored at preset intervals by *computerized equipment* at his bedside.

9. Mr. Johnson is diabetic and the nursing assistant took his blood sugar level before meals and at bedtime. She used a handheld piece of equipment called a glucometer that has *computer components* for testing blood and storing the readings.

10. Mr. Johnson's blood and urine samples were sent to the laboratory for computerized processing. As soon as the tests were completed, the results were entered and available on *computer* for the staff to review.

11. Mr. Johnson's charge nurse entered nursing notes about his care and condition directly into the *electronic health record system* that his health care team could access.

12. When Mr. Johnson was discharged, he was given instructions about diet and exercise that had originally been created with *word processing software*.

The health care professionals who provided direct care for Mr. Johnson or provided support services

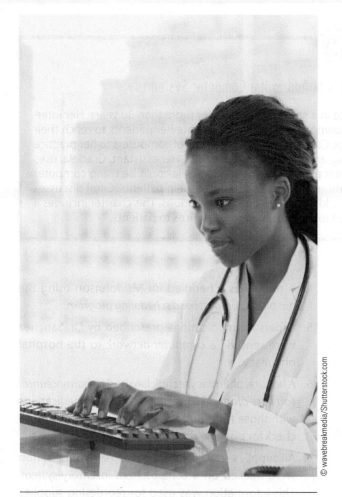

© wavebreakmedia/Shutterstock.com

FIGURE 18-1 Computer literacy is essential for today's health care professional.

needed to be **computer literate**. This means having the knowledge and skills to efficiently perform the computer tasks required of them, as well as a basic understanding of how computers work and what types of health care applications are currently available. (See Figure 18–1.) The type and number of computer-related tasks performed by health care professionals depend on their specific occupations and factors such as the size of the facility in which they work. Duties range from simple data entry to interpreting diagnostic test results. Employees in small facilities sometimes need to have a wider variety of computer skills than those in larger facilities, which have computer specialists on staff. For example, a dental receptionist in a single-dentist office may be asked to research and purchase a computer system to upgrade the administrative functions of the office. Large facilities, such as hospitals and groups of associated clinics, have information technology departments with specialized staff who purchase and maintain the computer systems. They may also design and program customized software. Figure 18–2 illustrates the flow of information in a medical practice management system.

Information Management

Keeping track of huge amounts of data is a challenge in the health care world. Having quick access to information is necessary for tasks such as selecting appropriate courses of treatment, preparing reports for regulatory agencies, and justifying insurance bills.

A **database** is a collection of information organized in a structured way. A small medical office might use a software program to develop a database of all active patients served by a specific insurance company. Many vendors today sell medical record and practice management software designed for small offices. Some have been created for particular specialties, such as pediatrics. Complex database management systems for large facilities have been created by a number of companies. See Box 18–1 for examples of health care databases.

The basic structure of a database is the key to its usefulness. Each collection of related data is called a **record**. For example, the data about each individual are grouped together in a separate record. These data are entered into **fields**. Suppose that a computerized patient record contains 15 pieces of demographic information, such as name, address, telephone number, occupation, and insurance company name. A collection of related records is a **file**.

Computerized databases have many advantages over paper filing systems. The following features make them especially useful in health care information management:

- Records can be retrieved quickly and easily.
- Records can be sorted, accessed, and reported in many ways. For example, patient records can be organized alphabetically by last name, grouped by zip code, grouped by insurance company, or listed chronologically by date of last visit.
- Information can be accessed by more than one person at the same time.

Box 18-1

Examples of Health Care Databases

Disease profiles
Insurance company records
Inventory management
Mailing lists
Patient records
Personnel records
Pharmaceutical records
Production reports
Research projects and results

FIGURE 18–2 Information flow in an integrated computerized management system for an ambulatory care setting.

Thinking It Through

Tyler is an occupational therapy assistant who works for Kelly Graziano, an occupational therapist with a private practice that specializes in hand therapy. In addition to assisting patients with their therapy and making splints, Tyler is helping Kelly computerize the administrative activities of the office. He wants to create a system to track the vendors used by the practice to supply equipment and materials. Answer the following questions to help him design a useful database:

1. How can the database be organized?
2. What data would be useful in each record?
3. How will the database make it easier to order supplies?
4. What reports might be useful for the practice? How often should they be generated?
5. How would such a system help Kelly with the financial management of her practice?

- Additions and changes can be entered easily.
- Reports can be generated as needed.
- Quality improvement studies can be conducted. (See Chapter 23.)

Accuracy is critical when entering data. Patient diagnoses, treatment plans, and billing are negatively affected by incorrect data. Carefully review and verify all input.

Electronic health records, made possible by database technology, are discussed in detail in Chapter 19.

Creation of Documents

The importance of accurate and professional-looking documents was discussed in Chapter 17. Computers are excellent tools to help create high-quality written material. Word processing software converts the computer into a "super typewriter" that gives the user the capability to create customized documents that are error-free. Written materials of all types—letters, reports, forms, and newsletters—can be produced with word processing software. See Box 18–2 for examples of word-processed documents found in health care. Software programs are available that enable the user to perform the following functions:

- Design the appearance of text and documents
- Edit, correct errors, and check spelling and grammar
- Store documents for later use
- Print and send documents by email, fax, or direct connection to other computers

Desktop publishing software is related to word processing software. It enables the user to easily combine text and graphics to create attractive newsletters, brochures, calendars, announcements, and so on. Presentation software carries documents a step further. Users can create slides to project from a computer, usually a laptop, onto a screen. Digital slides are commonly used for making professional presentations and for teaching.

Voice dictation software, a form of voice recognition software, converts spoken words to text. Increasing numbers of health care providers are using this technology for patient charting, reports, and standardized forms. Information that is dictated appears on a screen and the speaker can edit it as needed. Another type of software allows the speaker to complete the dictation and then sends the text to a professional medical transcriptionist for final editing. Voice dictation software has improved in accuracy over the past several years and has several advantages over traditional transcription services, which rely on handwritten documents from health care providers:

- It eliminates the problem of illegible or difficult-to-read handwriting.
- Reports tend to be more complete, as individuals can speak faster than they can write.
- The turn-around time for a complete, printed report is much faster.
- It is nearly as accurate, with one study showing it to be within 1.2 percentage points.
- The cost is considerably less.

Spreadsheets

Electronic spreadsheet software enables the user to perform high-speed calculations of numerical data. Spreadsheet software consists of intersecting rows and columns that form squares called cells. The user enters

Box 18–2

Using Word Processing in Health Care

Announcements

Business letters

Home care instructions

Information sheets for patient education

Medical reports

Memos

Newsletters

Payment collection notices

Research reports

numbers and formulas (instructions for performing calculations) into the cells. To create a simple budget using spreadsheet software, the amounts of income and expenses and the formulas for the desired calculations are entered. A formula may have several steps. The budgeting example would allow the user to calculate monthly income by adding all income and subtracting all expenses.

Electronic spreadsheets provide the basis for billing and accounting programs. In addition to speed and accuracy, these programs allow changes to be reflected throughout the spreadsheet. For example, if the cost of a clinic's rent increases, the effect on income can easily be calculated. All numbers affected by the change in rent will automatically be adjusted.

Computers have significantly changed patient billing methods. Amounts to be billed are not only calculated electronically, but they are also sent electronically to payers instead of being mailed. Starting in the year 2000, all Medicare and Medicaid claims had to be submitted electronically. Standardized codes have been developed that correspond to various diagnoses and treatment procedures. (See Chapter 22 for more information about medical codes.) The computer matches the codes for various procedures to a fee schedule and prepares bills. Additional numerical codes that identify specific insurance companies can be entered so that bills are automatically prepared in the proper format.

The high speed of computer calculations also enables the user to employ "if … then" scenarios to explore a variety of options. Questions such as the following can be posed:

- "If the number of patients visiting the clinic continues to grow at the current rate, how many full-time medical assistants will be needed next December?"

- "If we finance the purchase of new medical equipment at 6.5% interest, how much will the total cost be if the repayment period is three years? Five years?"

Electronic spreadsheet programs can also be used to create graphs and charts that illustrate numerical concepts and statistics. (See Figure 18–3.)

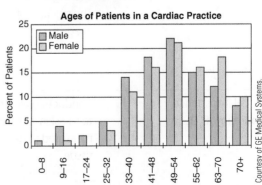

FIGURE 18–3 Graphs and charts can be easily created using computer software.

Thinking It Through

Ellie Myers has been entering patient billing data into the computer as part of her work as the administrative assistant and bookkeeper at Chandler Sports Medicine Clinic. The last week has been difficult for Ellie, because she has out-of-town relatives staying at her house and she is dealing with a variety of family problems. She is usually able to concentrate on her work but has been so tired the last few days that it has been difficult for her to fully focus on the details of data entry.

1. What might be the consequences if Ellie makes the following types of errors?

   a. Enters the wrong medical procedure codes on a bill to an insurance company

   b. Sends an appointment letter to the wrong patient

   c. Directs laboratory test requests to the wrong lab

   d. Enters the wrong numbers for expenses in the computerized accounting program

2. What would you recommend that Ellie do to protect against making mistakes of this kind?

As with databases, it is critical that data entered into the spreadsheet be accurate. One incorrect entry can affect hundreds of numbers. Carefully check all electronic spreadsheet entries.

Diagnostics

Many types of diagnostic tools are available as a result of the computer's capacity to manipulate data and perform high-speed calculations. This is an area in which technology has advanced rapidly.

Diagnostic Imaging

The computer's ability to mathematically convert thousands of measurements into images has encouraged the growth of technology that permits the viewing of soft tissues not possible with traditional X-rays. Safer and more efficient ways of seeing the inner workings of the body continue to be developed and implemented in modern medical facilities. (See Table 18–1 and Figures 18–4, 18–5, and 18–6.)

Dentistry has been improved by the introduction of safer methods of X-ray. Digital X-rays can now be taken, in which a small electronic chip is placed in the patient's mouth and an image sent to a computer. Viewed on the monitor, it can be enlarged, studied, and then stored in the patient's electronic record. The patient is exposed to a smaller amount of radiation than with traditional X-rays.

Remote Diagnostics

Technology enables information to be transmitted to nearly every corner of the earth, enabling health care providers to diagnose patients who cannot be examined by a health professional face-to-face. In addition, treatment advice and follow-up can be provided remotely. While this was developed to help patients in remote locations, clinics and hospitals now are using remote connections to diagnose and monitor patients in their homes.

Table 18–1 Diagnostic Imaging Techniques

Procedure	How it Works	Examples of Use
Computed tomography (CT)	X-rays are taken from many angles. Measurements of the density of tissues are converted to cross-sectional views.	Evaluate soft tissues for presence of disease and conditions, such as blood clots, fractures, and tumors
Magnetic resonance imaging (MRI)	Patient is placed in a magnetic field. The activity of hydrogen atoms in tissues is measured and converted into cross-sectional images.	View tumors clearly View brain structure and abnormalities See movement in the body, such as blood flow
Positron emission tomography (PET)	A radioactive substance is injected into the patient and detected by a scanner, resulting in three-dimensional images.	Determine how brain is functioning; used with Parkinson's and Alzheimer's diseases, epilepsy, cancer Can study effects of drugs on the brain and on some forms of mental illness
Ultrasonography	High-frequency sound waves hit tissues and organs and bounce back as echoes. The signals obtained are used to create images.	View movement Used when X-rays might cause harm, as with a fetus Examine organs Detect tumors, aneurysms, and blood vessel abnormalities
Electrical impedance tomography (EIT).	Conducting electrodes are attached to the skin. Electrical currents are measured to detect differences in tissue.	Proposed for: Monitoring lung function Detecting skin and breast cancer Producing images of the brain to locate hemorrhages, areas with inadequate blood supply, and sources of epileptic seizures

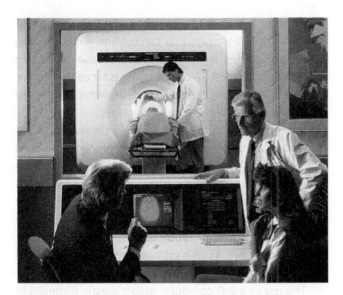

FIGURE 18–4 For magnetic resonance imaging (MRI), the patient is placed in the center of a large magnet.

FIGURE 18–5 MRI images of the brain.

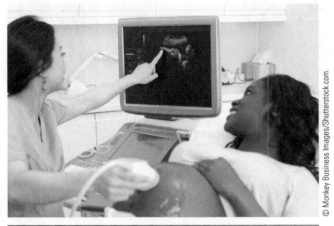

FIGURE 18–6 Ultrasonography is a safe procedure to use during pregnancy to determine the size, position, sex, and possible abnormalities of the fetus.

Examples of what is currently available include the following:

- Web-connected stethoscope that transmits heart and lung sounds
- Device that transmits data while a patient is sleeping at home to diagnose sleep apnea (disorder in which breathing stops and starts)
- Blood pressure cuffs that transmit information to a health care provider so medication can be adjusted if needed
- Blood glucose
- Sleep patterns

Medical Lab Testing

With computer technology, tests can rapidly be performed on tissue, blood, urine, and other body fluids. In addition, results can be analyzed and sent electronically to health providers. In addition to performing tests for patients, research labs make extensive use of computers. (See Figure 18–7.)

FIGURE 18–7 Computers are used extensively in medical labs for both diagnosing and research.

Fascinating Facts

Stephen Hawking, one of the world's most brilliant thinkers of the last several decades, was significantly paralyzed and lost his ability to speak due to a motor neuron disease. He continued to communicate with the world, including giving lectures, by means of computer technology that "read" his facial movements and created both text and speech through a synthesizer.

Treatment

Many new methods of treatment are based on sophisticated technology. **Fiber optics** is a technology that involves the use of hair-thin cables to transmit data. Their use for both viewing and working inside the body has increased the safety of surgery. A tiny camera, inserted through a narrow tube, projects images along the cable onto a screen, allowing the physician to see the inside of the body without having to make a large incision. When surgery is required, tiny instruments are introduced through other tubes and the procedure is guided by images on the screen. These micro-tools reduce healing time as well as the chance of infection.

Robotic surgery is made possible by fiber optics. An advanced method of surgery, it benefits patients by increasing accuracy and using minimally invasive procedures. As with expert systems, robots are not intended to replace humans. In fact, surgeons must receive special training and guide every movement made by the robot. The success of this type of surgery depends on the expertise of the "human partner." Sophisticated cameras provide surgeons with high-resolution, three-dimensional images. Sophisticated robots can be matched to the surgeon's voice and follow oral commands. This enables surgeons to perform procedures at a distance as they watch a monitor and guide the movements of the robot. Robotic surgery is currently used in many types of surgery, including cardiac, gynecological cancers, head and neck cancers, and urological procedures. (See Figure 18–8.)

Another treatment technology involves the use of **lasers**, focused light rays that can cut and remove tissue. Lasers are guided by computerized measurements to make precise incisions. A common use is for corrective eye surgery. Laser procedures are also used to remove diseased tissue and to treat bleeding blood vessels.

Image-guided surgery is based on a nearly three-dimensional mapping system that combines computed tomography (CT) with real-time information about the exact position of surgical instruments using infrared signals. This makes surgery more accurate and is especially useful when previous surgeries have changed the usual formation of a patient's body part, such as can happen with nasal surgery. As with robotic surgery, image-guided surgery tends to be less invasive and more accurate.

The use of a 3-D computer assists plastic surgeons in reconstructive and cosmetic surgery, and many dentists use computerized images to make perfectly fitting crowns.

Artificial intelligence is a very sophisticated technology that makes decisions based on real-life situations. Health care providers use these systems to help them diagnose and treat specific conditions. One of the first successful systems, MYCIN, was developed at Stanford University in the early 1970s. Although the system outperformed the diagnostic skills of the medical school faculty, it never had widespread use. This was because computer technology had not advanced sufficiently to support its use. Other concerns at the time involved ethics and legalities: If the system made an error, who would be responsible? The

© 2010 Intuitive Surgical, Inc.

FIGURE 18–8 Surgeons are now able to work with robotic equipment to perform procedures that are less invasive and safer for patients than traditional surgery.

example of MYCIN demonstrates how good ideas must sometimes wait until technology catches up.

Clinical decision-support systems (CDSS) in use today include:

- GIDEON (Global Infectious Diseases and Epidemiology Network): Support for diagnosis and treatment of infectious diseases

- TherapyEdge–HIV: Decision support system for treating human immunodeficiency virus (HIV)

Artificial intelligence, although intended to make computers behave like humans, is intended to *assist* health care professionals, *not* take the place of trained individuals. The reliability of expert systems varies, and they are not meant to be substituted for human input and decision-making.

Pharmaceuticals

More than 50% of Americans take prescription medicine regularly. It is significant, then, that computers have improved many aspects of the dispensing of pharmaceutical products. Drugs, including anesthetics, are accurately measured and dispensed through computer-controlled devices. The chance for error is decreased, as well as the potential for abuse by health care professionals.

Adverse drug incidents, estimated at one million annually, harm or cause the death of thousands of patients each year. These incidences include dosage errors, patient allergies, and dangerous drug interactions. One technology that shows promise to prevent these errors is the computerized physician order entry (CPOE) system. In this system, the prescribing provider enters medication orders into a computer that contains patient information, standard dosages, drug interactions, and so on. The system uses these data to check the appropriateness of an order before sending it to the pharmacy.

The FDA Adverse Event Reporting System (FAERS) is a database that contains information on adverse event and medication error reports submitted to the Food and Drug Administration. A system for tracking such errors has been developed and is involved in pilot testing in several states.

Telepharmacies allow the dispensing of drugs at sites other than pharmacies. Instructions for prescriptions are sent to a computerized dispensing unit. The unit prepares and releases the exact dosage. Safety features are built into the system to prevent incorrect types and amounts of drugs from being dispensed. This technology is especially useful in medical facilities that are located far from commercial pharmacies.

In some rural areas, telepharmacy technology provides services to customers from a pharmacist physically located at a central pharmacy site. Using video conferencing technology, the pharmacist communicates with the customer and a certified pharmacy technician who prepares the drug for dispensing. The pharmacist performs a drug utilization review, prescription verification, and patient counseling just as he or she would do if present in person. Several states have passed legislation that enable telepharmacies to serve outlying populations.

Rehabilitation

Computer technology has helped people with disabilities live more independently. Commands that can be activated with the touch of a button or pad, the voice, or simply by eye contact with the monitor allow the control of household functions. These include turning lights and appliances on and off, answering the telephone, and controlling room temperature.

Computer-aided design has contributed to improvements in prosthetic devices. For example, artificial legs can be designed that more exactly fit the physical characteristics of the individual. Tiny microprocessors can be inserted in prosthetics to improve their movement and to allow them to be better controlled by the user. In another application, computer technology enables the electrical stimulation of muscles that no longer receive stimulation from the brain through the nervous system. Scientists are even developing ways to enable brain function to operate prosthetic devices, thus enabling paralyzed individuals to move by using their thoughts.

Fascinating Facts

Mount Sinai Hospital in Toronto has taken advantage of iPhone® technology to develop an app called VitalHub that pulls together data from the hospital's 66 different applications. The new system includes patient records, test results, vital statistics, and medical research literature. Physicians use the system to quickly view all the information they need to make fast, accurate decisions about patient care. Using the iPhone®, everything can be accessed remotely, as well as on-site. For example, before arriving at the hospital a physician can review a patient's chart, see what drugs he is on, identify another drug that might benefit the patient, and then quickly check for possible drug interactions.

Patient Monitoring

Physiological monitoring systems employ computer technology to oversee critical body functions, such as heart and respiratory rates. Alarm systems may be connected to various types of monitoring systems to advise health care personnel when patients need intervention. (See Figure 18–9.) Obstetrical monitoring of the fetus during a woman's labor has become a standard procedure.

Computer systems also enable health care professionals to enter and track data for charting and recordkeeping. Bedside terminals and mobile computers enable keyboard entry of information, such as vital signs, dispensing of medications, fluid intake and output, and other information about care. This is known as **point-of-care charting**. Physicians who cannot get to the hospital can review patient data, look at X-rays and test results, and recommend treatments from anywhere in the world.

Computerized devices are also used by home health professionals, such as nurses and physical therapists, to record patient notes and progress. This information is then transmitted electronically into the patient's health record. Making sure that data are entered accurately when working in the field is extremely important.

Many specialized devices have been developed to assist health care professionals in tracking patient recovery. For example, a camera connected to a computer allows hand therapists to store and compare photographs of the patient's hand taken over time. This aids in evaluating the effectiveness of the treatment plan.

Research

Learning and keeping up-to-date with medical advances has been made easier by computerized resources. The National Library of Medicine, through MEDLINE/PubMed, contains millions of citations to journals and books.

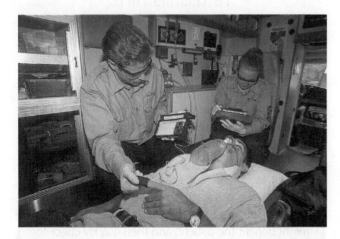

FIGURE 18–9 Pulse oximeters use computer technology to monitor a patient's pulse and determine the oxygen level in the blood.

Literature databases are like giant indexes, containing references to specific journal articles, books, and research reports. Each entry is accessible in various ways, such as the following:

- Preassigned key words that describe the content
- Words in the title
- Name of author(s)
- Name of journal
- Publication date

Other specialized databases are available in addition to MEDLINE. One of potential interest to health care students is the Cumulative Index to Nursing and Allied Health Literature (CINAHL). It contains indexes for more than 4,000 journals, including full-text availability for 1,300 journals. Two other large, specialized indexes of interest to health care students are the Educational Resources Information Center (ERIC) and PsychINFO.

In addition to providing published information, databases can serve medical researchers by their capacity to sort and match data. The term **bioinformatics** refers to the organization of biological data into databases applying information technology and computer science. Such databases make information easily available to scientists all over the world. Sharing information in this way contributes significantly to scientific progress.

The Human Genome Project is an example of bioinformatics. Begun in the late 1980s and completed in 2003, it was an international effort to collect the results of investigations relating to human genes (one of the biological units of heredity). The goal of the project was to identify all the approximately 20,000 to 25,000 genes in human DNA and store this information in an organized manner. Gene therapy is an exciting area of medical research that uses the results of the project. In this therapy, a "normal" gene is inserted into a cell to replace an "abnormal," disease-causing gene.

Pharmaceutical research has benefited from the computer's ability to sort and match the results of thousands of tests carried out to explore the effectiveness and safety of new drugs. Results can be obtained more

Fascinating Facts

The world's first computer, which was named the Z1, was invented by Konrad Zuse in 1936. His next invention, the Z2 was finished in 1939 and was the first fully functioning electro-mechanical computer.

rapidly and sent to the Food and Drug Administration for review. This is decreasing the time needed to obtain approvals for new products.

Education

Computers offer new ways to learn for students, health care professionals, and patients. Distance education over the Internet is widely available. This is a method of accessing courses enabling students to study at times and locations convenient for them and to proceed at their own pace. As discussed in Chapter 14, this is a way for health care professionals to earn continuing education units, as well as to keep up on the latest developments in their career fields.

The Internet allows storage of vast amounts of reference information. Entire sets of encyclopedias, reference books, and specialized dictionaries are available online. Wireless devices can hold thousands of pages, offering a convenient, mobile method for downloading and reading books in electronic form.

A.D.A.M. is an example of how the power of the computer can be harnessed to help students learn. Designed to teach anatomy, it is an interactive resource that contains a multimedia encyclopedia, more than 3,000 illustrations, and three-dimensional images that can be rotated (A.D.A.M. Education, 2017). A.D.A.M. is also available for consumer (patient) education.

Computerized simulations provide scenarios that allow students to interact. A realistic situation is presented, followed by questions and opportunities for students to suggest appropriate action. The computer responds to the student's input, either indicating its correctness or requesting more information.

Virtual reality technology, in which reality is simulated as closely as possible, enables health care providers to practice procedures before working on patients. These include inserting needles and performing surgical tasks. Surgeons can practice entire operations before working on actual patients.

Many professional licensing exams are now administered by computer. In the past, exams may have been offered only once or twice a year and graduates had to wait until they were scheduled. Some testing programs now individualize the exams by selecting each question based on the response given for the previous question. Test-takers who answer all or most questions correctly may pass the exam with fewer total questions. An example of this type of test is the National Council Licensure Exam (NCLEX), which is administered to registered nurse candidates.

Patients, too, can learn about their health conditions, self-care, and prevention techniques using the Internet. Credible, user-friendly websites, such as Medline Plus, offer dozens of articles, slide shows, and illustrations to inform health care consumers. Some hospitals make it possible for patients to obtain computerized health information.

Communication

Networks, computer systems linked together to share date, enable communication among the staff of one clinic or among a group of thousands of individuals the world over. An example of a simple networked system is five linked computers in a small medical office. Patient records are shared, and all staff members use the same printer. A large facility may have hundreds of computers linked together that carry out many of the functions described in this chapter. The Internet is the ultimate networked system, consisting of billions of computers located all over the world.

In addition to enabling health care professionals to communicate with each other, online websites now allow patients to view their personal health records using secure websites. Known as patient portals, they can be used by patients to access appointment dates, test results, reminders about vaccinations that are due, and much more. Securing this information is critical and records can only be accessed using an individual's login and password.

The Internet

The **Internet** began as a method for government authorities to communicate in case of nuclear attack. It has rapidly grown to become a principal means of communicating, conducting business, shopping, learning, securing needed information, and socializing.

Using the Internet for Research

Health care professionals can benefit from the Internet in many ways. Consider the case of Mark, a recently graduated nurse, who is hired by an orthopedic surgeon who specializes in joint replacements. Mark wants to learn more about these procedures and decides to see what he can find on the Internet. In one afternoon, he locates the following resources:

- Articles in medical journals
- Information produced by, and about, companies that manufacture artificial joints
- A newsgroup in which patients who have had joint replacement surgery share their experiences
- Articles in popular magazines, such as *Newsweek*
- A list of medical facilities and surgeons in the United States who specialize in joint replacement
- Government reports about the effectiveness of artificial joints
- Email addresses of university researchers who are experimenting with new types of artificial joints
- A medical bookstore that takes orders over the Internet

Mark started by using a search engine, a program on the Internet that looks through millions of documents. In his case, he entered the key phrases "joint replacement" and "artificial joint." Google and Bing are examples of general search engines. There are more targeted search engines, such as Google Scholar, PubMed, and Science Direct, that limit searches to non-commercial websites.

The major search engines allow you to be more specific by specifying phrases that must appear exactly as you enter them. In Mark's case, if he enters the words *artificial joint*, a search engine will find documents that contain both these words—but not necessarily together. (Search engines are becoming much better at recognizing these types of common phrases.) Using the advanced search function, or by enclosing the phrase in quotation marks, Mark increased his chances of finding useful websites.

It is important for students to remember that they must cite (give the source of) information taken from a website and used in a report or paper just as they would for material taken from a book or journal article. Copying information word for word from a Web source or using materials such as images without permission is plagiarism. There are several ways to correctly cite and list Web sources, just as there are different ways to organize a bibliography or reference list. Check with the appropriate style manual or your instructor to learn the preferred form.

Evaluating Internet Sources

At this time, material placed on the Internet is not regulated. Anyone can say anything and make any claims; therefore, not all information is reliable. Much of it consists of personal opinions or is motivated by the desire to sell products. Health care professionals must take care to determine the reliability of any information taken from the Web. The following guidelines can help you evaluate websites:

- Identify the source: Universities and government agencies tend to be reliable sources of information. Research and professional organizations, if not organized for the purpose of selling specific products, may also be reliable—for example, the American Heart Association and the American Association of Medical Assistants. The ending of a website address gives information about the sponsor. (See Table 18–2.) It should be noted here that commercial websites can be good sources of information. Many large corporations provide nonbiased information.

- Determine the author: Is the person an expert in the field? Does he or she have appropriate education and credentials? Is the purpose of the material to share information or report research findings? Or to persuade readers and sell ideas or products?

- Check for accuracy: Is a reference given for the information? Is the reference from a reliable source?

- Verify important data: Cross-check statistics and other numerical data.

- Look for signs of quality: Are the ideas well supported? Is the spelling accurate and vocabulary used correctly?

- Check for currency: Is the information recent and up to date?

Electronic Mail

Electronic mail (email) has become a standard professional communication tool. It provides a way to quickly send documents, such as memos, announcements, and reports to one or more persons. Some physicians and other health care providers are using email as an efficient means of communicating with patients.

It is important that email messages be clear and accurate, just as with any written material. The growing popularity of email means that some people receive dozens of transmissions daily. Keeping messages brief and to the point is considered a professional courtesy. Additional guidelines for professional health care emails include the following:

- State the email's purpose or content in the subject line

- Maintain a professional tone: avoid humor, sarcasm, and anything that might be misinterpreted

Table 18–2 Identifying Website Sponsors

Type of Sponsor	Website Address Extension	Example
Educational institution	.edu	University of Michigan, www.umich.edu
Government office or agency	.gov	National Institutes of Health, www.nih.gov
Professional organizations	.org	American Cancer Society, www.cancer.org
Businesses, corporations, and other commercial organizations	.com	Merck & Co., Inc. (pharmaceuticals) www.merck.com

- Include a greeting and a close that includes your contact information

- Do not use all caps (shouting) or all lower case (hard to read)

- Do not use abbreviations or emojis, such as those used in casual text messages

- Do not include confidential patient information (HIPAA rules are very strict - see Chapter 19)

- Proofread before sending, checking grammar, punctuation, and spelling

- When sending to more than one person, use BCC

Keep in mind that emails, like other written documents, reflect the professionalism of your organization.

In spite of the convenience of emails, there are times when a phone conversation is more appropriate. This may be true when the message is complex, difficult to explain, and might require a number of emails to complete; when an immediate response is needed; or when the topic is difficult or emotional, such as when a patient's test result is abnormal and a matter of concern.

Files created in other programs can be sent with an email message. For example, a report created in MS Word can be sent as an "attachment" to an email message without rekeying the document. This provides a convenient and economical way to send, review, revise, and return documents and share useful information. Suppose that two respiratory therapists in different states are working together to write a journal article. Using email attachments, they can send updated drafts of their work to each other for review. However, patient records and other documents containing personal health information should *never* be attached to an email.

A more recent development for sharing documents on the Internet is Google Docs which allow multiple users to edit a document with each able to immediately see the changes made by others.

It is not appropriate to conduct personal email correspondence or explorations on the Internet at work. Be aware that email messages may be stored in the form of backup files that belong to the employer. Employers have the right to read and monitor any messages sent through their computers by any employee. Many organizations have increased their monitoring of employee activity on the Internet.

Social and Professional Networking

Social networking websites, such as Facebook, have become a popular way for individuals to connect with friends and share personal news. By providing the means to easily stay in touch with family, friends, and former classmates, you can use social media network in your initial job search or when looking to change jobs throughout your career. A word of caution: Posting unflattering images of yourself, intended to be funny or entertaining, may be a harmful career move. This is because employers are increasingly checking social networking sites when considering applicants for employment. Showing yourself in a situation that demonstrates poor judgment, lack of respect for others, or other unfavorable characteristics could prevent you from being hired. In extreme circumstances, it can be cause for dismissal from a job.

In addition to Facebook, there are many networking sites that link people around the world who share common interests. One large specialty website is LinkedIn, which promotes professional networking. Members' profile pages emphasize their employment history and education rather than personal information. The company reports that many of its members are employment recruiters who use the site to look for and check on potential job candidates.

Virtual Communities

Virtual communities consist of individuals who use the Internet to communicate and share information. Both health care professionals and patients can share information and experiences about specific health conditions. Chronically ill, bedridden, and people with disabilities use the communication capabilities of the computer to break from the isolation that often results from these conditions. (See Figure 18–10.)

Telemedicine

The American Telemedicine Association defines **telemedicine** as "the use of medical information exchanged from one site to another via electronic communications to improve a patient's clinical health status." Transmission devices may include two-way video, smart phone, email, and various wireless tools. The medicine practiced by telemedicine is the same as that practiced in face-to-face consultations. Its major

Fascinating Facts

The first electronic computer ENIAC weighed more than 27 tons and took up 1,800 square feet of space.

© Belushi/Shutterstock.com.

FIGURE 18–10 Computers allow people with disabilities to more easily connect with the outside world and communicate with others.

advantage is that it provides expert medical help to patients in remote areas, such as farms far from towns, war zones, and wilderness areas. It is also increasingly used where convenience, rather than distance, is the issue. As discussed previously, patients can be monitored while remaining in their homes. A physician can send patient information to a colleague halfway around the world to obtain an opinion about a rare condition. Because images can be transmitted electronically, X-rays and other images can be sent for analysis. One hospital emergency department in Oregon sends CT scans of patients admitted during the night to Australia to be interpreted if there are no radiologists on duty at the hospital.

Telemedicine is especially helpful for the following functions:

- Allowing patient access to specialists who are located at a distance
- Communicating vital signs from home to allow monitoring at a health care facility
- Checking pacemaker function and performing ECGs over telephone lines
- Performing physical exams from a distance
- Providing more comprehensive emergency care by linking emergency medical professionals in the field and during patient transport with physicians

Although telemedicine has become an important part of health care delivery, there are three major obstacles to its expanded use:

1. Not all facilities, especially those in remote areas, have adequate infrastructure to support the necessary high-speed wireless technology.

2. State licensing laws sometimes prohibit the exchange of medical practice across state lines, even when done electronically.
3. Some physicians are not comfortable conducting examinations remotely.
4. Complex government regulations make it difficult or impossible for community based, non-profit, or public agencies that serve low-income patients to bill for telemedicine services.

In spite of these obstacles, telemedicine offers exciting possibilities for patients everywhere.

USING COMPUTERS EFFECTIVELY

You can increase the effectiveness of computers as work tools by using the following good work habits:

- Verify the accuracy of all data entered: When working on a large system, incorrect entries can negatively affect the work of others as well as the welfare of patients. Many medication errors in hospitals are the result of incorrect data entry.

Health care work demands accuracy to ensure high-quality patient care, as well as compliance with regulatory agencies.

- Always back up work using a backup system, such as an external hard drive or cloud storage service (services run on the Internet): Save work to the hard drive periodically. The workspace on a personal computer, called RAM, stores data only while the computer is on. If power is interrupted, any work not saved will be lost. Many software programs save work automatically at regular intervals. When a task or work session is completed, back up all files if not using an automatic storage system. Computers can break down, and emergencies can occur.

- Stay legal: It is against copyright law to install software that has been installed on another computer unless it is specifically allowed and stated by the manufacturer. Purchase and register needed programs. Site licenses that give permission to install software on more than one computer can be purchased for programs that will be loaded on more than one computer at a facility. Never bring personal software to load onto the workplace computer. (Some of these problems have been solved by software companies that now require you to purchase their programs directly online.)

- Keep up with advancements: Software is continually updated with new versions that offer additional features. Many updates are available at reduced prices for owners of previous editions. New websites, offering an increasing number of products and services, appear daily.

- Do not panic: Computers are still a relatively new technology, and the complexity of today's systems results in occasional glitches. It is almost impossible to damage computer hardware or software through normal use. If the computer does not understand a command, an error message will appear on the screen. These error messages can sound rather serious, but the worst thing that can usually happen is that work performed since it was last saved—either by the user or automatically by the program—is lost and must be redone. As discussed earlier, this can be avoided by regularly saving work. This said, entire system crashes do occur and thus there is the need to back up your files.

- Be flexible: When large facilities update or change their computer system, the transition can be stressful. During the first few days after "going live," it can seem as if the new system adds more work instead of more efficiency. It can take staff members time to learn and adapt to the changes. Fortunately, software analysis, design, and support are continually improving and making information technology easier for everyone to learn and use.

- Avoid injury: Prolonged use and improper positioning can result in physical injuries. See Chapter 9 for information about reducing the risk of workplace injuries, such as carpal tunnel syndrome, related to computer use.

COMPUTER SECURITY

The very characteristics that make computers useful in health care can also be a cause for concern. For example, the increased accessibility to patient records also increases the risk of breaching patient confidentiality. The need to protect privacy has been addressed by the federal government. Several major laws, such as the Electronic Communication Privacy Act of 1986, provide protection against unauthorized access or interception of data communications. The privacy of medical records is specifically addressed in the Health Insurance Portability and Accountability Act (HIPAA) implemented in 2003. (HIPAA and patient records are discussed in Chapter 19.) In spite of regulations, serious breaches of health care information have occurred when systems are hacked (broken into illegally).

There are precautions the health care professional can take to help ensure computer security. If assigned a password to gain access to a computer system, never give it to anyone else, even a coworker. Unauthorized users may be able to destroy or falsify data, add hours to their payroll records, or illegally transfer funds. Entries can often be tracked to the password used. The following practices will increase computer security:

- If passwords are chosen rather than assigned, do not use something obvious, such as a nickname.
- Close files containing private information before leaving the work area.
- Do not allow patients or other unauthorized persons to wander into the area where data entry is taking place.
- Shred discarded printouts before throwing them in the trash.

Computer viruses are programs that contain instructions to perform destructive operations, such as scrambling and erasing files and preventing the computer from operating normally. A common means of transmitting harmful programs is by clicking on links contained in emails from unknown sources or downloading "infected" material from the Internet.

It is not always obvious that a virus is present because the instructions may have been programmed to activate at a future date. All computers are susceptible to viruses. The following practices can help prevent viruses from infecting workplace computers:

- Do not open email messages or download files from unknown parties.
- Do not use your work email address for personal correspondence.
- Use purchased software to load application programs, not copies secured from friends or other outside sources; or download directly from the vendor's Internet site.
- Use antivirus software or an online service and keep it updated to protect against new viruses that are continually being created.

Wireless technology has its own security threats. When using public Internet access ("hot spots"), do not enter private passwords to websites or personal data, such as credit card numbers.

MAINTAINING THE HUMAN TOUCH

Although computers have become part of everyday life, there are still people who are not familiar or completely comfortable with this new technology. They complain that they feel like a number in a vast system over which they have little control. This perception may result in feelings of intimidation and annoyance. In fact, some physicians have resisted the implementation of EHRs because they have difficulty focusing on a patient, maintaining eye contact, and observing the patient's body language, while simultaneously entering data into a computer.

The health care professional should strive to provide a personal interface between patients and machines. Do not let the computer become a barrier. Those responsible for inputting patient data should extend a friendly greeting before beginning the data entry process. Look up and make eye contact periodically. If it is not obvious to the patient, explain what information you are entering and why. Make appropriate comments to convey a sense of caring to the patient. Communicate verbally and nonverbally that the patient is more important than the machine.

Thinking It Through

Stacey Petersen is the admitting clerk at a large urban hospital. The patients served come from a wide variety of cultural and economic backgrounds. Much of Stacey's work involves collecting and entering patient data into the hospital's computer system. Although most patients are comfortable with this procedure, some find it intimidating or are uneasy about "just what is being put into the computer." Of particular concern to Stacey are elderly patients from cultures in which health care is very personalized and where practitioners are well known to the patient.

1. What can Stacey do to help these patients feel more at ease?

2. How can a lack of understanding on the part of patients about the health care system affect the way they deal with health problems?

Health care professionals should also be prepared to respond to patients' concerns about the privacy of their medical records, identity theft, and the possibility of errors being entered on computers.

LEARNING MORE ABOUT COMPUTERS

Learning more about the capabilities and operation of computers can increase the efficiency and job satisfaction of the health care professional. Opportunities for promotion may be increased. The many ways to increase computer knowledge and skills include the following:

- Take classes
- Read the manuals (often online) for software
- Work through tutorials and help menus included with software programs
- Take tutorials available on the Internet
- Explore the various functions of software programs
- Read some of the many books that are available for all levels of users
- Research topics on the Web

Finding effective ways to learn about computers will help you keep up with a rapidly advancing technology that will continue to change the nature of health care.

SUGGESTED LEARNING ACTIVITIES

1. Find out what types of computer classes are available at your school and in the community that are appropriate for your needs.

2. Explore health-related websites such as Medline Plus, Web MD, and the Mayo Clinic. List the address and give a brief description of each. (Add these to the webliography started for Suggested Learning Activity 6 in Chapter 14.)

3. Visit a health care facility to learn about how computers are used for diagnosis, treatment, and administration.

4. Interview someone who is working in a health care field of interest to you. How are computers used in this field? How much work does this person perform using computers or computerized technology? What computer skills are considered essential to be successful in this occupation? Which skills will increase promotional opportunities? Write up a short report of your findings.

WEB ACTIVITIES

mHealth Intelligence

https://mhealthintelligence.com/news/complex-medicaid-rules-limit-fqhc-safety-net-telehealth-use

1. This article explains how government regulations are preventing the widespread use of telemedicine with low-income patients. Can you think of other areas of health care that are complicated or not easily accessible because of regulations?

2. How do you think this problem applying telehealth might be resolved in the future?

3. What are other ways that low-income Americans have difficulty gaining access to health care?

TelePharm

https://www.telepharm.com/how-telepharmacy-works/

This is an excellent video that explains how a telepharmacy works.

Medline Plus

https://medlineplus.gov/ency/patientinstructions/000880.htm

Patient Portals—an online tool for your health

1. What is a patient portal?

2. What are the contents on a patient portal?

3. How are patient portals used?

4. What are the benefits to patients who use them?

American Telemedicine Association

www.americantelemed.org

1. Choose three reports to read.

2. Write a short summary of each.

Medline Plus

https://medlineplus.gov/webeval/intro1.html

Evaluating Internet Health Information Tutorial

1. Read the 6-part tutorial.

2. Create a brochure or fact sheet explaining how to evaluate websites.

Health Care Cost and Utilization Project

https://www.hcup-us.ahrq.gov/news/exhibit_booth/hcup_fact_sheet.jsp

1. How are databases used to gather and organize data about hospital admissions?
2. How is this information used?

The Medical Futurist

https://medicalfuturist.com/ten-ways-technology-changing-healthcare

10 Ways Technology Is Changing Healthcare

1. Which change do you find most interesting? Why?
2. Have you personally been affected by any of these changes? Is so, which one(s)?
3. What change(s) do you think will most affect your career in health care?

Robotic Surgery at UAMS Using da Vinci Surgical System

https://www.youtube.com/watch?v=RJcRABevyCk

This video demonstrates how robotic surgery is performed.

IMPORTANT NOTE: This is a simulation for demonstration purposes—it is not being performed on a real patient. If it were, the woman changing the instruments would be wearing a mask and gloves and not touching the ends of the probes.

National Institutes of Health

https://report.nih.gov/nihfactsheets/ViewFactSheet.aspx?csid=45

Human Genome Project

1. How has health care benefited from this project?
2. What is the goal of the Cancer Genome Project? What do you think the effects of this project will be?

REVIEW QUESTIONS

1. Why is it important for today's health care professional to be computer literate?
2. List at least two computer applications for health care in each of the following areas:
   a. Information management
   b. Creation of documents
   c. Numerical calculations
   d. Diagnostics
   e. Treatment
   f. Rehabilitation
   g. Patient monitoring
   h. Research
   i. Education
   j. Communication
3. What are six guidelines for evaluating websites?
4. What are eight guidelines for writing professional emails?
5. What should be avoided when posting on social media sites?
6. What is telemedicine and what are five ways it is helpful in the practice of medicine?
7. What are four obstacles to the use of telemedicine?

8. What are six guidelines for using computers effectively?

9. How can health care professionals help ensure the security of computerized records?

10. How can health care professionals maintain the human touch when using the computer while working with patients?

11. What are three ways the health care professional can learn more about using computers?

APPLICATION EXERCISES

1. Refer to the Case of the Therapist Who Wants to Add to Her Computer System at the beginning of the chapter. Based on what you learned in the chapter, list new ways that Carol can use computer technology in her practice.

2. The students in an Introduction to Health Care class have just completed their study of the application of computers in health care. The course was an overview, and the students have been thinking about how they will use computer technology in their work. For each of the following students, suggest potential applications and the skills they should acquire for on-the-job success.

   a. Craig Kingman, paramedic

   b. Otis Brownwell, radiologic technician

   c. Christine Abbott, surgical technologist

   d. Marta Singh, registered nurse

   e. Jaime Bustamante, medical assistant

PROBLEM-SOLVING PRACTICE

Grace has been the medical assistant in a small clinic for many years. She performs both clinical and administrative duties. The two physicians in the clinic want to explore using telemedicine and other new technologies, as well as updating the office computer system. They have asked for Grace to be involved. She feels she has enough to do with the medical assisting duties and does not have time to help, nor is she really interested in having to learn a lot of new things. How can Grace use the five-step problem-solving process in this situation?

CHAPTER 19

Documentation and Medical Records

KEY TERMS

charting
chief complaint
electronic health records (EHRs)
electronic medical records (EMRs)
HIPAA (Health Insurance Portability and Accountability Act of 1996)
Joint Commission on Accreditation of Healthcare Organizations (JCAHO)
medical documentation
medical history
medical record
personal health records (PHRs)
plan
progress notes
SOAP

OBJECTIVES

Studying and applying the material in this chapter will help you to:

1. Define medical documentation, medical record, and charting.
2. List five examples of charting tasks performed by health care professionals.
3. List nine major purposes of medical documentation.
4. List five characteristics of good medical documentation.
5. List six possible negative consequences of poor medical documentation.
6. Explain the proper method for correcting errors on medical records.
7. Explain the source-oriented approach to recordkeeping and list the typical contents of a medical record.
8. Describe the content and explain the purpose of progress notes.
9. Describe problem-oriented charting, including its advantages and disadvantages.
10. Explain the meaning of SOAP including what the letters in the acronym stand for.
11. Describe narrative charting, including its advantages and disadvantages.
12. Describe charting by exception, including its advantages and disadvantages.
13. Define the following terms: electronic medical records (EMRs) and electronic health records (EHRs).
14. List three options a health care facility has when converting to an electronic health record system.
15. Give three examples of how an EHR system can be used in a physician's office.
16. List and explain ten advantages of an EHR system.
17. List and explain seven challenges of an EHR system.
18. Describe what information would be included in a personal health record (PHR) and explain why it is important for an individual to have one.
19. List the main features of the Health Insurance Portability and Accountability Act of 1996 (HIPAA), including the Privacy and Security Rules.
20. Provide methods for preventing hackers from stealing computerized data.
21. Explain how to properly send faxes and e-mails that contain protected health information (PHI).
22. Explain how to properly dispose of materials containing protected health information.

The Case of the Therapist Who Hates to Write

Joseph Lane, a respiratory therapist, enjoys working with patients and the technical aspects of his profession. But he has never enjoyed paperwork and dislikes writing documentation following the treatment he administers. His notes are hurriedly scribbled, and other health care professionals find them difficult, if not impossible, to read. In this chapter, the importance of accurate, complete, and legible documentation will be stressed. Inaccurate, incomplete, and illegible charting has consequences for patient care, jeopardizes regulatory compliance, and presents legal risks.

MEDICAL DOCUMENTATION AND RECORDKEEPING

Medical documentation consists of notes and documents that health care professionals add to the medical record. Examples of data contained in these records include patient statistics and information about care, results of tests performed, the patient's diagnosis written by a physician, treatments received, and medications prescribed.

A medical record is the collection of all documents that are filed together and form a complete chronological health history of a particular patient. A medical record is also commonly referred to as a medical chart, patient chart, or patient record. Recording observations and information about patients is known as charting.

Many health care professionals are responsible for some aspect of charting. Tasks may include the following:

- Recording demographic information about new patients
- Interviewing patients and filling in the medical history form
- Recording vital signs (e.g., temperature, blood pressure)
- Noting comments made by the patient
- Making notes on the patient's record as dictated by the physician, dentist, or other professional
- Recording any procedures performed
- Transcribing notes or dictation from other professionals into the medical records

Purposes of Medical Documentation

Complete and accurate medical documentation is critical in providing consistent patient care. It is the lifeline of communication that supports the coordination of care. This is especially important in today's health care environment in which many different health professionals may work with a single patient. Information included in the medical record is a significant source of data on which this variety of professionals can base their approach to the patient.

Good medical documentation and recordkeeping contribute to quality health care in the following ways:

- Improves the coordination and continuity of care.
- Reinforces decision-making capacities: Information contained in records provides health care providers with the information they need to make decisions about proper diagnoses, treatment options, etc.
- Helps enforce staff accountability: When information is "officially" noted in a record, the health care professionals making the notes can be held responsible for its content and any actions on their part.
- Achieves more accurate vital statistics: Information about deaths, disease outbreaks, etc., can be extracted from medical records rather than from oral reports that may be erroneous.
- Provides legal protection: Medical records are legal documents that are admissible as evidence in court. In the case of a malpractice lawsuit, for example, documentation provides proof of what has taken place with the patient. Only through written documentation can tests, procedures, and treatment be proven to have occurred. In the world of health care, "If it isn't documented, it isn't done."
- Helps ensure compliance with regulatory agencies: These include governmental bodies and the Joint Commission on Accreditation of Healthcare Organizations (JCAHO) an organization that accredits those health care organizations that meet its standards. Participation in certain programs, such as Medicare, requires that specific documentation guidelines be strictly followed.
- Improves cost control: Proper documentation prevents repetition and the performance of unnecessary procedures. It also helps ensure that appropriate

Thinking It Through

Ms. Shing Chun works in a clinic. The provider asks her to call Mrs. Yang and tell her the labs were normal and that a new medication has been sent to the pharmacy for her. When Ms. Chun calls, Mr. Yang answers and says his wife is not home, but he can take a message. Ms. Chun tells him to tell her the labs were normal and a new medication was sent to the pharmacy. Mr. Yang asks what tests were run and what medication was ordered. Ms. Chun declines to answer the questions by explaining that it is confidential information.

1. Did Ms. Chun break any HIPAA regulations?
2. If the labs had been abnormal, should she have handled it differently?

preventive measures, early intervention, and correct procedures are performed.

- Decreases denials from insurance companies: The need for care and proof that it is provided by appropriate personnel are supported by documentation.

- Provides data for investigation of errors and incidents: Errors do sometimes occur during surgeries, the administration of drugs, etc. Accurate records can assist in the investigation, analysis, and prevention of future errors.

By contrast, poor records can have the following negative consequences:

- Misinformed health care professionals and patients
- Increased legal risks
- Unnecessary repetition of tests and other investigations

Fascinating Facts

Subpoenas, in malpractice lawsuits, frequently arrive a year or more after the care was given and documented. When called to testify, most health care professionals do not even recall the patient or the care given and must rely entirely on their own documentation.

- Longer hospital stays
- Poor patient care
- Risk of repetition of serious incidents

Characteristics of Good Medical Documentation

- **Complete:** All requested information must be included. Each entry must include the date and signature of the appropriate health care personnel. Charting should be completed as soon as possible to prevent the omission of important information.

- **Concise and factual:** A lot of words are not better than a clear concise statement. Never use the chart to record guesses or opinions. State only what has been observed, done, or heard. If you are quoting a patient's statements, use quotation marks. For example, "I feel a sharp pain in my left leg every time I try to walk."

- **Properly identified:** The patient's name and identifying numbers should be visible on every page. It is critical that the record match the patient so that correct entries are made.

- **Legible:** Notes that cannot be read are useless. They do not serve their purpose of providing continuity of care. Furthermore, they present a liability and cause for negative legal and regulatory outcomes.

- **Uses correct spelling, terminology, punctuation, and grammar:** Poorly written documentation can be easily misinterpreted and gives the appearance of carelessness when the record is reviewed by others.

- **Clearly and objectively expressed:** Important details are correctly noted: temperature, size, amounts (fluids, drainage, medication, etc.). The words used are not subject to misinterpretation, such as "small," "a lot," and so on. Notes should be limited to what is observed. For example, write "ate 25% of the meal" rather than "ate poorly." Judgmental or humorous remarks about patients are unacceptable.

- **Does not duplicate findings:** Some facilities use graphic sheets on which the blood pressure, temperature, pulse, and respiratory rate are recorded. If so, it is not necessary to repeat this information in the written record. When a finding is abnormal, it may be repeated in the written record along with the associated action taken or treatment given to correct the problem. The record would then also include a follow-up assessment of how the patient responded to the action or treatment.

- **Uses abbreviations only if approved and listed in the facility's policy manual:** This reduces the possibility

Thinking It Through

Juanita is a registered nurse (RN) who works for a home health agency. She enjoys the work because she really cares about each of her patients and likes getting to know them as individuals. She tries to spend a little extra time on each home visit, chatting with them about their families, interests, pets, and so on. With more patients being released to their homes rather than to rehabilitation or other settings, her case load has increased. Juanita finds that sometimes she does not have time to complete all her charting until late in the evening. Sometimes she is not able to get to it until the following morning. She tries to complete it while eating breakfast before leaving for another day of rounds.

1. Discuss the possible consequences of Juanita's current work habits in terms of legal compliance and reimbursement.

2. Discuss any changes you would recommend.

of misunderstandings if the abbreviation used has several different meanings. For example, does "pt" stand for patient, prothrombin time, physical therapy, or part-time?

- Shows time and date of all entries: Accurate and chronological charting presents a picture of how the patient appears over time. If charting is not done in a timely manner, another health care professional may record an event with a time that occurred after the action that you intended to chart. The only option then is to write "late entry" and then chart, but this out-of-sequence information can still create confusion for others. (See Figure 19–1.)

- Signed by the proper person: Never sign for someone else or have anyone sign the charting you have done. Recording false information is a serious offense and should not be done under any circumstance.

Current date & time		Date & time of out-of-sequence note
10/10/15	1530	Late entry (10/10/15 - 1230)
		Skin appears slightly
		reddened and moist
		to the touch. Z. Hera RN

FIGURE 19–1 Sample of a late entry in charting.

10/15/15	0930	no complaint of pain. P. Zoe LPN
10/15/15	1030	ambulated independently
		50 feet with steady gait
		and no shortness of breath
		Z. Hera RN

Draw a line through empty spaces — Never leave a blank line in progress notes

FIGURE 19–2 Never leave empty lines in charting.

- Completed without leaving empty lines: All charting that begins after the previous signature and runs to the next signature belongs to the latter entry. If an empty space or line is left above the entry and signature of the health care professional, it is possible for someone else to chart information that now becomes part of the other health care professional's entry. (See Figure 19–2.)

- Never enter in advance of the medication or procedure: Chart only after the event has occurred, never before, in anticipation of doing it. For example, if a nurse charts that medications were given and then is suddenly called away, the other health care professionals will assume that the medications were given, and the patient will not receive the proper medications he or she needs for treatment.

- Written with black or blue ink (or as specified by the facility): Pencil is *never* acceptable.

Making Corrections on Medical Documentation

Medical records cannot be corrected in a way that covers up what was originally written. To do so can give the appearance that the records have been illegally altered and negates their value as legal records. Never use correction fluid (such as White-Out), erase, or use correction tape over errors. Observe the following practices:

1. Draw a single line through the error. The original entry must still be legible.

2. Write in the correct information where there is the most space: above, below, or following the original entry.

3. Note the error as required by your facility. For example, "M.E." may be used for "mistaken entry"; "correction" or "corr" may be acceptable. Be sure to learn the specific requirements for notations, and never create your own or assume that the facility will use the ones presented in textbooks. Regulatory

11/1/15	1400	Darvocet-N 100 ~~Percocet~~ i given for complaints error 11/1/15 ✓ of RUQ pain rated as 6 on a scale of 0 – 10. Z. Hera RN

FIGURE 19–3 Sample of how to make a correction in charting.

agencies differ in the terms accepted, and it is important to carefully follow their guidelines.

4. Date and initial the correction.

5. If an error is made while typing or word processing a document, you may correct it as you work. If it is discovered later, correct it by hand, following steps 1–4 as described here. (See Figure 19–3.)

6. If an error is made when entering data electronically, it cannot be deleted. Instead, there will be a special field in which to note the error.

CONTENTS OF THE MEDICAL RECORD

The medical record will be organized according to facility policy, and the health care professional is expected to maintain the integrity of the record by following all policies and procedures. Many physician offices will have a continuous chronological record format, but in large health care facilities there may be a *source-oriented* approach. This approach divides the record into different sections separated by tabs for each health care specialty. This has the advantage of making it easy to find specific information related to a specialty, but has the disadvantage of increasing the difficulty of seeing the overall view of the patient because many sections need to be referred to for the complete picture. In a source-oriented charting format, the chart may be separated into the following sections:

- History and physicals (H&P) and consultations: Typed or handwritten reports on the initial findings of all physicians seeing the patient. The primary physician will do a complete medical history, which includes a personal, familial, and social history. The personal history includes the patient's past medical problems and surgeries, allergies, current problems, assessment of each body system (see Chapter 20), and medications. The familial history lists medical problems of relatives that may indicate a tendency for the patient to develop these problems. The social history includes use of tobacco, alcohol, and illegal drugs. The suspected diagnosis and plan for further assessment and treatments are also included in

the medical history. Consultations occur when the primary physician asks another physician to see the patient for further evaluation of a specific problem. Some facilities have transcription services in which the physician dictates the detailed findings and then the transcriptionist types from the taped message. This is then placed in the chart for the physician to review and sign. (See Figure 19–4 for a sample medical history form.)

- Physician's orders: Written record of all orders for medications and treatments prescribed for the patient.

- Diagnostic tests: Any report that includes findings obtained in an attempt to diagnose or monitor the progress of patients, such as the results of laboratory tests, X-rays, and electrocardiograms (ECGs).

- Admissions: Completed forms and consents that deal with the admission process.

- Surgical procedures: Consents for, and reports related to, any surgical procedures performed.

- Graphics: A graphed format for blood pressure, temperature, pulse, and respiratory rate; may also have spaces for height and weight.

- Flow sheets: Forms for specialty needs, such as monitoring blood sugar levels or measurements of a wound as it heals. Many specialty fields create forms specific to their needs. (See Figure 19–5.)

- Medication record: Includes all medications administered by health care professionals at the facility.

- Photos: Some facilities allow the use of photos that document physical conditions related to dermatology, plastic surgery, orthopedics, etc. An example of their use is to document progress as treatment progresses.

- Progress notes: Written chronological statements about a patient's care. For example, each time a physician sees a patient he or she will make an additional note to update findings and plan for the care of the patient. Therapists (e.g., physical, occupational, and speech therapists) and other services (e.g., social workers, chaplain services) will note what was done and their assessment of results. Nurses will record what treatments they perform, the patient's response, any abnormal assessments, and plans for intervention. In large facilities, the physician, therapists, and nurses may have different sections of the chart in which to record their documentation.

When filing forms, reviewing charts, or charting, always verify that the correct form is in the chart by checking that the patient's name is on each document. An incorrectly filed form can lead to misunderstandings and errors. When

MEDICAL HISTORY FORM

Date _____
Patient's name _____

Age	Date of birth	Sex	
Address	City	State	Zip code
Phone ( )	Cell phone number	E-mail address	
Insurance company	Policy number		
Place of employment	Address		
Phone ( )	Job responsibilities		
Parent/Guardian if minor			
Address	City	State	Zip code
Phone ( )	Cell phone number	E-mail address	

Family History:

List family members: (mother, father, brothers, sisters, grandparents, etc.)—ages and health status (if deceased write their age at the time of their death and the cause). List allergies and/or any conditions or diseases they may have or have had, such as asthma, arthritis, tuberculosis, diabetes, cancer, heart disease, hypertension, kidney disease, mental illness, depression, or any other health problems that you know of in your family.

_____

_____

Patient's Past History: Mark the boxes to the right either "yes" or "no" for the following questions:*

Do you ever have or have you ever had any of the following: **(Yes) (No)**

SKIN
Rashes, hives, itching or other skin irritations ( ) ( )

EYES, EARS, NOSE, THROAT
Headaches, dizziness, fainting ( ) ( )
Blurred or impaired vision ( ) ( )
Hearing loss or ringing in the ears ( ) ( )
Discharge from eyes or ears ( ) ( )
Sinus trouble/colds/allergies ( ) ( )
Asthma or hay fever ( ) ( )
Sore throats/hoarseness ( ) ( )

CARDIOPULMONARY
Shortness of breath ( ) ( )
Persistent cough or coughing up blood or other secretions ( ) ( )
Chills and/or fever ( ) ( )
Night sweats ( ) ( )
Tuberculosis or exposed to TB ( ) ( )

Scarlet fever or rheumatic fever ( ) ( )
Chest pain ( ) ( )
Heart palpitations or rapid heart-beat or pulse ( ) ( )
High blood pressure ( ) ( )
Swelling of hands and/or feet ( ) ( )

GASTROINTESTINAL
Heartburn or indigestion ( ) ( )
Nausea and/or vomiting ( ) ( )
Loss of appetite ( ) ( )
Belching or gas ( ) ( )
Peptic ulcer, gallbladder or liver disease ( ) ( )
Yellow jaundice or hepatitis ( ) ( )
Diarrhea or constipation ( ) ( )
Dysentery ( ) ( )
Rectal bleeding, hemorrhoids (piles) ( ) ( )
Tarry or clay-colored stools ( ) ( )

GLANDS
Weight gain or loss ( ) ( )

Diabetes ( ) ( )
Thyroid or goiter ( ) ( )
Swollen glands ( ) ( )

GENITOURINARY
Kidney disease or stones, or Bright's disease ( ) ( )
Painful, frequent or urgent urination ( ) ( )
Blood or pus in urine ( ) ( )
Sexually transmitted disease (venereal disease) ( ) ( )
Been sexually active with anyone who has AIDS or HIV or hepatitis ( ) ( )

NEUROMUSCULAR
Problems with becoming tired and/or upset easily ( ) ( )
Nervous breakdown/depression ( ) ( )
Poliomyelitis (infantile paralysis) ( ) ( )
Convulsions ( ) ( )
Joint and/or muscular pain ( ) ( )
Back pain or injury/osteomyelitis/rheumatism ( ) ( )

Are you currently taking any medications? Yes ( ) No ( )
If yes, please list them_____
Have you ever had or been treated for cancer or any tumors? ( ) ( )
Are you anemic or have you ever had to take iron medication? ( ) ( )
Do you use tobacco? ( ) ( )
What type?_____
Do you use IV drugs or alcohol? ( ) ( )

WOMEN ONLY
Painful menstrual periods ( ) ( )
Pregnancy/abortion/miscarriage ( ) ( )
Vaginal infection or discharge/abnormal bleeding ( ) ( )

Last menstrual period_____
Birth control_____
List dates of all operations/surgeries, injuries, and illnesses that required hospitalization:

_____

_____

Did you ever receive benefits from a medical insurance claim due to illness or injury? Yes ( ) No ( )
Were you ever rejected from the military or for employment? ( ) ( )
Were you absent from school/work in the past 10 years because of illness or injury? ( ) ( )
Did you ever file a Workers' Compensation claim? ( ) ( )
Did you ever seek psychological or psychiatric treatment? ( ) ( )

*Please use the back of this form to explain any "yes" answers. Thank you.

FIGURE 19–4 A sample medical history form.

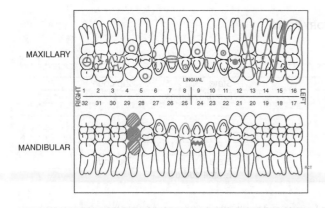

FIGURE 19–5 Sample dental form that uses symbols to record conditions as they occur over time with an individual patient.

filing or adding additional blank forms to the chart, always place them in the correct section in chronological order. The forms within each section will be chronological. The most current is usually on top, depending on facility policy.

If using paper charts, and the file becomes too thick, another file on the patient is started. This is referred to as "thinning a chart." A note is then made in the new chart that an older file exists for this patient. When requesting charts, always make sure that you have all the charts on the patient for review.

Progress Notes

The progress notes make up the written record of every aspect of a patient's relationship with the health care providers. They are the primary tool used to record, communicate, and coordinate the care given to the patient.

Thinking It Through

Sally Jones is an administrative medical assistant for Dr. Yin, an orthopedist in a single-physician office. Sally takes great pride in the appearance of all her work, particularly patient records. She neatly corrects any mistakes made with white correction fluid and is pleased at how tidy the files are. Sally is shocked when Dr. Yin is sued by a patient and loses the case. Dr. Yin's attorney reports that the patient's medical records were largely at fault for the loss of the case.

1. What do you think happened?

2. How might Sally's handling of patient records have contributed to the loss?

3. What recommendations would you make to avoid this type of problem in the future?

Careful documentation is a critical skill for the health care professional. Before charting, it is important for the health care professional to take a moment to organize his or her thoughts. For example, health care professionals can ask themselves what they observed while working with a patient, what has been done for the patient, and what the patient's response was to any interventions. It is important to always address the primary problem that required the assistance of health care services.

There are several ways to organize progress notes. It is the responsibility of health care professionals to learn the formats used at the facilities in which they work. Examples of common approaches are presented next.

Problem-Oriented Charting

Problem-oriented medical records are organized around the patient's health problems. After the initial assessment is completed, a list of problems and related plan of care are identified, and then all subsequent charting refers back to this problem list. If new problems develop, they are added to the list and dated. If a problem is treated and no longer exists, it is marked as resolved and dated. The advantage of this approach is that all health care professionals focus their charting on the same problems. The disadvantages of this approach are difficulties in keeping the problem list up to date and the possibility that patients may be seen more as problems to be resolved than as individual human beings.

The format for charting each problem is known as **SOAP**. These letters stand for the following components of the documentation:

S—Subjective: This is information that is sensed and reported by the patient. Known collectively as *symptoms*, they describe how the patient feels as a result of a disease or injury. It is best to record the patient's own words as closely as possible. Use quotation marks when noting exact words. The **chief complaint** is the reason the patient is seeking medical care and is included in the subjective section of the record. Significant patient behavior, such as missed appointments, failure to follow directions, and statements about discontent with treatments, should also be included in this section.

O—Objective: This information includes the observations made, and measurements taken, by health care personnel and are known as *signs*. Included are temperature and blood pressure; lab test results; description of a wound; color, temperature, and moisture of skin; and how a patient walks (gait).

A—Assessment: The assessment is the health care professional's impression of what is wrong with the patient, based on the signs and symptoms.

Problem List

Date Opened	No. Problem	Identified By	Date Resolved
1/15/15	#1 Angina related to coronary artery disease	B. Meed M.D.	
1/17/15	#2 Impaired mobility due to weakness of right lower extremity secondary to old stroke (1998)	Z. Hera RN	

Plan of Care

Date	Problem
1/15/15	#1 Angina related to coronary artery disease
	GOAL: Prior to discharge patient will be able to ambulate 300 feet with no angina
	PLAN: Gradually increase walking distance & pace after starting on new medication regimen

Progress Note

2/5/15	1700	Problem #1
		S: states "I had no pain in my chest when I walked twice around the floor."
		O: skin cool & dry. B/P 120/76 p. 84
		A: increasing walking distance with no angina
		P: continue to increase walking distance as long as stays angina free.
		Z. Hera RN

FIGURE 19–6 Sample of a problem-oriented progress note.

P—Plan: The plan documents the procedures, treatments, and patient instructions that make up the patient care. (See Figure 19–6.)

A variation of the SOAP charting is SOAPIE. The S, O, and A have the same meanings as just described. The P and the additional letters stand for the following:

P—Plan: What is planned for tests and treatment?

I—Interventions: What interventions are actually carried out?

E—Evaluation: Evaluation of the interventions. What were the results? Was the treatment effective?

Narrative Charting

Narrative charting includes detailed written notes on all aspects of care. It includes routine care, normal and abnormal findings, and any other information related to the patient's plan of care. The advantage of this approach is that the health care professional can use his or her own approach to describe the patient and the care given. The disadvantage is that it is often time-consuming and results in an extensive written record that is difficult to read through to find specific information. (See Figure 19–7.)

11/15/15	1800	Alert and oriented x3. No complaints of pain. Vital signs normal. Ate 100% of dinner. Z. Hera RN

FIGURE 19–7 Sample of a problem-oriented progress note.

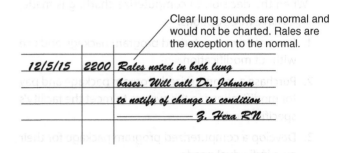

Clear lung sounds are normal and would not be charted. Rales are the exception to the normal.

12/5/15	2200	Rales noted in both lung bases. Will call Dr. Johnson to notify of change in condition Z. Hera RN

FIGURE 19–8 Sample of a problem-oriented progress note.

Charting by Exception (CBE)

Charting by exception is an abbreviated format. Only abnormal findings are noted. This requires a well-defined understanding of the normal findings that are used for a comparison. If no abnormal findings are found, then no written notes are required. The advantage in this approach is that it saves time and that the problems are easily identified by reviewing the notes. The disadvantage is that it is problem oriented, so the preventative or wellness aspects of care are not included. (See Figure 19–8.)

ELECTRONIC HEALTH RECORDKEEPING

In Chapter 18, the multiple uses of computers in health care were introduced. The impact of computers on health care professionals includes the trend toward computerization of medical records, the most significant change to date in patient care documentation. Facilities that do not currently have computerized systems will likely have them in the future as the hardware and software become more affordable. Computerized information and integration systems are replacing the written medical records systems that have been used for decades, kept in file folders, and filling rows of shelves and filing cabinets.

Electronic medical records (EMRs) are digital versions of the paper documents described previously. Electronic health records (EHRs) are designed to include information from all the health care professionals involved in a patient's care and enable information-sharing with other providers, such as laboratories and pharmacies (https://www.healthit.gov/faq/what-are-differences-between-electronic-medical-records-electronic-health-records-and-personal).

The U.S. government has promoted the use of computerized records as a way to make health care safer, more efficient, and more cost effective. In 2009, a federal economic stimulus package set aside grant money for physicians who accept Medicare and Medicaid patients to set up electronic medical record systems.

When the decision to computerize charting is made, facilities have three options:

1. Purchase a computerized program package and use without modification

2. Purchase a computerized program package and pay for modifications to the system to meet the facility's specific needs

3. Develop a computerized program package for their own individual needs

The choice of options is greatly influenced by identifying the needs of the facility versus the cost involved in the purchase and implementation of the program. These options are listed from least to most expensive. The most common decision by a facility is to choose option number 2. Most computerized programs are not specific enough for the individual needs of the facility, but trying to design a customized version is both very costly and time-consuming. In addition, many facilities do not have the in-house expertise to design such a sophisticated program. The software vendor and facility enter into a contract that details the cost of any modifications. The need to modify is likely to decrease in the future, as vendors are learning to create systems that more closely meet the needs of specific types of facilities, such as hospitals. (See Figure 19–9, A–C for examples of computerized records.)

Example of a Computerized System

EMRs and EHRs can go far beyond the core charting to include multipart systems that coordinate with laboratory, radiology, pharmacy, admission-discharge-transfer functions, and tools to allow data exchange. For example, for Ellen Nordstrom's visit with Dr. Stevens, the following transactions can take place:

- Ellen makes an appointment to see Doctor Stevens and the receptionist records the time and date.

- Before the appointment, Dr. Stevens quickly reviews Ellen's record to see the past history, current medications, and recent labs.

- Ellen arrives at the front desk, the receptionist records her arrival time in the computer, and the back office personnel are notified.

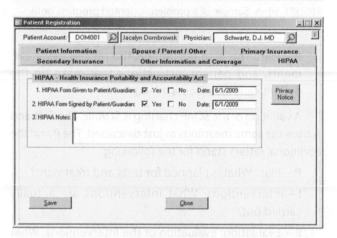

FIGURE 19–9 A—A sample computer database screen for statistical information. B—A sample computer database screen for insurance information. C—A sample computer database screen for HIPAA information.

- The medical assistant takes Ellen to the exam room, takes her vital signs, and enters them into her electronic medical record.

- During the visit, Dr. Stevens records his findings.

- Following the visit, Dr. Stevens can electronically order any new medications, labs, or other tests and place referrals.

- After the visit, Ellen can go to the lab, pharmacy, radiology, or other area where the orders will already be in the computer.

Advantages of Computerized Systems

As seen in the previous section, computerized systems can improve communication and efficiency in the medical facility. In addition, the following advantages that can improve patient care make the case for the switch to computerization:

- Reduction of errors: This is considered to be one of the most significant advantages of computerized recordkeeping. Handwriting can be illegible and transcription miscommunicated. These common errors are less likely to occur with the computer.

- Safety features: Many EMRs have flags or hard stops if an order is placed incorrectly, such as the wrong dosage of a medication.

- Easier access: Authorized health care professionals can access the patient's medical record from a variety of locations.

- Improved communication: Health care professionals can more easily exchange information, especially those who work in different departments or facilities. Also, systems can enable patients to view their own records, see upcoming appointments, and send e-mails to their providers.

- Standardization: Standard recordkeeping formats throughout the systems further improve communication between staff and departments.

- Improved privacy: Electronic records, if secured with passwords and encryption, are less at risk than paper records which are usually not stored in locked areas and may pass through many hands.

- Improved efficiency: Test results, for example, can be uploaded quickly and used by professionals immediately to make diagnoses and recommend treatment.

- Information sources: Extensive libraries of information can be accessed for provider research and clarification of recommended treatment protocols.

- Patient information and education: Documents that detail what has been ordered, future appointments, and any screening tests that are due can be printed out for patients to take home. If the system is tied to a patient education databank, educational materials can be printed out for patients to refer to later to reinforce information that may have been missed or forgotten when explained verbally at the visit.

- Addition of documents: Many systems can accept scanned documents. This allows for other forms of written material presented by the patient or a family member to be included in the computerized system, if they are deemed helpful.

Other helpful features a computerized system may have are "copy and paste" and "smart phrase" functions. These features have the ability, with only a few key strokes, to add extensive text to your document. Both features can save a great deal of time when charting commonly performed actions because much of the information does not have to be retyped. However, it can lead to problems if not used with caution. Information that is copied and pasted from a previous entry should be modified to demonstrate updated content with relevance for the current date. Although inserting a smart phrase that details the entire procedure you may be preparing to perform can be very advantageous, blanks frequently need to be filled and findings relevant to the process added to personalize the entry. Leaving the information unaltered, without modification, can misrepresent the patient's condition or the care provided during the encounter.

Challenges of Computerized Systems

In spite of the benefits to be gained from the computerization of health records and management, moving from paper to digital is a huge shift. A major challenge is the training of personnel. Change creates increased stress in an already stressful work environment. Time, training, support, and patience are required by everyone involved in the transition.

Some of the major benefits of computerization can also present problems, as seen in the following list of potential challenges:

- Cost: Purchasing a system can cost a small physician clinic hundreds of thousands of dollars; a system for a hospital or multifacility organization can cost millions of dollars. Including the initial cost, staff must be trained and the system must be maintained. For many individuals and organizations, these costs can be prohibitive.

- Cybersecurity: Some experts believe this to be the most serious threat to the computerization of health care information management. This is one reason for the passage of the Health Insurance Portability and Accountability Act of 1996, discussed later in this chapter. It is reported that in 2015, 113 million health records were compromised, 78.8 million of them in a single cyberattack. In response, cybersecurity budgets have increased, although it is reported that fewer than one third of U.S. health care organizations have a comprehensive cybersecurity program in place (https://www.hipaajournal.com/category/healthcare-cybersecurity/). According to *Becker's Hospital Review*, data breaches cost the health care industry $5.6 billion every year (https://healthinformatics.uic.edu/resources/articles/cybersecurity-how-can-it-be-improved-in-health-care/).

- Incompatibility of Systems: Many EMRs and EHRs have been developed by a variety of software companies. In the hurry to create systems for sale, many companies used variations of existing software. Adding to incompatibility of different systems is the competition between developers who do not want to share their data. As a result, it frequently happens that health care facilities cannot communicate with each other, leading to communication breakdowns, repetition of procedures, etc. This also leads to inconvenience for patients. For example, a patient may have an internist, a cardiologist, an ophthalmologist, and one or more other specialists involved in her care, with each using a different software system. This patient must set up a personal ID and password for each different computer system so she can access her health data or e-mail her provider. Some standards have been proposed to make systems more able to communicate seamlessly, but all parties must agree on what these are and this takes time. Some have proposed that it will take the collective effort of the government, providers, payers (Medicare and insurance companies), and patients to lead to true compatibility (also called *interoperability*) of EMRs and EHRs.

Providers' Concerns

- Barrier between them and their patients. Patients see their physicians staring at a computer screen instead of interacting with them. A related concern is that inputting data is cutting into the time providers would rather spend caring for patients.
- Technical malfunctions or software that does not meet all the requirements of the organization. A related problem is the start-up time needed when a new computer system is introduced, especially problematic in places such as busy hospital emergency departments where there isn't time for personnel to quickly learn the new system.
- Over-standardization that allows input only for the fields that have been entered into the system, making it difficult or impossible to enter lesser-used medications or treatments.

PERSONAL HEALTH RECORD

Personal health records (PHRs) are documents created and maintained by individual patients to help them communicate with various health care providers. Due to the mobility of individuals and the frequent changes in health care providers and insurance groups, it is recommended that each individual keep a PHR to ensure greater continuity of care. When patients bring their own PHR with them it benefits both the provider and the patient. It helps prevent the patient from forgetting information and also minimizes long delays on the provider's end in requesting the information from a prior source.

The type of information frequently provided in a PHR includes the following:

- Demographics, such as name, address, and contact information
- Emergency contacts
- Name, specialty, and contact information of previous health care providers
- Insurance provider(s)
- Medical directives, living will, organ donation, and so on
- General medical information: height, weight, blood type, vital signs, and so forth
- Allergies and drug sensitivities
- Current conditions and dates of diagnoses
- Previous surgeries, including date and results
- Medications (prescription and nonprescription)
- Immunizations and when last received
- Any relevant health care visits, such as hospitalizations, other specialists or therapists
- Pregnancies
- Medical devices
- Foreign travel
- Family history information

SAFEGUARDING HEALTH RECORDS

The health care professional must at all times be aware of and protect the privacy of the patient's record. Confidentiality of health information is both an ethical and legal matter. As discussed in the section, "Be Discreet" in Chapter 3, patient information cannot be released to anyone without the patient's written approval. Violating patient confidentiality, even if well intentioned, can result in a lawsuit and other serious consequences for the health care professional.

HIPAA

HIPAA (Health Insurance Portability and Accountability Act of 1996) is discussed in Chapter 3. But due to its importance, it is worth expanding on the provisions of this act that relate to medical records and documentation. Recall that HIPAA mandated significant changes in the legal and regulatory environment governing the provision of health benefits, the delivery of, and payment for, health care services, and the privacy and security of individually identifiable, protected health information (PHI) in written, electronic, and oral formats. It is the Privacy and Security Rules that are of greatest significance to medical records. The Privacy Rule gives the patient specific rights related to his or her medical record, such as the right to request:

- Access to and copies of the medical record
- An amendment to the medical record
- An accounting of disclosures of PHI
- A limit on information about himself or herself that is provided in a hospital directory

The Security Rule has administrative, physical, and technical safeguards. The following examples pertain to electronic PHI:

- Administrative safeguards: Developing security policies and procedures regarding use of electronic health records (EHRs); training the entire workforce on implementation of these policies and procedures
- Physical safeguards: Preventing unauthorized viewing of computer terminals by positioning them in appropriate locations, having screes that cannot be read from side angles, and not propping open doors that allow unauthorized access to private work areas
- Technical safeguards: Following good password policies and logging off the computer when stepping away

If you are working with paper charts, it is important not to leave them lying around where others can view them. Specific rules and regulations dictate who can be given copies of a chart and what procedure must be followed to request copies. Ask your supervisor for these guidelines and follow them without exception. If you are working with computerized records, your computer must be locked before leaving the station to prevent others from casually viewing the record. Many computers are located in traffic areas and a privacy screen placed over the monitor prevents others from reading the material unless they are directly in front of the monitor. Remember that patients' medical information belongs to them and them alone. No one else has a right to that information, regardless of the relationship, without the consent of the patient. If a patient is unable to handle his or her own health care decisions, then a power of attorney should be on file specifying who has the authority to receive information and make decisions. This limitation of access also applies to health care professionals. If you are not actively involved in a patient's care, you do not have a right to access that patient's chart. You also do not have a right to access a coworker's chart or a family member's or friend's chart. Breaking any of the HIPAA regulations could result in a lawsuit by the patient and/or corrective action that could include the following:

- Notification of the federal government if an incident involves a Medicare patient.
- Notification of the individual patient whose PHI was illegally accessed, used, or disclosed.
- Corrective action, up to and including termination, for the individual health care professional responsible for the incident.

Cybersecurity

As stated in a previous section, the widespread use of electronic health records has resulted in threats to the security of patient information. Social security numbers, personal IDs, and sensitive health facts have been reported stolen by hackers who demand huge payments for the return of the data.

The individual health care professional can help prevent these thefts by taking the following steps:

- Be aware of the importance of protecting patient data
- Practice good computer habits, such as closing programs when not in use
- Back up files
- Use strong passwords and change them regularly, following your facility's policies (A strong password consists of at least six characters, the more the better, that are a combination of letters, both uppercase and lowercase, along with numbers and symbols [@, #, $, %, etc.] if allowed.)
- Never share your password with anyone
- Secure your laptop to prevent it from being stolen

Sending Protected Information

Although sending information by facsimile (fax) is commonly used in all types of business and personal transactions, HIPAA Privacy and Security Rules consider it to be an unsecure method of transmitting data. Therefore, it should be used as little as possible and only by health care providers for treatment purposes, such as in an emergency when faxing is the best method to send or receive necessary information; or when the patient makes a written request that a fax be sent.

When a fax is sent, it should contain only the data necessary for the situation and be sent to a machine monitored by authorized health care personnel or the patient or a person designated by the patient. Include a cover sheet with a headline in bold type: **Confidential Health Information Enclosed.** As an additional safeguard, fax machines in health care facilities should be located in secure areas to avoid unauthorized access.

When available, *secure e-mails* should be used to send protected health information instead of faxes. These are transmissions that are encrypted, or scrambled, as they pass from the sender's to the receiver's computer. An exception is if a patient signs a form that explains the risks to confidentiality and gives you permission to send him or her unencrypted e-mails, A number of e-mail encryption services are available, but only one that supports HIPAA guidelines should be used by the health care facility. In non-urgent cases, it is recommended that PHI be sent by U.S. mail or a messenger.

Finally, there is the matter of disposing of anything that contains PHI. Paper records cannot be placed in waste baskets or dumpsters that are available to the public. They should be shredded, burned, or otherwise made unreadable. Prescription bottles with patient names should be stored in opaque plastic bags and picked up by a professional disposal vendor. Electronic records should be cleared or purged, using specialized software that makes the data inaccessible.

SUGGESTED LEARNING ACTIVITIES

1. If you are currently working in a health care facility, review some of the written or computerized documents and evaluate the documentation of records which you are authorized to view. Why are the examples good or poor? Can you get a real picture of that patient by reading the chart? *Remember to follow HIPAA guidelines and access only those records that you are working with as part of your designated work assignment.*

2. Create a patient who presents a specific health problem. Then write samples using the three formats of progress notes presented and check them against the characteristics of good documentation. If you make an error, remember to make the corrections according to accepted guidelines.

3. Work with another student to identify a specific situation that may occur in your health care specialty area. Then each of you should write a documentation. Compare your results.

4. Prepare a personal health record (PHR) with your health information following the guidelines presented in the text regarding the type of content to be included.

WEB ACTIVITIES

Seer Training Modules

Composition of a Medical Record

https://training.seer.cancer.gov/abstracting/record/

Review the material in this multipage training module, then write a summary of what you learn.

Capterra

Electronic Medical Record (EMR) Software

https://www.capterra.com/electronic-medical-records-software/#infographic

This site contains recommendations and reviews electronic medical records software. Choose two or three programs and view their profiles. Compare the features listed for each program and determine which one you feel would be the most helpful in the field you are interested in pursuing.

All Nurses

Nurses Notes: Guidelines on What Not to Chart

https://allnurses.com/nursing-issues-patient/nurses-notes-guidelines-913714.html

Identify three items not to chart that you previously did not know.

HIPAA Journal

https://www.hipaajournal.com/category/healthcare-cybersecurity/

Choose an article in this section on cybersecurity to read and then write a summary of what you learn.

Health IT Outcomes

Fixing the EHR Interoperability Mess

https://www.healthitoutcomes.com/doc/fixing-the-ehr-interoperability-mess-0001

After reading the article, create three lists:

1. Problems encountered by physicians when they cannot communicate over electronic EHR systems

2. Reasons for the incompatibility of systems

3. Suggestions for improving interoperability

Science Daily

When Hospitals Share Patient Records, Emergency Patients Benefit, Study Suggests

https://www.sciencedaily.com/releases/2014/01/140124101900.htm

After reading the news release, answer the following questions.

1. What advantage did the study find with hospitals that could access each other's records?

2. What do you think would be other benefits for patients if hospitals can share patient records?

3. What would be the probable impact on health care costs?

REVIEW QUESTIONS

1. What is the meaning of the following terms: medical documentation, medical record, and charting?

2. What are five examples of charting tasks performed by health care professionals?

3. What are nine major purposes of medical documentation?

4. What are five characteristics of good medical documentation?

5. What are six possible negative consequences of poor medical documentation?

6. How should errors be corrected on medical records?

7. What is a source-oriented approach to recordkeeping and what are typical contents of the medical record?

8. What are progress notes and what is their purpose?

9. What is problem-oriented charting and what are its advantages and disadvantages?

10. What is SOAP and what do the letters stand for?

11. What is narrative charting and what are its advantages and disadvantages?

12. What is charting by exception and what are its advantages and disadvantages?

13. What is the meaning of the following terms: electronic medical records and electronic health records?

14. What are the options a health care facility has when converting to an electronic record system?

15. What are three ways an electronic health system can be used in a physician's office?

16. What are ten advantages of an electronic health record system?

17. What are seven disadvantages of an electronic health record system?

18. What is contained in a personal health record (PHR) and why is it important for an individual to have one?

19. What are the main features of the Health Insurance Portability and Accountability Act of 1996 (HIPAA), including the Privacy and Security Rules?

20. What can be done to help prevent hackers from stealing computerized data?

21. When and how should faxes and e-mails containing protected health information be sent?

22. What is the proper way to dispose of materials, including those stored on computers, that contain protected health information?

APPLICATION EXERCISES

1. Refer back to the Case of the Therapist Who Hates to Write at the beginning of the chapter.

   a. What are the possible consequences of the therapist's approach to charting?

   b. What characteristics of good charting is he not following?

2. Ms. Henrietta Jenkins, a nursing assistant at an ambulatory clinic, is helping Mr. Wilkins off of the examining table. Mr. Wilkins suddenly feels faint, his legs give out from under him, and he falls to the floor. Ms. Jenkins notes that Mr. Wilkins never lost consciousness, but he is confused and asks where he is. She notes a 2- by 3-centimeter red mark on his forehead. His vital signs are B/P 100/60, T 98.6, P 92, R 20 (B/P, blood pressure; T, temperature; P, pulse; R, respirations). The physician examines Mr. Wilkins, finds no other injuries, and notes that he is no longer confused. Another set of vital signs are taken: B/P 124/80, P 78, R 18. Mr. Wilkins states he is feeling fine and leaves without further incident.

   a. What would be documented using problem-oriented charting?

   b. What would be documented using narrative charting?

   c. What would be documented using charting by exception?

   d. What additional information, if any, would be needed to complete the progress notes using each of the three charting formats?

PROBLEM-SOLVING PRACTICE

Katrina Cabrillo has always hated the idea of computers. She realizes that the Internet and e-mail are useful for other people, but thinks they are not necessary for her job. Recently she learned that her facility will be computerizing its charting, and she is horrified. She is so anxious that she has difficulty sleeping at night. Using the five-step problem-solving process, determine what Katrina can do about the fact that her facility will have computerized charting within the next year.

CHAPTER 20

Physical Assessment

KEY TERMS

afebrile
apnea
baseline
bradycardia
bradypnea
Cheyne-Stokes
dyspnea
eupnea
exhalation
febrile
hypertension
hypotension
inhalation
orthopnea
orthostatic (postural)
    hypotension
pulse deficit
pulse points
respiration
sphygmomanometer
stethoscope
tachycardia
tachypnea
vital signs

OBJECTIVES

Studying and applying the material in this chapter will help you to:

1. State the purpose of a history and physical (H&P).
2. List the information obtained in a complete H&P.
3. List the contents contained in a review of all body systems.
4. Define the term "baseline" and explain its importance.
5. Explain the meaning and significance of "variances from the normal."
6. Explain the difference between "assessment" and "data collection."
7. List eight examples of questions to use during the general survey of a patient.
8. List the components of, and questions to use when determining, the psychosocial status of a patient.
9. Define the following terms used during a physical assessment: inspection, auscultation, palpation, and percussion.
10. List the questions, observations, and actions to use when collecting information about the following systems and organs: musculoskeletal, integumentary, circulatory, respiratory, digestive, urinary, eyes and ears, nervous, endocrine, and reproductive (female and male).
11. Explain the purpose and value of using a pain rating scale.
12. Define "activities of daily living" and give five examples.
13. List the vital signs.
14. Describe what happens when the body gets too warm or too cool.
15. Describe the various types of thermometers for taking body temperature.
16. Explain the correct procedures for taking a temperature.
17. List the location of the body's major pulse points.
18. Explain the correct ways to take a pulse, including a pulse deficit assessment check.
19. Describe the two steps in the process of respiration.
20. Explain three observations to make when taking the respiratory rate.
21. State when the respiratory rate should be reported to your supervisor.
22. Explain the meaning of blood pressure, including the terms "systolic" and "diastolic."
23. Define the terms "hypotension" and "hypertension."
24. Give the blood pressure categories and corresponding numerical ranges for adults.
25. List possible effects of uncontrolled high blood pressure.
26. State the possible causes of hypotension and list the signs and symptoms.
27. Explain how to take a blood pressure reading.
28. List the factors that can affect blood pressure.

29. Explain the meaning of "white coat syndrome."
30. Explain the meaning and cause of orthostatic hypotension.
31. Describe conditions under which an arm should not be used for measuring blood pressure.
32. Explain how vital signs vary over the life span.
33. Explain why it is important to measure the height of older adults over time.
34. Explain why children and adolescents should regularly be weighed and measured for height.
35. Describe the various types of scales for weighing patients and how to use each.
36. Explain the meaning of the body mass index and how it is used.

The Case of the Unreported Observations

Mrs. Becker, age 83, arrives on time as usual for her appointment with Dr. Myers. Carrie Winsor, medical assistant, notes that Mrs. Becker seems unsteady as she walks across the room. When asked if she is all right, Mrs. Becker's answer is slightly garbled, but she states, "I must just be getting old." When Mrs. Becker speaks, Carrie notes a sweet, fruity smell that she thinks must be mouthwash. Carrie thinks Mrs. Becker seems depressed, but then thinks that she would be too if she had all the physical problems the patient has had with her diabetes, especially now that she has recently been diagnosed with renal failure and has started on dialysis. Dr. Myers is running behind with her appointments, and Carrie knows that it will be at least another 30 minutes and informs Mrs. Becker. Carrie continues with her other tasks, until she hears a sudden sound and finds Mrs. Becker on the floor and unconscious. This chapter will discuss how to objectively observe patients and how important it is for the health care professional to observe and promptly report abnormal findings to his or her supervisor so that early detection and treatment can be initiated.

GENERAL ASSESSMENT

The physician (or other primary care provider) takes a history and performs a physical exam on patients when they are seen for the first time or when they are admitted to the hospital. This is called the history and physical, commonly referred to as the H&P. As discussed in the previous chapter, the physician then either writes the findings in the patient's chart or enters them into the computer. If the facility is not computerized, the provider may have the option of dictating the notes for someone else to type up and place in the chart. When the typed information is placed in the chart, the physician must review it for accuracy and then sign the document.

An accurate and thorough H&P is very important because it provides the data on which the physician bases the initial diagnosis and treatment. The H&P consists of the following information:

- Date: The day on which the H&P is done.
- Demographic data: Includes age, sex, race, place of birth, marital status, occupation, and religion.

- Source of referral: Often one physician refers a patient to another because of that individual's expertise in a specific area; if so, it will be stated as such.
- Chief complaint(s): The primary problem from the patient's view—why the patient is seeking medical care.
- History of present illness: Includes when the problem first started; how frequently it occurs; how long it lasts; description, location, and severity of symptoms; if they are aggravated by any specific activities; if anything relieves the problem; if any treatments have been tried; and their effect on the symptoms.
- History: Includes the general state of the patient's health and any previous physical or psychological illnesses, accidents, injuries, surgeries, and hospitalizations.
- Current health status: Includes a list of allergies and immunizations; normal activity level and diet; current medications (prescription and over-the-counter);

if tobacco, alcohol, or illegal drugs are used; if any environmental or safety hazards are present; and if there are any sleep pattern disturbances.

- Family history of illness: Includes the age and health or cause of death of parents, siblings, spouse, and children. The physician will also ask if any family members have, or are experiencing, similar symptoms. The family history of specific diseases or conditions is also included (e.g., diabetes, heart disease, high blood pressure, cancer).

- Psychosocial history: Includes the home situation and support structure (family and friends) and any significant information that may affect the care of the patient.

- Review of all systems: Includes height, weight, vital signs, and a review of each body system. When a complete physical assessment is done, it is commonly referred to as a head-to-toe assessment, which indicates that all systems are being evaluated. It can also indicate a method that some health care professionals use to organize their assessment. The following survey is based on assessment of an adult patient. When working with children (pediatrics), the approach will vary depending on the child's age and condition (e.g., when assessing young children, it may be more appropriate to start with the feet instead of the head; also normal findings will vary based on the age of the child). After assessing orientation, the process would include an examination in the following order:

1. Head

2. Neck

3. Upper extremities

4. Chest (respiratory and cardiac systems)

5. Abdomen (digestive, urinary, and reproductive systems)

6. Lower extremities

The musculoskeletal, integumentary, nervous, endocrine, vascular, and lymphatic systems are relevant to the entire body and are assessed as one moves along the body.

The information obtained during the H&P is considered the baseline. The baseline information is important to determine how the patient is progressing in relationship to how he or she was at a particular point in time. It is important for the health care professional to review the H&P on the patient's subsequent visits because this information will increase the understanding of the patient's condition.

Noting Variances from Normal

A critical function of the health care professional is to be able to discriminate between normal and abnormal conditions and situations. Learning to observe patients, their symptoms, and their actions and asking appropriate questions provide vital information that can be used by other health care professionals and the physician in the care of the patient.

The observational skills needed are based on a thorough understanding of normal anatomy and physiology. When the meaning of normal is understood, it is an easy step to identify abnormal situations. A health care professional who observes an abnormal condition should immediately report the finding to his or her supervisor. Remember, though, that some patients begin with problems noted in the H&P. In this case, it is more valuable to compare a change in condition to this baseline.

Any change in a patient's condition may indicate a worsening of the condition, an improvement, a new problem developing, or a need for a change in treatment. The health care professionals who interact with, and observe, a patient over time may provide valuable information that the physician may not detect during relatively brief visits with the patient. It is for this reason that strong assessment skills are needed by all health care professionals whose responsibilities include interaction with patients.

Before continuing with the material presented in this chapter, it is important to note the distinction that is made when using the term *assessment* versus *observation* and *data collection*. In the health care workplace, the term *assessment* is restricted to activities performed by licensed health care professionals. When unlicensed health care professionals ask questions and make observations, it is called *data collection*. This distinction in no way negates the value of data collection. It is often the data collected by the unlicensed health care professional that guides licensed personnel to do further assessments.

General Survey

A problem with dividing the body into systems for the purpose of study is that health care professionals sometimes forget to look at the patient as a whole. To prevent this from happening, the health care professional should develop the habit of first performing a general survey of the patient. This means looking at and listening to the patient to secure an overall impression of presentation. It is important to note the normal findings in addition to the abnormal. How does the patient appear? What is the general impression you get from the patient? Another advantage of this approach is that it provides information about which area to focus on if time is limited. When doing

a general survey, the health care professional should look for answers to the following questions:

- What is the overall impression of the patient? Does he or she appear strong and healthy looking or weak and ill?

- What is the posture? Is the patient walking normally with a straight and erect posture or is he or she stooped or limping? Is there paralysis present?

- Are there any signs of distress? Is the patient moving and communicating freely or is there difficulty breathing, face wincing in pain, sweating or trembling, or holding part of the body (hand over area or rubbing area on body may indicate pain)?

- What is the body proportion and size? Is the body proportionate and normal in size or is there a noted disproportion, such as very thin or obese, tall or short?

- What is the color of the skin? Is the skin normal in tone or pale, flushed (reddish), jaundiced (yellow), or cyanotic (gray, dusty, or blue)? In non-Caucasian patients, the nail beds, whites of the eyes, and mucous membranes should be examined for color changes.

- Are any odors noted from body or breath? For example, is there a sweet or fruity smell to the breath (may be untreated diabetic or severe restriction of food intake)? Alcohol breath?

- What is the character of speech? Does the patient speak clearly and normally or is speech hesitant, slurred, fast, or slow?

- What are the vital signs (temperature, pulse, respirations, and blood pressure)? During these procedures, which are discussed later in the chapter, you will be touching the patient's skin. This provides the opportunity to note the skin for temperature changes and moisture (warm, cold, dry, moist); shaking the patient's hand upon greeting also provides an opportunity to note the skin temperature and moisture.

- What is the height and weight? Has there been a recent gain or loss?

- What is the level of consciousness? When patients have a diminished level of consciousness, it is necessary to note the extent of the problem, so comparisons can be made that indicate whether the patient is getting better or worse. Areas to note are:

  ○ Orientation: What is their best verbal response? Are they oriented to time (can tell you what day it is and what time), place (can tell you where they are), and person (can state their name)? Are they confused, inappropriate, or incomprehensible, or is there no response?

  ○ If there is no verbal response, note whether the eyes open spontaneously, or perhaps only to speech or to pain, or there is no response.

  ○ What is their best motor response—do they obey commands, move only in response to pain, or is there no response?

Using appropriate communication skills is necessary when working with patients. How we communicate verbally and nonverbally often determines the quality of the response we get when interviewing patients. Refer back to Chapter 16 to review special communication skills.

Psychosocial Observations

When performing a general survey, both the physical and psychological aspects of the patient need to be considered. When incorporating a psychosocial status of patients, along with a general survey, the following questions can guide the health care professional:

- Emotional status: What are the emotional responses? For example, is the patient anxious, angry, depressed, indifferent? Are the facial expressions appropriate to what is being discussed?

- Mental status: Is the patient's behavior appropriate for his or her age? What is the attention span? Does the patient ask appropriate questions? Can the patient recall information and incorporate new information?

- Appearance: Is the patient dressed appropriately for the weather? Well groomed? Does the patient have good personal hygiene? (This may give clues on emotional status or ability to care for self.)

Physical Observations

Skills frequently used during physical assessment are inspection, palpation, percussion, and auscultation.

- Inspection: Using the senses of vision, hearing, and smell for observation of patient condition.

- Auscultation: Listening to sounds inside the body with the aid of a stethoscope (e.g., lungs, heart, and bowel sounds).

- Palpation: Using the hands and fingers on the exterior of the body to detect evidence of abnormalities in the various internal body organs.

- Percussion: Using the fingertips to lightly tap on the exterior of the body to determine position, size, and consistency of underlying structures.

The preceding skills will be briefly introduced in the following sections as they relate to each of the systems presented earlier in Chapter 7. The health care professional

should chart the normal and the abnormal findings, so a complete picture of the patient can be documented. Palpation and percussion of the body will not be covered, as these are more advanced skills. As health care students progress through their educational programs, additional and more advanced skills will be introduced that are specific to their specialties. Examples of advanced skills that may be performed by licensed health care professionals will be listed, but not expanded on, because they are beyond the scope of this text.

Musculoskeletal

- Is there any discomfort with movement (pain, muscle spasms, stiffness)?
- Is the gait (manner of walking) normal or altered? Observe the posture.
- Observe muscle strength: Can the patient turn in bed without assistance; does the patient complain of weakness; is walking done with or without assistance?

Examples of advanced skills are inspection of joints for any swelling or deformity, assessment of the range of motion (ROM) of joints in which discomfort is experienced, and assessment of the amount of counter-resistance (pulling against an examiner's pull) to a force that a patient can maintain.

Integumentary

- Status of skin: What is the color and temperature (warm or cold), hair distribution? Note whether dry or moist.
- Are there any cuts, scrapes, swelling, rashes, incisions, or bruises on the skin?

Circulatory

- What are the vital signs?
- What is the weight? Has there been a recent unexplained gain or loss of weight?
- Is there any pain in the extremities? Where does pain occur; how is pain relieved (resting, elevation, or placing extremity in dependent position); does it occur at night; how far can the patient walk before leg pain occurs (claudication distance)?
- Palpate peripheral pulses for quality and strength. (Pulse points are presented later in this chapter.)
- Inspect extremities for swelling.
- Observe capillary refill: Pinch the patient's fingertip and let go, then watch how long it takes for the nail bed to become pink again. The nail beds of patients

with poor circulation to the extremities will take longer to return to a pink color. Use fingers/toes if nail beds are discolored or too thick to detect color changes.

- Inspect for neck vein distension: With the patient in erect or sitting position, inspect the neck for distension of the jugular veins; normally there is no distension of neck veins when in an erect position.
- Observe for activity intolerance: Does the patient report fatigue, palpitations (pounding felt in heart), or syncope (fainting) when engaging in any activities of daily living?

Examples of advanced skills include palpating the calf area for tenderness; using dorsiflexion (movement of the foot backward at the ankle) to check for pain in the calf, an indication of possible clots in the leg; auscultating breath and heart sounds, and using a Doppler probe if pulses are nonpalpable.

Respiratory

- What are the respiratory rate and rhythm?
- What colors are the skin and mucous membranes?
- Is there obvious difficulty with breathing? Is there any chest pain when breathing?
- Is there a cough? Productive (coughing up mucus) or nonproductive? If productive, what is the color (clear, white, yellow, green, red) and consistency (thin, thick, frothy) of the mucus?
- If the patient is experiencing difficulty breathing, when does this occur? Is there dyspnea (difficulty breathing) on exertion? Does the patient use accessory muscles to assist breathing (lifting shoulders on inspiration, retraction of abdominal muscles with respiration, flaring of nostrils)? Is the chest unusually large and rounded in shape? (This is called a barrel chest and may indicate an underlying chronic respiratory condition.)
- Check for cyanosis (bluish or purplish discoloration): Do the skin or nail beds appear cyanotic? The skin of a Caucasian patient who is receiving adequate oxygen is pink; in dark-skinned patients, a problem with oxygenation is noted by looking at the nail beds, lips, and mucous membranes of the mouth.
- Does the patient have orthopnea (i.e., does the patient breathe easier in a sitting versus a standing position)?

Examples of advanced skills are auscultation and percussion of the lungs, determining if the chest expansion is symmetrical or asymmetrical, and determining which accessory muscles are used for breathing.

Digestive

- What is the size and contour of the abdomen? Is the abdomen round, flat, or distended? Soft or hard?
- Has there been a change in bowel pattern or color or consistency of stools?
- When was the last bowel movement?
- Is there any abdominal discomfort? How is it relieved? What aggravates it?
- Have there been any sudden changes in weight and appetite?

Examples of advanced skills are auscultation of bowel sounds in all four quadrants and palpating for tenderness and masses.

Urinary

- What is the appearance of the urine (clear or cloudy, yellow or some other color)?
- Is there any burning when the patient urinates? Any urgency (sudden, strong desire to urinate), hesitancy (having the urge to urinate but difficulty getting started), or frequency (urinating more often than normal)?
- Does the patient have nocturia (the need to get up during the night to urinate)? If so, how often?
- Is the patient ever incontinent (unable to retain urine)? If so, does it occur all the time or only when coughing, laughing, or sneezing?

Examples of advanced skills are palpation and percussion of the bladder.

Eyes and Ears

Eye

- Are there any complaints of discomfort in the eye (pain, foreign body sensation, itching or irritation, fatigue)?
- Are there any complaints of visual disturbances—floaters or spots, loss of vision, tunnel vision (loss of peripheral vision), flashes of light, halos around lights, blurred vision, diplopia (double vision), curtain or veil over visual field, difficulty with color discrimination, photophobia (hypersensitivity to light)?
- Is there redness, swelling, drainage, tearing, or squinting when attempting to read printed material, or crusting of eyelashes?

Examples of advanced skills include using an ophthalmoscope to examine the internal structures of the eye, examining the movement of eyeballs and eyelids, and assessing the reaction of pupils to light (see later section).

Ear

- Is there any drainage from the ear?
- What is the patient experiencing (e.g., feeling of fullness; unusual sounds, such as popping or cracking when yawning or swallowing; heart beating in ear; tinnitus [ringing in the ears])? If a child is having discomfort in the ear, he or she is most likely to demonstrate it by rubbing the ear and crying.
- Does the patient use a hearing aid? Does the patient have a cochlear implant? The cochlear implant is an electronic device that can help provide a sense of sound to a person who is profoundly deaf or severely hard of hearing. The implant consists of an external portion that sits behind the ear and a second portion that is surgically placed under the skin.
- Hearing acuity: Is there difficulty hearing in one ear or both? Does the patient show behaviors consistent with diminished hearing, such as turning the head and leaning closer when spoken to or frequently asking for statements to be repeated? Many patients compensate for a hearing loss by reading the lips of the speaker. To prevent this from disguising hearing loss, the health care professional can speak while standing behind the patient or when the patient's back is turned.

Examples of advanced skills include using an otoscope to look inside the ear canal to examine the internal structures and conducting various hearing tests.

Nervous

- Is there any numbness or tingling?
- Many types of abnormal data already discussed may indicate a neurological problem, such as changes in skin temperature or color, impairment of mobility, and problems with emotional or mental status.

Examples of advanced skills are testing the reflexes, conducting a neurological exam to determine the strength and movement of extremities, and cranial nerve testing. Another commonly used assessment technique is to test the response of the pupil to light. Normally, the pupils are equal in size and shape and constrict symmetrically when exposed to a light source. Variances from this normal response may indicate neurological damage.

Endocrine

The endocrine system has such wide-ranging effects on the body that no additional questions are listed here. The most common problems with the endocrine system (i.e., diabetes and thyroid disorders) are usually identified in the evaluation of the other systems.

Female Reproductive

- Does patient menstruate? If so, how often, how long, and are there any problems related to this? When did menses (menarche) begin?

- Is there any pain, discharge, itching, or discomfort with the vagina or genitalia? Any lumps in the breasts or discharge from the nipples?

- Has the patient undergone any surgeries, such as hysterectomy (removal of uterus), oophorectomy (removal of ovary), mastectomy (removal of breast), or cesarean section (surgical delivery of the baby through an abdominal incision)?

Male Reproductive

- Is there any discharge from, or are sores noted on, the penis?

Pain Evaluation

Pain is subjective, and there is no test to confirm it in an objective manner. The best approach is to use a pain rating scale. Most facilities use this approach, and it helps to make the patient's level of pain easier to compare. The patient is asked to rate his or her pain on a scale of 0 to 10. Zero is no pain, and 10 is the worst pain the patient can imagine. (See Figure 20–1.) Each time a pain rating is done, the same scale is used. For example, if a patient reports pain to be 7 and then, after pain medication, reports it has dropped to 2, this is a good indication of the effectiveness of the medication. But if it has only dropped to a 5 or 6, this would indicate that the pain medication regimen needs to be reevaluated. It is also important to note any nonverbal cues that may indicate pain, such as limping, favoring an area, moaning, restlessness, and wincing.

If the patient is cognitively unable to rate his or her pain using a numeric scale, there are several visual representations that can be used. Refer to www.oucher.org and http://wongbakerfaces.org to view two such options.

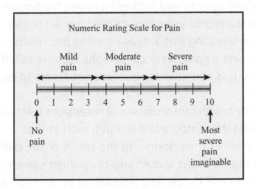

FIGURE 20–1 Visual analog scale for rating pain.

This is especially helpful for young patients (3 years or older) to communicate how much pain they are having as they can point to the face that best describes how they are feeling.

ADL Evaluation

Activities of daily living (ADLs) are the actions done on a regular basis to meet physical needs. These include bathing, eating, toileting, shopping, doing laundry, cleaning the house, paying bills, dressing, turning in bed, getting out of bed, and ambulating (walking). Conditions that affect the ability to perform ADLs may be temporary or permanent. For example, patients recovering from a recent surgery may temporarily not be strong enough to care for themselves, but a patient with a major and permanent spinal cord injury will never regain full function.

There are many diseases and conditions that diminish the patient's ability to perform these activities. When a patient is unable to perform his or her basic ADLs, help must be arranged. Family and friends are often able to assist, but if this is not possible, there are a number of agencies and facilities that will need to be evaluated to determine the best service for specific patient needs. This type of assessment is often performed by specially trained personnel (e.g., social workers, case managers, discharge planners) who are familiar with the various services available in the community. Chapter 2 presents information on some of the health care delivery systems available to assist patients to meet their health care needs.

VITAL SIGNS

The term **vital signs** refers to taking a patient's temperature, pulse, respiratory rate, and blood pressure. (See Table 20–1.) Taking the vital signs provides important information on the status of the patient. When referring to the temperature, pulse, and respiratory rate of a patient, it is common to use the abbreviation TPR. The abbreviation for blood pressure is B/P.

Vital signs have normal ranges. Readings that fall below or above normal may indicate a problem that needs further assessment. Comparing new readings with previous readings can provide information about whether the patient is improving or not. It is necessary to follow specific procedures to obtain accurate results; however, be aware that the procedures as outlined in this chapter may vary somewhat in different clinical settings. Never estimate or assume that the readings are the same as before, because inaccurate results can cause the wrong health care decisions to be made, which can jeopardize the patient's health.

Table 20–1 Vital Signs

Procedure	Purpose
Temperature	Measures how much heat is in the body. An elevation may indicate that an infection or other disease process is present
Radial Pulse	Measures how fast the heart is beating when felt at the wrist
Apical Pulse	Measures how fast the heart is beating by listening over the heart with a stethoscope
Respirations	Measures how fast the patient is breathing
Blood Pressure	Indicates how hard the heart is working to distribute blood to all parts of the body

Temperature

The body functions to maintain its temperature within a range that is best for maintaining homeostasis. If the body gets too warm, it will feel hot, begin to sweat, and cause a sense of thirst to be experienced. Sweating is a normal cooling system of the body. The intake of fluids assists in the sweating process, as well as in the replacement of lost fluids. If the body gets too cool, the skin will feel cool, and shivering will start as a way to increase metabolism through muscular activity. The normal average temperature varies with the route used to obtain the temperature. Readings obtained from the oral (mouth) and aural (ear) routes have the same range, but those from the rectal and temporal artery routes normally run a degree higher, and the axillary (under the arm) runs a degree lower. (See Procedure 20–1.) Other factors that affect the temperature are age of the patient (temperature control in younger patients is less stable and normal readings run higher than in adulthood), time of day (early morning readings are typically the lowest), and pregnancy (readings are higher). The temperature also varies depending on the temperature of the room, amount of clothes being worn, and number of blankets used while in bed. There are also normal variations among patients. Always refer to the patient's chart to review prior readings for comparison.

Electronic, tympanic (aural), chemical-dot, and temporal artery (infrared technology) are different types of thermometers available today. (See Figure 20–2a–d.) An *electronic thermometer* and *tympanic thermometer* will have a disposable plastic probe that is placed on the thermometer prior to use and discarded after each use. The temporal artery thermometer is rolled across the forehead and can be cleaned with alcohol between uses. There is also an infrared thermometer that does not require contact with the skin. It is swiped across the forehead and the reading appears within a second. Follow the manufacturer's instructions for the proper use, care, and cleaning of this equipment. When using *chemical-dot thermometers*, do not remove them from their protective covers in advance because they will begin to react to the room temperature. Be sure to follow directions supplied by the manufacturer. Always remember to follow standard precautions and facility policies regarding cleaning of equipment when working with patients.

Note: Glass mercury thermometers are not used in health care settings. They have been phased out due to concerns about mercury toxicity. Encourage your patients to switch to electronic thermometers for home use as there are a number of reliable, inexpensive brands on the market. Inform the patient that disposal of their mercury thermometers requires special handling and they should contact a hazardous waste collection facility for instructions. If they improperly dispose of products containing mercury, they may break and release mercury vapors. These vapors are harmful to their health and the environment.

When temperature is within the normal range, patients are said to be **afebrile**. When it is elevated above the normal range, they are **febrile**. An *intermittent fever* means that the temperature rises and falls. It can become elevated and then return to normal or even below normal. A *continuous fever* stays elevated over a prolonged period.

A fever is a defense mechanism against microorganisms. In an effort to kill the invading microorganisms, the body triggers the muscles to shiver, which increases metabolic activity and further increases the temperature. When the febrile episode subsides, it is accompanied by profuse sweating that acts as a cooling mechanism. When the sweating episodes occur at night, they are called night sweats. It is common for intermittent fevers to occur at night.

If the health care professional notes signs that may indicate that the temperature is rising, such as that the body feels warmer than normal to the touch or the patient is shivering, he or she should take the patient's temperature at this time. If the patient is sweating profusely, it means that the fever has broken and is coming back down to a lower temperature.

FIGURE 20–2a Electronic thermometers have a plastic probe that is placed on the thermometer and discarded after use. The temperature is read on a digital display.

FIGURE 20–2c Chemical-dot thermometers change color in response to the temperature of the skin.

FIGURE 20–2b Thermo-scan tympanic thermometer.

FIGURE 20–2d Temporal artery thermometer is used by sliding it across the forehead. The temperature is read on a digital display.

PROCEDURE

20–1

HOW TO TAKE A TEMPERATURE

Always Observe Standard Precautions

ROUTE

Oral

Normal Range (Adult)

97.6°F–99.6°F (36.5°C–37.5°C)

Procedure

1. You will need a clean electronic thermometer with oral probe and something to record the results on.

    Precautions: Do not use this route if the patient is a mouth breather; is unable to keep mouth closed around the thermometer; has had surgery or an injury to nose or mouth; is confused, unconscious, prone to seizures, has oxygen or a nasogastric tube; is too young; or is for any other reason unable or unwilling to follow directions.

2. Verify that the patient has not taken any food or fluid by mouth, smoked, or chewed gum in the last 30 minutes.

    Precautions: This will result in an inaccurate reading.

3. Clean with alcohol and, when dry, apply temperature probe sheath.

4. Ask the patient to open mouth.

5. Place thermometer under the tongue on either side, as close to the midline as possible.

(continues)

PROCEDURE

HOW TO TAKE A TEMPERATURE

(continued)

Precautions: The thermometer must be placed close to the fleshy area where the tongue attaches in order to get an accurate reading. If it is placed too far to either side, it may result in an inaccurate reading (low).

6. Instruct patient to close lips around thermometer but not to bite down on it.

7. Leave it in place until unit signals a final reading (see manufacturer's instructions).

8. Remove thermometer and read digital display.

9. Immediately record your findings.

10. Remove temperature probe sheath and dispose of properly. Clean thermometer with alcohol.

ROUTE

Axillary

Normal Range (Adult)
96.6°F–98.6°F (36°C–37°C)

Procedure

1. You will need a clean electronic thermometer, with oral probe and something to record the results on.

   Precautions: This is the least accurate method, but is often used when the oral route is not appropriate and an aural thermometer is not available.

2. Clean with alcohol and, when dry, apply temperature probe sheath.

3. Remove clothing from patient's shoulder and arm.

4. Ensure that axillary area is dry, wiping with dry towel if necessary.

   Precautions: Moisture can cause an inaccurate reading.

5. Place thermometer in the center of the armpit and place arm across the abdomen and close to side of body. (See Figure 20–3.)

6. Leave it in place until unit signals a final reading (see manufacturer's instructions).

7. Remove thermometer, read the digital display.

8. Immediately record your findings.

9. Remove temperature probe sheath and dispose of properly. Clean thermometer with alcohol.

ROUTE

Rectal

Normal Range (Adult)
98.6°F–100.6°F (37°C–38°C)

FIGURE 20–3 To take an axillary temperature, place the bulb of the thermometer into the center of the armpit and hold arm close to body.

Procedure

1. You will need an electronic thermometer with rectal probe (used only for rectal temperatures) and something to record the results on.

   Precautions: The rectal route is often inappropriate for infants and young children. Policies regarding its use vary among facilities.

2. Clean with alcohol and, when dry, apply temperature probe sheath.

   Precautions: Do not use this method if patient has diarrhea, has had recent surgery or injury to the rectum or prostate, or has had a recent myocardial infarct (heart attack).

3. Ensure that adults are in a side-lying position with top leg flexed forward.

4. Lubricate thermometer.

5. Insert thermometer into the rectum (1 inch for children, and 11/2 inches for adults).

   Precautions: Never force the thermometer into the colon.

6. Leave it in place until unit signals a final reading (see manufacturer's instructions).

7. Hold tip of thermometer while in place.

   Precautions: The thermometer must be held in place to prevent damage to rectal tissue or loss of thermometer into rectum.

8. Remove thermometer and read digital display.

9. Immediately record your findings.

10. Remove temperature probe sheath and dispose of properly. Clean thermometer with alcohol.

ROUTE

Aural (Tympanic)

Normal Range (Adult)

97.6°F–99.6°F (36.5°C–37.5°C)

Procedure

1. You will need an aural thermometer and something to record the results on.

2. Place disposable probe on the thermometer.

   Precautions: Follow manufacturer's instructions.

3. Stabilize the patient's head.

4. In children younger than 1 year, gently pull the ear straight back; in children older than 1 year and adults, pull the ear back and up.

5. Insert probe into ear canal until you obtain seal. (See Figure 20–4.)

6. Press scan button. (Results are obtained within seconds.)

7. Immediately record results.

8. Properly dispose of probe.

ROUTE

Temporal Artery (Infrared)

Normal Range (Adult)

98.6°F–100.6°F (37°C–38°C)

Procedure

1. You will need a temporal artery thermometer, alcohol wipes, and something to record the results on. Clean thermometer with alcohol and let dry before using.

   Precautions: Considered very accurate. Other sites that can be used are the femoral, axillary, and behind the ear; check manufacturer's directions regarding any restrictions.

FIGURE 20–4 Taking a patient's temperature with a tympanic (aural) thermometer.

2. Remove perspiration from forehead, remove hat, push back hair from forehead.

   Precautions: Moisture (perspiration) on the forehead causes cooling, which results in inaccurate results. Hair or hat on the forehead can raise the temperature and cause inaccurate results.

3. Center probe on the forehead (midline), press scan button and slowly move it across forehead to the temple area hair line.

   Precautions: Moving it too quickly can result in inaccurate results.

4. Immediately record results.

5. Clean probe with alcohol wipe, let dry, and return to holder.

   Precautions: Must be dry to work effectively.

Thinking It Through

Mr. Hulchanski calls the physician's office and speaks with Becky Smith, the medical assistant. Mr. Hulchanski has had recent surgery and was instructed to call the office in one week to report how he is doing. Mr. Hulchanski reports that he is feeling fine and that the surgical incision looks like it is healing well. He says the only thing that he has noticed is that when he awakens in the morning, his pajamas and linens are soaked. Becky asks if he has been running a fever, and he states that he has routinely taken his temperature several times during the day and it has been normal. In fact, he states that he is sure he is not having a fever because he actually feels chilled at times. Becky states that she is glad to hear that he is doing so well and to call back if any problems develop.

1. Becky documents "patient reports he is doing well and will call back if any problems develop." Is this the correct note to make in the chart? Why or why not?

2. Did Mr. Hulchanski report any variances from the norm?

3. What could possibly be happening to Mr. Hulchanski?

Fascinating Facts

- When you enter a cold environment the muscle fiber connected to your hair follicles tighten, then the skin surrounding the follicles sticks up and creates goose bumps.

- A raise in body temperature is a good sign that your body is working to fight off infection. It raises your body temperature and makes it harder for invading bacteria to survive.

- Your body temperature is usually lowest in the morning and highest in the evening.

Pulse

When the heart contracts and forces blood out of the heart and into the arteries, it creates a pulsing sensation that can be felt by the health care professional at certain points in the body. There are a number of locations where an artery comes close enough to the surface of the skin and where it passes over a firm surface (e.g., bone) that it can be felt. (See Figure 20–5.) These major **pulse points** are as follows:

- Temporal: Located on either side of the forehead.

- Carotid: Located on the front side of the neck on either side of the trachea (never massage this area or compress both carotids at the same time when taking a pulse; massages can trigger a sudden slowing of the heart rate, and compressing both carotids can decrease the blood flow to the brain).

- Brachial: Located in the inner side of the antecubital space (crease created when elbow is bent).

- Radial: Located in the wrist (thumb side); most commonly used site.

FIGURE 20–5 Location of pulse points that can be felt on the body.

- Femoral: Located in the inner aspect of the crease where the upper thigh joins the trunk of the body.

- Popliteal: Located behind the knee.

- Dorsalis pedis: Located on top of the foot arch.

When taking a pulse (Procedure 20–2), three observations are made:

1. Rate: The rate is the number of beats that occurs in 1 minute.

2. Rhythm: When the beats occur at even intervals, it is called a *regular rhythm*. If they do not occur at regular intervals, it is called an *irregular rhythm*. It is also

PROCEDURE   20–2

HOW TO TAKE A RADIAL PULSE

Always Observe Standard Precautions

STEPS

1. You will need a watch with a second hand and something to record the results on.

RATIONALE

As a health care professional, you should at all times have a watch with a second hand, a pen, and notepaper with you. A water-resistant watch with a large face for ease in reading is recommended.

(continues)

PROCEDURE

HOW TO TAKE A RADIAL PULSE

STEPS

2. Locate the radial pulse by gently but firmly pressing on the thumb side of the wrist until an indented area is felt. This is where the pulse is located. Use two or three fingers to feel the pulse. (See Figure 20–6.)

3. Place the patient's hand on his or her chest. (See Figure 20–7.)

4. Count the pulsations you feel in a 60-second period.

5. When you complete the procedure, leave your fingers on the pulse, and count the respirations.

6. Immediately record your findings.

RATIONALE

The health care professional always uses the fingers and never the thumb in taking a patient's pulse. The thumb has a pulse of its own, and if the thumb is used, the worker's own pulse may be mistaken for the patient's.

This makes it easier to count the respirations after the pulse is taken because the health care professional can feel the rise and fall of the chest.

Counting the heart rate for a full minute increases the accuracy of the result. If the pulse is strong, regular, and within the normal range, you can count the pulsations for 30 seconds and multiply times two for the 1-minute reading.

See Procedure 20–4.

Getting in the habit of writing down the actual numbers, instead of relying on your memory, will prevent errors.

FIGURE 20–6 To take a radial pulse, place two or three fingers in an indented area on the thumb side of the wrist.

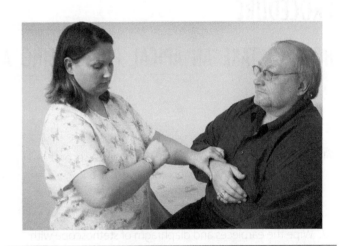

FIGURE 20–7 Positioning the patient's hand on his chest makes it easier to count pulse and respiration.

possible to have a recurring pattern with an irregular rhythm. For example, there may be a beat missed every two beats, and this happens consistently. This pattern is called a *regular irregular rhythm*. If there is no pattern to the irregular rhythm, then it is called an *irregular irregular rhythm*.

3. Pulse volume (strength of the beat): This describes the character of the beat. It may be described as weak, strong, thready (very fine and scarcely perceptible), or bounding (higher intensity than normal, then disappears quickly).

Another method for taking the pulse is to take an *apical pulse*. This method requires the use of a stethoscope. (See Figure 20–8.) A **stethoscope** is an instrument that amplifies sound and allows a health care professional to hear sounds from within the body. The stethoscope is placed over the apex of the heart, and the beats are counted as they are heard. The sound heard through the stethoscope as "lub-dub" represents one beat. (See Procedure 20–3.) The "lub-dub" actually includes the sounds of the various valves opening and closing as the blood flows through the heart's chambers. Sometimes the physician will order an apical pulse, but often this is not specified and the choice of pulse point is left up to the judgment of the health care professional. An apical pulse should be obtained when there is an irregular rate, on cardiac patients, when the radial pulse is difficult to palpate, and with infants and young children.

When the pulse rate is abnormally low, it is called **bradycardia**. For example, in an adult patient, a rate of less than 60 beats per minute would be called bradycardia. When the pulse rate is abnormally high, it is called **tachycardia**. For example, in an adult patient, a rate of more than 100 beats per minute would be called

FIGURE 20–8 The parts of a stethoscope.

tachycardia. The pulse rate is affected by many factors, including the age of the patient (Table 20–2), certain medications and disease conditions, physical activity, fever, and pregnancy.

PROCEDURE

20-3

HOW TO TAKE AN APICAL PULSE USING A STETHOSCOPE

Always Observe Standard Precautions

STEPS

1. You will need a stethoscope, a watch with a second hand, and something to record the results on.

2. Wipe the earpieces and diaphragm of stethoscope with alcohol wipes, and inspect the stethoscope prior to use.

3. Verify that the diaphragm side is where the sound will be heard.

4. If the diaphragm is cold to the touch, rub it against your clothing or hand until it is warm.

5. Place earpieces into your ears, with the earpieces pointing forward.

RATIONALE

As a health care professional, you should at all times have a watch with a second hand, a pen, and notepaper with you. A water-resistant watch with a large face for ease in reading is recommended.

If the earpieces have wax in them, remove wax prior to use, so the sound will not be diminished; do not use a stethoscope that has cracks or tears in the tubing because it may lead to inaccurate results.

The end of the stethoscope can be turned to switch between the diaphragm (high pitch) and the bell (low pitch) side (refer back to Figure 20–7); some stethoscopes have only a diaphragm, then no adjustment is needed.

A cold instrument placed on the skin creates a very uncomfortable sensation for the patient.

This directs the sound into the ear canal at the correct angle.

(continues)

PROCEDURE

HOW TO TAKE AN APICAL PULSE USING A STETHOSCOPE

(continued)

STEPS

6. Place the diaphragm of the stethoscope directly on the skin, over the apex of the heart, and hold it with gentle but firm pressure.

7. Instruct the patient to breathe normally.

8. Count the beats you hear in a 60-second period.

9. When you are done, leave the stethoscope in place and count the respirations.

10. Immediately record your findings.

RATIONALE

If placed over clothing, sounds caused by the stethoscope rubbing on the clothing may be misinterpreted as beats.

The patient may think you are trying to listen to their lungs and start to breathe deeply, which can alter the heart rate.

Counting the heart rate for a full minute increases the accuracy of the result. If the pulse is strong, regular, and within the normal range, you can count the pulsations for 30 seconds and multiply times two for the 1-minute reading.

See Procedure 20–4.

Getting in the habit of writing down the actual numbers, instead of relying on your memory, will prevent errors.

Table 20–2 Pulse Rates at Various Ages

Age	Average Pulse	Normal Range
Newborn	140	120–160
Infant	110	80–140
Toddler	105	80–130
Preschool Child	100	74–120
School-Age Child	95	70–110
Adolescent–Adult	80	60–90

FIGURE 20–9 To determine a pulse deficit, one person counts the apical pulse while a second person counts the radial pulse.

Another procedure that the health care professional may be asked to assist with is a pulse deficit assessment check. This requires two health care professionals. One will take the pulse at one of the pulse points (usually radial), and the other will simultaneously take the apical pulse. (See Figure 20–9.) This is always taken for a full minute and must be coordinated to start and stop at the same time. If there is a difference between the two readings, it is called the **pulse deficit**. For example, if the apical rate is 100 and the radial is 80, the apical–radial pulse deficit is 20 beats. The deficit represents the number of cardiac beats that do not reach the radial artery. Normally, there should be no pulse deficit.

An apical–radial deficit can be present in a number of cardiac conditions. For example, the heart may not contract with enough force for a pulse to reach the extremity, or the heart may be beating so rapidly that not enough blood can enter the heart on each beat. When doing an apical–radial pulse reading, the reading will be the same or the apical will be higher. It is not possible to get a radial pulse reading that is higher than the apical reading.

Respirations

Respiration refers to the process of moving air into and out of the lungs. When air is taken into the lungs it is called inhalation (inspiration), and there is a corresponding expansion of the chest as the lungs fill. When the air is expelled back out of the lungs, it is called exhalation (expiration), and there is a corresponding deflation of the chest cavity as the lungs empty. One full cycle (inhalation and exhalation) is called one respiration. Normal breathing is called eupnea and should be within the normal range, unlabored, and have an even rhythm. If the respiratory rate is above the normal range, it is called tachypnea, and if below normal it is bradypnea.

Three observations are made when taking the respiratory rate (Procedure 20–4):

1. Rate: This is the number of respiratory cycles that occur in 1 minute.

2. Rhythm: Both the respirations and the intervals between them should be evenly spaced; when there is a temporary absence of respirations, it is called apnea, and the length of the interval should be timed. Report any periods of apnea to your supervisor. Cheyne-Stokes is an abnormal breathing pattern with a period of apnea that can last for 10 to 60 seconds, which is then followed by a gradually increasing depth and frequency of respirations. It commonly occurs in patients with heart failure or neurologic diseases.

3. Respiratory effort: Breathing should occur through the nose, be unlabored, and be without sound; report to your supervisor if you note that the patient shows extra effort during breathing or if any sounds are heard (e.g., wheezing, gurgling, or other sounds). Also note the depth of the breathing, such as shallow, normal, or deep.

Many factors can affect the respiratory rate, but if the rate is outside the normal range (Table 20–3), has an irregular rhythm, or is labored, report it to your supervisor. Factors that can affect the rate are age, illness, drugs, exercise, and emotions. Because the respiratory rate can be consciously altered, it is important that the patient should not know when you are counting the respirations. The best approach is to place the patient's arm across his or her chest to take the pulse and then, when completed, leave your fingers on

---

PROCEDURE 20-4

HOW TO COUNT RESPIRATIONS

Always Observe Standard Precautions

STEPS	RATIONALE
1. You will need a watch with a second hand and something to record the results on.	As a health care professional, you should at all times have a watch with a second hand, a pen, and notepaper with you. A water-resistant watch with a large face for ease in reading is recommended.
2. After you finish counting the pulse, leave your fingers in position (if taking the radial pulse) or keep the stethoscope on the chest (if taking the apical pulse), and count the respirations.	Because the respiratory rate can be consciously altered, it is important that the patient should not know when you are counting the respirations. Do not tell the patient that you are now counting the respirations, or the rate may not be accurate. The health care professional can also feel the chest rise and fall by leaving the arm on the chest or the stethoscope in place.
3. Count the number of respirations taken in 1 full minute.	One respiration is a complete cycle that includes inhalation and exhalation.
4. Immediately record your findings.	Getting in the habit of writing down the actual numbers, instead of relying on your memory, will prevent errors.

Table 20–3 **Respiratory Rates at Various Ages**

Age	Normal Range
Infant	30–60
Toddler	20–40
Preschool Child	22–34
School-Age Child	18–24
Adolescent–Adult	16–20

the radial pulse while counting the respirations. This is also an appropriate time to note the color of the nail beds. They should be pink; if they are cyanotic (bluish or purplish), report this to the supervisor immediately.

Blood Pressure

Recall that the purpose of the circulatory system is to carry oxygenated blood to the tissues and organs throughout the body. The heart, a strong pump, creates pressure to move the blood and this results in pressure against the walls of the arteries, veins, and capillaries. This pressure consists of two forces: one occurs when the blood is pumped out of the heart; the second when the heart rests between beats. When blood pressure (B/P) is measured, both forces are noted: the first is the *systolic pressure* and is the highest pressure in the cardiovascular system. The second is the *diastolic pressure* and is the lowest pressure in the cardiovascular system.

Another way of correlating the reading of the B/P is to think of the sounds of the normal cardiac cycle. As previously described, when listening to the heartbeat, the examiner hears a "lub-dub" sound. The "lub" sound occurs as the heart chambers are contracting at their maximum force to push the blood out of the heart and into the arteries. This is the systolic phase of the heart. The "dub" sound is when the heart relaxes and is refilling with blood. This is the diastolic phase of the heart.

The two blood pressure numbers are separated by a slash. For example, 120/80 or 140/90. (See Table 20–4 for a definition of adult blood pressure categories.) If the patient's reading falls below normal, it is called hypotension. If the reading is above normal, it is called hypertension. Recent updates to guidelines from the American Heart Association and the American College of Cardiology changed the definition of high blood pressure or hypertension for most people. High blood pressure is now generally defined as 130 or higher for the first number, or 80 or higher for the second number (previously it was 140/90). Another change eliminated the differences in recommended numbers for people of different ages, including previous suggestions that people over 65 had higher thresholds for what is considered high blood pressure. At this time, the numbers given in Table 20–4 apply to all adults age 18 and older (https://www.health.harvard.edu/heart-health/reading-the-new-blood-pressure-guidelines).

Hypertension most often has no symptoms, but the increased pressure can damage and weaken the blood vessels causing them to narrow, rupture, or leak. Heart disease, stroke, and kidney failure are among the serious results of uncontrolled hypertension. Elevated and stage 1 hypertension can sometimes be lowered with lifestyle changes, such as losing weight; reducing salt, fat, and caffeine intake; and increasing physical activity. However, medication is necessary in many cases and usually prescribed for stage two.

Although hypertension is by far the most common problem, abnormally low blood pressure can be an indication of an underlying health problem, including dehydration, severe infection, and heart problems. Immediate medical attention may be required if the patient presents additional signs and symptoms:

- Dizziness or lightheadedness
- Fainting (syncope)
- Blurred vision
- Nausea
- Fatigue
- Lack of concentration

Table 20–4 **Blood Pressure Categories for Adults (18 Years of Age or Older)**

Category	Systolic (Top Number)	Diastolic (Bottom Number)
Normal	Less than 120	Less than 80
Elevated	120–129	Less than 80
Hypertension (High Blood Pressure)		
Stage 1	130–139	80–89
Stage 2	140 or higher	90 or higher
Hypertensive Crisis	Higher than 180	Higher than 120

Source: https://www.health.harvard.edu/heart-health/reading-the-new-blood-pressure-guidelines

Two pieces of equipment are needed to take a manual blood pressure: a stethoscope and a sphygmomanometer. A **sphygmomanometer** is an instrument that records the blood pressure in millimeters (mm) of mercury (Hg). The health care professional may encounter different types of recording devices. (See Figures 20–10a–c.) Some units show pressure on a circular dial and others as digital numbers. The circular dials are calibrated so that each mark represents 2 mm Hg. (See Figure 20–11.) Electronic sphygmomanometers (see Figure 20–10c) take the blood pressure and pulse automatically and display the readings on a digital screen. (After the cuff is placed on the arm, the machine can be programmed to automatically take readings at specific intervals.)

It takes repeated practice to master the skills for accurate manual blood pressure measurement. See Procedure 20–5 for the steps in taking a blood pressure reading.

When working with a manual sphygmomanometer, it is necessary to close the screw to inflate the cuff and to loosen the screw to release the air. Some health care professionals have difficulty remembering if turning the screw to the left or right will close or open the valve. It may be helpful to remember the saying "righty tighty, lefty loosey." This means that if you turn the screw to the *right* (as you look straight down at it) the valve will *tighten* and the cuff can be inflated. Turning the screw to the *left loosens* the screw, and air escapes.

FIGURE 20–10a Dial (aneroid) sphygmomanometer.

FIGURE 20–10c Electronic sphygmomanometer.

FIGURE 20–10b Digital sphygmomanometer.

FIGURE 20–11 The gauge of a dial (aneroid) sphygmomanometer. Systolic and diastolic readings are recorded as even numbers.

PROCEDURE

HOW TO TAKE A MANUAL BLOOD PRESSURE

Always Observe Standard Precautions

STEPS	RATIONALE
1. You will need a stethoscope, a sphygmomanometer, and something to record the results on.	To verify that the sphygmomanometer is calibrated correctly, check that the dial is resting at zero prior to use.
2. Verify that the cuff is the correct size for the patient and that the valve is closed to allow for inflation of bladder.	The bladder in the cuff needs to cover at least 80% of the circumference of the arm and clear the antecubital space by 1 to 11/2 inches to give accurate results.
3. Place the patient in a relaxed lying or sitting position, remove the clothing from the arm, and position the arm at heart level. Instruct the patient not to talk during the procedure.	Rolled-up sleeves can constrict the arm and alter the results; talking can interfere with hearing the readings correctly (it may also be necessary to turn off the television or radio).
4. Locate the pulse of the brachial artery in the inner aspect of the antecubital space, and place the arrows on cuff over this area.	Placing the stethoscope directly over the brachial artery will give the strongest sound.
5. Place your fingers on the radial artery and inflate the cuff until you can no longer feel the pulse. Note the reading and add 30 to it. For example, if the dial reads 120 when the radial pulsation ceases, add 30 to equal 150.	To get an accurate reading, it is necessary to pump the cuff to 30 mm Hg higher than the anticipated systolic pressure. This is the amount of inflation you will use when the blood pressure is taken.
6. Deflate the cuff by opening the screw. Wait at least 30 seconds.	Repeated inflation on the same arm in rapid succession will give inaccurate results.
7. Place the stethoscope in your ears and place the diaphragm over the brachial artery. Press gently.	The stethoscope diaphragm should be in full contact with the skin surface but not be pressed too hard.
8. Close the screw and inflate the cuff to the predetermined amount (from the example given earlier, this would be 150 mm Hg).	Never guess how high to inflate the cuff based on previous readings; check each time.
9. Slowly release the screw so the cuff deflates evenly (about 2 mm Hg at a time), and listen for the first sound of the pulse returning to the brachial artery. Make a mental note of the reading.	If the cuff is deflated too rapidly, the health care professional may not hear the first beat until a lower number is reached; the first sound heard from the brachial artery is the systolic pressure.
10. Continue allowing the cuff to deflate until you no longer hear any sounds from the brachial artery.	The health care professional will continue to hear a pulsing sound until it ceases, which is the reading for the diastolic pressure.
11. Continue to listen for any return of sounds from the brachial artery for an additional 20 to 30 mm Hg.	Some patients have what is called an auscultatory gap, where the beat of the brachial artery will again be heard. Note the new beginning and ending beats and chart the findings. For example, if you first heard beats at 170, the beats ceased at 120, then resumed at 100, then ceased again at 60, you would chart B/P 170/60 with auscultatory gap between 120 and 100.

(continues)

PROCEDURE

HOW TO TAKE A MANUAL BLOOD PRESSURE

(continued)

STEPS

12. Open the screw completely and let the cuff deflate rapidly.

13. Remove the stethoscope from your ears and the cuff from the patient's arm and immediately record your results in even numbers only (manual B/P) along with which arm was used.

14. If you are unsure of the blood pressure reading and want to recheck it, use the other arm or wait several minutes before using the same arm.

RATIONALE

The procedure is completed, and many patients do not like the tightness created by the cuff being inflated.

Getting in the habit of writing down the actual numbers, instead of relying on your memory, will prevent errors.

Repeated blood pressure attempts can cause inaccurate results.

The blood pressure cuff must fit correctly to get accurate results. Patients with very large or small upper arms may need a larger cuff or a pediatric cuff. An inflatable bladder is located within the outer covering of a cuff and should be long enough to cover 80% of the circumference of the arm. (See Figure 20–12.) The width of the cuff should fit comfortably below the armpit and extend no farther than 1 to 11/2 inches above the antecubital space.

Blood pressure is affected by many factors, including the age of the patient, certain medications and disease conditions, physical activity, the position of patient, and emotions. In fact, blood pressure is so variable in response to different factors that a diagnosis of hypertension is never made on just one reading. When patients visit the physician's office, they may feel anxious, and this causes the blood pressure reading to be higher than normal. Most physicians will want to see several high readings over time, when the patient is lying down in a resting position, before they conclude that the patient has high blood pressure.

White coat syndrome is a term that was coined to describe a situation in which patients' blood pressure readings are high in the provider's office but otherwise in the normal range. Even patients with diagnosed high blood pressure may have higher readings in the provider's office. The correlation is seldom this clear cut, however, the anxious emotions felt in the provider's office can also apply to other situations. If blood pressure is only occasionally high, it is not as dangerous as when it remains elevated most of the time. The patient may or may not actually feel anxious at the time (this mechanism appears to occur at a subconscious level). There are two concerns when considering white coat syndrome:

1. Patients may put themselves in this category and dismiss the need for treatment, as they feel it only occurs in that particular situation.

2. The high reading in the provider's office is assumed to be the patient's usual pressure and the patient is overtreated.

The best solution to this problem is for the patient to purchase his or her own blood pressure machine, take the blood pressure at home, and keep a record of all recordings. Taking this record to the next office visit will assist the health care provider in determining the best course of action.

When a patient's cardiovascular system is unable to make rapid changes to accommodate changes in position, he or she will experience a condition called **orthostatic (postural) hypotension**. Normally, when a person rises to a standing position, the blood vessels in the lower extremities constrict and the blood pressure increases to maintain adequate flow of blood to the brain. When that does not occur, the blood pools in the lower extremities and the blood pressure drops quickly, which results in a lack of oxygen to the brain. The patient experiences lightheadedness and may even pass out. This can also occur when a person has been on bed rest and is getting up for the first time, has recently had surgery, or is on certain medications. Patients with low blood pressure or low pulse rates are also prone to this problem.

FIGURE 20–12 The blood pressure cuff must fit correctly to get accurate results. The bladder should cover 80% of the circumference of the patient's arm. Position arrows on the cuff over the brachial artery.

When working with patients, always be on the alert and implement measures to ensure their safety. Have the patient get up slowly to allow more time for the cardiovascular system to adjust to the change in position. To assist the physician in diagnosing this problem, the health care professional may be asked to obtain a lying, sitting, and standing B/P. To do this, the health care professional takes a blood pressure reading with the patient lying down, then leaves the blood pressure cuff in place, instructs the patient to sit up, and rechecks the blood pressure. The same routine is repeated for the standing position. Check your facilities' policies because some specify the exact time interval required between the subsequent blood pressure measurements when performing this procedure. Also remember to ensure the patient's safety at the time of the test by monitoring during changes of position to prevent injury if he or she gets dizzy or passes out.

At certain times the arm cannot be used for blood pressure readings. Do not use the arm if surgery was performed on it, the patient has had a mastectomy on that side, a hemodialysis shunt (surgically created vascular access) is present in the arm, or if there is an intravenous (IV) infusion running into the arm (fluids running through

Thinking It Through

Ms. Sanchez is a nursing assistant at an acute care hospital in her hometown. Her supervisor has requested that she take Mr. Jordan's vital signs. When she enters the room, she introduces herself to Mr. Jordan and informs him that she will be taking his vital signs. He asks what she means by vital signs. He also tells her that he was hospitalized after having a myocardial infarction two days ago. She notes that he is receiving oxygen and has an IV line in his left arm.

1. What are vital signs?
2. Which arm should be used to take the blood pressure? Why?
3. What route should be used to take the temperature? Why?
4. Should the pulse be taken radially or apically? Why?
5. What three observations should be made when taking the pulse?
6. What three observations should be made when taking the respiratory rate?

Fascinating Facts

- The Centers for Disease Control and Prevention's National Center for Health Statistics reports that as many as 103 million Americans have hypertension. This number represents nearly *half* of all adults in the United States.

- Hypertension is called the silent killer because there are few if any symptoms, but if left untreated, it can lead to a heart attack, stroke, embolism, and kidney failure.

- In 90% to 95% of the cases, hypertension has no known cause. This type of high blood pressure is known as essential hypertension. However, hypertension has been linked to obesity. In rarer cases, high blood pressure can result from other illnesses, such as kidney or adrenal gland problems. That type of high blood pressure is called secondary hypertension.

a tube into a cannula placed in a vein). Patients who have a shunt for the purpose of dialysis can never have blood pressures taken on that arm. If neither arm is available for taking a blood pressure (e.g., burns to both arms), the popliteal artery can be used. A large blood pressure cuff will be required that fits around the thigh. Follow the same blood pressure procedure as with the brachial artery, but place the stethoscope behind the knee to use the popliteal artery.

HEIGHT AND WEIGHT

Height and weight measurements are routinely taken as part of the patient's chart when he or she visits the physician's office or is admitted to a health care facility. The height measurement for an adult does not need to be repeated once it is recorded in the patient's chart, because it will not vary. An exception to this is with older patients, many of whom lose height over time. This is because the discs between the vertebrae in the spine dehydrate and compress. The aging spine can also become more curved, and vertebrae can collapse (compression fracture) due to loss of bone density (osteoporosis). Loss of muscle in the torso can also contribute to stooped posture (http://www .berkeleywellness.com/self-care/preventive-care/article /why-you-shrink-you-age).

For younger patients, it is important to take both the height and weight. Growth charts used to record the measurements show the normal ranges for various ages. When the readings fall outside the normal ranges, it will alert the physician to potential problems requiring further evaluation. Refer back to the Suggested Learning Activities in Chapter 8 for the website that contains growth charts.

The weight will vary with a change in the patient's condition and with certain medications (e.g., diuretics). How frequently the patient is to be weighed is ordered by the physician or may be determined by your supervisor. Weight loss or gain may indicate a loss or gain of fat, muscle, or fluid. Patients with kidney or cardiac conditions often have problems with fluid balance and are weighed to determine the effectiveness of their medical regimen. When a patient starts to retain fluid, it will be seen on the scale long before it is visible on the body in the form of edema (swelling caused by excess fluid in the tissues of the body).

When a patient has edema or ascites (fluid accumulation in the peritoneal cavity), additional measurements may be indicated. Measuring the ankles or abdominal girth (around the abdomen) gives objective data on the patient's condition when results are compared to previous readings.

Various scales are available for measuring weight. Following are some of the most common:

- Standing balance scale: The scale must be balanced prior to use, and the patient must be able to stand upright in a steady position without holding on to anything or anyone. The weights on the bars are then moved until the bar balances at the center point. The height can be obtained at the same time by extending the height bar.

- Electronic standing scale: Patient stands on a platform as with the balance scale, but weight is shown on a digital read-out. Some electronic scales also measure height. (See Figures 20–13a–c.)

- Chair and wheelchair scales: Some chairs come equipped with a scale so the patient can sit while the weight is being taken. Another method is to place the patient in a wheelchair and then push it onto a scale, but in this case the wheelchair needs to be weighed while it is empty and its weight subtracted from the total weight of the patient in the chair to get the actual weight of the patient. (See Figure 20–14.)

- Mechanical lift scales (Figures 20–15a–b): Patients unable to move on their own can have a sling

FIGURE 20–13a The patient should stand unassisted on the scale, with the feet centered on the platform and slightly apart.

FIGURE 20–13b The patient should stand as erect as possible while height is being measured.

FIGURE 20-13c Adjust the weights on the balance bar until the bar balances at the center point. The combined total of the top and bottom bars is the weight of the patient.

FIGURE 20-15a Chair-style mechanical lift with scale.

FIGURE 20-14 Subtract the weight of the wheelchair from the total weight of the patient sitting in the wheelchair.

FIGURE 20-15b Bed-style mechanical lift with scale.

positioned under them and then be lifted off the bed to obtain their weight.

- Bed scales: Some hospital beds now come equipped with a scale. The advantage is that the patient does not have to be moved to take a weight. The patient lies in bed, and the scale is activated while a digital display shows the weight. Remove any excess items from the bed before weighing the patient.

Following certain guidelines when weighing patients will ensure more accurate results. These guidelines are listed in Box 20-1.

Box 20-1

Guidelines for Weighing Patients

- Weigh patients at the same time every day; the recommendation is to weigh patients first thing in the morning, after they empty their bladder and before they eat or drink.

- Use the same scale each time.

- Balance the scale before use, if indicated.

- Have the same amount of clothes on the patient each time and remove the shoes.

- Maintain the safety of the patient at all times by monitoring for signs of unsteadiness that could result in a fall.

If a patient is unable to stand for a height measurement, the measurement will need to be taken when the patient is lying down. Place the patient flat on the bed or examining table in a straight aligned position. Then place a mark at the top of the head and one at the bottom of the heels. Measure the distance between the marks and record it as the height. This method is also used with infants and children who are unable to stand.

Many facilities are now using a body mass index (BMI) to determine if the patient is at a healthy weight. The BMI measures the relationship between weight and height. BMI ranges are not absolute indicators but can serve as a guide to patients to demonstrate if they are at a health risk due to their weight. An inaccuracy occurs when the individual is very muscular or has lost a lot of muscle mass. See Figure 20–16 for BMI ranges for adults and Box 12–2 for the formula to calculate BMI.

ARE YOU AT A HEALTHY WEIGHT?

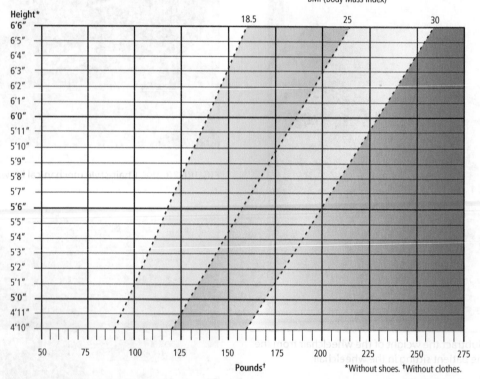

BMI measures weight in relation to height. The BMI ranges shown above are for adults. They are not exact ranges of healthy and unhealthy weights. However, they show that health risk increases at higher levels of overweight and obesity. Even within the healthy BMI range, weight gains can carry health risks for adults.

Directions: Find your weight on the bottom of the graph. Go straight up from that point until you come to the line that matches your height. Then find your weight group.

- **Under weight:** below 18.5
- **Healthy Weight:** BMI from 18.5 up to 24.9 refers to healthy weight.
- **Overweight:** BMI from 25 up to 29.9 refers to overweight.
- **Obese:** BMI 30 or higher refers to obesity. Obese persons are also overweight.

Source: American Academy of Nutrition and Dietetics.

FIGURE 20–16 Body mass index (BMI) chart.

SUGGESTED LEARNING ACTIVITIES

1. Identify the information included in a history and physical for yourself, a family member, or a friend, and write the information down in a chronological and organized manner.

2. Perform a head-to-toe evaluation on yourself and write the results in a narrative documentation format (refer back to Chapter 19).

3. Next time you experience pain (e.g., headache, stub your toe), assess your level of pain on a scale of 1 to 10. Then note how this level changes over time, until it is completely gone (level 0).

4. It will take time to develop the ability to feel a pulse, to hear the apical heartbeat, and to hear the blood pressure. Practice on yourself and your family to assist you in developing the needed sensitivity in your fingertips to feel these variations and in your ears to hear the sounds with a stethoscope. Closing your eyes to help focus all of your attention on your fingertips or ears may be a helpful technique to use when practicing.

5. Find all the pulse points on your body.

6. Calculate your BMI. (See Figure 20–16.) Based on this information, use the five-step problem-solving process to develop a plan for improvement, if necessary.

WEB ACTIVITIES

Wikipedia

https://en.wikipedia.org/wiki/Activities_of_daily_living

Activities of Daily Living

1. How does this site define ADLs?

2. Scroll down to see how the difference between Basic and Instrumental ADLs is defined and prepare a list of each.

3. Which of the ADLs can be assessed by observing a patient? Which would require information from the patient or another person, such as a caregiver?

4. How do the instrumental ADLs identified by the American Occupational Therapy Association differ from the seven listed in the previous section of the article?

5. What are the roles of occupational and physical therapists in helping patients regain their ADLs?

6. What types of tests are available for evaluating ADLs?

University of California, San Diego

https://meded.ucsd.edu/clinicalmed/vital.htm

A Practical Guide to Clinical Medicine—Vital Signs

1. What information can vital signs reveal about a patient's state of health?

2. Scroll down and read the section entitled "A few additional clinically oriented thoughts." What did you learn about blood pressure problems that were not covered in the text?

Medline Plus

https://medlineplus.gov/ency/article/004019.htm

Aging Changes in Vital Signs

List the changes in vital signs that can take place in aging adults.

Scientific American

https://www.scientificamerican.com/article/what-causes-a-fever/

What Causes a Fever?

1. Why does the body's temperature rise to fight infection?

2. What are other causes of fever?

3. What is the hypothalamus and how does it work to regulate body temperature?

4. Why is it best not to eat much when experiencing a fever?

5. What are the negative results of a very high fever?

Mayo Clinic

https://www.mayoclinic.org/diseases-conditions/high-blood-pressure/in-depth/high-blood-pressure/art-20045868

High Blood Pressure Dangers: Hypertension's Effects on Your Body

1. About how many people with untreated hypertension die of heart disease?

2. What is an aneurysm?

3. Describe the effects of hypertension on the heart, brain, kidneys, and eyes.

4. What is a high blood pressure emergency?

Mayo Clinic

https://www.mayoclinic.org/diseases-conditions/high-blood-pressure/in-depth/high-blood-pressure/art-20046974

10 Ways to Control High Blood Pressure Without Medication

1. Which of the ways also contribute to the prevention of cancer and heart disease?

2. Which ways can you incorporate into your own lifestyle habits?

3. What would be the advantages of making lifestyle changes instead of taking medication?

Mayo Clinic

https://www.mayoclinic.org/diseases-conditions/low-blood-pressure/symptoms-causes/syc-20355465

Low Blood Pressure (Hypotension)

1. What readings are considered low blood pressure?

2. What are the symptoms of low blood pressure?

3. What are some of the causes of low blood pressure not mentioned in the text?

4. Why does blood pressure tend to change throughout the day?

5. Why can a sudden drop in blood pressure be dangerous?

6. What are the four types of hypotension?

National Heart, Lung, and Blood Institute

https://www.nhlbi.nih.gov/health/educational/lose_wt/BMI/bmicalc.htm

Calculate Your Body Mass Index

1. Use the online calculator to determine your BMI.

2. Click on "Limitations of the BMI" to the right of the calculator. What are the limitations?

3. Is your BMI within the normal range? If it is above the healthy weight range, explore recommendations on the website for weight control. (If it is below, simply ensure you are intaking the proper amount of nutrients each day. See Chapter 12.)

REVIEW QUESTIONS

1. What is the purpose of a history and physical (H&P)?

2. What information is contained in a complete H&P?

3. What is contained in a review of all the body systems?

4. What does the term "baseline" mean and why is it important to know?

5. What does the phrase "variances from the normal" mean and why are variances important?

6. What is the difference between "assessment" and "data collection"?

7. What are eight examples of questions to ask during the general survey of a patient?

8. What are the components of the psychosocial status of a patient and what questions can be used to determine the status?

9. What is the meaning of the following terms: inspection, auscultation, palpation, and percussion?

10. What are the questions, observations, and actions used to collect information about the following systems and organs:

    a. Musculoskeletal

    b. Integumentary

    c. Circulatory

    d. Respiratory

    e. Digestive

    f. Urinary

    g. Eyes and ears

    h. Nervous

    i. Endocrine

    j. Reproductive (female and male)

11. What is the meaning and purpose of a pain rating scale?

12. What are activities of daily living? Give five examples.

13. What are the vital signs?

14. What happens to the body when it gets too warm or too cool?

15. What are the various types of thermometers used to take body temperature?

16. What are the correct procedures for taking a body temperature?

17. Where are the body's major pulse points?

18. What are the correct ways of taking a pulse, including a pulse deficit assessment?

19. What are the two steps in the process of respiration?

20. What three observations should you make when taking the respiratory rate?

21. When should you report a patient's respiratory rate to your supervisor?

22. What is the meaning of "blood pressure" and the terms "systolic" and "diastolic"?

23. What is the meaning of the terms "hypotension" and "hypertension"?

24. What are the blood pressure categories and corresponding numerical ranges for adults?

25. What are the possible effects of hypertension?

26. What are possible causes of hypotension? What are the signs and symptoms?

27. What are correct ways of taking a blood pressure reading?

28. What are the factors that can affect blood pressure?

29. What is the meaning of "white coat syndrome"?

30. What is the meaning and cause of orthostatic hypotension?

31. What are the conditions that would prevent you from taking a blood pressure on an affected arm?

32. How do vital signs vary over the life span?

33. Why is it important to measure the height of older adults over time?

34. Why should children and adolescents be weighed and measured regularly?

35. What are the various types of scales for measuring body weight and how is each operated?

36. What is the meaning and use of the body mass index?

APPLICATION EXERCISES

1. Refer back to The Case of the Unreported Observations and answer these questions.

   a. What variances from the normal was Mrs. Becker displaying?

   b. What are the possible outcomes of the patient losing consciousness and falling?

   c. How could Carrie have handled the situation differently?

2. Mr. Hussar, a 76-year-old patient, walks into the physician's office for his regular checkup. Mr. Hussar seems to be limping slightly as he approaches the desk to sign in for his appointment. Mrs. Jacobs, the receptionist, inquires how he is doing, to which he replies, "Fine." Mrs. Jacobs always looks forward to seeing Mr. Hussar because he is usually so cheerful and talkative, but she is disappointed when he just takes a chair in the waiting room to wait for the doctor. She notes that Mr. Hussar is not as neatly dressed as usual, nor as well groomed.

   a. Is there an alteration in the patient's gait?

   b. What value will being able to "note variances from the normal" provide? What knowledge is needed to be able to determine a variance from the normal?

   c. Are there any physical variances? If so, what are they?

   d. Are there any psychosocial variances? If so, what are they?

PROBLEM-SOLVING PRACTICE

Allen Burns gets a reading of 94/60 when taking a patient's blood pressure. Using the five-step problem-solving process, determine what Allen should do with this finding.

CHAPTER 21

Emergency Procedures

KEY TERMS

- anaphylactic shock
- cardiopulmonary resuscitation (CPR)
- closed fracture
- external bleeding
- first aid
- frostbite
- golden rule
- Good Samaritan Act
- hemorrhage
- hyperthermia
- hypothermia
- implied consent
- internal bleeding
- joint dislocation
- Medic Alert
- open fracture
- rescue breathing
- rescuer
- sprains
- strains (muscle)
- sucking wound
- victim
- wound

OBJECTIVES

Studying and applying the material in this chapter will help you to:

1. Explain the meaning of first aid and what is its goal.
2. State when cardiopulmonary resuscitation should be performed.
3. Explain the meaning and purpose of the Good Samaritan Act.
4. State the golden rule of first aid.
5. List the seven steps to follow that will protect both the victim and the rescuer when an emergency occurs.
6. List the signs and symptoms and describe the treatment for an allergic reaction.
7. List the signs and symptoms and describe the treatment for bleeding and wounds.
8. List the signs and symptoms and describe the treatment for bone, joint, and muscle injuries.
9. List the signs and symptoms and describe the treatment for facial injuries.
10. List the signs and symptoms and describe the treatment for burns.
11. List the signs and symptoms and describe the treatment for drug-related emergencies.
12. List the signs and symptoms and describe the treatment for poisoning.
13. List the signs and symptoms and describe the treatment for temperature-related illnesses.
14. List the signs and symptoms and describe the treatment for breathing difficulty.
15. List the signs and symptoms and describe the treatment for hyperventilation.
16. List the signs and symptoms and describe the treatment for chest pain.
17. List the signs and symptoms and describe the treatment for elevated blood sugar and low blood sugar (related to diabetes).
18. Describe the treatment for fainting.
19. Describe the treatment for fever.
20. List the signs and symptoms and describe the treatment for drowning.
21. Describe signs and symptoms and treatment for seizures.
22. List the signs and symptoms and describe the treatment for shock.
23. List the signs and symptoms and describe the treatment for stroke.
24. Describe the proper application of slings and spiral, figure-eight, and finger wraps.

The Case of the Out-of-Control Party

Josephine Robbins is a nurse at a local hospital. She lives in a nearby apartment complex and is trying to tune out loud noises coming from a party in the next complex. The noise seems to escalate, then she hears someone shout, "Oh my God, he stabbed him," and then there is silence. She calls 9-1-1, gets dressed, and goes to see if it is safe to offer assistance. After deeming it safe, she enters and sees the victim lying on the couch, unconscious. His respirations are shallow and rapid; his skin is pale and cold to the touch; and his lips, earlobes, and fingertips have a bluish tinge. The victim has a 2-inch cut on the left side of his chest where a knife is still inserted, but it is currently not bleeding. There is, however, a great deal of blood in the kitchen area, on the living room carpet, and on the victim's clothing. Josephine does her assessment, gives first aid, and monitors the victim's condition until the paramedics arrive. When the paramedics arrive, she introduces herself and gives them a report of observations and care given. The paramedics continue the care and transport the victim to the hospital. In this chapter, you will learn how to approach emergency situations and how to give appropriate first aid measures to assist victims.

EMERGENCY SITUATIONS

First aid refers to providing emergency care to an accident victim or to someone who has suddenly become ill. The goal of first aid is to provide care to minimize the effects of the injury or illness until the victim can be treated by a physician.

The American Red Cross recommends that all persons take a first aid and safety course. The course covers what to do in an emergency, how to give first aid, and how to prevent accidents and injuries. The American Red Cross and the American Heart Association (AHA) recommend that everyone be trained in giving **cardiopulmonary resuscitation (CPR)**. CPR is administered when someone is not breathing and does not have a pulse. The ARC and AHA believe that many lives would be saved if more people were trained to give emergency care. More people trained in emergency care increases the chance that an injured person can start to receive care immediately rather than it being delayed until medical help arrives.

To encourage individuals to get involved in helping victims during an emergency, all states and the District of Columbia have passed a **Good Samaritan Act**. This is a law that protects individuals from liability when they stop to assist someone who has been hurt or is ill. This protection covers acts that are within the ability of the person to provide as long as there is no gross negligence or willful intent to harm the victim. The Good Samaritan laws vary between states. You should request specifics from your local police department, library, or attorney. You can also search for your state's law on the Internet. (See Box 21–1 for an example.)

The **golden rule** in providing first aid is to "do no further harm." When a person goes into health care as a career, it is because of a desire to help others. When an emergency

Box 21–1

Example of Good Samaritan Law: Arizona

Any health care provider licensed or certified to practice as such in this state or elsewhere, or a licensed ambulance attendant, driver or pilot as defined in section 41-1831, or any other person who renders emergency care at a public gathering or at the scene of an emergency occurrence gratuitously and in good faith shall not be liable for any civil or other damages as the result of any act or omission by such person rendering the emergency care, or as the result of any act or failure to act to provide or arrange for further medical treatment or care for the injured persons, unless such person, while rendering such emergency care, is guilty of gross negligence.

situation arises, it is natural to want to do anything and everything possible to assist the victim. The best way to be ready for this situation is to learn as much as possible about first aid and CPR. But it is also just as critical not to attempt anything you do not have the skills to perform. If the procedure needed is beyond your skill level, then immediately seek help. Getting the appropriate help for the victim can save a life.

Many people fantasize about having the ability to assist someone in an emergency. The thoughts are that the intervention performed saved a life, the rescuer is declared a hero or heroine, and the victim recovers and is very grateful. This indeed may be the situation, but another reality can also occur. Perhaps there is little that can be done to help, the victim is uncooperative, or all attempts at first aid fail, and the victim dies. Some accident sites can be extremely upsetting, and the images and sounds can continue to emotionally upset the Good Samaritan for some time after the event. Even if the outcome of assisting someone is less than ideal, then take satisfaction in knowing that you did the best you could to assist in a very difficult situation.

When an Emergency Occurs

When approaching an injured or ill person, there are certain steps to follow. These steps include actions that will protect the **rescuer** (person giving care), as well as the **victim** (person requiring care).

Assess the Environment

Before approaching the victim, assess the situation to determine if it is safe to approach. If there are loose electrical wires, the potential for a sudden fire or explosion, the smell of gas, or any other hazards that would put the Good Samaritan at risk, the appropriate course of action is to not approach, but to call for help immediately. If the victim is conscious, inform him or her that you will call for assistance and stay with them until help arrives. Most states have emergency medical services (EMS) that are reached by dialing 9-1-1 on a telephone. The person answering has been specially trained and will ask questions that should be answered as accurately as possible. EMS will want to know the name and location of the victim, what the nature of the emergency is, and what, if any, treatment has been given. The EMS personnel will send services as deemed appropriate, such as an ambulance, a fire engine, and/or the police. They may also be able to advise you on what to do to further assist the victim. Remember that your first priority is to keep yourself safe. If you take a risk and become a victim, too, then there is no one to call EMS. Assessing a situation is not done only once; the situation must be continually monitored. For example, if there is smoke in the immediate area, is the amount increasing?

Obtain Consent to Treat

When approaching a stranger, state your name and level of training and ask if you may help. If the victim is responsive, ask questions to better understand the situation. (See Box 21–2.) Explain what you think is wrong and what you plan to do. If the victim is conscious, permission must be obtained prior to administering care. If the victim is a child, determine if a parent or guardian is present to obtain consent for care. If the victim is unconscious, consent is implied (known legally as **implied consent**) and first aid can be administered. Implied consent also applies when a minor needs emergency medical assistance and the minor's parent or guardian is not present. Remember that

---

Box 21–2

Interview the injured or ill person or bystanders, if necessary, using the mnemonic SAMPLE to get a better understanding of the situation and the nature of the person's injury or illness.

S = Signs and symptoms

A = Allergies

M = Medications

P = Pertinent medical history

L = Last food or drink

E = Events leading up the incident

---

victims have the right to refuse care, and this request must be respected. If consent for care is not given or consent revoked during care, but it is obvious that care is required, do not touch or give care. Instead, call EMS if it has not already been notified.

Try to Determine What Happened

Do not assume what might have occurred. If the victim is conscious, ask for information. Look around the environment for any clues that can assist in determining what care is needed. For example, if there is an empty bottle of pills or chemicals that may have been ingested, note what they are and inform EMS, because they may be able to give you directions on how to treat the victim immediately. Many people with specific medical conditions wear necklaces or bracelets or carry cards with them that contain important information that can assist you in determining what care to consider and also in informing the EMS about what type of help to send. This form of identification is called **Medic Alert**, and it may specify if the victim is diabetic, epileptic, or has specific heart problems. There may also be information about specific allergies that will be helpful for the personnel from EMS to know before administering medications. Another thing to determine is if there are other victims. Perhaps someone was thrown from the car or is in a different area than where you are located.

Follow Standard Precautions

Following standard precautions is essential in all situations in which the rescuer may come into contact with body fluids. It is a good idea to be prepared at home, in the car, and at work for medical emergencies. Carry disposable gloves to put on prior to contact. Another valuable item to carry at all times is a barrier device for giving mouth-to-mouth resuscitation. These resuscitation devices have a mouthpiece with a one-way valve attached to a plastic

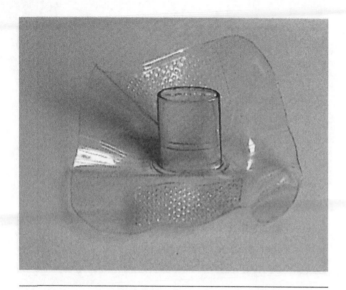

FIGURE 21–1 Portable barrier device to protect rescuer during resuscitation.

shield that prevents the rescuer from getting saliva, blood, or vomit in his or her mouth. (See Figure 21–1.) Some of these devices are small enough to fold into a small pouch that is attached to a key chain. Information about the contents of a first aid kit can be obtained from the American Red Cross. A first aid kit can be kept in the home, car, or office for ready access when needed.

Enlist the Help of Bystanders

Determine if there are others in the area who can assist in the care of the victim. If you are the most experienced person, then stay with the victim and instruct someone else to call EMS. Instruct those willing to help to do other tasks, such as rerouting traffic, keeping onlookers away from the scene, looking for clues as to what happened, or tending to other victims.

Never Move a Victim

A neck or back injury can be made worse or result in permanent paralysis if the victim is moved. The only exception to this rule is if the victim's life is in immediate danger if he or she is not moved. When it is absolutely necessary to move the victim, make every attempt to keep the spine in straight alignment. When turning a victim with a neck or back injury, turn the body as a unit to prevent spinal cord injury. If you move an injured extremity, support it during the move to prevent further vessel or nerve damage.

Stay Calm

A calm, reassuring manner in treating a victim will decrease the stress of the situation for the victim, others in the area, and you. Many people who feel they cannot handle certain situations are quite surprised to discover how effectively they can think and act in an emergency situation. If the scene is more than the rescuer can handle, the best thing to do is to call EMS immediately.

CARDIOPULMONARY RESUSCITATION (CPR)

An expectation of most health care employers is that all health care professionals will attend classes to maintain a current certification for performing CPR. These classes provide theory and hands-on practice for assisting a victim in the following situations:

- Obstructed airway: Perform the Heimlich maneuver, a method that uses pressure to expel material that is stuck in the throat, preventing the victim from being able to inhale air.
- Not breathing: Perform **rescue breathing**, which is a technique in which the rescuer breathes for the victim.
- Not breathing and has no pulse: Perform CPR, which includes rescue breathing and doing compressions to the chest to stimulate cardiac blood flow for the victim.

Because the specific guidelines for CPR may be revised annually and the best approach to learning this material is to receive training from a CPR-certified instructor, the specific procedures are not presented in this text. It is highly recommended that every person be certified in CPR. It is of particular importance that all health care professionals and students obtain and maintain CPR certification.

Advanced certificates are also available. Advanced cardiac life support (ACLS) is available for health care professionals who take care of adults, and pediatric advanced life support (PALS) is offered for those working with children. Employers may require these classes as a condition of employment for physicians, specialty nurses, respiratory therapists, emergency technicians, and paramedics but they can also be taken by others. ACLS and PALS usually include a review of CPR, but their primary focus is advanced life support measures, such as interpretation of cardiac rhythms and the determination of the medications to administer for treatment in cardiac emergencies.

FIRST AID PROCEDURES

When approaching any victim to administer first aid, the first step is always to determine whether the victim is breathing and has a pulse. If not, CPR should be started.

CPR is always the first priority in an emergency. If the victim does not require CPR, then the next step is to assess the victim for any other problems that may need attention. Implementing proper first aid procedures can prevent further injury and assist in the recovery of the injured person. Discussed in the following sections are a variety of first aid procedures that are commonly used in medical emergencies.

Allergic Reactions

Allergic reactions can range from mild to life threatening. The reaction is the result of the body's defense mechanism being triggered by a normally harmless substance. An allergic reaction can be triggered by skin contact (e.g., lotions, poison ivy); ingestion (e.g., certain foods and drugs); inhalation (e.g., sprays and pollen); or injection (e.g., venom from insect and snake bites). Once an allergy has developed, it may become more severe with each re-exposure, depending on the type of reaction. In the most extreme case, a condition called anaphylaxis occurs, in which the respiratory system swells to such an extent that air is prevented from entering the lungs. This is called anaphylactic shock, and if it occurs, death will follow if it is not treated immediately.

See Procedure 21–1 for first aid related to allergic reactions.

PROCEDURE 21–1

FIRST AID FOR ALLERGIC REACTIONS

Always Observe Standard Precautions

CONDITION AND SIGNS AND SYMPTOMS	PROCEDURE	RATIONALE
Mild to Moderate Reaction *S/S*: Itching, hives, and flushed face. Swelling may involve the eyes, face, or tongue. The victim may be weak and dizzy and have nausea and vomiting.	• Be calm and reassuring in approach to victim. • If there is an itchy rash, apply anti-itch lotion (e.g., calamine lotion) and cool compresses.	• Anxiety increases the allergic reaction. • Soothing the itch makes it less likely that the victim will scratch the area, which not only increases the intensity of the rash but may also cause an infection.
	• Try to determine the source of the allergic reaction. • A physician may recommend an over-the-counter medication (e.g., Benadryl). • Call EMS if the condition worsens.	• The victim can avoid it in the future. • Taking an antihistamine can decrease the effect of an allergic reaction. • It may advance to a severe reaction.
Severe Reaction *S/S*: The mild to moderate reactions may be present, but they can quickly become more severe. In the worst cases that lead to anaphylaxis, there is difficulty breathing, wheezing, and tightness of the chest. The victim may have difficulty swallowing and become unconscious. Untreated anaphylaxis can lead to death.	• Call EMS. • If the victim has emergency allergy medication, help him or her administer it. • Do not give the victim anything by mouth if he or she is having difficulty breathing. • Do not place a pillow under the victim's head.	• Severe reactions can lead to anaphylactic shock. • Victims with known severe allergies may carry a kit for administering an injection to stop a reaction. • It may enter the lungs and cause further breathing difficulties. • Elevating the head may close off the airway.

(continues)

PROCEDURE

FIRST AID FOR ALLERGIC REACTIONS

CONDITION AND SIGNS AND SYMPTOMS	PROCEDURE	RATIONALE
Bites and Stings (e.g., insects, spiders, scorpions, and snakes) *S/S:* Localized reaction to bite or sting may be seen, such as redness, pain, and swelling. There may be an obvious bite mark. An allergic reaction may occur as noted in the section on allergic reactions.	• Try to identify what bit or stung the victim.	• This will assist EMS personnel to treat victim.
	• Kill it if there is no risk to the rescuer, and keep it for identification.	• The rescuer's safety comes first, or there will be two victims and no one to call EMS.
	• If there is a stinger (e.g., from a honeybee), remove it by scraping it with your fingernail or a credit card.	• Do not use tweezers because it may force more venom into victim.
	• Promptly remove a tick using a fine-tipped, pointed tweezers with a smooth inside surface. Grasp the tick at the head as close to the skin as possible. Pull upward slowly and steadily without twisting until the tick releases its hold. Wash the area with soap and water and apply antibiotic wound ointment if no known allergies or sensitivities to the ingredients. If you think that the tick's mouth parts are still embedded in the skin, the person should see a health care provider.	• This decreases the chance of mouth parts remaining in the victim. • Ticks carry pathogens, such as Lyme disease and Rocky Mountain spotted fever. Also the longer the mouth part is embedded, the more likely an infection can develop.
	• Call EMS immediately if a poisonous spider, scorpion, or snake has bitten the victim.	• The victim must receive the appropriate injection of antivenom without delay.
	• If an allergic reaction occurs, treat it as noted for allergic reactions.	• Same as for allergic reactions.
	• Stay with the victim for at least an hour.	• Sometimes reactions are delayed.
	• Clean the area with soap and water and apply antiseptic ointment.	• Cleaning helps to prevent infection.
	• Remove any confining clothing or jewelry.	• Clothing and jewelry act as a constricting band if swelling occurs.
	• Apply a cold compress.	• This can decrease pain, swelling, and the spread of venom.

(continues)

PROCEDURE

FIRST AID FOR ALLERGIC REACTIONS

CONDITION AND SIGNS AND SYMPTOMS	PROCEDURE	RATIONALE
Bites and Stings *(continued)*	• Have the victim lie still and keep the bite area below heart level. • Do not apply a tourniquet. • Consult with a physician to determine if any additional preventive measures should be taken. • Instruct the victim to observe for infection (e.g., increased pain, redness, or swelling; discharge from the site, swollen glands, fever, flu-like symptoms, or red streaks coming from the site) and get medical help immediately if symptoms occur.	• Lying still slows the rate at which the venom spreads. • A tourniquet cuts off blood to the extremity, may result in damage to tissues, and could result in the need for an amputation. • The victim may need additional treatment to prevent disease that may have been contracted through the bite or sting (e.g., tetanus, Lyme disease). • Infections require follow-up care and treatment by a physician.

Bleeding and Wounds

Bleeding occurs when a blood vessel is damaged. Heavy bleeding is called a **hemorrhage**. Damage to the soft tissue of the body from violence or trauma is called a **wound**. **External bleeding** occurs when blood drains to the outside of the body through a break in the skin. If there is bleeding that occurs inside the body, it is called **internal bleeding** and is more difficult to detect. Suspect internal bleeding if the victim has a broken bone or has been hit forcibly (e.g., a car accident in which the victim hits the dashboard or steering wheel, is struck by an object, or receives other types of trauma to the head or body). If internal bleeding is suspected, the victim must have a medical evaluation.

When giving first aid to a victim who has a wound, the rescuer must clean the wound and protect it from further damage. If there is external bleeding that does not stop spontaneously, first aid will be required to stop the bleeding before the victim loses too much blood.

Bleeding can occur from a vein or an artery. *Arterial bleeding* is a brighter red and comes out in spurts with each heartbeat. This is a life-threatening situation and must be stopped as soon as possible. *Venous bleeding* flows evenly and can also result in a great deal of blood loss. Remember to follow standard precautions when caring for victims with wounds and bleeding.

A tourniquet (tight band placed around an arm or leg to stop bleeding) is rarely used in emergency care because it too often does more harm than good. It is used only as a last resort to save a life because it can result in the loss of the limb below the injury. See Procedure 21–2 for first aid related to bleeding and wounds.

Bone, Joint, and Muscle Injuries

When a bone is broken, it is called a fracture. An **open fracture** is when the broken bone protrudes through the skin. A **closed fracture** is a broken bone that does not break the skin. When a joint becomes disconnected from its socket, it is called a **joint dislocation**.

Strains result from the sudden tearing of muscle fibers during exertion and are often referred to as pulled muscles. **Sprains** are torn ligament fibers that result in a loosening of the joint.

PROCEDURE

21–2

FIRST AID FOR BLEEDING AND WOUNDS

Always Observe Standard Precautions

CONDITION AND SIGNS AND SYMPTOMS

External Bleeding

S/S: Blood coming from a wound. Weakness, confusion, or a decreasing level of consciousness may indicate excessive blood loss. Loss of function distal to the wound indicates damage to tendons or muscles. Loss of sensation distal to the wound indicates damage to the nerves.

PROCEDURE

- Call EMS if you suspect internal bleeding or if there is heavy external bleeding or other serious injuries.

- Apply cold compresses to bruised areas.

- If there is bleeding from the leg or arm, elevate it above heart level (unless contraindicated by neck or back injury, or discomfort).

- Do not use a tourniquet.

- To stop bleeding, apply direct pressure with a clean cloth or sterile dressing over the area. (See Figure 21–2.) If the rescuer needs his or her hands free to do additional first aid, a pressure dressing can be applied to decrease the bleeding. (See Figures 21–3a–e).

- When the dressing becomes soaked with blood, do not remove it; instead place the new dressing on top.

- Do not look under the dressing to see if the bleeding has stopped.

- Do not apply pressure over an embedded object, the eye, or on a head injury if a skull fracture is suspected.

- If bleeding from an arm or leg does not stop after 15 minutes of direct pressure, then use pressure-point bleeding control. (See Figures 21–4a–b.)

RATIONALE

- The victim will require medical evaluation and intervention.

- Bruising can be decreased as the cold constricts the blood vessels.

- Elevation of the extremity will decrease the pressure in the vascular system of the arm or leg and thus decrease bleeding.

- Cuts off blood to the extremity, resulting in damage to tissues and the possible need for an amputation.

- Pressure slows the blood flow so body can use its natural clotting mechanism.

- Removing the dressing may reinitiate or increase bleeding.

- Lifting the dressing may reinitiate bleeding.

- This may cause further damage.

- This technique will decrease the flow of blood to the affected area.

(continues)

PROCEDURE

FIRST AID FOR BLEEDING AND WOUNDS

(continued)

FIGURE 21–2 By using direct pressure and elevation, most severe bleeding can be controlled.

FIGURE 21–3c Split the end of the bandage into two strips.

FIGURE 21–3a Maintain direct pressure and elevation when applying a pressure dressing. Do not remove previous dressing, but apply the pressure dressing over the previous dressing.

FIGURE 21–3d Tie the ends tightly into a knot right over the wound.

FIGURE 21–3b Wrap the roller bandage or long strip of cloth firmly around the wound. Overlap each rotation partially over the previous one to hold it securely in place.

FIGURE 21–3e Check for circulation to verify that the dressing is not too tight. If there is no pulse or the fingers are turning bluish, loosen the dressing and rewrap it.

(continues)

PROCEDURE

(continued)

FIRST AID FOR BLEEDING AND WOUNDS

CONDITION AND SIGNS AND SYMPTOMS

Internal Bleeding

Abdominal injuries can cause internal bleeding.

S/S: Blood in the vomit, urine, or stool, or from the vagina; distended abdomen; nausea; abdominal tenderness; signs and symptoms of shock. (See shock under Other Conditions.) Weakness, confusion, or a decreasing level of consciousness may indicate bleeding inside the skull that is causing pressure on the brain.

Wounds

S/S: Tear or open area anywhere on the body.

PROCEDURE

- Call EMS

- Do not give the victim anything to eat or drink.

- Place the victim on his or her back and elevate the knees with a pillow or blanket if there is abdominal discomfort.
- Keep the victim still and treat him or her for shock as needed.
- Stay with victim until medical assistance arrives.
- Do not try to clean a large wound or remove any embedded objects.

- Remove any obvious loose debris from the wound.
- If an object is protruding from the body, do not remove it. (See Figure 21–5.)

RATIONALE

- The victim must be evaluated and treated by medical personnel.
- The victim may need surgical intervention; food or drink may cause vomiting.
- This position relaxes the abdominal muscles and decreases pain.

- This is to prevent further injury.

- Give rescue breathing or CPR as needed.
- Cleaning can increase the bleeding and cause additional damage.
- This decreases contamination of wound.
- Removing the object may cause further damage or initiate bleeding.

FIGURE 21–4a For an arm wound, the pressure point is on the brachial artery. It is located between the large muscles (biceps and triceps) on the inside of the arm. Press firmly with your fingers, until you no longer feel a pulse.

FIGURE 21–4b For a leg wound, the pressure point is on the femoral artery. It is located in the groin at the bend of the leg. Press firmly with the palm of your hand (or use both hands for more pressure) against the pelvic bone, until you no longer feel a pulse.

(continues)

PROCEDURE

21–2

FIRST AID FOR BLEEDING AND WOUNDS

(continued)

CONDITION AND SIGNS AND SYMPTOMS

Sucking Wounds

S/S: Bubbling from any wound of the neck or chest; difficulty breathing.

PROCEDURE

- If the chest or neck has been punctured or if there is an object protruding from the chest or neck, note if there is any bubbling from the wound. If so, this is called a **sucking wound**, and it needs to be sealed as soon as possible.

- With a sucking wound, apply an airtight dressing (e.g., plastic wrap, tin foil, plastic bag, or other nonporous material) over the site. If you do not have nonporous material, you can use a regular gauze pad or clean cloth coated with petroleum jelly (i.e., Vaseline).

- When applying an airtight dressing, leave one edge untaped or unsealed.

- Do not move the patient unless absolutely necessary.

- Do not give the patient anything by mouth.

RATIONALE

- Bubbling is caused by air passing through a wound that has penetrated the respiratory system. The victim will be experiencing difficulty with breathing because air is escaping as he or she breathes.

- An airtight dressing prevents the escape of air from the respiratory system.

- This allows trapped air to escape.

- Movement may cause further injury.

- Surgery may be required.

FIGURE 21–5 Never remove an object protruding from the body. Immobilize the object by placing dressings around the object and taping the dressing in place.

(continues)

PROCEDURE

FIRST AID FOR BLEEDING AND WOUNDS

CONDITION AND SIGNS AND SYMPTOMS	PROCEDURE	RATIONALE
Amputations *S/S*: Part of the body severed from its attachment (e.g., all or part of a finger, toe, arm, leg, nose, or ear).	• If an amputation of a body part occurs, save the severed part. • After giving the appropriate first aid to the victim, try to locate the part if it is not in the immediate area. • Once the body part is found, rinse it off, wrap it in a moistened cloth, and place it in a plastic bag or other container. • If ice is available, place the bag in a container with ice and water. Do not place the part directly on ice. • Write the name of the patient and the time of the accident on the container with the body part. • Make sure the amputated body part remains with the victim when he or she is transported to the hospital.	• It may be possible to reattach the amputated part after reaching the hospital. • First aid for the victim is the first priority. • A clean, moist body part is more apt to be successfully reattached. • Lowering the temperature of the body part will extend the amount of time for successful reattachment. Direct contact with the ice will cause freezing and damage the tissue. • This assists medical personnel at the hospital who will decide if reattachment is possible. • This prevents unnecessary delays in locating the part.

A helpful mnemonic for treating bone, joint, and muscle injuries is RICE:

- R = rest—limit use of the injured body part
- I = immobilize—stabilize the injured body part with an elastic bandage or a splint to limit motion
- C = cold—apply cold pack wrapped in a thin, dry towel to the area for no more than 20 minutes at a time, then wait at least 20 minutes before applying the cold pack again
- E = elevate—prop the injured part up to help to reduce swelling. Do not do this if raising the injured part causes more pain

See Procedure 21–3 for first aid related to bone, joint, and muscle injuries.

Injuries to Facial Structures

Injuries to the eyes, ears, and nose are common. Any eye injury should always be taken very seriously because it can involve the loss of vision. A blow to the ear can cause loss of hearing.

See Procedure 21–4 for first aid related to injuries of the facial structures.

Burns

Burns can occur from heat, radiation, chemicals, or electrical current. The severity of the burn is determined by the size, depth, and location of the burn. Minor burns are referred to as *superficial* or *first-degree burns* because only the top layer of the skin (epidermis) is involved. If the burn continues and extends beyond the superficial layer to the dermis, it is a *partial-thickness* or *second-degree burn*. (See Figure 21–7.) If the burn continues even deeper, it is a *full-thickness* or *third-degree burn*. (See Figure 21–8.) The amount of pain the victim reports does not necessarily reflect the severity of the burn because deeper burns can destroy nerve endings and be painless. (See Figure 21–9.)

Fascinating Facts

The National Center for Environmental Health (NCEH; www.cdc.gov/nceh/), which is part of the Centers for Disease Control and Prevention (CDC), reports the following statistics:

- Unintentional injuries were the fifth leading cause of death for all ages.

- Poisonings were responsible for 25% of the injury deaths, followed by motor vehicle traffic accidents at 17.5%, and firearms at 17.4%.

- There were 34.4 million medically attended injury and poisoning episodes in the noninstitutionalized population.

- Home was the leading place of injury occurrence, accounting for 42% (24% in the home and 18% outside the home) of the respondent-reported nonfatal, medically attended injury episodes.

Thinking It Through

Marlow Barrons is a nurse on vacation in Alaska. After fishing all day, she and her friends are unloading their boat when an emergency call comes to the Coast Guard. She overhears them discussing that a professional fisherman has amputated his arm in the gears of his boat. She tells them she is a nurse and offers assistance. Her offer is accepted, she boards the Coast Guard boat, and they speed off to the site of the accident.

1. What signs and symptoms can Marlow anticipate seeing based on the report of the accident?

2. What type of first aid should she anticipate the victim will need?

3. Are there special considerations regarding the amputated arm?

PROCEDURE

21-3

FIRST AID FOR BONE, JOINT, AND MUSCLE INJURIES

Always Observe Standard Precautions

CONDITION AND SIGNS AND SYMPTOMS	PROCEDURE	RATIONALE
Fractures and Joint Dislocations *S/S*: Pain, swelling, and loss of function. In an open fracture, a bone protrudes through the skin, creating a wound. If the joint is dislocated, the joint will appear deformed. Deformity may also occur with fractures.	• Immobilize the broken bone or dislocated joint using a splint or sling. (See Figures 21–6a–c). Do not move the victim until the affected limb is immobilized, unless there is no other option. If no medical supplies are available, look around for items that will work as an alternate splint (e.g., a thick twig or board could be used on each side of a leg or arm and attached with strips of cloth; a sweater could be used to make a sling for the arm).	• This prevents further injury.

(continues)

PROCEDURE

FIRST AID FOR BONE, JOINT, AND MUSCLE INJURIES

(continued)

CONDITION AND SIGNS AND SYMPTOMS	PROCEDURE	RATIONALE
Fractures and Joint Dislocations *(continued)*	• Do not attempt to realign a misshapen bone or joint. Do not test for function.	• This may cause further injury to the tissues. For example, it could cause hemorrhage, nerve damage, or an embolus (a mass that travels through the body and can cause damage elsewhere by obstructing blood flow).
	• Do not give anything by mouth.	• The victim may require surgical repair of the bone.

FIGURE 21–6b Some air splints are inflated by blowing into a nozzle. Care must be taken to avoid overinflating any splint. Always check for a pulse distal to the splint.

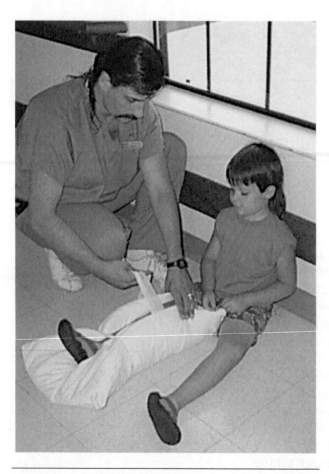

FIGURE 21–6a Splints should be long enough to immobilize the joint above and below the injured area.

FIGURE 21–6C Commercial slings usually have a series of straps that extend around the neck and the trunk of the body.

(continues)

PROCEDURE

FIRST AID FOR BONE, JOINT, AND MUSCLE INJURIES

(continued)

CONDITION AND SIGNS AND SYMPTOMS	PROCEDURE	RATIONALE
Fractures and Joint Dislocations *(continued)*	• If there is an open fracture, cover it with a dressing prior to immobilizing the area. Do not wash or attempt to remove anything from the area.	• The dressing prevents further contamination of the wound. Washing or removing anything from the area can result in further damage.
	• When immobilizing an area, leave it in the position in which you found it and make sure that the area above and below has extra support, so the injured area is immobilized.	• This prevents further injury.
	• Check for circulation below the injury to ensure that the splint is not too tight.	• Lack of circulation can result in damage to, and death of, the tissues.
Muscle Strain (Pulled Muscle) *S/S:* Sudden tearing sensation felt during exertion, followed by pain and swelling.	• Remove any constricting clothing or jewelry.	• Clothing and jewelry act as a constricting band if swelling occurs.
	• Apply cold compresses as soon as possible for no more than 20 minutes at a time, then wait at least 20 minutes before applying the cold pack again.	• This decreases swelling.
	• Do not place ice directly on the skin.	• Freezing the skin causes tissue damage.
	• Elevate the limb.	• This decreases swelling.
	• Contact a physician if the pain is severe, if there is loss of function or impairment of circulation below the injury, or if the area is misshapen.	• The injury will need medical evaluation and treatment.
	• A physician may also recommend an over-the-counter anti-inflammatory medication.	• This decreases inflammation and swelling.
	• Rest the injured area for at least 24 hours. Do not use the injured area if pain occurs with movement.	• Rest allows the injury to heal and prevents further injury.
	• If there is no improvement, seek medical assistance.	• The injured area needs further evaluation.
Sprain *S/S:* Pain and swelling; loosening of the joint. Unless there is a complete tear, the joint will still function.	• Same as for muscle strain.	• Same as for muscle strain.

PROCEDURE

FIRST AID FOR FACIAL INJURIES

Always Observe Standard Precautions

CONDITION AND SIGNS AND SYMPTOMS	PROCEDURE	RATIONALE
Eye Injuries *S/S*: Tearing, redness, stinging, burning, or pain in or around the eye; sensitivity to light; and rapid blinking. Blows to the eye can cause internal bleeding and damage to the tissues.	• Do not press on the eye or allow the victim to rub the eyes. • If a foreign object is irritating the eye, flush the eye with a large amount of water. • Do not use cotton swabs (e.g., Q-tips) or any instruments (e.g., tweezers) to try to remove objects from eye. • If the object is not flushed out and is embedded, do not attempt to remove it; instead cover both eyes with a dressing and await medical assistance. • If there has been a blow to the eye, lay the victim flat, cover both eyes, and call for medical assistance. • If a "black eye" is forming, apply a cold compress to the area.	• This prevents further injury. • Loose particles will wash away in the water. • Cotton sheds fibers that will get in the eye. Sharp instruments can cause further damage. • Trying to remove the object can create more damage. Covering both eyes decreases movement of the injured eye. • Laying the victim flat decreases loss of fluid from the eye. Covering both eyes decreases movement of the eyes. • A cold compress decreases bleeding by causing vasoconstriction (constriction of blood vessels).
Ear Injuries *S/S*: Bleeding or drainage from the ear, loss of hearing, earache, redness, bruising, or swelling around the ear. Ruptured eardrum causes severe pain.	• Do not block bleeding or drainage from the ear. If possible, lay the victim on his or her side with the injured ear down. • Do not attempt to clean inside the ear. • If an object is in the ear and clearly visible, place the victim's injured ear downward and gently wiggle the object with tweezers. • Do not attempt to remove an object that is not visible. Seek medical assistance. • If ruptured eardrum is suspected, place a dressing over the ear. Seek medical assistance.	• Promoting drainage will prevent buildup of pressure in the ear that can cause more damage. • This prevents further injury and contamination. • This may dislodge the object, and it will fall out as a result of gravity. • This may push the object farther into the ear canal. • This prevents contamination of the ear.

(continues)

PROCEDURE

FIRST AID FOR FACIAL INJURIES

CONDITION AND SIGNS AND SYMPTOMS	PROCEDURE	RATIONALE
Ear Injuries *(continued)*	• If an insect is in the ear, do not allow the victim to poke a finger into the ear. Have the victim hold his or her head with the ear pointing up. If medical assistance is not immediately available, the victim is very uncomfortable, and you are sure it is only an insect, place several drops of room-temperature oil into the ear (e.g., cooking oil, baby oil, and mineral oil). Seek medical assistance.	• Putting an object in the ear may cause an insect to bite or sting. The insect may climb out on its own if given an opportunity. Oil will drown the insect, but can dangerously expand other objects that may be in the ear.
Nose Injuries Most nosebleeds (epistaxis) stop on their own, but if not, first aid may be needed. *S/S*: Blood coming from the nostrils or running down the back of the throat. If the bleeding is from the back of the nose, there may be a feeling of fullness in the ears, coughing up blood, gagging, or choking due to blood in the back of the throat. A broken nose may look crooked.	• If there is an object lodged in the nostril, attempt to remove it by having the victim hold the other nostril and blow out the nostril with the object, or have the victim sniff some pepper to induce a sneeze. If this does not work, get medical help.	• This increases pressure behind the object to propel it out.
	• Do not put anything into the nostril to try to grab hold of the object.	• This may push the object in farther.
	• Instruct the victim to breathe through the mouth and not inhale through the nostril.	• This decreases the risk of blood entering into lungs.
	• If the nose may be broken, have the victim sit down, lean forward, and apply a cold compress.	• Leaning forward helps prevent blood from running down the back of the throat. A cold compress decreases bleeding by constricting blood vessels.
	• Do not attempt to straighten a broken nose, but seek medical assistance.	• This may cause further damage.
	• If the nose is not broken, attempt to stop the bleeding by instructing the victim to sit down and lean forward while applying pressure on the soft part of the nose. Maintain the pressure for at least 15 minutes, then release. If there is still bleeding, repeat the procedure for 15 more minutes. Then, if it has not stopped, seek medical assistance.	• Leaning forward helps prevent blood from running down the back of throat. Applying pressure decreases the blood flow and encourages clotting. If you cannot stop the bleeding, medical evaluation and treatment are needed.

Courtesy of the Phoenix Society of Burn Survivors, Inc.

FIGURE 21–7 Second-degree or partial-thickness burn: The skin is wet, red, swollen, painful, and blistered.

Courtesy of the Phoenix Society of Burn Survivors, Inc.

FIGURE 21–8 Third-degree or full-thickness burn: All layers of the skin, plus the fat, muscles, bone, and nerve tissues, are destroyed.

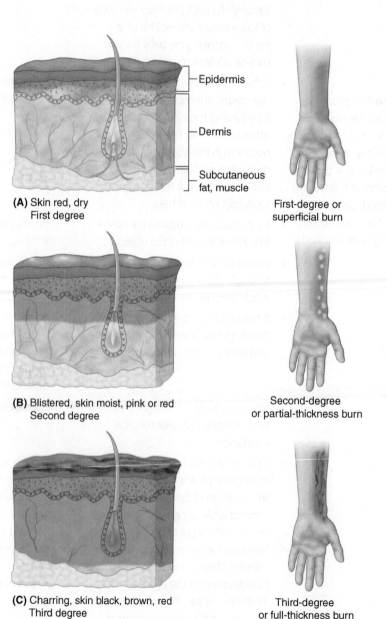

— Epidermis

— Dermis

— Subcutaneous fat, muscle

(A) Skin red, dry
First degree

First-degree or
superficial burn

(B) Blistered, skin moist, pink or red
Second degree

Second-degree
or partial-thickness burn

(C) Charring, skin black, brown, red
Third degree

Third-degree
or full-thickness burn

FIGURE 21–9 Types of burns.

When caring for burns, remember the following three steps:

1. Stop the burning.
2. Cool the burned area.
3. Cover the burned area with clean, dry dressings (apply loosely).

See Procedure 21–5 for first aid related to the various sources of burns.

When treating burn victims, always assess them for the possibility of damage to the respiratory system through inhalation of smoke or fumes from chemicals. The damage to the respiratory system can cause swelling that will prevent the victim from breathing properly. Look for discoloration around the nostrils or mouth as a possible indication. If it is likely that the victim has inhaled smoke or fumes (was in a smoky room, exposed to chemical fumes, or has discolored nostrils) but is not experiencing difficulty in

PROCEDURE

21–5

FIRST AID FOR BURNS

Always Observe Standard Precautions

CONDITION	PROCEDURE	RATIONALE
Heat (e.g., flames, hot liquids, or grease)	• Extinguish the fire (e.g., if the victim's clothing is on fire).	• This stops the burning.
	• Move the victim to a well-ventilated area if smoke is present. Move accident victims only when it is necessary to protect them.	• This protects the victim from damage to respiratory tract due to smoke inhalation.
	• When moving victims, maintain their body alignment.	• This prevents further damage in the event they may have a neck or back injury.
	• Run cool water over the burned area for several minutes or immerse the area in cool water (use a cool, wet cloth on areas that cannot be immersed and rewet as necessary by pouring additional cool water onto the cloth).	• This cools the burned area. Cooling should not be done if a burn is major or covers an extensive area, because it can dangerously lower the body temperature.
	• Do not apply ice except on a minor burn, such as a finger burned on the stove.	• This can freeze tissue and cause further damage.
	• Remove clothing from the burn area if possible, but if it is stuck to the burn, do not use force.	• Forcibly removing clothing will increase damage to tissues.
	• Do not break blisters.	• Blisters form a natural sterile protection to the area.
	• Cover the burn with a clean, dry cloth (use sterile, nonadhesive dressings if available).	• This covers the burned area to prevent contamination.
	• Do not apply any ointments to a severe burn.	• Ointments can hold the heat in, increasing the severity of the burn.
	• Apply a bandage loosely.	• This prevents pressure on the burn.
	• Do not use cotton as a dressing.	• Cotton adheres and leaves small fibers embedded in the wound.
	• Prevent chilling.	• Chilling is common with burns.

(continues)

PROCEDURE

FIRST AID FOR BURNS

CONDITION	PROCEDURE	RATIONALE
Radiation (e.g., sunburn)	• Move the victim so he or she is no longer exposed to the sun.	• This stops the burning.
	• Cool the burn as discussed earlier.	• Same as for heat burns.
	• Apply a dressing as discussed for heat burns.	• Same as for heat burns.
	• Prevent chilling.	• Same as for heat burns.
Chemicals Numerous household and environmental products cause burns when in contact with skin.	• Prevent any further contact of the victim with the chemical.	• If any chemical remains on the victim's clothing, it will continue to burn the victim; if possible, remove any clothing and jewelry exposed to the chemical.
	• Move the victim to a well-ventilated area if fumes are present. Move accident victims only when it is necessary to protect them.	• This protects victim from damage to the respiratory tract due to inhalation of fumes.
	• When moving victims, maintain their body alignment.	• This prevents further damage if the victim has a back or neck injury.
	• Flush the burn with large amounts of cool water and continue to do so until EMS arrive.	• This cools the burn.
	• Always flush away from the body.	• This prevents the chemical-laden water from touching unexposed areas of the skin.
	• If there is any chemical in the eyes, flush them continuously with cool water.	• Eyes are very sensitive to chemical burns, and vision may be lost if chemicals are not completely removed.
	• If only one eye is affected, flush from the inner aspect of the eye to the outer. (See Figure 21–10.)	• This prevents the chemical from getting into the other eye.
Electrical Current (electrical cords or lines and lightning)	• Do not touch the victim if he or she is still in contact with a live electrical wire (have the power turned off first).	• As the rescuer, you must protect yourself first. If you are unable to touch the victim, call EMS.
	• Do not cool the burn.	• Burns are not on the surface.
	• Apply a clean, dry dressing.	• This prevents contamination.
	• Prevent chilling and do not move the victim if possible, because other injuries may be present.	• There will usually be only a small burn area noted on the surface, but extensive internal damage can be present, caused by the current as it traveled through the body (look for an exit burn also).

(continues)

PROCEDURE

FIRST AID FOR BURNS

(continued)

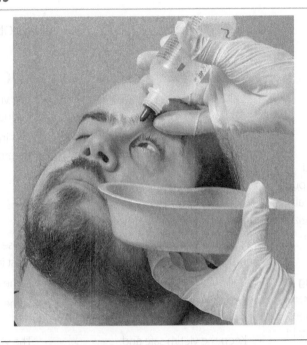

FIGURE 21–10 To flush an eye, hold the eyelid open and run the water (use sterile saline if available) from the inner part of the eye toward the outer part.

breathing, do not dismiss the problem because the effects can be delayed for up to 24 hours.

Drug Abuse

"Drug abuse" refers to the misuse or overuse of any drug. These drugs may be legal or illegal, prescription or over the counter, and include any substance that alters how the body functions. For example, prescription and over-the-counter medications, caffeine, alcohol, nicotine, or any illegal drug preparation can cause life-threatening situations.

The opioid crisis in the United States prompted researchers to find ways to counteract overdoses of this type of drug. As a result, the medication *naloxone* has been developed and approved by the FDA to rapidly reverse opioid overdose. Although considered to be a prescription medication, in many states it can be purchased at a pharmacy without a prescription from a physician.

Another condition that can cause the need for medical intervention is when an addictive drug is taken and the body develops a craving for more of the drug. If the drug is not continued, the body will go through a process of withdrawal that can create life-threatening situations.

See Procedure 21–6 for first aid related to drug overdose and withdrawal.

Poisoning

Poisoning most commonly occurs through ingestion and inhalation. Poisons that come in contact with the skin are treated similarly to burns that occur when caustic (destructive to living tissue) chemicals come into contact with skin. The procedure is to perform lots of flushing to remove the poison, while taking care not to get it on the victim's uncontaminated areas or on the rescuer's skin.

If you suspect poisoning, do not wait for signs and symptoms to develop; instead seek medical assistance immediately. Do not rely on the label's directions, because they may be incorrect. Instead call the poison control center (National Poison Help Hotline 1-800-222-1222) or EMS (9-1-1) because they can supply you with the information needed to immediately and most effectively treat the poison victim.

Identifying the source of the poison is important in determining the proper treatment for the victim. If the victim is unable to give any information (is a child, unconscious, or confused), look around for any clues as to the source of the poison (e.g., empty bottle or other container, source of fumes, traces of powders or liquids in the area, poisonous plants, and bystander information).

The most critical component of poisoning first aid is prevention. Because young children are the frequent

PROCEDURE

FIRST AID FOR DRUG-RELATED PROBLEMS

Always Observe Standard Precautions

CONDITION AND SIGNS AND SYMPTOMS	PROCEDURE	RATIONALE
Drug Overdose *S/S*: Behavioral changes, such as overexcitation, hallucinations, and agitation. There may be difficulty breathing, drowsiness, tremors, and excessive sweating. The size of the pupil is often smaller or larger than normal. Nausea and vomiting may occur. Seizures and unconsciousness may develop.	• Call EMS. • Try to determine what was taken, when, how much, and which route (e.g., oral, inhalation, injection). Be aware that it may have been more than one type or also combined with alcohol or other substances. • If possible, collect samples of the drug and of any vomit for analysis.	• The victim needs medical evaluation and intervention. • This information will assist in determination of treatment. • These samples can be analyzed to assist in determination of treatment.
Withdrawal from Addictive Drug *S/S*: Behavioral changes, such as extreme restlessness, hallucinations, depression, anxiety, and agitation. Tremors and cold sweats may occur. Nausea and vomiting may occur. Seizures may develop. The main focus of the victim may be to find some of the drug he or she is withdrawing from in order to alleviate the discomfort.	• Call EMS. • Try to determine what drug the victim has been taking. • Keep the victim safe and comfortable until medical assistance arrives.	• Same as for drug overdose. • Same as for drug overdose. • The victim may harm himself or herself when experiencing severe behavioral changes or if seizures occur.

victims of accidental poisoning, it is essential to keep all harmful substances locked in cabinets or out of the reach of children. Remember that children can be quite inventive in using furniture to climb up to reach desired objects, so using a locked cabinet is the preferred approach.

Poisoning by ingestion can be caused by many common products found around the home, such as cleaning agents, yard care products, cosmetics, medications, paints, plants, car fluids, personal care items, and spoiled food or contaminated water. Inhalation dangers include sources of poisonous fumes, such as gas leaks, automobile exhaust, and chemical fumes.

See Procedure 21–7 for first aid related to poisoning.

Temperature-Related Illness

Exposure to excessive cold can cause cold-related injuries. If the skin begins to freeze, it is called frostbite. **Frostbite** occurs most commonly on the extremities or exposed areas, such as fingers, toes, nose, cheeks, and earlobes. If the body temperature drops below normal, it

is **hypothermia**. Hypothermia can occur inside and outside the home, depending on a number of conditions. These conditions include extreme cold, wet clothes, and being immersed in cold water. Newborns, the elderly, and those in poor health can become hypothermic in an underheated room.

At the other extreme, exposure to excessive heat can cause heat-related injuries. Being outside in high temperatures and humidity can cause the body temperature to increase above normal (**hyperthermia**), and a loss of body fluids by excessive perspiration can result in the loss of salt and subsequent dehydration. Certain medications and medical conditions can aggravate the problem. Newborns, the elderly, and those in poor health can become hyperthermic in an overheated room with poor ventilation. Other contributing factors are obesity, excessive exercise, and ingestion of alcohol. The heat-related illnesses from least to most severe are heat cramps, heat exhaustion, and heat stroke.

See Procedure 21–8 for first aid for temperature-related illnesses.

PROCEDURE

FIRST AID FOR POISONINGS

Always Observe Standard Precautions

CONDITION AND SIGNS AND SYMPTOMS

Ingestion (swallowing)

S/S: Vary widely depending on the substance ingested and how it affects the various systems. For example, gastrointestinal (GI) symptoms may include nausea, vomiting, diarrhea, abdominal pain, or loss of appetite. The skin may be pale, and the victim may feel dizzy, weak, irritable, or drowsy. There may be pain while swallowing or burns or residue around the mouth. There may be seizures or complete loss of consciousness.

Inhalation (breathing)

S/S: Vary depending on the substance inhaled. May be similar to the signs and symptoms listed for ingestion.

PROCEDURE

- The goal of immediate treatment is to get the poison out of the body, but do not administer any food, fluids, or home remedies or induce vomiting unless directed to do so by medical personnel.
- If the victim does vomit, make sure the vomit is cleared from the mouth.
- Save any vomit.

- Keep the patient safe and comfortable until help can arrive.
- The goal of immediate treatment is to get the victim into fresh air.
- Before entering an environment where poisonous gases may be present, apply protective breathing gear. If no protective breathing gear is available, place a wet cloth over your nose and mouth, and then take several deep breaths of fresh air before entering to remove the victim.
- If there is a visible cloud of fumes, keep your head above or below it.
- If possible, open windows and doors and turn off any source of fumes.
- Do not light any flames or flip any switches.
- When the victim is in fresh air, the poison control center or EMS can be called.
- The victim should be kept safe and comfortable until help arrives.

RATIONALE

- Getting the poison out of the body will prevent further absorption of the poison, but inducing vomiting for a substance that burned the GI system on the way down will also burn it on the way up.
- This prevents it from blocking the airway and from entering the lungs.
- It can be analyzed to identify the source of the poisoning.
- This prevents further injury and decreases anxiety.

- This prevents further inhalation of poisonous gas.

- The rescuer must protect himself or herself against becoming the second victim of the fumes.

- The cloud will contain the highest concentration of fumes.

- This decreases the concentration of fumes in the area.

- Fumes may ignite.

- You will need further directions on care and the victim may need medical intervention.

- This prevents further injury and decreases anxiety.

PROCEDURE

21–8

FIRST AID FOR TEMPERATURE-RELATED ILLNESSES

Always Observe Standard Precautions

CONDITION AND SIGNS AND SYMPTOMS	PROCEDURE	RATIONALE
Frostbite *S/S:* Initially the skin is red and painful; then as the skin begins to freeze, it loses feeling (numbness), then becomes hard and white and blisters. In severe frostbite, the blood vessels freeze and the skin becomes black due to the death of tissues from lack of oxygen.	• Do not thaw out the area unless it can be kept thawed. • Do not massage the area. • Do not use direct heat to thaw the area. • Remove any constricting clothes or jewelry. • To thaw the frozen area, place it in warm water or apply a warm cloth; keep water or cloth warm (not hot) until area softens and color and sensation return; as the area thaws, pain and swelling can be expected. • After thawing, apply a sterile, dry dressing. • If fingers or toes are frostbitten, place a dressing between them. • Move the thawed area as little as possible. • Discourage smoking or drinking alcohol.	• Refreezing will increase damage. • This increases damage to tissues • This thaws the area too quickly. • This increases circulation. • This thaws the area slowly. • This prevents contamination. • This keeps them separated. • This minimizes damage to tissues. • Both constrict the blood vessels and decrease circulation to the affected area.
Hypothermia *S/S:* In mild cases there is shivering, skin is cold to the touch, and there is confusion and lack of coordination. In severe cases the shivering stops; coordination problems increase, along with slurred speech and problems with vision; the heart rate slows; and the victim becomes drowsy and just wants to be left alone. The victim can become irrational and uncooperative. If untreated, the victim will progress to coma and death.	• If frostbite and hypothermia are present, treat the hypothermia first. • If respirations are below 6 per minute, begin rescue breathing. • If possible, gently move the victim to a shelter. • Remove wet clothes and replace them with dry ones. • Remove constricting clothes and jewelry. • Do not use direct heat. • Apply warm packs (towels or linens) to the neck, chest, and groin. • If the victim is able to drink, give him or her warm, sweet fluids.	• Hypothermia is the most life threatening. • This supplies the victim with needed oxygen. • This removes the victim from further exposure. • Wet clothes increase the cooling of the body. • This increases circulation. • It may burn the victim. • These packs warm the body. • This warms the body internally and supplies some calories.

(continues)

PROCEDURE

FIRST AID FOR TEMPERATURE-RELATED ILLNESSES

(continued)

CONDITION AND SIGNS AND SYMPTOMS

PROCEDURE

RATIONALE

Hypothermia *(continued)*

- Wrap the victim in a space blanket (contains an insulating material that prevents heat from escaping) or aluminum foil, including the neck and head; the rescuer can also place his or her own body next to the victim to warm him or her.

- This assists in rewarming the victim.

HEAT-RELATED CONDITIONS

Heat Cramps

S/S: Muscle cramps in the abdomen and legs, lightheadedness, and weakness may occur when excess salt and fluid are lost from the body (heavy perspiration). If the problem progresses to heat exhaustion, the skin may appear pale or red, cool to the touch, and moist; the victim may complain of headache, thirst, weakness, and dizziness; the pupils will be dilated (larger than normal), and nausea and vomiting may occur; behavior may be irrational or the victim may be unconscious.

- Do not give liquids that contain alcohol or caffeine.

- The victim needs water and electrolytes to replenish what was lost.

- Do not give any medication used to lower the temperature (e.g., aspirin or Tylenol).

- This does not treat the underlying problem.

- Do not give salt tablets; instead use a salt-and-water solution or an electrolyte drink (e.g., Gatorade or Pedialyte).

- Salt-and-water solutions replenish fluid and electrolytes.

- Fan the victim.

- Cools by increasing evaporation.

- Move the victim to the shade or a cooled room and elevate the feet if not prohibited (e.g., it causes difficulty breathing; there is a head, neck, spine, or leg injury; or it makes the victim uncomfortable).

- It is important to begin the cooling process immediately.

- Apply cool water to the body (do not use alcohol rub); wrap the victim in cool towels and turn on a fan.

- This aids in cooling by increasing the evaporative process.

- Apply cold towels to the back of the neck, on the groin, and under the arms.

- This cools the major areas where blood vessels are close to the surface.

- When the temperature lowers to 100°F, the cooling effort can be stopped, but monitor the victim closely for the next 2–4 hours.

- The victim may relapse even after apparent recovery.

Heat Stroke

The skin will be dry, hot, and red; confusion, weakness, and seizures may occur; pupils will be constricted (smaller than normal), pulse rapid and weak, and breathing rapid and shallow; the body temperature will be markedly increased (above 102°F); the victim may be unconscious.

- Call EMS.

- This condition is life threatening.

- Do not give liquids to a victim with heat stroke.

- Fluids may enter the lungs. EMS will start an IV when they arrive.

- If EMS is not immediately available, immerse the victim in cold water, but monitor his or her alertness, pulse, and respirations closely.

- This starts the cooling process.

Thinking It Through

John Street is a health care student and is feeling the need to get away from the stress and routine of studying. He decides to take a hike in the local mountains with his friends. As they ascend the mountain, it gets cooler and begins to rain. One of the hikers, Paul, starts to lag behind. Paul has always been a slower climber, so they continue on. A little while later, John turns around to see how Paul is doing and can no longer see him. John backtracks and finds Paul sitting beside the trail. He is shivering and his skin is cold to the touch. Paul says he is just very tired and needs to rest for a while and that he will catch up later.

1. Should John leave Paul to rest by himself?

2. What may be happening to Paul?

3. What first aid, if any, should be given to Paul?

Other Conditions

A number of other commonly occurring conditions may require the assistance of someone trained in first aid. They may be seen separately or in conjunction with other conditions. Knowledge of these conditions will prepare the rescuer to take the appropriate actions when they occur. See Procedure 21–9 for first aid related to these conditions.

Bandaging

Knowing how to apply slings and wraps can be very useful when working with a variety of injuries that require first aid. See Procedures 21–10 through 21–13 for applying a triangular sling and three wraps, commonly used with musculoskeletal injuries.

PROCEDURE 　　　　　　　　　　　　　　　　　 **21–9**

FIRST AID FOR OTHER COMMON CONDITIONS

Always Observe Standard Precautions

CONDITION AND SIGNS AND SYMPTOMS	PROCEDURE	RATIONALE
Breathing Difficulty Problems with breathing can be caused by many sudden illnesses, injuries, or worsening medical conditions. *S/S:* Shortness of breath, coughing, audible sounds (wheezing, gurgling, whistling) coming from respiratory system, and exaggerated use of chest muscles to breathe. If the victim is not getting enough oxygen, the mouth and fingertips may be pale or bluish in color.	• Do not place a pillow under the victim's head. • Loosen any constricting clothing and assist the victim into the most comfortable position, unless neck or back injury is suspected. • Ask the victim if there is any medication he or she takes for the problem (e.g., asthmatics may have an inhaler with them). • Call EMS and keep the victim safe and comfortable until help arrives.	• This may close off the airway. • Constricting clothing may prevent the victim from breathing deeply. • Symptoms may be alleviated with their medication. • The victim may need evaluation and treatment.

(continues)

PROCEDURE

FIRST AID FOR OTHER COMMON CONDITIONS

(continued)

CONDITION AND SIGNS AND SYMPTOMS

PROCEDURE

RATIONALE

Hyperventilation

Rapid breathing that causes the carbon dioxide level in the blood to fall too low. The most common cause is anxiety, but it may also be caused by illness, injury, or certain medications.

S/S: Fast, shallow respiratory rate, followed by the sensation of numbness around the mouth and in the hands and feet. Blood pressure may fall, and fainting can occur.

Chest Pain (Angina)

Chest pain is associated with a lack of oxygen to the heart muscle. Damage to the heart muscle from a lack of oxygen is called a heart attack or myocardial infarction.

S/S: Pain is described as dull or crushing (victim may state that "it feels like an elephant is sitting on my chest"). The pain may radiate to the shoulder, arm, or jaw. Angina can also be felt in atypical locations (especially in females), such as jaw, back, or underarms. There may be difficulty breathing and heart palpitations. Often the victim will perspire heavily and feel nauseated and anxious, and the skin will be pale or bluish and moist.

- Have victims breathe into a paper bag, hold one nostril closed (make sure the mouth is closed) while breathing, or have them cup their hands over their mouth and nose while breathing.
- The victim will need a calm and reassuring approach. Encouraging the victim to talk is often helpful.
- Always call EMS immediately.

- Have the victim stop any activity he or she was doing.
- If the victim has medication for angina, assist him or her in taking it.

- Do not give the victim anything to eat or drink.

- Loosen any constricting clothing and keep the victim warm.
- Stay with the victim until help arrives.

- Start rescue breathing if he or she stops breathing, or give full CPR if the heart stops.

- These techniques are effective in returning the carbon dioxide level in the bloodstream to normal.

- This condition is often caused by, or worsened, with anxiety.

- Many victims deny that they are having a heart attack and instead explain it as indigestion. They may be correct, but any chest pain needs to be evaluated medically to determine if the victim had a heart attack.
- This decreases the demand on the heart.
- Many people with recurring chest pain have a medication called nitroglycerin that is placed under the tongue.

- This increases demand on the heart, and the victim may develop nausea and vomiting.
- This encourages full deep breathing and circulation.
- If the condition worsens, the victim may need rescue breathing or CPR.
- Brain damage occurs in as little as 3–5 minutes when the brain is deprived of oxygen.

(continues)

PROCEDURE

FIRST AID FOR OTHER COMMON CONDITIONS

CONDITION AND SIGNS AND SYMPTOMS	PROCEDURE	RATIONALE
Diabetes Lack of adequate insulin production results in elevated blood sugar; if too much medication is taken to correct this condition, the blood sugar may become too low. *S/S: High blood sugar* (hyperglycemia) develops gradually and is characterized by excessive thirst, hunger, and urination. There may be vomiting, flushed skin, rapid breathing, and a fruity smell to the breath. The victim may be confused and resist your attempt to assist. If left untreated, the victim will go into a diabetic coma. *S/S: Low blood sugar* (hypoglycemia) develops more rapidly and is characterized by sweating, hunger, confusion, pale skin, and poor coordination. This is referred to as an insulin reaction and if left untreated may result in coma and death.	• If victims state that their blood sugar is too high and they need to have an insulin injection, assist them with the administration of the medication. • Get medical help and stay with the victim to monitor his or her condition. • If the victim is conscious, give him or her unsweetened liquids. • If the victim states that his or her blood sugar is too low, immediately give something sweet (e.g., fruit juice, sugar in water, candy). If this is the problem, the victim should improve within 5–15 minutes after administration of the sweet. • When recovered, the victim should eat some protein and carbohydrates (e.g., crackers and cheese or peanut butter and bread). • If the victim does not recover or is unconscious, call EMS. • If in doubt as to whether it is high or low blood sugar, treat it with something sweet.	• Many diabetics are very familiar with the signs and symptoms and know how to treat it. • The condition may worsen and further assistance will be needed. • Liquids with sugar will make the problem worse, so use unsweetened liquids as they will combat the dehydration that occurs with hyperglycemia without increasing the blood sugar. • Many diabetics are very familiar with the signs and symptoms and know how to treat it. Sweetened items increase the blood sugar. • This prevents further insulin reaction because the quick-acting sweets are digested and eliminated quickly. • The victim needs further evaluation and treatment. • If it is low blood sugar, the victim should recover quickly, and if high blood sugar, the additional sweet will not significantly affect the problem.

(continues)

PROCEDURE

FIRST AID FOR OTHER COMMON CONDITIONS

(continued)

CONDITION AND SIGNS AND SYMPTOMS

Fainting (Syncope)

S/S: Brief loss of consciousness that comes on quickly, perhaps due to low blood sugar, standing too long, or low blood pressure when arising too rapidly from a lying or sitting position. Sometimes there are warning signs (dizziness, nausea, weakness, and blurred vision), but not always. A loss of consciousness after a head injury is not fainting, but a concussion.

Fever (Hyperthermia)

S/S: An increase in body temperature, usually caused by the body's attempt to combat infection. (For elevated temperature related to exposure to heat, see hyperthermia under Temperature-Related Illnesses). Children are particularly susceptible to high fevers when an infection is present. The fever can rise quickly and result in seizures. The younger the child, the more sensitive he or she is to an increase in temperature.

PROCEDURE

- If you are present when the victim is falling, assist him or her gently to the floor.
- Place the victim on his or her back and elevate the legs 8–12 inches.
- Do not place a pillow under the head.
- Loosen any constricting clothing.

- Do not attempt to awaken the victim by throwing water on him or her, shaking, or slapping the face.
- If vomiting occurs turn the head to the side.

- Call EMS if the victim is not alert within approximately 5 minutes, is elderly, or other signs and symptoms are noted that may indicate another problem.
- Remove excess clothing and blankets.
- Gently cool the child by sponging him or her with lukewarm water.
- Call the physician at once for further instructions, such as giving medication to bring the fever down (e.g., acetaminophen). Never give aspirin to an infant or child who has a fever or other signs or symptoms of a flu-like or other viral illness.
- Even lower fevers that persist over 24 hours need to be evaluated.
- Call EMS if the child is having difficulty breathing, has unusual skin color, a stiff neck, or appears ill.

RATIONALE

- This prevents injury from the fall.

- This increases blood circulation to the brain.
- This may obstruct airway.

- This allows for deeper breathing and better circulation.
- This is not an effective technique and may injure victim.

- This prevents vomit from obstructing airway and entering the lungs.
- The victim needs further evaluation and treatment.

- Excess coverings can increase body temperature.
- This lowers the body temperature.

- Aspirin given to infants or children can result in Reye's syndrome, an extremely serious and life-threatening condition.

- The cause needs to be determined.

- This may indicate a serious underlying condition requiring immediate treatment.

(continues)

PROCEDURE

FIRST AID FOR OTHER COMMON CONDITIONS

CONDITION AND SIGNS AND SYMPTOMS

PROCEDURE

RATIONALE

Drowning

Unconsciousness and death result from the lack of oxygen to the body as water enters the respiratory tract. Drowning can occur in only a few inches of water if the victim is a child or is injured. The most common causes are accidents, sudden illness, cramping, alcohol consumption, and getting into areas where the person is not a strong enough swimmer to return to safety.

S/S: Skin cold and pale. Lips, earlobes, and fingernails are a bluish color. The victim may not be breathing.

- Be on the alert for irregular swimming strokes, when only the head is above the water, and if the person is fully dressed.
- Call EMS.

- Rescue the drowning victim if you can do so without endangering yourself. It is best not to enter the water, but to extend a stick, life preserver, or some other object for the victim to grab and then pull him or her to safety.

- Do rescue breathing and treat the victim for hypothermia as needed. Do full CPR if no pulse is present.

- Drowning victims usually cannot call for help.

- The victim will need evaluation and treatment.

- If the rescuer enters the water, he or she may become hypothermic or the victim may panic and pull the rescuer under too.

- If the water is quite cold, the victim may still be able to be revived, even if submerged for longer than 3–5 minutes.

Seizures (Convulsions)

Seizures are caused by irregular brain activity such as that seen in someone with epilepsy, or they can be caused by a sudden change in a medical condition. Many of the other first aid emergencies discussed in this chapter can result in seizures.

S/S: Sudden falling and loss of consciousness with drooling or frothing from the mouth. There may be loss of bowel or bladder control. Grunting or groaning may be heard. Some people experience a perceptual disturbance, called an *aura*, before the onset of a seizure. This may be a strange light, unpleasant smell, or confusing thoughts. (Auras also commonly occur before and during a migraine, a recurring type of headache.) There are three common types of seizures:

- If the victim is falling, support the victim as he or she falls.
- Remove any sharp objects in the area.
- Loosen tight clothing.
- Do not place anything into the mouth, try to restrain the victim, move the victim (unless in danger), or perform rescue breathing during a seizure.

- Do not try to keep the victim awake, but place him or her on the stomach or side (if you suspect neck or back injury, roll the body as a unit to a side-lying position, while keeping the spine in straight alignment). Protect the airway if vomiting occurs.

- This prevents injury to victim as he or she falls to the floor.
- This protects the victim from injury.
- This eases the ability to breathe.
- Most seizures last less than a minute, and the main role of the rescuer is to keep the victim safe from harm.

- After the seizure, the victim may go into a deep sleep after regaining consciousness momentarily and will probably be confused.

(continues)

PROCEDURE

FIRST AID FOR OTHER COMMON CONDITIONS

(continued)

CONDITION AND SIGNS AND SYMPTOMS	PROCEDURE	RATIONALE
Seizures (Convulsions) *(continued)* 1. Petit mal—brief unconsciousness, followed by confusion 2. Focal—localized twitching in one part of the body (e.g., face or arm) 3. Grand mal—generalized strong muscle spasms of the entire body	• Call EMS.	• The victim may need further evaluation or treatment.
Shock Shock occurs when there is a disruption in the flow of blood to the cells throughout the body. Any medical emergency can cause shock. *S/S:* The victim may feel weak, dizzy, restless, or confused. The skin is pale, cold, and clammy. Lips, earlobes, and fingertips may be bluish. The respirations are shallow and rapid. Nausea, vomiting, and chest pain may be present. The victim may experience numbness and paralysis or be unconscious.	• Call EMS. • Place the victim in the shock position if there is no neck or back injury. (See Figure 21–11.) • Turn the victim's head to the side if there is vomiting or drooling.	• The victim needs further evaluation and treatment. • Elevating the lower extremities increases blood flow to the brain. • This prevents blockage of the airway.

FIGURE 21–11 Place emergency victims in the shock position, unless they have neck, back, or lower limb injuries. Do not use the position if it is uncomfortable for the victim or if he or she has breathing difficulty.

(continues)

PROCEDURE

FIRST AID FOR OTHER COMMON CONDITIONS

CONDITION AND SIGNS AND SYMPTOMS	PROCEDURE	RATIONALE
	• Do not elevate the head.	• You want maximum flow of blood to the brain to prevent brain damage.
	• Loosen restricting clothes and keep the victim warm.	• This eases breathing and maintains blood flow.
	• Do not give the victim any liquids or food.	• The victim may vomit and block the airway.
	• Give first aid for any underlying illness or injury.	• Shock is normally secondary to another problem.
	• Do not use the shock position if it is uncomfortable.	• The victim may have another injury or illness.
	• Do not use the shock position if the victim has a sting or bite in the lower limbs.	• This increases the release of venom into the system.
	• Stay with the victim and assist as needed until medical help arrives.	• If the condition worsens, the victim may need rescue breathing or CPR performed.
Stroke or Cerebrovascular Accident (CVA) Caused by a ruptured or clogged artery in the brain resulting in death to the affected brain cells. *S/S:* Sudden onset of weakness, dizziness, headache, and unsteady coordination, followed by weakness or paralysis of the face, arm, and leg or one side of the face. Speech may be slurred or garbled, or absent, and vision may be affected. If the signs and symptoms are temporary and disappear within 24 hours, it was not a stroke, but a condition called a transient ischemic attack (TIA). Sometimes called a mini-stroke, a TIA is a temporary lack of oxygen to brain cells. It is a very serious sign and warns of a potential future stroke.	• Call EMS	• Quick response may prevent death or decrease damage as there is a medication that can be administered if the stroke is caused by a clogged artery. But it must be administered within a specified timeframe to be of value.
	• Help the victim get into a comfortable position.	• This eases breathing and anxiety.
	• Give no liquids or food by mouth.	• The victim may vomit and block the airway.
	• Stay with the victim and assist as needed until medical help arrives.	• If the condition worsens, the victim may need rescue breathing or CPR performed.

(continues)

PROCEDURE

FIRST AID FOR OTHER COMMON CONDITIONS

(continued)

CONDITION AND SIGNS AND SYMPTOMS

Unconsciousness

Any medical emergency can result in the victim losing alertness and awareness of the surroundings. This state can range from a brief period, such as fainting, to a prolonged coma.

S/S: The victim may drift in and out of consciousness, varying from feeling drowsy, restless, and unable to orient himself or herself or make sense when speaking to not moving or speaking at all.

PROCEDURE

- Call EMS if the victim does not quickly regain consciousness (i.e., simple fainting) or if illness or injury is evident.

- The goal of the treatment of the unconscious victim is to maintain the airway.

- Do not give anything by mouth.

- Keep the victim warm.

- If there is no neck or back injury, place the victim in the recovery position by turning the head to the side, or turn the entire body to the side or onto the abdomen.

- Gently tilt the victim's head back.

- If neck or back injury is suspected, leave the victim in the position in which he or she is found unless there is difficulty in breathing. If the victim is having difficulty breathing or is choking or vomiting, roll the entire body as a unit to a side-lying position while keeping the spine in straight alignment.

- Enlist the assistance of bystanders, if possible, when moving the victim to ensure the head, neck, and back stay in a straight line.

- Give first aid for any underlying illness or injury.

- If the victim becomes restless, you may have to gently restrain him or her.

- Stay with the victim until medical assistance arrives.

RATIONALE

- The victim needs medical evaluation and treatment.

- The victim is unable to cough, clear the throat, or turn the head to drain vomit or drool from the mouth when the airway becomes obstructed.

- The victim may choke on fluids or vomit and obstruct the airway.

- This maintains good circulation.

- This prevents obstruction of the airway if the victim vomits.

- This maintains the airway.

- This prevents further injury to the neck or back.

- It is easier to maintain body alignment when there are more people for turning in unison.

- Unconsciousness is usually a result of another illness or condition.

- This prevents the victim from injuring himself or herself.

- If the condition worsens, the victim may need rescue breathing or CPR performed.

PROCEDURE

21–10

APPLYING A TRIANGULAR SLING

Always Observe Standard Precautions

USAGE

It is used to support an injured shoulder, collarbone, or arm. If the arm is broken, apply the splint first to immobilize the broken bone, and then place it in the sling.

A sling can be made from a large triangular cloth, a sweater, a pillowcase, or other materials that can be cut to the appropriate size.

PROCEDURE

(See Figures 21–12a–c)

1. Support the injured part and slide the sling under the arm on the victim's injured side.

2. Place the top corner over the victim's uninjured shoulder.

3. Pull the bottom corner of the sling up past the victim's chin and over the shoulder on the injured side. Leave the fingers showing.

4. Tie the sling around the victim's neck, placing it a little to one side.

5. Fold over the extra cloth at the victim's elbow and secure it with a safety pin.

6. Check for circulation.

RATIONALE

Always support the injured arm when applying a sling to prevent further injury.

Creates a cross-body support to secure the other end with a knot.

Leaving the fingers exposed allows for convenient circulation checks.

Placing the knot a little to one side prevents the knot from pressing on the back of the neck.

Creates a cradle to secure the elbow.

Always check for circulation when applying splints and slings to ensure there is adequate perfusion of the extremity.

FIGURE 21–12a Support the injured part and slide the sling under the arm on the victim's injured side. Place top corner over the victim's uninjured shoulder.

FIGURE 21–12b Pull the bottom corner of the sling up past the victim's chin and over the shoulder on the injured side. Leave the fingers showing.

(continues)

PROCEDURE

APPLYING A TRIANGULAR SLING

FIGURE 21–12c Tie the sling around the victim's neck, placing it a little to one side so the knot does not press on the back of the neck. Fold over the extra cloth at the victim's elbow and secure it with a safety pin.

PROCEDURE

APPLYING A SPIRAL WRAP

Always Observe Standard Precautions

USAGE	PROCEDURE	RATIONALE
A spiral wrap can be used on arms, legs, and the trunk of the body.	(See Figures 21–13a–b) 1. Start wrap at distal end.	Enhances circulation and decreases swelling.
	2. Anchor the bandage by leaving a corner exposed. The corner is then folded down and covered when the bandage is circled around the limb.	Holds the end in place to prevent slippage.
	3. Overlap each rotation over the previous one by approximately half the width of the previous layer.	Holds the wrapping securely in place.
	4. Place your hand between the bandage and the victim's skin if inserting a pin; can also secure with tape.	To prevent accidental injury to the patient.
	5. Verify circulation in the fingers and toes if the wrap is used on the arm or leg.	Always check for circulation when applying wraps to ensure there is adequate perfusion of the extremity.
	6. Verify ease of breathing if the wrap is on the trunk.	A too-tight wrap will restrict chest movement during respirations.

(continues)

PROCEDURE

21–11

APPLYING A SPIRAL WRAP

(continued)

FIGURE 21–13b Place your hand between the bandage and the victim's skin if inserting a pin; can also secure with tape.

FIGURE 21–13a Always start wrap at distal end. Anchor the bandage by leaving a corner exposed. The corner is then folded down and covered when the bandage is circled around the limb. Overlap each rotation partially over the previous one to hold it securely in place.

PROCEDURE

21–12

APPLYING A FIGURE-EIGHT WRAP

Always Observe Standard Precautions

USAGE

A figure-eight wrap can be used to bandage a joint, such as an ankle, an elbow, or a wrist, because it secures both sides of the joint. Using a spiral wrap is not effective for wrapping joints, because the wrap tends to slip off easily.

PROCEDURE
(See Figures 21–14a–b)

1. Anchor the bandage at the instep and wrap several times around the instep. Then bring the wrap up diagonally over the foot.

RATIONALE

Holds the wrapping securely in place.

(continues)

PROCEDURE

APPLYING A FIGURE-EIGHT WRAP

(continued)

USAGE	PROCEDURE	RATIONALE
	2. Bring the bandage around the back of the ankle and then down over the top of the foot and back under the instep.	This creates a figure-eight pattern.
	3. Repeat the figure-eight pattern, moving the wrap out in both directions (up the leg and toward the toes) with each repeat of the pattern while overlapping approximately half of the previous layer.	Partially overlaps the previous layer to hold it securely in place.
	4. When completed, wrap around the ankle several times and secure the end.	Holds the wrapping securely in place.
	5. Check circulation distal to the wrap.	Always check for circulation when applying wraps to ensure there is adequate perfusion of the extremity.

FIGURE 21–14a Anchor the bandage at the instep and secure by wrapping several times around the instep. Then bring the wrap up diagonally over the foot.

FIGURE 21–14b Bring the bandage around the back of the ankle and then down over the top of the foot and back under the instep. This creates a figure-eight pattern. Continue this process, moving the wrap out in both directions (up the leg and toward the toes) with each repeat of the pattern. Partially overlap the previous one to hold it securely in place.

PROCEDURE

APPLYING A BANDAGE TO A FINGER

Always Observe Standard Precautions

USAGE

A wrap for a finger can be made from a thin strip of gauze or cloth. It is used to support the finger and decrease movement. If the finger is broken, apply the splint first, using small twigs, pencils, or popsicle sticks on both sides, then wrap the finger.

PROCEDURE

(See Figures 21–15a–d)

1. Place the end of the wrap at the bottom of one side of the finger and fold it over the tip of the finger and down to the bottom of the other side of the finger. Repeat this three to four times.

2. Start at the bottom of the finger and spiral the wrap up and down the finger.

3. Secure by doing several figure-eight wraps around the wrist.

4. When the figure-eight wrap is complete, circle the wrist several times. Split the wrap and tie in a knot.

5. Monitor patient. If any signs of decreased circulation occur, loosen the wrap immediately.

RATIONALE

Creates a recurrent dressing.

Holds recurrent wrap securely in place.

Anchors wrap to prevent it from falling off the finger.

Secures wrap to wrist.

Swelling may occur that will increase the tightness of the wrap and compromise circulation.

FIGURE 21–15a Place the end of the wrap at the bottom of one side of the finger and fold it over the tip of the finger and down to the bottom of the other side of the finger. Repeat this three to four times.

FIGURE 21–15c Secure by doing several figure-eight wraps around the wrist.

FIGURE 21–15b Start at the bottom of the finger and spiral the wrap up and down the finger to hold securely in place.

FIGURE 21–15d When the figure-eight wrap is complete, circle the wrist several times. Split the wrap and tie in a knot or secure with tape or safety pin.

SUGGESTED LEARNING ACTIVITIES

1. If you do not already have a CPR certification, arrange to attend a class for certification. You can locate classes by calling your local health facilities, community colleges, the American Red Cross, or the American Heart Association.

2. Contact the American Red Cross and plan to attend their next first aid and safety class, if it is not part of your program of study.

3. Evaluate your home environment for potential hazards and risks for injuries.

4. Practice the four types of slings and wraps on family, friends, or classmates.

WEB ACTIVITIES

Very Well Health

https://www.verywellhealth.com/do-all-states-have-good-samaritan-laws-1298836

Do All States Have Good Samaritan Laws?

1. In most states, under what circumstances are caregivers protected from prosecution for medical mistakes?

2. Why is it difficult to determine if a caregiver's mistake is *reasonable*?

3. Who makes the final decision of what is reasonable?

4. Do all states protect everyone from liability, whether they are medically trained or not?

5. Are untrained persons required by law to help victims of medical emergencies?

6. What are the actions for which there is never any liability?

Mayo Clinic

https://www.mayoclinic.org/first-aid

Choose a topic not covered in your text and summarize the information.

American Heart Association

https://www.heart.org/en/about-us/heart-attack-and-stroke-symptoms

Heart Attack and Stroke Symptoms

1. What are the symptoms of a heart attack?

2. What are the symptoms of a stroke?

American Red Cross

www.redcross.org

1. How can a person donate blood in your area?

2. What are the donor guidelines?

REVIEW QUESTIONS

1. What is the meaning of first aid and what is its goal?

2. When should cardiopulmonary resuscitation be performed?

3. What is the Good Samaritan Act, and how does it protect the rescuer?

4. What is the golden rule of first aid?

5. What are the seven steps to follow when an emergency occurs that will protect both the victim and rescuer?

6. What are the signs and symptoms and treatment for an allergic reaction?

7. What are the signs and symptoms and treatment for bleeding and wounds?

8. What are the signs and symptoms and treatment for bone, joint, and muscle injuries?

9. What are the signs and symptoms and treatment for facial injuries?

10. What are the signs and symptoms and treatment for burns?

11. What are the signs and symptoms and treatment for drug-related emergencies?

12. What are the signs and symptoms and treatment for poisoning?

13. What are the signs and symptoms and treatment for temperature-related illnesses?

14. What are the signs and symptoms and treatment for breathing difficulty?

15. What are the signs and symptoms and treatment for hyperventilation?

16. What are the signs and symptoms and treatment for chest pain?

17. What are the signs and symptoms and treatment for elevated blood sugar and for low blood sugar (related to diabetes)?

18. What is the treatment for fainting?

19. What is the treatment for fever?

20. What are the signs and symptoms and treatment for drowning?

21. What are the signs and symptoms and treatment for seizures?

22. What are the signs and symptoms and treatment for shock?

23. What are the signs and symptoms and treatment for stroke?

24. What are the four common types of slings and wraps used to treat musculoskeletal injuries and how are they applied?

APPLICATION EXERCISES

1. Refer back to the Case of the Out-of-Control Party:

   a. What would have been appropriate first aid measures for the stabbing victim?

   b. Should Josephine remove the knife from the chest? Why or why not?

   c. If there is bubbling coming from the chest wound, what would this indicate? What additional first aid measures would be necessary?

   d. Which organs are located in the left side of the chest that may have been damaged by the knife?

2. One hot day William notices his neighbor John mowing the lawn. He notes that John looks flushed and is sweating profusely, but he is overweight and out of shape and it is awfully hot and humid outdoors to be doing yard work. Thirty minutes later, John's wife frantically knocks on the door saying John is having chest pain. She is very frightened. She says he has a heart condition and that she has called 9-1-1.

   a. What is the most likely cause of John's chest pain?

   b. What actions can William take until EMS arrives?

PROBLEM-SOLVING PRACTICE

Michael Huang is a health care student and a single father with two small children at home. He is very concerned about the safety of his active and inquisitive children and is wondering if there are any potential hazards in his home environment. Using the five-step problem-solving process, determine what Michael can do to identify and correct any hazards at home. (Note: Students can use their own home for this problem-solving assignment.)

CHAPTER 22

Paying for Health Care

KEY TERMS

account payable
account receivable
capitation
coinsurance
copay
cost of money
Current Procedural Terminology
    (CPT) codes
deductible
diagnostic-related groups
    (DRGs)
exclusive provider organization
    (EPO)
expenditures
fee-for-service
financing
gatekeepers
health maintenance
    organization (HMO)
International Classification of
    Diseases (ICD-10) codes
managed care
Medicaid
Medicare
negotiated fees
point of service (POS)
preauthorization
preferred provider organization
    (PPO)
premium
prepaid plans
primary care providers (PCPs)
profit
reimbursed
Veterans Health Administration

OBJECTIVES

Studying and applying the material in this chapter will help you to:

1. List the factors that are contributing to the high cost of health care.
2. List the six categories of wasted health care dollars.
3. Explain how the attitudes and behaviors of many Americans contribute to the high cost of health care.
4. Describe the negative consequences the high cost of health care has for many Americans.
5. Identify the three categories of health care institutions based on their source of funding.
6. Describe how methods for paying medical costs have changed over the years.
7. Describe the three most common methods patients use to pay for their health care.
8. Explain the purpose of Medicaid, who it covers, and how it is administered.
9. Explain the Medicare system, including Parts A, B, C, and D.
10. Describe the Veterans Health Administration.
11. Define the terms "deductible" and "coinsurance."
12. Define DRGs and explain their purpose.
13. Explain the purpose of managed care systems and list their goals.
14. Describe the following types of managed care plans: HMO, PPO, EPO, and POS.
15. Explain how a prepaid health plan works.
16. Define the term "negotiated fees."
17. Explain the meaning and purpose of "primary care provider."
18. Explain the meaning and purpose of "preauthorization."
19. Explain the Affordable Care Act and state its major purpose.
20. List major components of the Affordable Care Act.
21. List three methods enacted to cover the costs of the Affordable Care Act.
22. Identify the four major areas of expenditures incurred by a health care delivery system.
23. Define "account receivable," "account payable," and "the cost of money."
24. Describe seven ways that the health care professional can help control facility costs.
25. Describe the ICD-10 and CPT codes and explain their purpose.
26. Describe ways that health care professionals can improve their personal efficiency
27. Explain what is meant by "acting with thought."

The Case of the Inefficient Office

Constance Madison has seen many changes in her career working in medical records. Although computerization has helped organize recordkeeping, it has also brought feelings of disorder during periods of transition. Constance sometimes feels overwhelmed and frustrated with what seems to be endless paperwork, lack of support, duplication of effort, and insufficient time to do what needs to be done during the day. Her knowledge of the changes in health care delivery and the needs of the system keep her focused on doing her best to make a positive contribution during stressful times. She has made several suggestions to her supervisor that have been adopted by her department. In this chapter, you will gain an understanding of why there is a tremendous amount of change occurring in the health care environment and how you can look for ways to improve efficiency, rather than focusing on the problems. By learning how individual employees can contribute to the efficiency of the organization, you will be able to make a positive impact. Identifying areas of inefficiency and waste enables you to work toward correcting them and creating a more enjoyable and productive work environment.

THE RISING COSTS OF HEALTH CARE

A major concern in the United States today is how to effectively control health care costs that have dramatically risen over the past few decades. While every type of product and service has steadily increased in price over the years, health care costs have grown at a faster rate than almost anything else. It is estimated that in 2017, health care cost $3.5 trillion in the United States, up 4.6% from 2016. This amount represents almost 18% of the country's gross domestic product (the total value of goods produced and services provided in a country during one year).

Although there is disagreement among experts about which factor is most responsible for the high cost of health care in the United States, there are a number of factors with which most agree:

- Prices are high for everything from medical equipment to doctor's fees. Prices in the United States tend to be higher than in other countries. For example, in 2013, the average cost for coronary artery bypass graft surgery was $75,345, while the same surgery cost $15,742 in the Netherlands and $36,509 in Sweden (Blumberg, 2018).

- Administrative costs, which some estimate to be from 20% to 30% of total health care costs, are extremely high. Most of these costs are related to insurance: the existence of multiple companies requires dealing with different processes for claim submission. Coding requirements for various diagnoses and procedures, discussed later in this chapter, add to the personnel and time needed for these tasks. (See Figure 22–1.)

- Drug costs are especially high, compared with other products. And being the most widely used method of treatment, they contribute significantly to the cost

FIGURE 22–1 Administrative costs account for up to 30% of health care spending in the United States.

of health care. It is estimated that it can cost as much as $1 billion to develop a new drug, so pharmaceutical companies charge high prices to regain their investments and make a profit.

- Defensive medicine, meaning the use of multiple tests by doctors to avoid being sued, adds to the cost. It is estimated that as much as $650 billion annually can be attributed to defensive medicine (Epstein, 2019).

- Technological advances have created more expensive equipment and treatments. While some advances produce better results, this is not always the case: many new and expensive treatments reportedly are ineffective or no better than existing methods.

- Overuse of specialists who charge more than primary care physicians, adds to the cost of health care. Experts believe there are many conditions that primary care doctors can treat just as well, or even more effectively because they have a more comprehensive knowledge of the patient.

Two other factors that contribute to high health care costs are waste and fraud. In 2012, the Institute of Medicine reported that about 30 cents of every dollar, or $765 billion, spent annually on health care is wasted on unneeded care, huge amounts of paperwork, and fraud (Alonso-Zaldivar, 2012). The report broke this amount into six categories of waste:

$210 billion	Unnecessary services
$190 billion	Excess administrative costs
$130 billion	Inefficient delivery of care
$105 billion	Inflated prices
$75 billion	Fraud
$55 billion	Prevention failures

The report suggested that health care costs could be better controlled without decreasing the quality of care. Reforms suggested included demanding greater accountability from hospitals and major medical groups and encouraging more collaboration among medical professionals (Alonso-Zaldivar, 2012).

Although we spend more per person on health care than any other country, our care results and patient satisfaction are below those of many other countries (further discussion of this issue appears in Chapter 23).

The high costs of health care may increase at even a faster rate in the future due to the growth of our aging population, who use the most health care services, and the decreasing health of the young. The nation's youth are showing an alarming increase in obesity, poor diet, and lack of physical fitness, which is resulting in an onset of chronic conditions at a very young age.

The United States currently has the highest rate of diagnosed diabetes, a disease related to obesity, among all other developed countries, costing our country $327 billion in 2017 (http://www.diabetes.org/advocacy/news-events/cost-of-diabetes.html). This trend clearly underscores the importance of preventive measures to provide a long and healthy life, as well as decreasing the amount spent on health care. Heart disease and certain forms of cancer are other conditions that may be prevented by weight control and physical exercise. Unfortunately, studies have shown that many Americans prefer drugs and other "quick fixes" to lifestyle changes which would prevent much suffering and expense. The many drug commercials on television and in magazines are designed to make drug therapies look easy, featuring people using the medications as healthy and enjoying life.

Although total health care costs currently average close to $10,345 per person, these costs are not evenly distributed among all patients. In fact, about 10% of patients incur 80% of the costs. It is estimated that about 75% of total health care costs come from patients with chronic conditions.

Impact of Costs on Individuals

The high cost of health care has a negative effect on millions of Americans. Although efforts have been made to make insurance available to more Americans (discussed later in this chapter), medical expenses are reported to cause the largest percentage of bankruptcies in the United States, perhaps as high as 26%. In 2016, the number was estimated to be 770,846. Of these, it is believed that 50% were the result of hospitalizations.

In addition to bankruptcies, one report states that up to 40% of Americans have medical debt at any given time and at least 25% of those under age 65 struggle to pay medical bills. Unexpected debt and bankruptcies are experienced even by people who have health insurance. This can happen when they

- Mistakenly believe their insurance covers the services they receive
- Don't expect the high deductibles and co-pays
- Are unaware that the hospital or service is not covered by their insurance plan

HEALTH CARE INSTITUTIONS

A wide variety of health care institutions exist—from hospitals to home health agencies, medical offices to long-term care facilities, and everything in between. But all of these types of service institutions can be grouped into three categories, based on the type of funding they receive:

- Nonprofit institutions: This category operates as a charitable agency and any net earnings must be reinvested into the organization. They are granted tax-exempt status by the Internal Revenue Service. Donations to a nonprofit organization are often tax deductible to the individuals and businesses making the contributions.
- Proprietary (for-profit) institutions: These operate in the same manner as any for-profit business and pay local, state, and federal taxes.
- Government institutions: They are referred to as public health care facilities. Most of their funding comes from local, state, or federal sources. Examples include Veterans Administration (VA) hospitals and state mental and rehabilitative facilities.

HISTORY OF HEALTH CARE REIMBURSEMENT

In the past, patients paid the physician's asking price for services provided. For those who could not pay cash, payment might be fresh vegetables from the garden or a load of wood. As health care became more sophisticated and costly, insurance companies became the preferred method of covering costs. Patients made regular, agreed upon payments to the insurance company, each one called a premium. When medical care was needed, patients would visit the physician of their choice and the physician would order tests, prescribe medications, admit the patient to the hospital, or perform surgery. The physician determined what actions to take and the insurance companies paid for the services. This was known as fee-for-service.

As costs rose in recent decades, insurance companies and other payers questioned the efficiency of fee-for-service as a pricing method. Rather than encouraging savings, they argued, it rewarded the providers who prescribed the most services, such as lab tests and diagnostic procedures. Payers believed that the providers of health care—physicians, hospitals, and other professionals and facilities—should be held accountable for costs. Duplication of services, unnecessarily long stays in hospitals, and expensive brand name drugs are examples of practices labeled as "wasteful." The approach to lowering costs while maintaining quality of health care will be addressed more fully in Chapter 23.

HEALTH CARE PAYMENT METHODS

Three methods for payment are commonly used in the United States:

1. Direct pay: In this method, the patient pays for health care costs using his or her own money. This approach may lead to a more judicious use of health care services, but it is catastrophic when costs exceed the patient's financial ability to pay.

2. Private insurance: Individuals purchase their own insurance policy or it can be part of a benefits package from employment. Employers are able to purchase policies less expensively than an individual because the costs are spread over a group, some of whom will not need care. These policies may include stipulations whereby the employee incurs part of the cost. There are many private insurance plans available with different levels of coverage.

3. Government plans: Funded by a government agency, examples of these plans include military health care for active personnel and their families, as well as

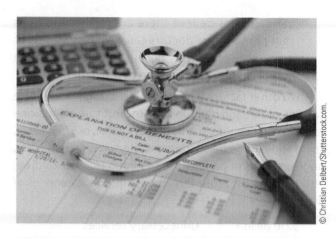

FIGURE 22–2 Explanation of Benefits are sent to Medicare recipients to let them know which of their health care expenses Medicare has covered.

the Veterans Administration hospital system. There are other government plans, too, the largest ones being Medicaid (low-income) and Medicare (over 65 years of age or disabled). Government programs are discussed in greater detail in the next sections. (See Figure 22–2.)

GOVERNMENT PROGRAMS

Medicaid is a public health insurance program that plays a major role in the U.S. health care system, accounting for 20% of health care spending in the United States. Regulated and partly funded by the federal government, it is administered by the states which determine who and what services are covered, delivery models of care, and methods for paying health care providers and hospitals. Governed by Section XIX of the Social Security Act, two thirds of Medicaid coverage is provided by private managed-care plans that contract with the states to provide services.

The purpose of Medicaid is to help certain categories of low-income and low-asset people and covers 20% of Americans, including children, parents of eligible children, pregnant women, disabled persons, and elderly persons who need assistance paying their portion of costs not covered by Medicare. The 2010 Affordable Care Act expanded the program by extending covered care to non-elderly, low-income adults. (See Box 22–1.) Coverage is quite comprehensive and includes expenses not covered by Medicare, such as eyeglasses and dental.

Nursing home care is not covered by Medicare (some is covered but with limitations and strict requirements) which accounts for Medicaid paying the costs for a large percentage of nursing home residents. At the same time, not all nursing homes accept Medicaid for payment, just

Box 22-1

Who Are Medicaid Recipients?

- 50% of mothers giving birth in a typical state
- 83% of poor children (poor as defined by family income)
- 48% of children with special health care needs
- 45% of non-elderly adults with disabilities
- 60% of nursing home residents
- 20% of Medicare beneficiaries

Source: Kaiser Family Foundation. https://www.kff.org/medicaid /issue-brief/10-things-to-know-about-medicaid-setting-the-facts-straight/

as not all health care providers will see Medicaid patients. However, a growing number of service providers are now accepting Medicaid.

Medicare was established by Congress in 1965. It is part of the Social Security Administration and provides health insurance for people aged 65 and older and others, such as the severely disabled, who qualify for social security.

On December 8, 2003, President George W. Bush signed into law the Medicare Prescription Drug, Improvement and Modernization Act (MMA) of 2003. This legislation provides seniors and people living with severe disabilities with a prescription drug benefit, more choices, and better benefits under Medicare. This was one of the most significant improvements in senior health care since the inception of Medicare in 1965.

Medicare is administered by the Centers for Medicare and Medicaid Services (CMS) and consists of four parts:

1. Hospital insurance (Part A) helps pay for inpatient care in a hospital or skilled facility (following a hospital stay), some home health care, and hospice care. The premium for Part A has already been paid through payroll taxes.
2. Medical insurance (Part B) helps pay for outpatient services and many other medical services and supplies, such as physicians' fees, diagnostic tests, and physical and occupational therapy. Part B is voluntary and if coverage is elected, there is a monthly premium deducted automatically from the person's social security payment.
3. Medicare advantage (Part C) plans are available in many areas. People with Medicare Parts A and B can choose to receive all of their health care services through a provider organization, such as a health maintenance organization (HMO) or a preferred

provider organization (PPO). (HMOs and PPOs are described under managed care, later in the chapter.)

4. Prescription drug coverage (Part D) helps pay for medications prescribed for treatment. There is a monthly fee for this coverage, although it is included in some Medicare advantage plans.

Many people assume that Medicare is free and covers all medical expenses, but this is not correct. Medicare has a monthly premium along with deductibles and coinsurance amounts. A **deductible** is an amount required to be paid each year by the insured before benefits become payable. **Coinsurance** is a cost-sharing provision stipulating that the insured is to assume a percentage of the costs of covered services. Under Medicare Part B, the beneficiary pays coinsurance of 20% of allowed charges. In a Medicare prescription drug plan, the coinsurance will vary. For more specific information refer to www.medicare.gov.

Because Medicare has a deductible and coinsurance that must be paid out-of-pocket, many individuals elect to purchase a supplemental insurance policy from a private insurance company or enroll in an HMO. The private insurance supplement is called a Medigap policy. Medigap policies vary in price and coverage. If an individual is enrolled in Medicare and has a Medigap policy, then each plan will pay its share of covered health care costs.

Veterans Health Care

The **Veterans Health Administration** is the largest integrated health care system in the United States serving nine million veterans in 1,250 health care facilities, including 172 medical centers and 1,069 outpatient sites (https:// www.va.gov/health/). All veterans with a service-related disability rating are entitled to VA health care. Eligibility for other veterans is based on many factors, including active duty service; type of military discharge; and disability and health conditions incurred during active duty. Veterans can fill out a questionnaire provided by the VA to see if, and for what, they qualify.

Medicare and Medicaid Reimbursement

By providing funding, the government has assumed a leading role in regulating both the costs and quality of health care provided under Medicare and Medicaid. A major move to control costs was the development of **diagnostic-related groups (DRGs)** by Congress in 1983. The typical, expected hospital costs of all common diagnoses were determined. Providers of care for Medicare patients receive that amount, regardless of the actual cost of care. For example, if two hospitals perform a hip replacement surgery on a Medicare patient, they are **reimbursed** (paid back) the amount that Medicare approves, not what they charge. Different facilities may receive a different percentage of the amount charged depending on factors such as their location, population served, and if they serve as a teaching hospital. Hospitals that can do the procedure for less than the amount reimbursed are allowed to keep the extra money. Hospitals that spend more must make up the difference themselves. Exceptions to this policy are made when there are documented complications or additional diagnosed problems.

Government Regulations

The actions of the government have had a significant impact on the health care system because Medicare patients make up a large portion of the patient population. Health care facilities that bill Medicare or Medicaid for reimbursement of costs related to the care of a patient who is covered by one of these programs must be certified prior to incurring costs in order to receive compensation. Health care professionals who provide services for Medicare and Medicaid patients must understand and follow all regulations and requirements in order to ensure compliance and reimbursement. This actually extends to almost all facilities because most insurance companies state that organizations must have Medicare approval for their policies to be in effect.

MANAGED CARE

One response to rising costs has been the development of **managed care** plans, which contain specific built-in cost controls. These plans incorporate business concepts designed to increase efficiency by giving health care providers incentives to cut costs. Simply stated, the goals of managed care are to do the following:

- Provide health care that patients can afford
- Ensure high-quality care
- Discourage unnecessary costs
- Eliminate duplication of procedures
- Earn a **profit** (amount of money remaining after all costs of operating a business have been paid) for both health care providers and insurance companies (or, if nonprofit, ensure that income covers all costs)

Types of Managed Care Plans

Several variations of managed care plans are in use today:

- **Health maintenance organization (HMO)**: Provides insured health care limited to care from providers who work for or contract with the HMO. These providers have agreed to charge less for their

services while meeting quality standards. Patients who enroll in these programs must use in-network providers except in emergencies and must see a primary care physician, or "gatekeeper," before seeing a specialist (who must also be in the HMO). Many HMOs provide integrated services and focus on prevention and wellness. HMOs have lost popularity in recent years due to the restrictive requirements and use of gatekeepers, also known as primary care providers (PCPs). These are health care professionals, often physicians, who serve as the patient's first contact when entering the health care system. The PCP evaluates patient complaints and determines the appropriate level of care. Today HMOs cover only 14% of American workers under employer health care plans.

- **Preferred provider organization (PPO)**: Health plan more flexible than an HMO, but potentially more expensive. Providers contract on a fee-for-service basis with employers, insurance plans, or other third-party administrators. Patients pay less if they use providers in the plan's network, but for an additional cost, can use hospitals and services outside the network without a referral. Patients do not need to see a primary care physician before going to a specialist. PPOs cover the highest percentage of American workers at 48%.

- **Point of service (POS)**: An HMO and PPO hybrid in which members can see an in-network provider for a reduced rate or out-of-network provider for a higher rate. Patients do need a referral to see a specialist. Ten percent of American workers have POS plans through their employers.

- **Exclusive provider organization (EPO)**: Another hybrid of an HMO and PPO in which services are covered only if providers and hospitals are in the plan's network, except in emergencies. An advantage to this type of plan is that patients are not required to see their primary care provider before seeing a specialist. EPOs enable employers to create benefit packages specific to their company's needs.

All managed care systems employ several methods in an effort to achieve the goals listed in the previous section. Examples include prepaid plans, negotiated fees, primary care providers, and review of services using preauthorization.

Prepaid Plans

A major attempt to reduce costs has been the development of **prepaid plans** in which health care providers are paid *before* rather than *after* services are performed.

This payment method is based on the idea that providers can be motivated to be more efficient. Let's look at an example of how these plans work.

1. A health insurance company signs up 10,000 customers, known as *enrollees*.

2. Each of the 10,000 pays a monthly amount known as a *premium* to the insurance company.

3. The insurance company contracts with a health care service group that agrees to provide medical services to the enrollees. The physicians are paid a set amount for each enrollee. This is the only payment they receive, regardless of the type or number of services provided to the patients. This method of payment is called **capitation**.

4. Enrollees must use the physicians who have contracted with the insurance company. Depending on the plan, they may be required to pay a set amount for each service provided. This is called a **copay**.

5. The goal is that costs will average out. Some patients will require more care than the set amount covers, whereas others will not seek any services.

Although the practice of prepayment has been shown to increase efficiency in many cases, the method has opponents. Some argue that cost containment goals conflict with quality care goals. They worry that the number and quality of services will have to be sacrificed in order to increase profits. Several movements are underway at both the state and federal levels to pass laws to protect patient access to appropriate care.

Negotiated Fees

Another method for paying health care providers is by pre–agreed-upon amounts that are negotiated between health care providers and insurance companies, to pay for specific services. These are known as **negotiated fees**. They may cover all or only a percentage of the provider's actual charges. Depending on the type of plan, the patient pays the difference or the physicians accept as payment in full the amount paid by the insurance company.

Primary Care Providers

One of the most important control mechanisms is the use of **primary care providers (PCPs)**, also known as **gatekeepers**. As explained previously, they are the first point of contact for patients in HMOs. Diagnostic procedures and treatment plans must be approved by PCPs in order to be covered by insurance. They provide the referrals that patients must have before seeing specialists.

An advantage of the use of PCPs is that they provide consistency in patient care. They have a global picture of their patients' history and overall health care needs.

A disadvantage is that patients must go through them when they may already know that they need to see a specialist. It adds time and expense to the process of receiving necessary care. For example, Dan O'Riley has been seeing a dermatologist for the past five years for treatment of a chronic skin condition. His employer changes insurance companies, and Dan enrolls in the new HMO. He discovers that in order for the insurance company to pay for his skin treatments, he must choose and visit a PCP to get a referral to see his dermatologist.

Review of Services

Many insurance companies use review procedures to determine which costs they will cover. Diagnostic tests, treatments, hospitalizations, and so forth are reviewed to determine medical necessity and cost effectiveness. Insurance companies will not pay for certain nonessential medical services and referrals to specialists that have not been preapproved. Securing these approvals is known as **preauthorization**, and it is essential that health care professionals know when preauthorizations are necessary.

Thinking It Through

Josephine Copley arrives at work late, having had little sleep the night before. She hopes she can get caught up on some of her personal calls and still get the insurance forms sent out on time to meet the deadlines for submitting claims for reimbursement. She is working intently when approached by a patient who is very confused by her Medicare claim statements. The patient has questions on some of the supplies she was charged for. She does not know what they were used for or why.

Josephine is feeling quite stressed and is curt with her, saying, "I am sure all the charges are correct. Besides, Medicare doesn't pay like they used to anyway, so it doesn't matter. I'm just too busy to deal with this right now. It seems that patients want more and Medicare wants to pay less."

1. What are the possible consequences of Josephine's comments?

2. Was it appropriate that Josephine make negative comments about the patient's health care plan?

3. How could she have handled this situation differently?

4. What external circumstances may have contributed to Josephine's behavior?

Fascinating Facts

By 2021, it is expected that spending on health care will reach *$4.8 trillion*. It is estimated that as much as 30% of health care dollars are wasted each year.

Source: *https://meritagemed.com/surprising-facts-united-states-health-care/*

PROVIDING AFFORDABLE HEALTH CARE

Private health insurance coverage is based on the concept of spreading the risk. For example, the sellers of car insurance assume that not everyone who buys coverage will use it. There will be some accidents and stolen vehicles that must be paid for, but most people who are covered will never make a claim. Health insurance is based on the same principle. Although some people will suffer serious health problems and cost more than the amount of their premiums, others will use much less. In order for this system to be profitable, health insurance companies tried to reduce the number of people who required expensive care. This was accomplished in several ways:

- Requiring applicants for insurance to pass physical exams
- Not selling insurance to people who had certain preexisting conditions, such as heart disease
- Selling policies to people with preexisting conditions, but not covering the costs related to these conditions

Although these methods helped insurance companies improve their cash flow, it left many people who were most in need of health care without coverage. This challenge was one of several that prompted calls for a system of national health care that would provide coverage for everyone, regardless of health condition or economic status.

In response to this problem, President Obama signed into law the Patient Protection and Affordable Care Act in 2010 (commonly called the Affordable Care Act [ACA] or "Obamacare"). This legislation was planned to provide easier access to health care by making insurance available to, and affordable for, all Americans. The first regulations went into effect in 2014, and the rollout of new regulations were scheduled to continue until 2020. Some highlights of the bill included:

- Health insurers could not deny children or adults health insurance because of preexisting conditions.
- Businesses with fewer than 50 employees received tax credits covering up to 50% of employee premiums. Those with more than 50 employees had to provide health care coverage.
- Everyone except certain low-income individuals had to purchase health insurance or face a $695 annual fine (called the *individual mandate*). Low-income individuals received government subsidies to help them purchase insurance.
- Medicare drug coverage was improved for seniors and the disabled.
- Young adults could be covered by their parents' health insurance until age 27.
- Preventative care without copays would be in effect by 2018.
- No health care plan was required to offer abortion coverage. If offered, it had to be paid for separately by the individual.
- Insurance companies would no longer be able to cancel an enrollee's coverage when he or she gets sick.
- Chain restaurants were required to provide a "nutrient content disclosure statement" alongside their menu items.
- Websites were developed to make it easier for Americans in any state to seek out affordable health insurance options.

As with any extension of coverage, the question of how to pay for it has been vigorously debated. Among the changes implemented to help create the necessary revenue to cover the costs of the ACA are the following:

- In 2012, the Medicare payroll tax was expanded to include unearned income (investment income) for families making more than $250,000 a year ($200,000 for individuals).
- Insurance companies were scheduled to pay a 40% excise tax on so-called "Cadillac" high-end insurance plans worth over $27,500 for families ($10,200 for individuals) starting in 2018.
- A 10% excise tax was assessed on indoor tanning services.

This list is by no means comprehensive, but highlights some of the provisions supporting the new legislation.

Controversy about the ACA has continued as the bill is applied and, with the change of administrations in 2016, efforts were made to repeal the entire Affordable Care Act. Although these efforts were unsuccessful, some key parts have been repealed or delayed. One key component that was repealed in late 2017 was the individual mandate, considered essential to funding the government subsidies to help lower-income Americans purchase health insurance. The means of providing health care is a highly political issue, and at the time this book is published, there will surely have been more changes on how it is organized and paid for in the United States.

The main intent of the ACA was to provide better access to health care and it is reported that since 2010, at least 20 million more Americans have health insurance. At the same time, it has been pointed out that very little was done to control the cost of health care.

CONTROLLING ORGANIZATIONAL COSTS

The effects of managed care, insurance restrictions, and government regulations have greatly affected all types of health care organizations. Facilities must focus on controlling expenditures. Expenditures refer to any money that is spent in the process of doing business. The expenditures are the cost of resources required to maintain a health care delivery system. These costs occur in four major areas. (See Figure 22–3.)

1. Financing
2. Technology and supplies (pharmaceuticals and equipment)
3. Facilities
4. Personnel

Financing refers to the source of money used to run a business. Financing resources for a health care facility come primarily from a variety of health insurance companies (federal or private), although loans from banks are another source of funds. Other financing resources may be individuals who pay for their own care or donations that individuals and corporations give to nonprofit facilities.

Insurance plans have their own sets of rules, procedures, and paperwork to be completed before payments for patient services are sent to the facility. The key factor here is to be as efficient as possible in completing the paperwork correctly and completely, so the payment can be received as soon as possible for services provided. For example, the CPT codes described later in this chapter must be accurate. When services have been given and the payment not received, the amount owed is recorded in what is called an account receivable. A sound business practice is to keep the accounts receivables as low as possible. Keeping the accounts receivables low is an important part of financial management and relates to the cost of money. The cost of money refers to the value that could be earned on money if it were received by the facility and invested. For example, if a facility has $1 million in accounts receivables and a 10% interest rate could be earned on that money, the facility is losing $274 for each day the payment is delayed ($1,000,000 × 10% ÷ 365 days/year). The facility may also be paying interest on loans that it cannot pay off until the receivables are in the account. When money is owed to others for services, supplies, or equipment received, it is recorded as an account payable.

Technology and supplies refer to the cost of equipment and supplies that are used in the process of giving health care services to patients—for example, diagnostic equipment, medications, catheters, beds, and linens. Computerized systems, described in Chapter 19, have become a major expense.

Facilities are the physical buildings and the land they stand on and the cost of maintaining them—for example, the painting, repairing, and remodeling of the buildings; landscaping; electricity; garbage removal; and maintenance of parking areas.

Personnel (labor costs) refers to the individuals who work in all areas associated with the functioning of the health care delivery system. They include both the direct care workers and those in support roles. Examples include nurses, physical and occupational therapists, medical assistants, X-ray and lab technicians, accountants, admissions staff, managers, pharmacists, dieticians, coders,

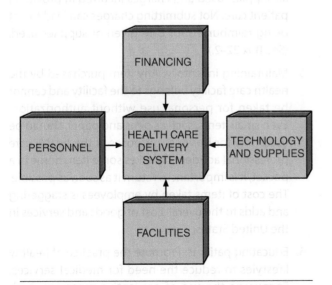

FIGURE 22–3 Resources required to maintain a health care delivery system.

administrators, and maintenance workers. *The total cost of the salaries of all the health care professionals is often the largest cost incurred by a facility.*

HEALTH CARE PROFESSIONALS' IMPACT ON COSTS

The career success of the health care professional will depend, to a great degree, on his or her ability to contribute to the control of rising costs. Every health care professional must take fiscal (financial) responsibility for his or her performance. The need for efficiency and accountability on the part of everyone in the system cannot be overemphasized. The question that must be asked is, "How can I help reduce unnecessary costs?" It is easy to dismiss the consequences of one person's impact on the finances of a health care facility, but when totaled up over time and multiplied by the number of health care professionals who are very concerned with efficiency, the cost savings can be quite significant.

There are many ways health care professionals can contribute to the efficient and cost-effective functioning of the facility:

1. Practicing personal efficiency: This refers to the health care professional's performance and how each worker contributes to overall efficiency. For example, when workers arrive late or take excessive breaks, it affects their coworkers' workloads and their ability to perform their duties efficiently. This results in a decrease in patient satisfaction. The costs of poor-quality care are often related to the following problems:

   • Duplicated work between departments

   • Loss of time due to inefficient task performance

   • Loss of staff due to job dissatisfaction

   • Recruitment and training of new employees

   • Expenditure of energy and time in the investigation of complaints

   • Lawsuits (litigation) and malpractice settlements

   • Employees repeatedly making the same errors in tasks, despite instruction

   • Time wasted reporting and correcting errors

   • Expenses related to overutilization of diagnostic tests to avoid malpractice

2. Focusing on the job: When at work, 100% of the health care professional's attention must be focused on the duties at hand. The needs of patients and the organization/employer must have top priority.

3. Carefully using supplies and equipment: Damage or loss of supplies and equipment can add significantly to the cost of operations. Always use supplies only as needed and avoid waste by taking only that which is needed to complete the task. Handle equipment carefully and follow the manufacturer's instructions on the proper use and care of all equipment.

4. Billing and coding correctly and not misplacing charges: The **International Classification of Diseases ICD-10 codes** assign numbers to diseases and conditions, also known as diagnoses. **Current Procedural Terminology (CPT) codes** were developed by the American Medical Association in 1966 to document and report all types of services, including surgical and radiological procedures, rehabilitation treatments, and lab tests. Thousands of standardized codes are in use to provide the information on which insurance claims are based. Codes are contained in the following reference books, available in both print and electronic versions: *Current Procedural Terminology (CPT)* and *Classification of Diseases, 10th Revision; Clinical Modification (ICD-10-CM).*

   Health care professionals who have responsibility for submitting codes for reimbursement must learn to properly use these references. Special training is recommended and many employers require certification. Coding is very specific to the particular diagnosis or procedure. Improper coding can lead to various problems, ranging from a loss of income for the provider to charges of fraud for overbilling. All health care professionals need to be sure to note all supplies used and charges incurred in providing patient care. Not submitting charges can lead to not being reimbursed for care given or supplies used. (See Box 22–2.)

5. Maintaining inventory: Any item purchased by the health care facility belongs to the facility and cannot be taken for personal use without authorization. Even small items, such as pens and paper, should be used only for business purposes. If the health care professional accidentally takes some item home in a pocket, it is important to return it as soon as possible. The cost of items taken by employees is staggering and adds to the overall cost of goods and services in the United States.

6. Educating patients: Promote the practice of healthy lifestyles to reduce the need for medical services. Encourage the use of preventive measures, such as immunizations and prenatal care, to reduce the

---

Box 22-2

ICD-10 Code Examples

S93.4 Sprain of ankle

S93.401 Sprain of unspecified ligament of right ankle

S93.402 Sprain of unspecified ligament of left ankle

S93.409 Sprain of unspecified ligament of unspecified ankle

Required seventh digit to identify the encounter:

A—Initial

D—Subsequent

S—Sequela

Notice the specificity for just this diagnosis. If the code is not specific and does not match the other documentation, the charge will be declined and revenue lost (or delayed until further clarification can be obtained).

---

need for more expensive care later. Clearly explain patient self-care practices to prevent unnecessary office visits.

7. Being willing to cross-train: Cross-training means learning skills outside those traditionally expected in a given occupation. Health care professionals who have a variety of skills and can perform many tasks are more cost effective than employees who have a limited number of skills. Cross-trained health care professionals can fill in as needed, eliminating downtime and delays in delivering patient care or completing department tasks. Examples include respiratory therapists who learn to draw blood and transcriptionists who can perform insurance coding and billing. Being willing to acquire additional skills, learned and practiced under proper supervision, can significantly increase the health care professional's value to an employer and create career opportunities.

Personal Efficiency

Employees who have difficulty performing efficiently on the job often have poor organizational skills, are confused about their priorities (what is most important), and may be slow in making decisions. Efforts to make personal changes may be necessary. Each individual must do a self-evaluation to identify areas that need improvement.

There are numerous books, blogs, and other websites that help with personal assessment by presenting principles to follow in the process of change. Browsing the business and self-improvement sections in a bookstore or on the Internet may assist you to identify an author or website that relates the material in a manner that addresses your particular concerns and can assist you in your efforts to improve. The drive for personal effectiveness is a lifelong pursuit, but if developed can lead to personal and career success. Certain behaviors form a foundation for such improvement:

- Use the problem-solving process identified in Chapter 1 to assist in determining what areas in your life, if improved, would create the most dramatic changes for the positive. This is where the greatest effort and time should be spent.

- Assume responsibility for your life and your decisions. Remember, not making a decision is a decision. Procrastination is a decision too—the decision to postpone the issue.

- Don't just let life pass you by as you passively look at the world. Take action, make decisions, and initiate changes after a sound evaluation of what is needed. Be willing to accept the consequences of any actions you do or do not take.

- Don't allow yourself to get sidetracked with the minutiae (trivia) of life. The details of daily life and the related interruptions can seem compelling, but don't forget to focus on the big picture of what you have identified as central to your well-being.

- Expect setbacks in your progress, but do not use this as an excuse not to continue.

- If you feel you do not have enough time, monitor how your time is spent and then evaluate and eliminate the unimportant time wasters. (See more about time management in Chapter 12.)

- Communicate clearly and honestly with others when a conflict arises. Look for solutions that will satisfy all involved (this may require creative decision-making). Make sure you understand what the other person is truly saying; do not just argue your side. If you are listening empathetically, you will not be planning what you will say next when the other person is speaking.

- Look at your life from a holistic perspective. You and those around you have physical, social, emotional, and spiritual needs. Individuals who address all these areas function better.

If the health care professional is unable to find personal satisfaction, there is a greater likelihood of also having a dissatisfying professional life. Achieving maximum personal effectiveness enables the health care professional to make contributions that lead to an efficient and high-quality organization.

Acting with Thought

The importance of thinking has been emphasized throughout this text. In order to control costs, all health care personnel must pay attention to their actions. The question presented earlier in this chapter, "How can I help reduce unnecessary costs?" should prompt additional questions, the answers to which will guide one's work:

- What are the facts?
- What is the best course of action?
- What is the right thing to do?
- What is the probable impact of my actions?

Applying the problem-solving model introduced in Chapter 1 will assist the health care professional to carefully review situations, gather necessary information, and make sound decisions.

Thinking It Through

James de Melendez has been a respiratory therapist for 22 years. He enjoys working with patients and administering therapies. Although James keeps up with the continuing educational requirements of his profession, he is resistant to learning skills that he considers to be outside the practice of respiratory therapy. James wants to move to a small town and applies for a position in the town's only hospital. He is surprised when he is not hired. When he follows up with the supervisor who interviewed him, he is told that due to cost-control measures, the hospital is focusing on hiring multiskilled professionals who can perform duties in various departments.

1. How has James failed to keep up with trends in health care delivery?
2. What can he do to improve his future employment opportunities?
3. What are the implications for your future career?

SUGGESTED LEARNING ACTIVITIES

1. Consider your own financial situation and determine if there are any accounts receivables (any money due to be paid to you: money you have lent; a paycheck for the last two weeks' work; payments you have made in advance for services, such as newspaper or magazine delivery). Do you have any accounts payables (do you owe money)? How do these compare?

2. If you have worked or currently work, identify ways in which your performance has affected the cost of doing business. Review the areas listed under the section "Health Care Professionals' Impact on Costs."

3. Look for articles on the Internet or in news magazines about the rising cost of health care. Are any solutions offered? Do you agree or disagree with the solutions proposed? Explain why.

WEB ACTIVITIES

Meritage Medical Network

21 Surprising Facts about United States Health Care

https://meritagemed.com/surprising-facts-united-states-health-care/

1. Which of the facts did you find most surprising?
2. Which was the least?

3. Check the facts given in items 6 and 7 with other sources, such as the World Health Organization. Have these statistics changed?

4. Why do you think the United States has poorer outcomes than many other developed countries?

Health Affairs

Health Care Cost Control: Where Do We Go from Here?

https://www.healthaffairs.org/do/10.1377/hblog20180705.24704/full/

1. Who benefits from the high prices of health care products and services?

2. Who suffers most from high health care costs?

3. What is "targeted regulation"?

4. Which groups (employers, consumers, etc.) need to take action to help control health care costs? What are these actions?

5. Why is the control of health care costs in the United States so complex?

Michigan Today

Drugs versus Lifestyle Medicine: Combating Chronic Disease

https://michigantoday.umich.edu/2015/02/14/drugs-versus-lifestyle-medicine/

1. What is the meaning of "fix-it medicine"?

2. Do you agree with what the author writes about why people don't change their lifestyle habits? Why or why not?

3. If more people made more healthy choices, how might this affect health care costs in the United States?

American Diabetes Association

The Cost of Diabetes

http://www.diabetes.org/advocacy/news-events/cost-of-diabetes.html

1. List the direct and indirect costs of diabetes in 2017.

2. What is the average expenditure per patient?

3. Which group of patients with diabetes has fewer doctor visits and fewer prescribed medications?

4. Which four states have the highest populations with diabetes?

Statistica

Distribution of U.S. health care expenditure from 2014 to 2018, by payer

https://www.statista.com/statistics/237043/us-health-care-spending-distribution/

1. Which type of payer paid the most for health care in 2018? The least?

2. What percent of health care was covered by government plans?

3. Which payers' percentages have increased from 2016 to 2018?

Medicare

https://www.medicare.gov/

After exploring the different sections of the website, answer the following questions:

1. Who is eligible to receive Medicare free Part A?

2. How much was the premium for Medicare Part B in 2018?

3. What services are covered by Part A? By Part B?

4. What are examples of services not covered by Medicare?

5. How can eligible patients get Part D, Medicare prescription insurance?

Medicaid

Eligibility

https://www.medicaid.gov/medicaid/eligibility/index.html

1. How many Americans currently have Medicaid coverage?

2. Which groups of people are currently covered by Medicaid?

3. How did the Affordable Care Act alter Medicaid?

4. What are the financial guidelines for determining eligibility?

5. What is a "medically needy program"?

6. What recourse do individuals have if they are turned down for Medicaid?

Children's Health Insurance Program (CHIP)

https://www.benefits.gov/benefit/607

1. What is the purpose of CHIP?

2. Who administers the programs?

3. Is the CHIP program the same in every state?

4. What does CHIP cover?

University of Washington

https://depts.washington.edu/bioethx/topics/manag.html

Read the information on managed care and then click on "Case 1" and read the scenario.

1. What are your thoughts on this topic?

2. Click on "Discussion" and read the comments.

3. Do you agree with the information provided? Why or why not?

National Conference of State Legislatures

The Affordable Care Act: A Brief Summary

http://www.ncsl.org/research/health/the-affordable-care-act-brief-summary.aspx

Identify two features of the new law that you agree with and two with which you have concerns. Explain why.

AAPC Coder

https://coder.aapc.com/cpt-codes/

1. Click on several categories to get an idea of how specific CPT codes are.

2. Explain why it is important to take great care when choosing and entering codes when billing insurance companies.

World Health Organization

http://www.who.int/news-room/detail/18-06-2018-who-releases-new-international-classification-of-diseases-(icd-11)

WHO releases new International Classification of Diseases (ICD 11)

1. When was the ICD 11 released?

2. When will it come into effect?

3. What are the major changes from ICD 10?

4. Do you think these changes will make it easier for health care professionals to use the classification system?

Snacknation

31 Things People Do to Increase Their Productivity at Work

https://www.snacknation.com/blog/increase-productivity-at-work/

1. Read through the suggestions.

2. Are there any you think might help you become more efficient and productive?

3. Choose one or two to try for a couple of weeks. Were they helpful?

REVIEW QUESTIONS

1. What factors contribute to the high cost of health care?

2. What are the six categories of wasted health care funds?

3. How do the attitudes and behaviors of many Americans regarding their own health habits contribute to the high cost of health care?

4. What negative consequences are experienced by many Americans as a result of the high cost of health care?

5. What are the three categories of health care institutions based on their source of funding?

6. How have methods for paying medical costs changed over the years?

7. What are the three most common methods that patients use to pay for their health care?

8. What is the purpose of Medicaid, who does it cover, and how is it administered?

9. Who is covered by Medicare? What services are covered?

10. What is the Veterans Health Administration and who does it cover?

11. What do the terms "deductible" and "coinsurance" mean?

12. What are DRGs and what is their purpose?

13. What is the purpose of managed care? What are its goals?

14. How do the following types of managed care plans work: HMO, PPO, EPO, and POS?

15. How does a prepaid health plan work?

16. What is the meaning of "negotiated fees"?

17. What is the meaning and purpose of a "primary care provider"?

18. What is the meaning and purpose of "preauthorization"?

19. What was the major purpose of the Affordable Care Act?

20. What are the major components of the Affordable Care Act?

21. What are three methods enacted by the government to pay for the Affordable Care Act?

22. What are the four major areas of expenditures incurred by a health care system?

23. What is the meaning of the following terms: "account receivable," "account payable," and "the cost of money"?

24. What are seven ways that health care professionals can help control the costs of their facilities?

25. What are ICD-10 codes? CPT codes? What is their purpose?

26. What are ways that health care professionals can increase their personal efficiency?

27. What is meant by "acting with thought"?

APPLICATION EXERCISES

1. Refer to the Case of the Inefficient Office at the beginning of the chapter. What suggestions would you offer to your supervisor if you were in Constance's position?

2. It is a particularly busy day for Aubrey Casein as she rushes to assist several physicians as they perform patient procedures. It seems to her that the requests for supplies are coming in faster than she can meet the demand. She knows that the inventory tags on each of the items must be placed in the appropriate location for the charge to be billed to the correct patient's insurance. But today she decides to perform this task later when it slows down and places the inventory tags in her pocket. The day continues at the same fast pace, and Aubrey arrives home to discover numerous charge tags still in her pocket.

   a. What are the possible financial implications of Aubrey's actions?

   b. What are the ways she can use to identify which inventory tag goes with which patient?

   c. What are the possible consequences if she charges the wrong supplies to a patient?

PROBLEM-SOLVING PRACTICE

Patricia Leonard is trying to find health care coverage for herself, her husband, and her two children. Using the five-step problem-solving process, determine what Patricia can do to evaluate different options in health care insurance.

CHAPTER 23

Quality Control and Customer Service

KEY TERMS

adverse drug events

advocate

Agency for Healthcare Research and Quality (AHRQ)

constructive criticism

external customers

internal customers

Patient Care Partnership

quality improvement

The Joint Commission (JCAHO)

utilization review (UR)

The Case of the Angry Patient

Mr. Ramirez has been hospitalized for the last six days following orthopedic surgery. He is experiencing discomfort and is anxious about not being able to go home and be with his family. When Carolina Mims, physical therapy assistant, enters Mr. Ramirez's room to assist him with his exercises, he lets her know how unhappy he is about how he is being treated. The food is bad, it took "forever" for the nurse to respond to his call button, and the portable urinal has not been emptied. "It's disgusting," he tells Carolina and then asks, "Who's in charge here, anyway?" The

(continues)

OBJECTIVES

Studying and applying the material in this chapter will help you to:

1. Describe how the United States ranks in quality of care compared with comparable countries.
2. Explain the meaning of quality in health care.
3. Describe three approaches to measuring quality of care, including their limitations.
4. Explain the challenges of comparing patient outcomes when measuring quality of care.
5. State the overall goal of health care.
6. Explain what is meant by quality improvement.
7. Explain the role of the Centers for Medicare and Medicaid regarding health care quality.
8. Describe the Partnership for Patients and its goals.
9. Describe The Joint Commission and its safety goals.
10. Describe the Agency for Healthcare Research and Quality and its goals and activities.
11. List the 12 patient rights adopted by the American Hospital Association.
12. Describe a utilization review.
13. List the actions that health care professionals can take to help reduce the incidence of medical errors.
14. Explain the meaning of an "adverse drug event."
15. List the eight reasons for the occurrence of adverse drug events.
16. State the "Five Rights" of medication safety.
17. Identify the internal and external customers in a health care setting.
18. Give examples of questions to check the level of customer service in a health care facility.
19. Explain the major reasons that patients file lawsuits against health care providers and facilities.
20. Explain what it means to be an advocate for patients.
21. Describe the methods that health care businesses use to determine customer satisfaction.
22. Describe the steps to use when working with unhappy customers.
23. Explain how to maintain good relationships with internal customers.
24. Describe the characteristics of constructive criticism.
25. Discuss how a health care professional can view destructive criticism in a constructive manner.

fact is, there have been numerous complaints about the quality of the food, and unfortunately, the nursing staff is shorthanded because two nurses have called in sick. Carolina takes a few minutes to listen to Mr. Ramirez, demonstrates empathy for his discomfort, and tells him that she will report his complaints to the nursing supervisor. She is then able to proceed with the exercise session.

Knowing how to effectively handle complaints and work to make improvements in the system can make the difference between a high-quality patient care delivery system and one that fails. Understanding the principles of patient satisfaction will help you resolve problems that could lead to complaints and lawsuits.

QUALITY OF CARE

Finding the balance between maintaining high-quality patient care and controlling costs is a major struggle for modern providers of health care. Although the United States spends more on health care than any other country, it ranks lower in life expectancy and patient satisfaction and higher in infant mortality than many other industrialized countries:

- Life expectancy is 26th among comparable countries
- Infant mortality is 30th out of 40 countries
- Patient satisfaction is 4th at 89.33% after Sweden, Finland, and Norway (https://www .beckershospitalreview.com/quality/where-does-the-us-rank-internationally-in-patient-satisfaction .html)

Discussions about improving the quality of care and raising patient satisfaction begin with two very difficult questions:

1. What is quality of care?
2. How can quality of care be measured?

Quality can be defined as a measure of the degree to which delivered health services meet established professional standards and judgments of value to the consumer. Quality may also be seen as the degree to which actions taken or not taken maximize the probability of beneficial health outcomes and minimize risk and other negative outcomes. There are various methods of measuring for quality of care.

Approaches to Measuring Quality of Care

Measuring quality of care may seem straightforward, but it is not an easy task. Let's look at several approaches and the problems inherent in each.

1. Patient satisfaction: If this criterion is used, then we need to look at what patients want and would rate the highest. Patients are concerned with the following:

- Easily accessible and available services
- Timely and safe delivery of care
- Coordination between services and continuity of care
- Effectiveness of services—that is, the delivery and outcome of care

Unfortunately, if these concerns were addressed without regard to costs, they would lead to prohibitive health care costs.

2. Lowest costs: Using this criterion, the health care facilities that spent the least would be measured as the most effective. This is obviously an inadequate tool because it means that those providing the least care are rated as the best.

3. Patient outcomes: This criterion is based on how well patients recover or manage their ailments. This may seem an obvious choice for measuring the success of a health care experience. Did the patient recover to the prior state of health? This method also has limitations though, because it ignores the value of the time spent in the health care system and only focuses on the end result. For example, if a patient received no education about an upcoming surgery prior to the procedure but recovered and returned to an active and normal life, is this really quality of care? Perhaps the patient stayed in the hospital a few days longer because he or she was not being prepared for the care requirements needed to return home earlier. Could this be classified as a positive outcome?

Another challenge in comparing patient outcomes is the tremendous number of variables that exist among patients with similar procedures. For example, if two patients undergo the same surgical procedure and have no complications, should they both be expected to be discharged from the hospital within the same time frame? On the surface, the answer may be yes, but other factors must be considered. What if one patient is 30 years old and the other is 90 years old? What if one has a preexisting condition (e.g., diabetes or heart disease) and the other does not? What if one lives alone and the other has family and friends willing to come in and assist with the care?

If the patient outcomes for one health care facility are compared with those of another as a measurement of quality, another concern arises in this approach. What if one hospital shows a much higher death rate than another? Is this an indication that the first is giving worse care than the second? Perhaps the first hospital is located where there is a large elderly population and the other in a neighborhood with many young families. How would this affect the statistics?

Currently, there are no absolute answers when discussing such complex issues. These issues are far from being resolved and will continue to be central to health care in the foreseeable future. The focus of this text is not on solving these complex issues facing health care, but on assisting the health care professional in developing the skills and behavior needed to perform at the highest level and deliver the highest possible quality of care. Health care professionals must ask themselves what they can do to best meet the needs of the organization, their coworkers, and patients.

In health care, the goal is 100% correct care with no errors, because anything less can have serious consequences for both patients and health care professionals. This may seem unrealistic, but when viewed from a personal perspective, it becomes real. For example, how would you feel if you were among those who had the wrong surgical procedure performed on them? Or what would be the consequences to you and your family if you contract hepatitis B from a needle stick? Everyone must continually strive to provide competent, conscientious, and appropriate care.

QUALITY IMPROVEMENT

In the past, the belief was that if more was done, the result would be an increase in quality of care. It is now believed that the focus must be on *improving quality of care and on cost containment*. The processes used to find ways to preserve or improve quality of care while decreasing costs are called **quality improvement**. There are a number of agencies, both public and private, working to improve the quality of health care and patient safety.

Centers for Medicare and Medicaid Services

The Centers for Medicare and Medicaid Services (CMS) is a federal agency within the U.S. Department of Health and Human Services (DHHS). Programs for which CMS is responsible include Medicare, Medicaid, the Children's Health Insurance Program (CHIP), the Health Insurance Portability and Accountability Act of 1996 (HIPAA), and the Clinical Laboratory Improvement Amendments (CLIA). The CMS promoted the development of internal monitoring (within health care organizations) and evaluation processes. These were designed to identify the changes needed to decrease costs while still *maintaining* quality.

The CMS requires all health care facilities to establish a quality assessment and performance improvement (QAPI) program that is committed to ensuring high-quality and cost-effective care. Medicare contractors are required to prepare and submit a QAPI report to the CMS in order to receive reimbursement for any of the CMS programs. This report has many components. Being a Medicare contractor is vital to the functioning of any health care facility, not just those that care for patients aged 65 and older. This is because most private insurance companies, and also certifying agencies, require that a health care facility be a Medicare contractor.

Partnership for Patients

The Partnership for Patients is a public-private partnership, under the umbrella of the CMS, working to improve the quality, safety, and affordability of health care for all Americans. Members consist of physicians, nurses, hospitals, employers, patients and their advocates, and federal and state governments. Specific goals include a 20% reduction in hospital-caused harm to patients and a 12% reduction in 30-day hospital readmissions.

The Joint Commission

The Joint Commission is an independent, not-for-profit organization that accredits and certifies health care organizations in the United States. Its mission is to improve patient safety and each year it sets goals to achieve this mission. Its hospital safety goals for 2018 include the following:

- Identify patients correctly
- Improve the effectiveness of communication among caregivers
- Improve the safety of using medications
- Reduce the risk of health care–associated infections
- Prevent patients from falling

The Joint Commission certification is recognized as a symbol of quality and currently applies to 21,000 organizations. All health care professionals should be aware of these goals and strive to contribute to meeting them in their work.

Agency for Healthcare Research and Quality

The **Agency for Healthcare Research and Quality (AHRQ)** is an agency within the United States Department of Health and Human Services. (The current federal administration has proposed that it be merged with the National Institutes of Health, so this may have occurred by the time this textbook is published.) The goals of AHRQ are to enhance the quality, appropriateness, and effectiveness of health care services and access to care by

- Conducting and supporting research, demonstration projects, and evaluations
- Developing guidelines
- Disseminating information on health care services and delivery systems

Research results and tools are available to assist facilities and professionals evaluate their quality of care. For example, the Child Care Quality Tool Box contains definitions of, and methods for, measuring child care quality (https://www.ahrq.gov/professionals /quality-patient-safety/quality-resources/tools/chtoolbx /understand/index.html#useda). And the Nursing Home Survey on Patient Safety Culture was developed to solicit staff opinions about safety and health care quality in their nursing homes (https://www.ahrq.gov/sops/quality-patient-safety/patientsafetyculture/nursing-home/index.html).

American Hospital Association

In 1973, the American Hospital Association adopted the Patient's Bill of Rights which was recently renamed the **Patient Care Partnership**. The 12 rights, in abbreviated form, are as follows: Patients have the right to:

1. Considerate and respectful care
2. Obtain information concerning their diagnosis, treatment, and prognosis
3. Make decisions about their care plan
4. Have an advance directive (described in Chapter 3)
5. Every consideration of privacy
6. Confidentiality of their records
7. Review their records
8. A reasonable response from the hospital to his or her request for care and services
9. Ask and be told the business relationships among the hospital and other businesses and organizations
10. Consent or decline to participate in medical research studies
11. Expect reasonable continuity of care
12. Be informed of hospital policies and practices that relate to their care

(The Patient Care Partnership is also discussed in Chapter 3.)

Internal Monitoring

Each health care facility develops its own programs to evaluate the facility, identify areas for measurement, and perform reviews. These programs are designed by the health care facility to meet its internal needs. The assumption is that all areas can be improved (Box 23–1) and that this improvement will result in a higher quality of care and cost efficiency. This approach is based on data and uses a scientific approach to collect and analyze information and processes. The focus is on long-term system improvements.

Another process frequently used by health care facilities is called **utilization review (UR)** or utilization management (UM). This is an evaluation of the necessity, appropriateness, and efficiency of the use of health care services, procedures, and facilities. UR can be done by a peer review group (see Figure 23–1) or a public agency. It is a method of tracking, reviewing, and rendering opinions regarding care provided to patients. Usually UR involves the use of protocols, benchmarks, or data with which to

---

Box 23–1

Three Primary Areas to Examine When Evaluating a Health Care Facility for Quality Improvement

1. Organizational structure: How is the facility structured? What is the management style? How is communication encouraged? What changes would increase efficiency and accessibility?

2. Health care professionals: How do the health care professionals function as a team? What processes could be changed to increase efficiency and employee satisfaction?

3. Patient outcomes: Is the patient satisfied with the care? Was the outcome of his or her health care problem resolved in an efficient and appropriate manner with minimal suffering and confusion? Was the care provided in a coordinated manner to decrease duplication of services and minimize confusion?

FIGURE 23-1 Quality improvement issues are identified by conducting studies of facility performance.

compare specific cases to an aggregate set of cases. (See Box 23–2.) Managed care organizations sometimes refuse to reimburse or pay for services that do not meet their own sets of UR standards. UR involves the review of patient records and patient bills primarily, but may also include telephone conversations with providers. The practices of precertification, recertification, retrospective review, and concurrent review all describe UR methods. UR is one of the primary tools utilized by health plans to control overutilization, reduce costs, and manage care.

Box 23-2

Utilization Review Example

Problems are identified by the health care facility (e.g., a seemingly high rate of urinary infections in patients with a Foley catheter). These problems are called key indicators of quality care and are quantified (e.g., a chart review is done to determine how many patients with a Foley catheter have developed a urinary infection during a specified care time frame). The result is compared to industry standards to see if it exceeds the expected rate of such problems. If it is determined to be a problem area, education or other interventions are done to correct the identified problem. Then the study is repeated for subsequent periods (usually on a quarterly basis) to determine whether or not improvements have occurred as a result of the intervention. The results are used as measurements to determine if the quality of care is improving or declining. The focus is on individual performance, deviation from standards, and problem solving.

So far in this chapter, we have discussed the need to increase quality while decreasing costs. These may at first appear to be contradictory goals, but they are not. The following real-life examples demonstrate how the quality of care can be improved while costs are decreased.

- Not prescribing broad-spectrum antibiotics: Past practice was to order a broad-spectrum antibiotic when prescribing antibiotics for a patient. The philosophy was that the broader acting drug would "get whatever was there." But as more was learned about the development of bacterial resistance when unnecessary antibiotics are prescribed, it was determined that performing a culture (a test to see what bacteria are present) and using a more specific antibiotic was the best treatment choice for the patient. This had the advantage of decreasing the risk of resistance developing and rendering the drug ineffective when it was really needed. The cost advantage in this case is that the more specific antibiotics are often less expensive than the broad-spectrum antibiotics.

- Ordering disposable bibs: Health care professionals in a hospital would often use a towel as a bib when feeding patients to prevent the gown from being soiled. The administration conducted a study that demonstrated that the cost of sending the towels to the laundry was more than that of purchasing disposable bibs. The disposable bibs were purchased, and much to the delight of the staff, were more effective for their intended purpose, as well as costing less.

REDUCING MEDICAL ERRORS

A critical aspect of quality improvement in health care is the effort to reduce medical errors. A study by Johns Hopkins' safety experts reported that as many as 250,000 patients die annually as a result of medical errors, making this the third leading cause of death in the United States (https://hub.jhu.edu/2016/05/03/medical-errors-third-leading-cause-of-death/). The report emphasizes that these deaths are not due to "bad doctors," but to systemic errors that include poorly coordinated care and fragmented insurance networks.

Although some errors are the result of problems with the system—that is, at a higher level than that of the individual health care professional—there are actions the individual can take to help prevent errors that result in patient harm or death:

1. Act with thought. An emphasis in this text has been on *thinking like a health care professional:* observing, reflecting, and drawing on prior knowledge.

2. Take care when communicating patient information to others, as when leaving a shift and informing your replacement.

3. Do not rely on your memory to retain important information. Take notes when there is much to remember.

4. When making a decision regarding patient care, stop and ask yourself "Are you sure?" before proceeding.

5. Report to your supervisor if your schedule (hours worked, amount of work expected) is causing you fatigue that affects your effectiveness at work.

6. Report conditions that affect worker effectiveness, such as noise, poor lighting, heat, and clutter.

7. Work on improving your communication skills to prevent misunderstandings between you and your patients, coworkers, and supervisor.

8. Ask for assistance if you are unsure of how to perform a procedure, use equipment, or handle a patient situation.

9. Listen to patients if they have doubts about the treatment they are receiving or the medication they are taking, and report these concerns to their physician or other provider.

(List adapted from *https://www.medaptus.com/13-systems-principles-reduce-medical-errors-hospitals/*)

Medication Errors

Medication errors can occur anywhere between a prescription and when the patient receives the medication. Many, although not all errors result in **adverse drug events** (ADEs), defined as "harm experienced by a patient as a result of exposure to a medication." According to the AHRQ, each year ADEs account for almost 700,000 emergency department visits and 100,000 hospitalizations (https://psnet.ahrq.gov/primers/primer/23/Medication-Errors-and-Adverse-Drug-Events). Some sources report even higher numbers, including tens of thousands of deaths.

Medication errors can be due to numerical misidentification, as discussed in Chapter 4, but there are many other reasons why they occur:

- Improper dosing of drugs, especially dangerous with certain high-risk drugs such as intravenous heparin (decreases blood's clotting ability). The proper amount of this drug relies on careful measurement of the patient's weight and frequent monitoring of the blood's clotting ability to prevent severe bleeding.

- Taking too much or too little of a medication. It is important that dosage is clear in prescriptions and on drug container labels so the health care professional knows how much to administer. Patients may not understand about proper dosages to take at home. Studies have shown that caregivers, such as parents,

as well as patients, make many drug administration errors (https://psnet.ahrq.gov/primers/primer/23/Medication-Errors-and-Adverse-Drug-Events).

- Confusing medications with similar names. Drugs may have difficult spellings and similar names, making them easy to confuse. A couple of examples are *oxycodone and oxycontin* and *sulfadiazine and sulfasalazine.*

- Problems tracking drug use. The opioid epidemic and resulting deaths discussed in Chapter 2 has resulted in part from patients being able to get multiple prescriptions from different providers.

- Failing to understand how and when to take drugs. This is particularly problematic with those elderly patients who have difficulty remembering events of the day, such as when they last took their medications.

- Negative interactions of drugs. This can occur when patients use different providers to get prescriptions and a variety of pharmacies for the dispensing of drugs.

- The prevalence of *polypharmacy*, meaning taking more drugs than medically necessary. The AHRQ states that this is likely the strongest risk factor for ADEs. The preference of many Americans is to take a pill rather than make lifestyle changes and they pressure their providers who are often willing to write a prescriptions.

Most ADEs are caused by commonly used drugs. In fact, four medications—account for more than 50% of emergency department visits: (1) antidiabetic agents, such as insulin; (2) anticoagulants, such as warfarin; (3) antiplatelet agents, such as aspirin; and (4) opioid pain medications.

Health care professionals who participate in administering medications should be aware of the "Five Rights" of medication safety: Administer the Right Medication, in the Right Dose, at the Right Time, by the Right Route, to the Right Patient. If something does not seem correct about an order, it is correct for the health care professional to question it. For example, if a dosage doesn't seem logical, the provider who ordered the medication should be asked to verify. "Just following orders" is not a justification and the health care professional who administers an incorrect medication may be held just as accountable as the provider who ordered it.

CUSTOMER SERVICE

Satisfactory customer service is essential to the success of health care business in today's competitive market. When the term *customer* is used, it refers to both internal and external customers. **Internal customers** are those who work in the health care industry. For example, health care professionals from other offices, outside suppliers of medical and pharmaceutical supplies, and coworkers are internal customers who are affected by the behavior of those they work with on a day-to-day basis. **External customers** are those who come to the health care provider for services. They may be referred to as customers, patients, consumers, or clients.

Patients come to health care providers for a variety of reasons. (See Box 23–3.) They may hope to have a specific problem cured and their prior level of health restored. The visit may involve a request for a routine evaluation to confirm the patient's level of health or to obtain information on preventive measures that will help to prevent future problems. Or a sudden illness or emergency situation may develop that requires immediate attention. Whatever the reason for patients' contact with the health care facility, there is always the expectation that high-quality professional service will be delivered. (See Figure 23–2.)

When a patient evaluates the service received, it is not just the outcome that is important, but the entire experience. For example, two patients can have the same diagnosis, receive the same treatment, and return to their prior level of health within the same time frame, but one may be satisfied and the other very upset with the care received. It is necessary to review more than simply the medical problem that was presented. All aspects of contact with the patient must be examined when checking for quality. Examples of questions to ask about patient service include the following:

- If the initial contact was made by telephone, how was the patient treated? Was he or she placed on hold? Disconnected? Was the health care professional courteous and did he or she express interest and concern?

- When the patient arrived for the appointment, was he or she greeted in a friendly, yet professional manner? How long did he or she wait before being seen by the health care professional? Was the patient kept informed of any delays?

- Was the patient required to wait for procedures and tests once they were scheduled?

- Was he or she given clear instructions and were all questions answered? Was the patient given information about how to have future questions answered?

- Were all procedures explained and consent obtained?

Box 23–3

Services Sought by Patients through the Health Care System

1. Prevention
   - Education: Examples include nutrition and exercise, prevention of heart disease, smoking-cessation programs, how to manage diabetes
   - Routine physical exams
   - Screening tests: Examples include mammogram, sigmoidoscopy/colonoscopy, Pap smear, blood pressure check, PSA (screening test for prostatic cancer), fecal blood, cholesterol and lipids blood tests

2. Emergency and Urgent Care Services
   - Illnesses and injuries that need immediate attention

3. Inpatient Services
   - Surgery
   - Illnesses and injuries requiring continuous acute care
   - Specialized treatments
   - Rehabilitation

4. Long-Term Care
   - Nursing homes
   - Assisted living

5. In-Home Care
   - Nursing
   - Therapy
   - Homemaking

6. Psychological/Psychiatric Services
   - Counseling
   - Medication

7. Dental Services
   - Preventive care
   - Treatment and restoration

8. Pharmaceuticals and Medical Supplies and Equipment
   - Medications and other items needed to restore or maintain health

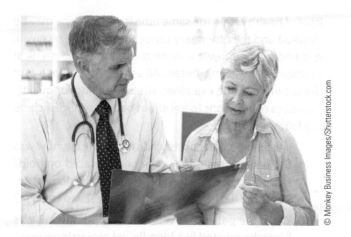

© Monkey Business Images/Shutterstock.com

FIGURE 23–2 Patients expect high-quality care. Their satisfaction must be one of the goals of every health care professional.

- Were all personnel courteous and compassionate when delivering care? Or was the care rough and abrupt and not considerate of the patient's needs?
- If the patient was in the hospital, what was the temperature and quality of the food? Was it quiet at night so he or she could sleep with a minimum of interruptions? Was he or she able to get prompt assistance when needed?

As health care professionals, it is sometimes easy to slip into a routine of just doing the job and forgetting that this may be a very frightening or stressful experience for the patient. When working with patients, use the time to learn more about their thoughts, concerns, and learning needs. This is not the time for the health care professional to share the exciting weekend trip or the fun date from the night before. Avoid engaging in social conversation with other health care professionals and ignoring the patients. They are there for service, and the focus must be concentrated on their needs. Social interactions with coworkers should be saved for breaks or after-work hours.

At the same time, health care providers should not interpret being professional as working with a "stone face" without expressing friendliness or emotion. Giving warm and focused attention to a patient can make a positive difference. An actual example is the case of a patient who had eye surgery and had to lie on her stomach for several days. Most of the caregivers simply spoke to her back; however, one bent down so the patient could see her face. The patient reported later that she felt gratitude for this thoughtful gesture because it made her feel valued.

Most people are surprised to learn that lawsuits brought by patients are more closely related to whether the patient does or does not like the health care professionals than to any other factor. In the past, it was common to have life-long relationships with physicians, based on mutual trust

Thinking It Through

Dr. Arthur has maintained a successful orthopedic practice in Midtown for many years. He has a good reputation for providing caring service. In recent months his medical assistant, Nathan Alberts, has received an increasing number of patient complaints about having to wait to see Dr. Arthur when they arrive for their appointments.

1. How should Nathan respond when patients complain about the delays?

2. Using the problem-solving process, what steps would you recommend Nathan take in order to resolve this problem?

and respect. Today, it is more common for patients to be treated by strangers. Changes in health care plans may require that new health care providers be chosen. If a referral to a specialist is required, the referring physician may have to be chosen from a list of approved specialists. Health care professionals must take advantage of every patient contact to create positive relationships and provide the highest quality care possible.

It is a common belief that if a lawsuit is filed, there must be good cause. Someone must have made a mistake. This is not necessarily true. Lawsuits may be filed as a result of emotional responses to perceived wrongs. Or they may concern matters of little importance, known as frivolous lawsuits. Keep in mind, though, that any lawsuit filed, whether it seems legitimate or not, will cause a great deal of stress for everyone involved. The amount of time and money spent in addressing a lawsuit can be overwhelming. Many lawsuits can be avoided by working to ensure that all patients are satisfied customers.

Taking Responsibility for Quality

Because this is an introduction to health care text, we have repeatedly emphasized the importance of reporting to, or checking with, your supervisor. This is important, but providing quality care involves more than this. You have a depth of responsibility that goes beyond just being a subordinate employee. Each individual health care professional should take his or her role very seriously. Everyone reports to a boss but that does not exempt them from maximizing their contribution to the organization. Even those who run large corporations that make widgets have an accountability. They report to the board of directors and frequently are accountable to shareholders if the corporation is listed on the stock exchange.

In health care, it is more important than ever to assist in efforts to give quality care and decrease costs. Your job is not just making widgets; how you conduct yourself affects the well-being of another person. It is not enough to just turn the problem over to someone else or hope it goes away. You need to ask yourself, "Have I done everything I can to resolve this problem?" If you need to refer a problem to someone else, then you can ask, "Is there some way I can expedite this issue?"

Sometimes it will be necessary to be an **advocate** (one who supports or promotes the interests of others) for the patient or draw attention to an ongoing problem that is not being addressed. Your supervisor may be busy or perhaps does not immediately see the issue that you do. In this case, it will be necessary to use your communication skills to get the proper attention the problem needs. Good quality health care means doing the right thing at the right time, in the right way, for the right person; and getting the best possible results.

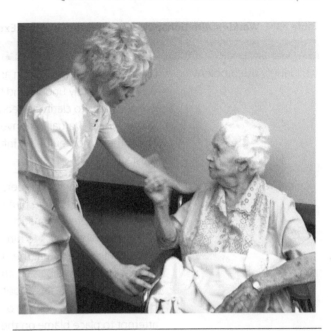

FIGURE 23–3 Good listening skills are essential when handling a patient complaint.

Customer Satisfaction

The "3 to 11 rule" of customer satisfaction states that for every good thing that happens to us we tell three people. For every bad thing that happens we tell 11 people.

One approach that many health care businesses use to determine how satisfied their customers are is to conduct customer surveys. These can be done in two ways:

1. Mailing out questions that customers answer and return by mail

2. Calling customers and asking them to respond to questions over the telephone

Some health care facilities maintain a log listing all complaints, what was done to address the complaint, and if the resolution was satisfactory. If the results are made available to staff, it is worth the health care professional's time to review the comments. The areas of concern may be very different from what is expected and can lead to changes in performance that will create greater customer satisfaction.

When working with unhappy customers, it is critical to fully understand their view of the situation. (See Figure 23–3.) To accomplish this, it is necessary to listen without interrupting and to not display signs of defensiveness. The guidelines in Table 23–1 will assist in handling this type of interaction.

Remember that each health care professional is responsible for patient satisfaction. The cost of an unhappy patient is much more than the loss of that one patient because he or she will probably tell family, friends, and coworkers.

It is also important to recognize that satisfaction is a subjective perception. Therefore, a health care professional must listen carefully and constantly to determine if the patient has any concerns. The patient may have a positive outcome to his or her medical treatment but may be unhappy with the experience due to a cold food tray, a delay in answering a call light, waiting for tests, delayed treatments, an unemptied bedpan, delayed pain medications, or an unfriendly or curt caregiver. Patients can be dissatisfied if they perceive that their problems are not seen as important.

Internal Customers

It is just as important to maintain good relationships with internal customers as with external ones. One of the common mistakes made when working with coworkers is to quickly point out errors but not take the time to stress what they do well. Praising coworkers for a job well done, a courtesy extended, or a quick response to a situation can build trusting and mutually satisfying working relationships. Everyone wants to do well on the job, to contribute to the effectiveness of the office or facility, and to have a sense of self-satisfaction with their contributions. When people take pride in their work, they will work harder and more cooperatively than they will if they feel that others are being overly critical.

Good relationships also require that criticism be given when appropriate. **Constructive criticism** is based on optimism. The intended message is that setbacks or failures are due to circumstances that can be changed for the better. It holds out the hope of improvement and suggests the beginning of a plan for doing so. (See Figure 23–4.) On the other hand, *destructive criticism* has the effect of creating helplessness, anger, and rebellion. The person is immediately put on the defensive and may no longer be receptive to suggestions for improvement. When

Table 23–1 Working with Unhappy Customers (Internal and External)

Steps	Comments
1. Identify the problem	• Listen to the complaint with an open mind. • Try to completely understand the customer's side of the situation. • Ask questions to clarify as needed, but do not interrupt needlessly. • Do not display verbal or nonverbal defensiveness. • Thank the customer for the information, because the goal is to always obtain customer satisfaction.
2. Seek resolution	• If the problem is with you personally, it is appropriate to apologize, thank the customer for the feedback, and assure him or her that you will do your best not to repeat the error. • If you need more information before the problem can be resolved, let the customer know when you will get back to him or her. • Provide information that the customer may be lacking. Make sure the customer is open to hearing what will be said and that it is phrased in a nondefensive manner. For example, if a customer complains about having had to pay for parking on the last visit, this could be addressed in a defensive or nondefensive manner. A defensive approach usually is an attempt to place blame on the customer, whereas a nondefensive approach does not. Consider these statements: Defensive—"Well, if you had just asked about it, we would have validated the ticket for you." Nondefensive—"I am sorry, we should have informed you that we validate parking tickets for patients. Do you have your ticket with you so we can validate it for you today?" • If you do not have the authority to deal with the problem, refer the customer to the proper person or ask the person with the authority to contact the customer.
3. Verify satisfaction	• Does the customer feel the problem has been resolved satisfactorily?

individuals are led to believe that their failures are due to personal faults that cannot be changed, they lose hope and stop trying. For example, a medical assistant is just starting a new job. In her haste to try to manage too many duties in order to make a good first impression, she inadvertently forgets to log two patient appointments. The result is that three patients are scheduled for the same time with the same nurse practitioner. The medical assistant's supervisor addresses the situation: Constructively: "While I know how overwhelming all the duties you have to accomplish are, it is important that you accurately accomplish each duty. Until you feel more comfortable with all your duties, try to concentrate on one duty at a time (e.g., answer one phone call; finish the scheduling of a patient's appointment prior to answering another phone). Destructively: "You messed up! The nurse practitioner will not have a chance for a break, and the whole day's schedule is behind." Box 23–4 contains effective guidelines for giving constructive criticism.

It is difficult to hear criticism, especially if it is not presented as constructive criticism. When receiving destructive criticism from someone, the health care professional can change it into a more positive experience by implementing the suggestions in Box 23–5.

FIGURE 23–4 The goals of constructive criticism are to encourage improvement and to resolve problems.

Box 23-4

How to Give Constructive Criticism

- Be concise and clear during conversations. If the other person does not understand exactly what you mean, it increases the chances of misunderstandings. Giving specific examples that illustrate the issue is a great way to increase clarity.

- Never use vague, general, or harsh terms. It is frustrating to hear that you are doing something wrong or not performing well and not understand exactly what can be done to correct the situation.

- Include positive comments of what the other person is doing well. Using positive and negative comments is sometimes referred to as the "sandwich technique." Start and end the conversation with positive feedback and then incorporate (sandwich in) the area(s) that need improvement.

- If the problem directly affects you, state how it makes you feel. For example, if a coworker is not completing his or her tasks before leaving the workplace, state that you feel taken advantage of and rushed by having to complete the extra tasks.

- Show a respectful attitude toward the other person. Always strive to preserve the other person's self-respect. Everyone makes mistakes or has areas that need improvement.

- Demonstrate a cooperative attitude. Give ample opportunity for the other person to ask questions and seek clarification about what is being stated. Offer positive suggestions for improvement.

- Be sensitive as this may be difficult for the other person to hear. No one likes to confront their faults. If the reaction is defensive, do not respond defensively in turn. Acknowledge the reaction and attempt to redirect to a more positive exchange.

- Provide time for face-to-face communication that is done in private. It is uncomfortable giving a criticism, but distancing oneself by using impersonal messages or memos creates greater discomfort and prevents the opportunity for the other person to respond or seek clarification.

- Use empathy when communicating. Stay aware of the impact on the person of what you say and how you say it.

- Never complain to others about the performance of a coworker. Communicate directly with him or her privately and confidentially.

Box 23-5

Responding to Destructive Criticism

- Look for the "kernel of truth" in the statement.
- Be aware of your emotional response and set it aside in an effort to benefit from the exchange.
- Do not attack the other person. You may feel that you have information about his or her own performance, attitude, or practices, but now is not the time to share these thoughts.
- If the situation becomes too emotional, ask to take a break and negotiate a time to resume the conversation later. This gives you an opportunity to put things in perspective.

- Even if you do not agree with what is being said, be open to trying to understand it from the other person's point of view.
- If the feedback is valid, take responsibility and initiate the needed changes in behavior.
- Look at the experience as an opportunity to develop stronger team relationships with coworkers and to improve communications. Work with the person giving the criticism to solve the perceived problem.
- Ask for specific examples if you are unclear about what is being said.
- Ask for suggestions about how you might improve.

Fascinating Facts

- A business hears from only 4% of its unhappy customers. The other 96% go elsewhere for service.

- Sixty-eight percent of the unhappy customers leave because of an attitude of indifference toward them.

- Seventy percent of complaining customers will do business with you again if you resolve the complaint in their favor. This increases to 95% if the complaint is resolved on the spot.

Positive relationships with coworkers provide the foundation for making efforts as an organization to offer high-quality service to all customers. *Employee satisfaction leads to customer satisfaction.*

Thinking It Through

Carstyn Franklin is a certified occupational therapy assistant (COTA) working in a busy hand therapy clinic. She and the other two assistants work with patients, make splints, and teach the use of adaptive devices so that patients can learn to perform homemaking and self-care practices as independently as possible. Brandon Williams, one of the other assistants, has the habit of leaving equipment, tools, and supplies wherever he last used them instead of putting them away. This results in delays for the other assistants because they must locate needed items before they can do their own work.

1. Describe in detail how Carstyn can speak with Brandon about his work habits.

2. What should be the goal of her communication?

3. How can she present the problem in order to increase the chances of resolution?

4. How can she respond if Brandon reacts defensively?

SUGGESTED LEARNING ACTIVITIES

1. Survey friends and family members about their health care experiences. Were they positive or negative, and why? What did they want from health care professionals? Did they receive it?

2. Spend some time thinking about how you would want to be treated as a patient. What would be most important to you?

3. Watch for examples of good customer service as you shop and go about your other activities. Describe what you believe makes them good.

4. Try using the suggested constructive criticism method the next time you need to discuss a problem or behavior concern with someone. What methods did you use? What was the result?

5. Pay attention to how you receive criticism. Do you usually find it to be a learning experience? A confrontation? A waste of time?

WEB ACTIVITIES

Agency for Healthcare Research and Quality

Understanding Quality Measurement: Child Health Care Quality Toolbox

https://www.ahrq.gov/professionals/quality-patient-safety/quality-resources/tools/chtoolbx/understand/index.html

After reading the material, write a paper that summarizes the information, including definition of quality and the components involved in measuring quality of health care for children.

Stanford Health Care

About Us: Quality

https://stanfordhealthcare.org/about-us/quality.html

1. Read Stanford's information for patients regarding how they define and measure quality: Overview and Measuring Quality.
2. What questions do they recommend that patients ask to assess the quality of care at Stanford?

University of Michigan

Drugs versus Lifestyle Medicine

https://michigantoday.umich.edu/2015/02/14/drugs-versus-lifestyle-medicine/

1. Do you agree with the author's view of Americans' preferences?
2. Do you see examples of the behavior he describes among your friends, family members, and others?
3. If many Americans made lifestyle changes, how might this affect the quality of health care? The cost of health care?

The Joint Commission

2019 National Patient Safety Goals

https://www.jointcommission.org/standards_information/npsgs.aspx

Click on links to facilities in which you might work in your career. Then click on "Simplified Version." What actions could you take as a health care professional to help achieve the goals listed?

The White House

Fact Sheet: Medicare Prescription Drug, Improvement, and Modernization Act of 2003

https://georgewbush-whitehouse.archives.gov/news/releases/2003/12/20031208-3.html

1. Do you believe the changes to Medicare brought about by this Act increased the quality of care for senior Americans?
2. Why or why not?

Pharmacy Times

Look-Alike, Sound-Alike Drug Names

https://www.pharmacytimes.com/publications/issue/2010/december2010/medicationsafety-1210

Read through the list, then list the suggestions that follow for avoiding mix-ups with drugs.

Online Search

Search for "customer service guidelines."

1. Review one of the samples.
2. What is your opinion of these guidelines?
3. How do they compare to the ones where you have worked? (If you have never been employed, then use the school as the comparison.)

Becker's Hospital Review

10 Strategies to Provide Patients with Superior Customer Service

https://www.beckershospitalreview.com/hospital-management-administration/10-strategies-to-provide-patients-with-superior-customer-service.html

1. Do you agree with the suggestions given?
2. Can you practice any of these strategies in your daily life?
3. How might you apply these suggestions in your future career?

REVIEW QUESTIONS

1. How does the United States rank in life expectancy, patient satisfaction, and infant mortality when compared to other countries?
2. What is the meaning of quality in health care?
3. What are three approaches to measuring the quality of care?
4. What are the challenges when comparing the quality of patient outcomes?
5. What is the overall goal of health care?
6. What is meant by quality improvement?
7. What is the role of the Centers for Medicare and Medicaid regarding the quality of health care?
8. What is the Partnership for Patients? What are its goals?
9. What is the Joint Commission? What are its safety goals?
10. What is the Agency for Healthcare Research and Quality? What are its goals and activities?
11. What are the American Hospital Association's 12 patient rights?
12. What is a utilization review?
13. What actions can health care professionals take to help reduce the incidence of medical errors?
14. What is the meaning of an "adverse drug event"?
15. What are eight reasons for an adverse drug event to take place?
16. What are the Five Rights of medication safety?
17. Who are internal and external customers in a health care setting?
18. What are examples of questions that can be asked to help determine the level of customer service in a health care facility?
19. What are the major reasons that patients make the decision to sue their health care provider and/or facility?
20. What does it mean to be an advocate for patients?
21. How do health care businesses determine customer satisfaction?
22. What steps should be followed when working with unhappy customers?
23. How can the health care professional maintain good relationships with internal customers?
24. What are the characteristics of constructive criticism?
25. How can the health care professional view destructive criticism in a constructive way?

APPLICATION EXERCISES

1. Refer to the Case of the Angry Patient at the beginning of this chapter. How would Carolina respond to Mr. Ramirez's criticism constructively? Destructively?
2. Alicia has just about had it at work. As a respiratory therapist, she loves working with patients. She knows that breathing difficulties create great anxiety, and she likes knowing that her work helps patients resolve more than just their physical problems. But Alicia is distressed by the disarray in the hospital department where she works. Her schedule is often changed, sometimes with very little notice. This causes problems with her child care arrangements. Equipment is not always put away where it should be, and supply inventories are often depleted. Alicia decides to discuss the situation with her supervisor.

She recently took a workshop on quality improvement and believes that what she learned could be applied to resolving her department's disorder.

a. How can Alicia present her concerns in a positive way to her supervisor?

b. What can she share about quality improvement that might be helpful?

c. What kinds of processes might be put in place to help resolve the department's problems?

PROBLEM-SOLVING PRACTICE

Refer to Box 23–2, Utilization Review Example. Compare this example with the five-step problem-solving process described in Chapter 1. Is the complete process being used?

CHAPTER 24

Job Leads and the Resume

KEY TERMS

chronological resume
cold calling
cover letters
functional resume
networking
objective
resume
school career service
traits

OBJECTIVES

Studying and applying the material in this chapter will help you to:

1. State the number of hours that experts recommend devoting to the job search.

2. Explain why having a positive attitude is important when searching for a job.

3. Explain the purpose of preparing an inventory of your employment skills and personal traits that are of value to an employer.

4. List eight common workplace preferences job seekers should consider.

5. Describe ways to organize a workplace for your job search.

6. Describe two ways to project a professional image.

7. List seven sources of job leads and job search assistance.

8. List the three types of networking.

9. Explain how to use the Internet effectively in your job search.

10. Explain three ways to avoid employment scams on the Internet.

11. State the purpose of a resume.

12. List and describe the contents of each section of the resume.

13. Describe the organization and purpose of chronological and functional resumes.

14. List ten characteristics of an effective resume.

15. Explain the purpose and characteristics of effective cover letters.

The Case of the Unprepared Applicant

Jenny Nguyen recently passed her state exam to become a registered dental assistant and is seeking her first job. Jenny did well in her training, but has not had much experience applying for jobs. The career services counselor at Jenny's school calls her on Tuesday morning to tell her about a job opening with Dr. Chambers, a well-respected dentist in her area. A job in his dental clinic would be an excellent opportunity for a new dental assistant. Jenny is interested in the position but has put off completing her resume and needs a few more hours to finish it. She is also nervous about her interviewing skills and delays calling Dr. Chambers. When she finally calls on Friday afternoon, she learns that the job was filled that morning. In this chapter, you will learn how to be prepared for job opportunities and avoid experiencing disappointments like Jenny did.

OVERVIEW OF THE JOB SEARCH

The job search can be an exciting and challenging experience for the health care graduate. The purpose of this chapter and Chapter 25 is to help students and graduates plan and carry out the activities necessary to secure satisfying employment.

It may surprise you to learn how much the job-seeking process is like a job in itself. You should plan to devote at least 20 hours each week to your job search. Some employment professionals even recommend that you spend up to 40 hours. That may sound like a lot, but think about it. Health care students spend a lot of time, money, and effort completing an education. Furthermore, a large percentage of waking hours are spent at work. It makes sense to devote the time necessary to find a job you like and that makes the best use of your education. Job satisfaction is an important factor in a person's quality of life. Investing time and effort in the job search will pay off in the future.

Developing a positive attitude will help make the job search more successful. Almost everyone feels nervous or apprehensive about approaching potential employers in the hope of being hired. Job seekers often see themselves as powerless, but this is not true. You can increase your self-confidence if you understand that graduates who offer the skills and **traits** (personal characteristics) that employers need, and the positive, can-do attitude that they want, are a welcome addition to their staff. Employers want to hire people who meet more than the position's minimum qualifications.

What Do You Have to Offer?

A common problem for new graduates is that they don't realize how much they have to offer employers. You may be concerned that your lack of health care experience will make it difficult for you to find a job. Graduates are often surprised to discover just how many qualifications they really have. The first step in a successful job search is to identify these qualifications. For example, your technical skills are up to date and fresh in your mind. This is a plus. However, these skills are only part of what makes an effective employee. The traits that will most likely determine your success in securing and maintaining employment include professionalism, enthusiasm, willingness to learn, a positive attitude, and reliability.

Spend some time creating a personal inventory of both your technical and nontechnical skills. The technical skills are the most obvious and can be collected by reviewing textbooks, class and lab materials, and clinical evaluations.

Three of the most important non-technical skills are the ability to:

1. Communicate: Listen carefully to others. Organize thoughts and speak clearly at a level appropriate for the listener.
2. Problem-solve: Identify problems, gather necessary information, consider alternatives, and use good judgment when choosing a solution.
3. Work as a team member: Help others, work cooperatively, manage conflict.

Other personal characteristics of value to health care employers include the following:

- Integrity: Be honest, maintain confidentiality, choose the right way rather than the easy way.
- Responsibility: Work without constant supervision, know when to ask for help.
- Dependability: Follow through on obligations without being reminded. Complete all assigned tasks. Always be on time and rarely be absent.
- Organization: Be accurate and efficient. Use time well. Prioritize your tasks.
- Consideration: Be friendly, polite, empathetic, and patient. Work well with diverse populations.
- Willingness to learn: Ask questions, acquire new knowledge and skills, and keep up to date in the field.

Think about what you have learned in your roles as a parent, student, volunteer, group member, and employee. Life is rich with experiences to draw from. Use your self-inventory to boost your self-confidence and prepare to write an effective resume and present yourself well at interviews. This will provide a strong foundation on which you can build a successful job search.

What Are Your Expectations?

Before starting the job search, it is important to identify your employment preferences. There are many types of working environments, and finding the one in which you work best is an important factor in determining career success. Consider the following when thinking about the type of facility in which you want to work:

- Size of facility
- Pace and speed of work
- Amount of time spent working with others and working on your own
- Amount of supervision
- Hours of work

- Type of patient population
- Type of professional specialty
- Location
- Orientation and training offered

Identifying appropriate job leads is easier when you have thought about your preferences.

At the same time, remember that recent graduates are usually qualified for *entry-level* positions. More job opportunities will open up as you gain experience. A good career move may be to compromise some of your preferences in exchange for starting out with an employer who offers you opportunities to learn and grow professionally.

It is also important to be aware of your financial needs. Track your current expenses for a few months and calculate the minimum amount needed to cover your cost of living. Consider the following basic expenses:

- Housing and associated costs: Rent or mortgage, insurance, utilities, phone, repairs, cleaning supplies, child care
- Transportation: Vehicle, fees, insurance, gas, repairs, loan payments
- Clothing and grooming supplies
- Health care, including insurance
- Food
- Child care
- Student loan payments
- Entertainment

Organizing Your Time

Planning your time structures your job search and ensures that you focus on activities that are most likely to bring results. Decide how many hours you can devote to your search each week and make weekly and daily to-do lists of tasks. A typical list would include the following:

- Making phone calls
- Revising your resume to target specific employers
- Writing and sending thank-you letters
- Searching the Internet for information and job leads
- Following up on leads

Be prepared to take advantage of, and follow up on, every opportunity. If at the last minute you learn about a chance to attend an interview, you want to be ready. Have your resume, interview clothing, and reliable transportation available at all times during your job search. Career services personnel that many graduates lose job opportunities because they don't act fast enough on leads.

Organizing Your Space and Supplies

A good way to keep yourself organized is to devote a specific area in your home to your job search. Keep all the supplies and materials you will need together so they are easy to find. Don't take the chance of losing the phone number of a potential employer because you wrote it on a little scrap of paper in the kitchen. You will find the following items helpful in conducting an effective job search:

- Appointment calendar, either electronic or paper.
- System for recording information, such as potential employers, the names and addresses of people who might provide assistance with the job search, and questions you want to ask potential employers. Apps for phones are available to help you organize your job search. Other ways to maintain this information include electronic files, a three-ring binder, or index cards in a small file box.
- Good quality paper and matching envelopes for resumes, cover letters, and thank-you notes. White or off-white is a good choice for the health care field.
- Computer supplies. Keep an extra print cartridge on hand.
- Dictionary, either electronic or printed: Anything you send to a potential employer must be completely free of spelling errors.
- Street maps of your area or access to electronic maps or a GPS/navigation system

Projecting a Professional Image

You may be receiving calls or emails from your school, people who have contacts, and potential employers. Be sure that these contacts are handled in a manner that reflects well on you. If you have a shared phone at home, review proper phone manners and message-taking with everyone who answers the phone. You don't want to miss a possible interview because you don't have the return phone number or the caller was put off by rude manners. A family member who answers incoming calls with a hostile "Yeah?" may damage your efforts before you even have a chance to take the call. If you have an answering machine with a recorded message or a cell phone with voicemail, be sure the message is not off-color or too cute. Remember that what the caller hears represents you as a potential employee.

Recall from Chapter 18 that anything posted online, including social networking sites, should be in good taste. If you use a social networking site such as Facebook, use it to your advantage by posting information and photos of yourself performing volunteer work, helping with a

community project, or other activities that portray you in a positive light. Increasing numbers of employers report checking social networking sites for all job candidates. Also, your email address should be appropriate for someone seeking a career in health care.

It is important that you look and act professional during all job search activities in which you have any contact with an employer. Professionalism is a way of life, not behavior saved for "special occasions." For example, show courtesy and respect to receptionists when you call or go to an office for an interview. Their opinion may be valued by the people doing the hiring.

FINDING JOB LEADS

Finding an employer whose needs match your qualifications can take up most of your job search efforts. There are many ways to locate job openings, and the chances of finding the right job are increased by using as many of these sources as possible.

School Career Service

Many graduates find employment as a direct result of working with the staff in the **school career service**. (This may have another name, such as "employment assistance.") This office may provide help with the following:

1. Resume writing
2. Interview practice
3. Internet access
4. Dressing for success
5. Current information about local employers:
   - Major health care facilities
   - Directories of physicians and other health care professionals
   - Hiring practices
   - Who is most likely to hire recent graduates

Although it is *your* responsibility to become employed, it is a mistake not to take advantage of the help that is available.

Many employers depend on schools to provide them with prequalified applicants for job openings. Schools may be notified before jobs are advertised. (See Figure 24–1.) Make a commitment to follow up on all leads and attend any interviews that are scheduled for you. An unhappy event for the school staff is to receive a call from an employer with the news that a graduate who was given a lead did not contact the employer or show up for the interview. Always follow up, even if the job does not seem to be exactly what you want. When referred individuals

FIGURE 24–1 Seek the help of the career services staff in your school.

fail to show up, it damages the credibility of the school and may hurt its future relationship with the employment community. And the job may turn out to be the right one, after all. Even if it is not the right job, the experience will provide practice for interviewing skills, and the employer may provide a connection to another job that *is* a match.

Keep the school informed of your job search progress and advise them of any changes to your contact information (phone and address). Job leads can be lost when schools cannot locate graduates. Also, it is important to let your school know when you accept a job. Some states and accreditation agencies require schools to report on the employment status of their graduates.

Community Career Centers

Government agencies have organized resource centers for job seekers. The U.S. Department of Labor sponsors Career One Stop. Its website, www.careeronestop.org, contains links to state and local career offices all over the United States.

Networking

Networking means meeting and interacting with people who might be helpful with your job search. Ideally, you can return the help in some way. Networking is considered by many experts to be the most effective way of securing employment, much more so than answering job postings on the Internet which are seen by thousands.

There are three types of networking contacts. The first consists of everyone you know. Tell as many people as possible that you are in the job market. A friend at church may know that his dentist is looking for an assistant. The pharmacist at the local drugstore may have a colleague who needs a pharmacy tech. Project professionalism and enthusiasm about starting a health care career.

The second type of networking contact is a health care professional or employer. In addition to being potential sources of job leads, they can provide general information about the field and tips on getting ahead. Professional networking contacts include the following:

- Instructors
- Other school staff
- Guest speakers
- Attendees at professional meetings, conferences, and workshops
- The supervisor and staff at your clinical site
- Professionals at job fairs
- Your personal physician, dentist, and other health care providers

Don't be shy about approaching people who might be able to help. Smile, introduce yourself, and tell them that you are preparing to enter the health care field. In addition to being a source of job leads, professional contacts can provide valuable information. Here are some questions to ask:

- What skills are most important for succeeding in this career?
- What personal traits are most important?

Thinking It Through

Jasmine is feeling discouraged. She completed a nursing assistant program 2 months ago and still has not found a job. Joe Dorland from her school's placement office called this morning wanting to know if she had followed up on the job opening he gave her last week. She told him she hadn't, because the job was on the other side of the city and it would take her at least 40 minutes to get there on the bus. Joe had called with other leads that she hadn't cared to follow up on. They either sounded pretty boring, were in parts of town she didn't know, or didn't pay enough. Jasmine really thinks that the school should do more to help her get what she wants in a job.

1. Does Jasmine have realistic expectations about the job search?
2. Is she likely to continue receiving help from the school's career services office? Explain your answer.
3. What would you suggest that Jasmine do to increase her chances of finding a job?

- What qualities do employers look for when hiring for this occupation?
- What are the major duties?
- Which hospitals, facilities, companies, physicians, or dentists are good to work for and why?
- What is your best advice for someone who wants to work in this field?
- Can you recommend anyone else I can talk to about working in this field?

The third type of networking is through the Internet, described in the next section.

Keep accurate records of networking contacts. Create an electronic file or a section in your notebook or use index cards to keep track of names, titles, addresses and phone numbers, where you met, and any planned follow-up action.

Send a thank-you note to anyone who meets with you or provides information. The importance of this simple act of courtesy cannot be overemphasized. Let them know when you are hired and keep in touch. Networking should become a habit maintained throughout your career. It is a way to stay current in the field, develop friendships with other professionals, and add to the enjoyment of work. (See Figure 24–2.)

Internet

Use the Internet as an important, but not exclusive, job-search tool. There are a growing number of ways to use it in the job search:

- Learn job search techniques: Excellent information is available about finding job leads, resume writing, interviewing, and many other topics. Job-search websites change rapidly; a good one that is current as of this writing is www.job-hunt-org
- Get information about specific facilities: Most health care providers, such as clinics and hospitals, have their own websites. These are excellent sources of information and often contain job postings and information about how to apply. Many include application or resume forms that you can fill out on the screen and submit electronically. In fact, some employers now accept only electronically submitted applications and resumes. Search by name for facilities in your area. Many employers have Facebook accounts on which you can learn about the organizations. LinkedIn is a good professional social networking organization that you can use to connect with others who work in the field or for your targeted employers. By joining, you can also view employer profiles and view job postings. (See Box 24–1 for information about using social media.)

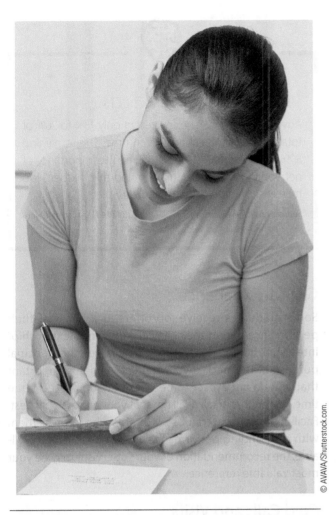

FIGURE 24–2 When networking, it is important to send a thank-you note to anyone who helps you.

- Find job openings: Some websites collect job openings from sources across the country. Jobs are classified by category, and you can restrict your search to a specific geographic location. Examples include www.indeed.com, simplyhired.com, www.monster .com, and http://us.jobs. Other websites specialize in health care, such as www.healthjobsnationwide.com. Some of these job banks have apps for your phone. Craig's List includes job openings, but be cautious as it is more susceptible to scams.

- Post your resume: Many websites have been designed to allow job seekers to post their resumes online. Health care employers are beginning to review these sites when looking to fill positions. Some schools allow graduates to use the school's phone number as the contact so that inquiries can be screened. Take care when placing your resume online, especially if there is a fee involved. *Never* submit personal information, such as your social security number. If you do decide to put your resume online, be sure that it is perfect. Many people are likely to see it. Because so many individuals post their resumes online, there is tremendous competition for actually securing a job. These websites should *not* be your main source of job leads.

- Check out professional organizations: In addition to general information about the profession, some have job banks available to members. See Appendix 1 for a list of many health care professional organizations.

Box 24-1

Using Social Media in the Job Search

According to a survey conducted by Career Builder, 70% of employers use social media to screen applicants during the hiring process.

What to avoid on social media:

1. Job candidate posted provocative or inappropriate photographs, videos, or information: 40 percent

2. Job candidate posted information about them drinking or using drugs: 36 percent

3. Job candidate had discriminatory comments related to race, gender, religion, etc.: 31 percent

4. Job candidate was linked to criminal behavior: 30 percent

5. Job candidate lied about qualifications: 27 percent

6. Job candidate had poor communication skills: 27 percent

7. Job candidate bad-mouthed their previous company or fellow employee: 25 percent

8. Job candidate's screen name was unprofessional: 22 percent

9. Job candidate shared confidential information from previous employers: 20 percent

10. Job candidate lied about an absence: 16 percent

11. Job candidate posted too frequently: 12 percent

Source: https://www.businessnewsdaily.com/2377-social-media-hiring.html

The number of websites available for job seekers is growing daily. They tend to change names and addresses, discontinue operations, or merge with other sites. A few make unrealistic claims, such as having more job postings than they actually do. Others may publish misleading job search information or even scams. The following are ways to avoid scams:

- Be suspicious of jobs listed that are too good to be true. For example, a high salary is offered for a job that generally does not pay that much.

- Verify the job listing. If not on an employer's website, check with the employer either online or with a phone call to make sure the job opening actually exists.

- Do not respond to offers you receive from "employers" you have not contacted, especially if you are pressed to make an immediate decision, asked to send money, and/or are asked to submit personal information, such as your social security number.

(See Figure 24–3.)

FIGURE 24–3 The Internet is a valuable source of help during the job search, but should be combined with other methods.

Fascinating Facts

Advertised job openings represent only 15% to 20% of total available jobs at any given time. The remaining *80%* are never published anywhere. The importance of networking and researching to find this "hidden" job market cannot be overemphasized.

Source: https://www.npr.org/2011/02/08/133474431/a-successful-job-search-its-all-about-networking

Clinical Experience

Some graduates receive job offers as a result of their performance during their clinical experience (externship/internship/fieldwork). This is *not*, however, the principal purpose of this part of your training, and it is important that you *do not expect* to be offered a job. At the same time, conduct yourself at all times at your professional best. Facilities have created jobs for interns who impress them with outstanding performance. Even if a job is not available, the recommendation of your supervisor may be your most valuable reference.

Cold Calls and Visits

Cold calling refers to calling or visiting employers to make the first contact. The purpose is to identify possible job openings and to inform the employer that you are looking for employment. Because the majority of jobs are not advertised, this can be a good way to locate openings. Cold calling requires self-confidence and good communication skills. It is essential to be courteous and considerate when making contacts.

It is most efficient to visit buildings or complexes that have many offices. Be sure to dress professionally and take copies of your resume. (If possible, send your resume in advance of your visit.) Smile, introduce yourself, inquire about openings, and leave a resume. Do not ask for an interview, however, when dropping in without an appointment. Whether calling or visiting in person, be brief, be appreciative, and be on your way.

Job Fairs

There are many types of gatherings that employers attend to recruit employees. Although interviews are not usually conducted nor job offers made, employers provide valuable information to job seekers and may collect their resumes.

Take advantage of these activities. Dress professionally and take copies of your resume. Check your area for the following types of opportunities to meet employers:

- Career fairs sponsored by your school: The employers who attend these are sending the clear message that they hire recent graduates. Ask lots of questions and collect brochures, business cards, and any other handouts offered. Learn as much as you can. After the event, organize the information you have collected. Write notes about whom you met, application procedures, and whom to contact for an interview. Keeping good records is especially important if it will be a while before you are ready to start the formal job search.

- Career fairs sponsored by chambers of commerce and government organizations: Check the bulletin board in the career service center at school and the Internet.

- Career orientations and information meetings sponsored by employers: Some large health care facilities conduct open meetings to recruit applicants and explain their hiring process. Contact the human resources department at organizations in which you are interested. You may be encouraged to submit a resume in advance.

- Professional conventions and conferences: Some employers recruit at these meetings. (See Appendix 1 for a list of professional health care organizations.)

THE RESUME

A **resume** is a written summary of professional qualifications. Its purpose is to convince employers to interview you and consider you for employment. Therefore, your resume must represent you well and convince employers that you are the kind of person they need.

Fascinating Facts

Seven in ten employers use social networking sites to research job candidates during the hiring process. Nearly half of employers check up on current employees on social media. A third of employers have reprimanded or fired an employee based on content found online.

Source: http://press.careerbuilder.com/2018-08-09-More-Than-Half-of-Employers-Have-Found-Content-on-Social-Media-That-Caused-Them-NOT-to-Hire-a-Candidate-According-to-Recent-CareerBuilder-Survey

Some students choose to have someone else, such as a professional resume preparer, write their resume. Or they use a standard template they find on the Internet. They may be unsure about what to include or have weak word processing skills. While it is a good idea to seek advice from employment professionals and essential to have someone qualified proofread your resume, there are several important reasons why *you* should determine the content and organization:

- It must accurately represent your skills: It is essential that they are neither exaggerated nor minimized.

- It is important to include the personal traits, such as good teamwork skills, discussed earlier in this chapter: Only you know what these are.

- Canned resumes should be avoided: They tend to look insincere and give the impression that they were put together without much thought.

- You must know exactly what your resume says: It often serves as the basis for questions at interviews.

Resume Contents

Resumes contain several sections and each has a specific purpose. It is essential that all content be written accurately and completely.

Heading

This section includes your name and contact information (address, phone number, and email address) and is placed at the top of the resume. Make it easy for potential employers to contact you by listing a current phone number, along with the area code. If necessary, include an alternate number where messages can be left. Do not be one of those people who loses opportunities because interested employers cannot find them. Center the heading at the top of the page and highlight your name by using capital letters. It is not necessary to use the label "Resume," because the content and format makes it easy to identify.

Introduction

Traditionally, the next part of the resume is the **objective**, a statement of your job goal. It is written as a simple job title or includes additional information about your qualifications and preferences. Here are a few examples:

- *Job title only*: Position as a medical assistant

- *More specific*: Position as a front-office medical assistant

- *Include information about your qualifications*: Position as an administrative medical assistant in which I apply my computer skills and organizational ability.

- *Include information about your preferences*: Position as a clinical medical assistant in a pediatric office.

Today, employment specialists recommend that job applicants use a different approach. The objective, they point out, focuses on what the applicant *wants*, rather than what the applicant can *offer* the employer. Therefore, experts suggest that the resume begin with a list of qualifications for the targeted job or lists them immediately following the objective so the employer knows for what position you are applying. This list highlights the important skills and traits that directly relate to the needs stated by the employer.

Here is a sample *summary of qualifications* for a pediatric medical assistant applicant who has a background teaching in a preschool:

- Certified medical assistant
- Up-to-date administrative and clinical skills
- 13 years of experience working with children in a variety of settings
- 5 years of experience teaching disabled children
- Bilingual, English–Spanish
- Ability to communicate with people of all ages
- Maintained perfect attendance while attending medical assisting program and working part-time
- Ability to work well under pressure and manage priorities

Notice how a variety of abilities and experiences are used to describe the applicant as a unique and well-qualified candidate. They can come from previous work, school, or personal experience.

Education

This is an important section for graduates who are new to the health care field. In fact, it may be the section you want to be most detailed and listed at the beginning of your resume because recently acquired skills are the major qualifications for employment in entry-level positions. (See Figure 24–5 for an example of a resume that highlights the education section.) List the schools attended, starting with the most recent. Include high school only if graduation or a GED is a job requirement or is where you acquired your health care training. For each school, list the dates attended or the date the certificate, diploma, or degree was awarded. The following items can also be added to this section:

- Special training, such as cardiopulmonary resuscitation (CPR) or computer classes that are related to the job objective
- Honors or awards earned
- Cumulative grade point average (GPA) if it is 3.0 or higher
- Special school projects that are related to the targeted job

- Facts that demonstrate such traits as initiative, ability to manage time, and persistence
- Summary of what you learned. List the courses taken or prepare a list of skills acquired. This is especially helpful for the employer if the program included an unusual variety of skills or if the occupational outcome is a relatively new job title. Here are two examples showing how to write the education section:

Example 1 Associate in Applied Science Degree, Medical Assisting, 2019

Healthcare College, Lincoln, NE

- Completed CPR and first aid training
- Honor Roll all semesters
- Earned 3.7 of a possible 4.0 GPA

Example 2 Diploma, Patient Care Assistant Program, 2018

BeWell School of Medical Careers, Philadelphia

- Received Perfect Attendance Award
- Served as chairperson for annual all-school diversity picnic
- Completed program while working part-time and raising two young children
- Knowledge and skills acquired include:
  - Medical terminology and body systems
  - Computer keyboarding and data entry
  - Medical and surgical asepsis
  - Nursing assistant skills
  - Home health aide skills
  - Rehabilitation aide skills
  - Unit clerk skills
  - Phlebotomy
  - Electrocardiograms

Certifications and Licenses

Include this section only if they are not listed in another section, such as education. Examples:

- Certified Medical Assistant
- Licensed Vocational Nurse, California License #1234568910
- Current CPR certification
- Registered Dental Assistant

Work Experience

This section can also be called Employment History. List your previous jobs starting with the most recent. Include the name and location of each employer, along with the dates worked and the titles of all positions held. Create a bulleted list of phrases, using action verbs, to describe your duties and achievements. Do not use complete sentences or the word "I." Think about how you contributed to the success of your previous employers. Were you extremely reliable? Did you increase sales? Develop a more efficient system for organizing the office? Don't worry if your work history does not seem very impressive. Completing a health care educational program demonstrates the ability to set and meet new career goals.

It is appropriate to include clinical experience (e.g., internship, externship, or fieldwork, etc.) in either the work experience or education section. Give the name and location of the facility, as well as a list of the duties performed. Be sure to label these appropriately as "internship," "externship," "fieldwork experience," and so on. To imply that it was a paid position is dishonest. Examples of work history section:

Example 1 Sales Associate 2015 to Present

Hercules Men's Store, Gary, IN

- Assist customers
- Close out cash register each night
- Maintain perfect attendance
- Increased sales by 17% in first year employed
- Consistently earn highest top-volume sales associate award each quarter

This job, although not related to health, demonstrates the ability to communicate, motivation to succeed, honesty, and reliability. Every employer is looking for these qualities.

When listing your job duties, use the past tense for jobs you no longer hold and present tense for jobs at which you are currently employed.

Example 2 Medical Assistant Externship June 2018–September 2018

Caring Community Clinic, Charleston, SC

Performed back-office duties under the supervision of Dr. Emilio Jimenez

- Took medical histories
- Took vital signs
- Prepared patients for examinations and procedures
- Assisted physician with procedures and minor surgeries
- Administered medications
- Applied principles of infection control
- Received highest ratings (5 on scale of 1 to 5) in all areas on final externship evaluation

Optional Sections

The following are optional sections to include on your resume if they add important information not mentioned elsewhere:

- Special skills: Skills other than what would normally be expected from your training. For example, a medical assistant applicant with the ability to troubleshoot and correct computer problems.
- Languages: Languages other than English can be listed here or under special skills. It is customary to indicate the ability level—for example, "Spanish: Speaking and comprehension good, writing ability fair."
- Awards and honors: If applicable. List only those not already included in the education section. Provide brief explanations if it is not clear how they were earned.
- Community service and volunteer work: List the duties performed and events in which you participated.
- Memberships in professional organizations: These demonstrate commitment and interest in keeping up to date. Serving as an officer or member of a committee demonstrates willingness to accept responsibility, practice leadership, and take an active role in organizations.
- Hobbies and interests: List any that support your bid for the job. For example, sports such as swimming or tennis demonstrate that you value good health and recognize the importance of exercise.

Formatting the Resume

"Formatting" refers to the arrangement of the content in the resume. Two commonly used formats are the chronological and the functional. The **chronological resume** features a work experience section in which the duties and accomplishments of previous jobs are listed. This is a good choice for someone who has a strong, steady work history, especially one in which jobs held required increasing amounts of responsibility. It is also recommended for applicants who have work experience in health care. Figure 24–4 contains an example of a chronological resume.

The **functional resume** highlights clusters of skills and abilities gathered from a variety of experiences. Job titles are listed in the work experience section without detailing duties and accomplishments. Functional resumes are recommended for people who are changing careers and have a variety of skills and experiences that can be transferred to the new field. Three clusters are usually recommended. See Figure 24–5 for an example of a functional resume.

LISA GRAZIANO
8407 Wentworth Ave.
Manchester, NH 03103
(603) 123-4567

Medical Transcriptionist

QUALIFICATIONS

14 years full-time experience working as a medical transcriptionist
Ability to prepare reports for all major medical specialties
Keyboarding speed of 97 wpm

WORK EXPERIENCE

Medical Transcriptionist   2003–Present
Chatsworth Medical Center, Manchester, NH
- Transcribe patient's medical reports as dictated by physicians
- Distribute reports to appropriate departments
- Obtain charts for physicians
- Received Employee of the Quarter award four times (based on reliability, cooperation, and efficiency)

Medical Transcriptionist   2005–2007
St. Claire Hospital, Boston, MA
- Transcribed daily reports for surgical department
- Copied records for billing
- Answered telephone and transferred calls

Administrative Assistant   2002–2005
Dr. Patrice Tibere, Boston, MA
- Word processed all correspondence and research reports
- Located and gathered reference materials as requested
- Handled mail, answered telephone, maintained Dr. Tibere's schedule, made travel arrangements

EDUCATION

AA Degree, Medical Transcription, 2005
Lawrence Medical College, Boston

Word Processing Certificate, 2002
Regal College, Boston

MEMBERSHIPS

American Association for Medical Transcription
Lawrence Medical College Advisory Board

FIGURE 24–4 Example of a chronological resume. This is usually a good choice for applicants who have a strong work history and/or experience working in health care.

KELLY CISNEROS
9125 Soledad Avenue
El Paso, TX 79907
(915) 123-4567

OBJECTIVE	Position as a **Clinical Medical Assistant** in a pediatric office
EDUCATION	AS Degree, Medical Assistant, 2019 Caldwell Technical College, El Paso • Perfect Attendance Award three semesters out of four • Earned 3.7 of a possible 4.0 GPA • Externship at Valley Pediatric Center, El Paso • "Excellent Rating" for overall externship performance
EXPERIENCE WITH CHILDREN	8 years providing private day care in home 3 years teaching disabled preschoolers Cub Scout leader Volunteer tutor at Sanchez Elementary School
ORGANIZATIONAL SKILLS	Maintained state-approved day care facility Secretary of PTA at children's school Coordinate scheduling and activities for local junior soccer team
COMMUNICATION SKILLS	Make presentations to local organizations about child safety issues Write articles for Sanchez Elementary School parent newsletter 5 years experience as telephone receptionist in a busy insurance office Speak, read, and write Spanish fluently
WORK HISTORY	Cisneros Quality Day Care 2010–2018 Owner of home-based day care for up to six children SpecialCare Preschool 2007–2010 Teacher Calderon Insurance Agency 2002–2007 Receptionist

FIGURE 24–5 Example of a functional resume. This is usually a good choice for applicants who have no experience working in health care.

Resume content can be organized in a variety of ways. The fact is, there is no "best way" that everyone should use. The important thing is that the resume be reader-friendly and highlight the qualifications that best support the targeted job. These qualifications should be placed closest to the top of the page. For example, an applicant for a transcriptionist position with outstanding keyboarding speed and accuracy could list these in a qualifications section. A bilingual medical assistant applicant in an area with a large Hispanic population could highlight the ability to speak Spanish in the qualifications section.

Important Resume Guidelines

Although there are a variety of ways to organize the content, there are a few guidelines that should *always* be followed:

- Be accurate: Check for perfect spelling, correct grammar, and accurate dates. This is important for all professions, but especially when applying for a job in health care, which depends on accuracy for the well-being of both patients and workers.

- Be conservative: This is a characteristic of the medical field. Choose good quality paper in white or a very light gray or beige.

- Be neat: Have no corrections, smudges, or creases.

- Make it easy to read: Don't crowd the information; leave some white space. Margins should be at least one inch on all sides.

- Keep it professional: Don't include personal information such as age, marital status, and number of children.

- Do not include information that is best discussed in person: This includes why you left previous jobs, salary information, or special conditions, such as having a physical disability.

- *Do not include your social security number.*

- Use proper spacing: Double-space between headings, then single-space within each section.

- Use special features for highlighting: Capitalize all major words in the headings. Or you may want to bold all words in headings.

- Keep it concise: Limiting it to one page is recommended, unless you have more relevant information than will fit on one page without crowding.

- Have someone qualified review and proofread your resume. This is the most important written document in your job search efforts, so keep working on it until it is error-free and represents you at your best.

Thinking It Through

Greg Berglander recently graduated from a radiological technologist program and has passed his state's licensing exam. He's ready to begin applying for jobs. The problem is that he doesn't have a resume prepared. Although Greg can use a computer, he does not keyboard quickly and has poor word processing skills. He believes that the career services center at his school should be more helpful and put something together for him. After all, they know the courses he took and probably have access to his grades. And he can tell them anything else they need to know.

1. Do you agree with Greg? Why or why not?

2. What action would you recommend that he take?

Recent Resume Trends

- A common practice until recently was to state "References Available Upon Request" at the bottom of the resume. The current practice is to omit this statement. (But you *do need* to have at least three references listed on a separate piece of paper.)

- Internet posting: Some employers have standard resume forms that you can fill out on the screen and send electronically. Take extra care when filling these out. Once the send key is pressed, there is no chance to correct information.

- Electronic scanning: Employers who receive large numbers of resumes and do not have time to review them all are using scanners to enter them into a computerized data bank. The computer looks for key words that match the words in job descriptions. When there is a job opening, all resumes matching its requirements are recalled for review. If an employer indicates that resumes will be scanned, it is important to include descriptive words in your objective and throughout the resume. Read postings and job descriptions carefully to identify key words. Avoid staples, folds, or special features, such as bolding or fancy fonts. These are difficult for the computer to read.

COVER LETTERS

Cover letters are sent with resumes as a way to introduce yourself and inform the employer why you are sending a resume. Customize your letters as needed for the following situations:

- When responding to an advertised opening: In your letter refer to the job posting and state that you are interested in the position. Explain briefly how you meet the stated requirements. Do not simply repeat the specific information listed on your resume, but refer the employer to it for more detailed information. Request an interview and thank the employer for his or her time and consideration. See Figure 24–6 for an example of a cover letter responding to an advertised position.

AD:

DENTAL ASSISTANT. Excellent verbal, scheduling and collection skills. Full-time. Front and back office as needed. Computer literate with good work ethic. Commitment to high-quality patient care.

1357 Keystone Drive
Chicago, IL 60606
July 23, 20—

Dr. Harold Mims
1842 Grand Avenue
Chicago, IL 60606

Dear Dr. Mims:

This letter is in response to your ad for a dental assistant. I recently graduated from Harrison Dental College and believe that I fulfill the requirements stated in your ad.

Providing **high-quality patient care** was emphasized throughout the dental assisting program at Harrison. I would welcome the opportunity to begin my dental assisting career in an environment where patients are the top priority.

The program at Harrison emphasized the need for good **verbal skills** in the workplace. We were given many opportunities to practice them. In the skills lab students were required to explain all procedures orally to "patients" before and during hands-on work. I also received grades of "A" in my communication courses, which included Oral Communication and Interpersonal Relations for the Health Care Professional.

I understand the need for a smooth-running **front office** and enjoyed the administrative and **computer training** portion of my training. Performing duties in both the **front and back office** would allow me to apply my organizational skills. My previous jobs, outlined in the enclosed resume, required me to be responsive to the needs of my employers.

My **strong work ethic** is demonstrated in my excellent attendance records, both at school and work, willingness to complete all assigned tasks, and commitment to doing my best at all times.

I would appreciate the opportunity to meet with you to further discuss how I might contribute to the success of your practice. I can be reached at (312) 123-4567. My email address is kbosner@goodmail.com

Thank you for your consideration.

Sincerely,

Kelly Bosner

Kelly Bosner

FIGURE 24–6 Cover letter responding to an advertised position. Note how the key words in the ad are bolded in the letter.

- Sending the resume to be considered for an unadvertised position: State the purpose of the letter, who told you about the opening (be sure you have that person's permission), or simply say that you understand there is an opening for which

you might qualify. Briefly state your qualifications, explain why you are interested in the job, and then close with a request for an interview and a thank you. See Figure 24–7 for an example of this type of letter.

1357 Keystone Drive
Chicago, IL 60606
July 25, 20—

Ms. Tasha Jefferson, Office Manager
Compton Dental Clinic
6397 Flanders Street
Chicago, IL 60606

Dear Ms. Jefferson:

I am a recent graduate of Harrison Dental College. The Employment Coordinator at Harrison, Ms. Juanita Sanders, recommended that I contact you about a possible opening at Compton Dental Clinic. She believes you would be interested in an applicant with my excellent attendance record and academic achievements.

The dental assistant program at Harrison was rigorous and I feel well prepared to perform both front and back office skills. I developed good work habits during my training as well as at my previous jobs, which are listed in my resume. In addition, I had the opportunity to develop good communication skills and am committed to becoming a contributing member of a dental care team.

I would appreciate the opportunity to meet with you to further discuss the needs of Compton Dental Clinic and my qualifications. I can be reached at (312) 123-4567. My email address is kbosner@goodmail.com

Thank you for your consideration.

Sincerely,

Kelly Bosner

Kelly Bosner

FIGURE 24–7 Cover letter responding to an unadvertised position.

- You are moving to a new location and sending letters of inquiry in advance: Inform the employer that you are relocating to the area. Explain the type of work you are seeking. Include a brief statement of your qualifications and when you will be available for an interview. Ask to be considered for any appropriate openings and state that you will follow up with a phone call. Conclude with a thank you. (See Figure 24–8.)

---

900 Peach Blossom Lane
Atlanta, GA 30326
September 24, 20—

Sarah Masterson, RHIA
Director—Health Information Management Department
Blackwell Rehabilitation Hospital
2106 S.W. River Street
Portland, OR 97423

Dear Ms. Masterson:

The purpose of this letter is to inquire about possible openings for a Registered Health Information Technician at your facility. I graduated from Caprio Health Care Institute in Atlanta in June and am relocating to the Portland area in November.

My training at Caprio was comprehensive and I feel confident that my training has prepared me to work competently in the health information field. I work well with others, have strong computer skills, and look forward to contributing to the success of my future employer.

I will contact you the week of November 12 after my arrival in Portland. In the meantime, I can be contacted at (404) 123-4567 or by email at g.hayes@goodmail.com

Sincerely,

Glenda Hayes

Glenda Hayes

FIGURE 24–8 Cover letter for a graduate moving to a new location.

Writing Good Cover Letters

Cover letters, like the resume, represent you and influence whether you are invited for an interview. Here are some guidelines for writing winning letters:

- Word process
- Be sure that grammar and spelling are perfect.
- Use the same paper as for the resume.
- Address the letter, if possible, to a specific person. Call the facility and ask to whom it should be directed. Check for the correct spelling of the name.
- Send individualized letters for each employer or position, matching them to the targeted position.
- Do not write more than one page. Busy employers don't have time to read more than that.
- Use a standard business letter format (see Chapter 17).

SUGGESTED LEARNING ACTIVITIES

1. Talk with successfully employed friends and family members about how they got their jobs.

2. Review the Internet, newspaper, news magazines, and professional journals regularly for articles about health care trends, facilities, and employment-related topics.

3. Check out the websites suggested in this chapter and use available links to learn what information is available for job seekers.

4. Visit your school's career service and find out what resources are available. Introduce yourself to the people who work there, if you don't already know them.

5. Find a Web posting, printed ad, or job description for a health care job in which you are interested.

   a. List the skills and traits that you think would be required.

   b. Prepare a summary of qualifications.

   c. Create an appropriate resume and cover letter to apply for the position.

WEB ACTIVITIES

The Balance Careers

https://www.thebalancecareers.com/how-much-time-to-spend-on-a-job-search-2062204

How Much Time Should You Spend on a Job Search

1. What factors determine how many hours a person should spend on their job search?

2. What activities does the article recommend you spend time on during your job search?

NPR (National Public Radio)

https://www.npr.org/2011/02/08/133474431/a-successful-job-search-its-all-about-networking

A Successful Job Search: It's All About Networking

1. Why is networking so important?

2. What percent of jobs are published?

3. Why is submitting a resume or application not as effective as networking?

4. According to the article, how many contacts should job-seekers make each month?

5. What should be emphasized in a cover letter?

Job-Hunt

https://www.job-hunt.org/jobsearchmistakes.shtml

The "Dirty Dozen" Online Job Search Mistakes

1. Read the article and think about your own job search.

2. List any suggestions you weren't aware of.

Indeed

https://www.indeed.com/

1. Explore jobs of interest in your area. (Note: entering the zip code along with the city name helps refine the search.)

2. Is the search function easy to use?

3. How much information was given about each job?

The Balance Careers

https://www.thebalancecareers.com/how-to-make-a-successful-job-search-cold-call-2062610

How to Make a Successful Cold Call in a Job Search

List the suggestions for making a successful cold call.

Monster

https://www.monster.com/career-advice/article/avoid-the-top-10-resume-mistakes

The 10 Worst Resume Mistakes to Avoid

1. After reading the article, check the list against your resume.

2. Did you find any suggestions that will improve your resume?

3. If so, make any changes necessary.

Michigan State University: Career Services Network

https://careernetwork.msu.edu/resources-tools/resumes/action-verbs.html

139 Action Verbs to Make Your Resume Stand Out

See how many of the verbs listed can help you in preparing the Work History section of your resume.

Purdue Online Writing Lab

https://owl.purdue.edu/engagement/job_search_resources/cover_letters/index.html

1. Read the sections about writing good cover letters.

2. Did you learn anything new?

3. If so, how can you apply what you learned to writing cover letters to accompany your resume?

REVIEW QUESTIONS

1. How many hours do experts recommend you spend on your job search each week?

2. Why is having a positive attitude important during the job search?

3. What is the purpose of developing a personalized skill inventory as a first step in your job search?

4. What are eight factors that you should consider when identifying your workplace preferences?

5. How should you organize a workplace dedicated to your job search?

6. What are two ways to project a professional image?

7. What are seven sources of job leads and job search assistance?

8. What are the three types of networking?

9. What are the ways to effectively use the Internet in your job search?

10. What are three ways to avoid employment scams on the Internet?

11. What is the purpose of a resume?

12. What are the major sections of a resume and what are the contents of each?

13. What is the difference between a chronological and functional resume?

14. What are ten characteristics of a successful resume?

15. What are the purpose and characteristics of an effective cover letter?

APPLICATION EXERCISES

1. Refer to the Case of the Unprepared Applicant at the beginning of the chapter. Describe what Jenny could have done differently to avoid missing the opportunity to interview with Dr. Chambers.

2. Omid Riazati is starting his last month of classes at PrepWell College. He will then have an eight-week externship before completing his medical laboratory technician program. He is not sure where he wants to work when he graduates, but wants to get started on investigating employment possibilities and plan his job search activities. Create a job search to-do list and schedule for Omid to begin now and follow until he finds employment.

PROBLEM-SOLVING PRACTICE

Gerardo has completed his training to be a medical equipment technician, but he is concerned about starting the job search because he believes his writing skills are poor. He is not sure how to go about writing a good resume, cover letter, and thank-you note. How can he apply the five-step problem-solving process to get started on a successful job search?

CHAPTER 25

Interview, Portfolio, and Application

KEY TERMS

behavioral questions
illegal questions
job interview
letters of recommendation
portfolio
references
reference list
situational questions

The Case of the Modest Applicant

Sam Kingsley is seeking his first job as a phlebotomist. He has enjoyed his training and is eager to apply it in the workplace. While he went to school, Sam waited tables in a local family restaurant. Regular customers always liked to sit in Sam's section because of his friendly, helpful attitude. Many of the customers were older and especially liked Sam's respect-ful attitude toward them. Sam's first interview was at a medical laboratory that works with large numbers of walk-in patients. He felt that he handled the questions

(continues)

OBJECTIVES

Studying and applying the material in this chapter will help you to:

1. Explain why it is important to learn about the employer before a job interview. List ways to obtain this information.
2. Explain how job candidates can prepare to present their technical and non-technical qualifications at job interviews.
3. Give five examples of appropriate questions to ask at job interviews.
4. Give three examples of questions you should not ask at a job interview.
5. Give two examples of each of the following types of questions you may be asked at an interview: general employment, behavioral (situational), and health-care specific.
6. Explain how to answer difficult questions about sensitive issues.
7. Give five examples of questions that are illegal for employers to ask at a job interview.
8. Describe three ways to handle illegal questions asked by employers.
9. Describe an appropriate interview appearance for a man and a woman.
10. Explain the role of references in a job search and give three examples of people who would be appropriate references.
11. Define "letters of recommendation" and explain their purpose.
12. Explain the purpose of a professional portfolio.
13. List eight items that can be included in the health care applicant's professional portfolio.
14. List five items to take to a job interview.
15. Describe ways to practice interviewing skills.
16. Give examples of positive actions to take before a job interview starts.
17. List ten key points to help you do well during an interview.
18. List four recent interview trends.
19. List six actions to take after an interview to increase your chances of being hired.
20. List five pieces of information an employer can require of a potential hire.
21. Explain how to accept and decline job offers properly.
22. Explain how to deal with being rejected for a job following an interview.
23. List seven guidelines to follow when filling out a job application.

well by emphasizing his recent technical training. After all, he did not have any other experience that related to work in phlebotomy. When Sam did not get the job, he learned that the employer did not believe he had presented himself as a strong candidate. This chapter explains how students can draw on all kinds of experiences to best present themselves to potential employers.

THE JOB INTERVIEW

The **job interview** is a conversation between an applicant and a potential employer. It is an opportunity for applicants to present their qualifications in person. Securing this interview has been the goal of all job search activity to this point. The purpose of this chapter is to help make interviewing as productive and pleasant as possible, resulting in an offer for the job you want.

Consider the interview as an opportunity for you and the employer to get to know each other and see if you fit each other's requirements. Keep in mind that interviews can be stressful for employers, too. A position must be filled, and the vacancy may be causing extra work. Interviewers want to hire employees who can help solve problems, not create new ones.

The Importance of Proper Preparation

Many job applicants are nervous about the idea of meeting face-to-face with an employer. The key to overcoming nerves is to prepare well and practice thoroughly.

Being prepared will enable you to focus on learning about the employer's needs and responding appropriately to the questions you are asked.

Not being prepared is the single best way to set yourself up for failure. The things you must do before attending an interview are discussed in the following sections.

Learn About the Employer

It is essential to know something about the employer and the position you are applying for. Having some background information will enable you to:

- Show the employer that you are motivated, interested in the job, and have self-initiative
- Create appropriate examples from your experience to demonstrate qualifications for the job
- Prepare your own questions about the employer and the job

Sources of information vary, based on the size of the facility. To learn about major organizations, use the Internet, as discussed in Chapter 24, or call the human

resource office. Ask for the URL (web address), written materials, announcements about job fairs (if a large organization), and any other sources of information. Watch for articles about health care facilities in the local newspaper, typically the business section. If the employer does not have a website, it may be necessary to call or stop by to observe and ask a few questions. Even if you are not there for an interview, dress professionally. Every contact you have with a potential employer is part of the job interview. The receptionist is often a good source of information. The following are examples of appropriate questions to ask:

- How long has the facility or office been in business?
- What is the professional specialty?
- What are typical ages and types of patients served?
- What is the pace of the work?

Try to get a job description before the interview. Use it to prepare targeted examples that match your qualifications to the needs of the employer. If skills are required that you do not have but can learn, be prepared to explain to the employer how you plan to acquire them.

It is also important for applicants to demonstrate knowledge about the health care field in general. Keep informed about trends and issues of concern to employers, such as those discussed in Chapter 2. The Internet, newspapers, news magazines, and professional journals contain articles about health care topics that affect health care careers. You should also stay current on the ethical and legal issues facing health care providers. Employers want to hire people who can help them deal with the growing number of regulations and constant changes that affect the delivery of health care today.

Prepare to Demonstrate Your Qualifications

College employment professionals report that one of the main reasons students do not get hired is that they fail to sell themselves. Many graduates fail to realize how much they have to offer an employer and therefore do not explain fully how they can be of benefit. This is the reason for creating the personal inventory that was recommended in Chapter 24. Review your list and create examples that illustrate your mastery of them. Start with your technical skills:

- What procedures and tests can you perform?
- At which skills are you most proficient?
- On which skills have you received compliments from patients or classmates or good evaluations from instructors or supervisors?
- In which classes did you receive the highest grades?
- Which skills and procedures were you able to practice most during your clinical (externship/internship /fieldwork) experience?

Now recall some experiences that support your skills and think about how to present them. Here are a few examples:

"I'm very efficient at performing blood draws. My classmates always wanted to work with me in the lab because …"

"I've worked hard to learn to do insurance coding accurately. I received top grades on all my assignments. The manager who supervised my externship allowed me to do more coding than externs are usually allowed to do because …"

"I enjoy word processing and reached a keyboarding speed of 83 words a minute. I also find medical terminology very interesting. Even more important for medical transcription, I'm very accurate …"

Here are two examples that show how to illustrate your non-technical skills:

"I'm good at calming people who are afraid of the dentist. For example, when I was on my externship, there was a woman who was really nervous and I helped her by …"

"My time management skills are strong. During the two years of my nursing program, I maintained part-time employment and still made sure that my three children and I arrived on time for school every day."

Prepare Your Questions

The interview is an opportunity for the applicant to find out about the employer and get the information needed to make an intelligent decision if a job offer is received. Asking appropriate questions also shows that you are a motivated, thinking person who is sincerely interested in the job. Here are some examples of appropriate questions to ask:

- What are the specific duties and responsibilities of this position?
- May I have a copy of the job description?
- I see on the job description that I would be required to _____. Can you tell me more about that?
- Could you describe a typical day for a person in this position?
- Is there a training program for new employees? How does it work?
- What equipment would I be working with?
- What do you think are the most important qualifications for a person to succeed in this position? What qualities in an employee are most important to you?
- Who would I be reporting to? Can you tell me about that person?
- How would I be evaluated?
- If I performed well, would there be opportunities for advancement?

Be sure that the questions are appropriate for the situation. For example, a private physician's office with four employees is not likely to offer opportunities for promotion. To ask about them indicates a lack of knowledge about the employer. It might also give the impression that you will leave for a larger facility after acquiring a few months of experience.

Questions to Avoid

Showing more interest in personal gain than in contributions to the employer is one sure way to lose employment opportunities. The following questions should be avoided until a job has been offered:

- How much is the pay?
- Do you provide medical insurance? Dental insurance?
- How many vacation days will I get?
- How long are the lunch hours and breaks?
- Can we leave early on Fridays?
- What are the paid holidays?

Some of this information may be needed before making a decision on whether to accept the job. First, however, concentrate on learning about the job itself and presenting yourself as the right person for it.

Anticipating an Employer's Questions

Certain kinds of questions are popular with interviewers everywhere. Avoid being caught off guard. Be prepared with answers to the following common questions, including examples to support your answers.

General Employment Questions

- *Tell me about yourself*, or, *Describe yourself*. Give a brief personal history that focuses on why you want to work in health care. Include your education and any experiences that have reinforced your interest and qualifications for this job.

- *Why do you want to work here?* Explain how the facility matches your work goals and qualifications. Describe how you believe you can make a positive contribution. Explain why you are interested in the particular type of work being performed there. (Note: This is why you research the organization in advance.)

- *Why do you think you are qualified for this job?* Explain how you meet the specific duties of the job. If necessary, ask the interviewer to explain them more fully. This will give you information on which to base your answer.

- *What can you contribute to this facility?* As with the previous question, explain how you can help the employer based on what you understand his or her needs to be. This is a good opportunity to use examples from your training and past experience.

- *What are your strengths and weaknesses?* Give examples of strengths that relate to the job. Describe a specific situation that illustrates the quality. Weaknesses should be handled honestly. You can name a skill or personal characteristic, along with your plans for improving it. Or you can describe a previous weakness and how you have corrected it. It is best not to volunteer a weakness that is a major requirement for the job. You may decide on your own that you are not qualified for the job, but it is not necessary to disqualify yourself immediately. The only exception is if the interviewer asks you directly about your level of competency in specific areas. Do *not* claim a skill that you do not have or great expertise in something in which you are a beginner. And do not state that you have no weaknesses, as you will come across as less than honest or at best, without good self-knowledge.

- *What did you like best about your last job? Least?* Again, try to focus on areas that are related to the job under discussion. Choose something you liked that is required on this job. Good answers, if they are true, to "liked least" would be that you did not have enough responsibility, the work was not challenging, and so forth. Avoid answers such as "There was too much work," or "The place was a mess." When answering this kind of question, *never* make negative remarks about previous employers. This will cause employers to wonder what you might say about *them* in the future.

- *Which classes did you like best? Least?* Be honest, but again, avoid saying that your least favorite class covered some of this job's major duties! Use this information when deciding if this job is a right choice for you.

- *What are your short and long-term employment goals?* This can be a tricky question. You do not want to appear to lack professional goals or ambition. On the other hand, employers do not want employees who are only interested in staying for a short time to gain experience. Employers invest considerable time and money into hiring and training new employees. A stable staff also contributes to the quality of a facility. Let the employer know that you want to apply what you have learned in your program and welcome the opportunity to learn more. Your goal is to develop your skills and become an excellent and professional dental assistant, radiology technician, practical nurse, and so on.

Behavioral and Situational Questions

The purpose of behavioral questions and situational questions is for the interviewer to learn about how you have dealt with—or would deal with—common workplace circumstances, such as working under stress, getting along with others, and solving problems without the help of a supervisor. You might be given a scenario and asked how you would handle it or be asked to provide an example of a real situation from your own experience. The best way to prepare for these types of questions is to mentally review your employment history for examples of typical workplace problems. If your work history is limited, think about situations related to school, volunteer work, or family responsibilities. (Take care, however, not to discuss highly personal problems at the job interview.)

Examples of the kind of information to include in responses:

- Handling stress by practicing good time management, prioritizing, delegating, taking care of your health, engaging in physical activity

- Describing the successful planning and completion of a project

- Working well with others on a sports team, committee, or class project

- Handling an interpersonal conflict by applying good communication skills, including listening and compromising

Health Care Specific Questions

Questions may be asked that deal specifically with the job under consideration. These require a good understanding of the chosen occupation and might include examples such as the following:

- What coping skills do you use during an emergency with a patient?

- What is the biggest issue facing nursing today?

- What would you do if you believed a coworker was stealing narcotic medications from the supply cabinet?

- How do you feel about the risk involved with radiation?

- What would you do if you had a stroke patient who was having difficulty getting dressed?

- Tell me what you know about the equipment you need to operate on this job.

- How would you deal with a mistake you made on a lab test that's already been reported?

- How do you deal with uncooperative patients? Suppose, for example, that you needed to draw blood twice in a sitting. How would you explain this to the patient?

(*Source:* Adapted from *Resumes for the Health Care Professional*, 2nd ed., by K. Marino, 2000, New York: John Wiley & Sons.)

Difficult Questions

Some questions are difficult to answer, especially if something in your history might be of concern to an employer. If it is necessary to explain past problems, stay calm and confident, be honest, and let the employer know that previous difficulties will not affect your ability to perform the job.

- *Have you ever been fired from a job?* If you have, be honest. *Do not* blame or badmouth a previous employer. If true, you can say that you disagreed on issues. If you were in the right, explain the facts of the situation. ("I wasn't comfortable being asked to perform duties that were outside my scope of practice.") If you were at fault, explain how you have corrected the situation. ("I have improved my time management skills and have arrived at work on time every day for the past 18 months.")

- *Why have you changed jobs so often?* If the jobs were part-time or intended to be short-term while attending school, state this. If there were other reasons, try to show how this will no longer be a problem. For example, if previous jobs were routine and not challenging, explain that this is what prompted you to become trained in health care. You have now found an area to which you can commit yourself.

Illegal Questions

It is illegal for employers to use certain facts about job applicants when making hiring decisions. **Illegal questions** during an interview require the disclosure of information about these kinds of facts.

Here are examples of some illegal questions an employer might ask:

- How old are you? What is your date of birth?

- Are you married?

- Do you have children?

- Have you ever been arrested?

- Where were you born?

- Do you own your home?

- Do you have a disability or handicap?

- Have you ever filed for workers' compensation insurance?

These questions may be asked by employers who do not realize they are illegal. Or they may be asked in an attempt to learn about characteristics such as the applicant's dependability and trustworthiness.

Applicants have the right to refuse to answer questions believed to be illegal. They may inform the employer that specific questions are illegal. If you want the job and believe the employer is not deliberately breaking the law, there are two strategies that may be more effective:

1. Ask how the questions relate to the job requirements. This allows you to directly respond to the employer's concern. For example, a question about where you live may be asked by an employer who has had difficulties with employee attendance. The issue is arriving on time, not financial status.

2. Incorporate answers to possible but unasked questions. For example, if you are a female in the age range likely to have small children, explain how you have arranged reliable child care to ensure that you will not miss work.

In the unlikely event that questions are offensive, such as those that are sexual or racial in nature, it is appropriate to refuse to answer and leave the interview. Report the incident to the career services office at your school.

Creating a Professional Appearance

The interviewer's first impression will be based on your appearance. If it is negative, chances for hire may be lost before the formal interview even starts. Give yourself every advantage by creating a look that says, "I'm a professional who will fit easily into a health care environment."

In Chapter 13, the elements of a professional appearance for the health care professional were discussed. The following summary highlights interview essentials:

- Make sure that everything about you is clean. This includes hair, fingernails, teeth, breath, clothing, and shoes. Bathe or shower and use a good deodorant.

- Demonstrate your knowledge of what is appropriate in the health care setting. Do not use products that have fragrances. Scents from perfumes, body lotions, hair spray, and other personal care products can be offensive when people are ill or have allergies. Do not take the chance of clinging tobacco odors by smoking on the way to the interview. Remove nose, lip, tongue, and other visible piercings. Cover tattoos with long sleeves. (Some employers are becoming more lenient regarding tattoos and piercings, but until you learn the specific policies, it is best to be conservative.) Refrain from activities that result in hickeys being visible at the time of the interview. (Health care employers have mentioned this as a problem with applicants.)

- Wear conservative attire. Women should choose a simple dress, suit, blouse and skirt, or pantsuit. Avoid anything low cut and revealing or sexy in any way. Men should wear slacks and a white or light-colored shirt.

- If you are unsure about what to wear, ask an instructor or career services for advice. Some schools recommend that job applicants wear their school scrubs or lab coat, but this should be discussed with career services to find out if the employer with which you have the interview approves of this practice. If you are on a tight budget, ask if the school has interview clothes to lend to their students. Thrift and second-hand shops often have appropriate clothes at reasonable prices. Some cities now have special shops and services that provide job seekers with free clothing and accessories, along with good advice about how to dress appropriately.

- Avoid jeans, T-shirts, sunglasses, hats, athletic shoes, and anything symbolic of gangs, religious groups, or political organizations.

- Keep jewelry simple. Men should remove earrings and women should wear only one pair.

- Women should avoid heavy makeup and colored nail polish. Long hair should be tied back or pinned up.

- Men with facial hair should trim it neatly. Men should tie long hair back. (These fashions are acceptable to employers in many parts of the country. Your area might be an exception.)

FIGURE 25-1 Make a strong, positive statement with professional dress and grooming.

A professional appearance tells the employer that you take work seriously and consider the interview to be an important occasion. (See Figure 25-1.)

Securing References

References are people who will vouch for your qualifications and character. They are willing to be contacted by potential employers to answer questions about you. References should not be family members, relatives, or friends. Good examples are former supervisors, instructors, clergy, or professionals who know you well.

Applicants should have between three and six references. Ask only those people whom you believe will give you a good recommendation. *Never* give anyone's name as a reference if he or she has not given you permission in advance. Keep your references informed about the jobs for which you interview and tell them the name of the person who might call.

Create a **reference list** that can be given to prospective employers upon request. Use the same paper used for your resume. Label it "References" and put your own name, address, phone number, and e-mail address centered at the top of the page. Then list the name, title, address, phone number, and e-mail address of each reference. It is also helpful to add the relationship you have with each person, such as employee, coworker, or student. Be sure to give accurate phone numbers. People who are difficult to locate or have numbers that are not in service do not appear credible and may do you more harm than good.

Letters of recommendation are statements written on your behalf by former employers and other professionals who know your work. Ask for a letter from any job that you leave on satisfactory terms. Keep the original letter and make copies to give to future potential employers.

Thinking It Through

Cathy Nazerian is hoping that she will finally find an employer who understands what it is like to be a single mother. Before enrolling in the medical assistant program, she had to change jobs six times in the previous 14 months. Cathy found her employers to be very unsympathetic about things that really were not her fault. She couldn't control her unreliable babysitter, old car, and the fact that working while caring for three children tired her out so much that she couldn't always make it to work. Fortunately, she was able to maintain good attendance while in school because her mother had just retired and agreed to help her out temporarily with the kids.

1. How should Cathy respond to employers who ask about her frequent job changes?

2. What changes, if any, should Cathy make in her attitude about employers?

3. What would you suggest she do to reduce the need to change jobs so frequently?

Creating a Portfolio

A **portfolio** is an organized collection of written documents that you can show to employers. Its purpose is to support claims about your qualifications and, according to career professionals, it can give you an advantage over other candidates.

The following documents are examples of appropriate contents for health care graduates:

- Copy of your diploma or certificate of program completion

- Copy of your professional license, certification, or registration

- Certificates that demonstrate competencies: keyboarding speed, cardiopulmonary resuscitation (CPR), course completions, and so on

- Documentation of accomplishments and service: awards, letters of appreciation, and so on

- Positive evaluations from your clinical experience and previous employment

- Class assignments that demonstrate proficiency in the tasks related to the job target: completed insurance forms, business letters, charting samples, and documents created with medical management software (Be sure that anything included is absolutely perfect.)

- A list of your technical skills and competencies (Organize them by work categories: administrative, clinical, patient care, computer, and so on.)

- Letters of recommendation from previous employers and others who can vouch for your character

To assemble the portfolio, group similar materials together and place them in a logical order. If there are many items, make a table of contents. Insert the papers in plastic page protectors and place them in a three-ring binder that has a nicely finished cover in a conservative color. A presentation binder containing page protectors can also be used.

Do not send the portfolio with the resume. Take it to interviews to demonstrate your competencies. (You do not leave it with the employer.) For example, if the employer asks if you know current procedural terminology (CPT) coding, an accurately completed coding assignment would be an appropriate exhibit. You may not have an opportunity to show the portfolio at every interview. Use it only when it can support responses to questions or if the employer asks to see it.

Start early in your educational program to collect items for a portfolio. Keep them neatly stored together so you can find them when needed. Focus on completing all class assignments correctly and neatly, so that they not only fulfill class requirements but can also serve you in the job search.

Today, it is possible to create an online portfolio on services such as LinkedIn. This might be something to check into if you have the time and computer expertise.

What to Take to an Interview

Demonstrate your organizational skills and ability to plan ahead by having everything you might need at the interview. This will also prevent you from feeling flustered when you cannot find a pen to fill out an application. Use the following checklist as a guide:

- Extra resumes

- Application, if you filled it out at home

- Reference list

- List of important facts: driver's license and social security numbers, and details about employers that are not listed on your resume but might be requested on an application

- Portfolio

- Copies of letters of recommendation

- Copies of licenses and certifications

- Pen and notepad

- Appointment calendar, electronic or paper

Getting to interviews on time while fulfilling other responsibilities can be challenging. If you will be going directly from school or work, take along appropriate emergency supplies for your situation, such as breath mints and a clean shirt. Take steps to avoid feeling rushed and unprepared; this will help you be at your best.

Practice, Practice, Practice

Practice is the best way to do well at every interview. Ask a friend, family member, or classmate to play the part of the employer. Practice smiling, introducing yourself, and shaking hands. You may feel silly practicing such simple actions, but the basics are important. A surprising number of job offers are lost because of lifeless handshakes and poor eye contact.

Give your "employer" a list of commonly asked questions and practice answering them. Practice your closing (described in the next section) and leaving the interview on a positive note.

Participate in any mock (pretend) interviews offered by your school. If possible, have your interview recorded so that you can critique yourself. Listen and watch carefully. Did you do the following:

- Maintain eye contact?
- Speak clearly using a pleasant voice?
- Avoid using meaningless words like "uh" and "you know"?
- Sit calmly with good posture?
- Show enthusiasm?
- Answer questions fully but without rambling on?
- Appear to be interested in the other person?
- Support your answers with examples?

Practice as often as possible so that when it is time for actual interviews, you feel more relaxed. You would never think of performing a procedure on a patient without sufficient practice. Prepare for job interviews in the same way.

Starting Off on the Right Foot

Do everything possible to avoid being late for an interview. Do not lose a job opportunity before even having the chance to present your qualifications. Plan to arrive about 15 minutes early. This gives you time to check your appearance in the restroom and fill out any necessary paperwork. If you are unfamiliar with the area where the facility is located, try to make a dry run before the day of the interview.

Attend job interviews alone. Bringing a friend or family member can demonstrate a lack of self-confidence. Bringing your children, rather than arranging for childcare, demonstrates disorganization. If someone gives you a ride, have the person wait outside or in another part of the building.

Turn off your cell phone, if you have one with you, before you arrive at the interview location. Allowing your phone to ring during the interview is not only extremely poor manners, it may cost you the job.

Be courteous and pleasant with *everyone* you meet, including the receptionist. Do not show impatience or comment negatively if you had trouble finding the location, must wait for the interviewer, or encounter other difficulties. Demonstrate the same professionalism expected of you on the job. The interview is composed of much more than just the time spent sitting with the employer in a formal setting. It starts with the first contact, whether that is a phone call, a resume submitted, or a personal visit.

When you are introduced to the interviewer, smile, establish eye contact, and return the handshake firmly. Wait to sit down until you are offered a seat or the interviewer has sat down. (See Figure 25–2.)

Here are some key points to help you do well during the discussion portion of the interview:

- Keep your purpose in mind: to sell yourself and your qualifications.

© vgstudio/Shutterstock.com.

FIGURE 25–2 Greet the employer with a smile, eye contact, and a firm handshake.

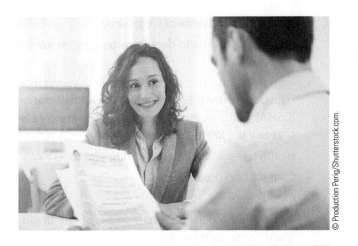

FIGURE 25–3 Listening carefully to the employer is essential for a successful interview.

FIGURE 25–4 You may be asked to take a written test as part of the job-application process.

- *Listen* carefully to the employer. (See Figure 25–3.) What are the employment needs and concerns or problems? What is he or she looking for in an employee?
- Answer questions in ways that show how you are qualified for the job.
- Answer questions fully, but do not talk too long or give out information that was not requested.
- Show interest in the job by asking questions when invited to do so or when you have the opportunity.
- Balance warmth and friendliness with professionalism. *Employers hire people they like.*
- Never share gossip or make negative remarks about previous employers or anyone else. Do not discuss your personal problems.
- Do not place anything on the employer's desk unless invited to do so. And *never* read papers or appear to be snooping in any way.
- Project positive nonverbal communication. Sit up straight in the chair or lean forward slightly to show interest, maintain eye contact, and speak clearly using good expression and enthusiasm. Do not chew gum, and avoid nervous habits, such as twisting your hair or jiggling your leg.
- *Never* lie. You should be prepared to answer difficult questions honestly. If a lie is discovered after you are hired, it can be grounds for dismissal.

In addition to asking you questions during an interview, some employers give a written test or have applicants complete a task. In these cases, draw on what you have learned, try to relax, and do your best. (See Figure 25–4.)

When the employer indicates that the interview is drawing to a close and you are unsure of the next step in the process, ask what it is. Is there anything you need to send to the employer? When will applicants be notified of a hiring decision? Do not be afraid to ask these questions. At the same time, do not take too much time if it is obvious the employer needs to end the interview. Whether you are interested in the job or not, express appreciation for the opportunity to interview and leave courteously.

Recent Trends in Interviews

- Peculiar or unexpected questions designed to help the interviewer understand how you think
- Group interviews, in which there may be more than one job applicant or more than one interviewer with one applicant
- Video and phone interviews
- Psychometric tests (e.g., reasoning tests, personality profiles, ability assessments, and motivation questionnaires)

After the Interview

Think of the interview as a process that continues until the job is filled, either by you or by someone else. Here are some follow-up activities that can tip the scale in your favor:

- *Send a thank-you letter.* This is one of the most overlooked ways to demonstrate consideration for the interviewer and interest in the job. It never fails to make a positive impression. Do it immediately after the interview, even if you decide that you are not

Fascinating Facts

More than one in five hiring managers report that they are less likely to hire candidates who do not send a thank-you note after the interview. Some will actually dismiss an applicant for consideration because it shows a lack of follow-through or sends the message that the applicant is not serious about the position.

Source: CareerBuilder, "More Than One-in-Five Hiring Managers Say They Are Less Likely to Hire a Candidate Who Didn't Send a Thank-You Note, Finds New CareerBuilder Survey." www.careerbuilder.com /share/aboutus/pressreleasesdetail.aspx?id=pr631&sd=4/14/2011 &ed=04/14/2011.

qualified for or interested in the job. This employer may have a more appropriate job in the future or may know another employer whose needs match your skills. If you want the job, restate your interest. If you have applicable qualifications you did not discuss at the interview, mention them now in your letter. Figure 25–5 contains an example of a post-interview thank-you letter. Note that this communication is more than simply a thank-you note; it is, in fact, an additional opportunity to sell yourself to the employer. (Note: The majority of hiring managers report it is acceptable to send the thank you by email.)

- Send in any requested information, applications, or other items.
- Advise all references that they may be called.
- Review your impressions of the employer and facility. Be prepared to either accept or reject the position if it is offered.
- Place a follow-up telephone call if you do not hear by the date you were told you would be contacted. Let the employer know that you are still interested in the job and ask if a hiring decision has been made. If not, ask when it is expected to be made.
- Continue your job search activities, even if you believe the interview went well.

Additional Requirements

Many health care facilities have special requirements as part of the hiring process in response to social problems and public health concerns. The following may be encountered in the job search or after a job has been accepted:

- Tests for the presence of illegal drugs
- Psychological tests to determine tendencies toward violence
- Immunizations, such as the hepatitis B vaccination (The Occupational Safety and Health Administration [OSHA] requires employers to give these free of charge if the job involves exposure.)
- Health screening tests, such as those for tuberculosis
- Criminal background check
- Credit check
- Disclosure of social security number, if not already given (for tax withholding)
- Information about family, such as number of children (for insurance purposes)
- Proof of right to work legally in the United States

ACCEPTING THE JOB

Congratulations! Your hard work and persistence have paid off, and you have received a job offer that you want to accept. If you accept the offer verbally, such as over the telephone, follow up with a letter in which you

Thinking It Through

Wayne Blackman is applying for a position as a radiologic technologist at an imaging center. He feels very confident about his qualifications. After all, he graduated with honors and passed the state licensing exam with high scores. Wayne is unhappy with the interview he had this morning at the center. After hurrying to get there on time, he had to wait 20 minutes for the director, Ms. Rodriguez. Before the interview started, he told her that he thought it was rude to have kept him waiting. During the interview there were two phone calls and some kind of urgent situation with a patient that Ms. Rodriguez had to attend to. This made it difficult for him to fully inform her about his qualifications and spend the time necessary to show off his portfolio. Wayne feels pretty sure he can get the job, though, if Ms. Rodriguez can take the time to look at his academic and test records.

1. Do you agree with Wayne that he will probably be hired? Explain your answer.
2. Should Wayne have done anything differently? Why or why not?

1357 Keystone Drive
Chicago, IL 60606
July 31, 20—

Ms. Tasha Jefferson, Office Manager
Compton Dental Clinic
6397 Flanders Street
Chicago, IL 60606

Dear Ms. Jefferson:

Thank you very much for giving me the opportunity to interview for the position of dental assistant at Compton Dental Clinic. I enjoyed talking with you and learning more about the needs of the clinic.

Compton impressed me as being committed to providing high-quality patient care and developing its patient education programs. I believe that my experience as a peer tutor during my studies at Harrison Dental College would help me contribute to your educational efforts. I may not have mentioned during the interview that I am proficient in desktop publishing software and enjoy creating informational materials.

I am very interested in the position and would be pleased to have the opportunity to join the Compton team. Thank you again for your consideration.

Sincerely,

Kelly Bosner

Kelly Bosner

FIGURE 25–5 Follow up *every* interview with a thank you letter.

express your thanks for the offer, the fact that you accept it, and what you understand to be the title, salary, and start date.

If you are not sure about whether to accept a position, ask the employer if you can respond in one or two days. Do not take longer than that. It may not be possible for the employer to extend the extra time if it is urgent that the vacancy be filled.

DECLINING THE JOB

Just as with the acceptance, respond in writing even if you decline the job in a phone call. Thank the employer for the time spent and confidence in your abilities. State simply that you have decided not to accept the offer. It is not necessary to explain your decision. *Never* ignore a job offer. Remember that this employer may have an extensive network in the health care community. Lack of courtesy in rejecting an offer can damage your chances with other employers.

DEALING WITH REJECTION

All jobs are not meant for all people. If you are not offered a position, it can be for many reasons: You did not have all the required qualifications, someone with the "perfect" combination of skills and experience applied for the same job, or your preferred work style was not a fit. Not being selected for a job should not be taken as a personal rejection. Talking with someone supportive can help you deal with disappointments encountered during the job search.

If you find that you repeatedly fail to receive an offer, review your interviewing skills and ask career services or your instructor for advice. Some employment professionals recommend that you ask the employers with whom you have interviewed for feedback and suggestions. Do *not* approach them in a hostile manner, demanding to know why you did not get the job. Explain that you want to improve your job-seeking skills and would appreciate their help. Some employers have a policy of not answering this kind of question. Therefore, do not be insistent or express anger if they are not willing to discuss the reason why you were not hired.

FILLING OUT APPLICATIONS

You may be asked to fill out an application at any time during the job search, either in printed or electronic form. (See Figure 25–6 for an example.) Some organizations that do not have current openings allow applicants to submit an application that is kept on file for future openings. Others have applicants fill them out at the time of the interview. Be sure to have all necessary information, including dates and locations of your education and previous employment. You also need the names and phone numbers of all references. Regardless of when the application is completed, here are a few important guidelines:

- Read the entire application *before* filling it in. Then start back at the beginning and answer each question completely. In the employment section, do not write, "See resume." If you are hired, your application can serve as a legal document, and it must be filled in completely to be valid.

- Type or print neatly using a black pen. The way you fill out an application tells the employer about your ability to follow directions and your attention to detail. If the application is filled out electronically, take care to check for mistakes before pushing the "enter" or "send" key. (Be aware that some employers today accept only applications that are submitted electronically.)

- Be sure that all your facts are accurate. Check that all dates and numbers are correct, especially your phone number.

- Write "N/A" (not applicable) if a question does not pertain to you, so the reader will know that you did not miss the question.

- Write "negotiable" in the salary section, unless you have already been told what it is.

- Include your signature and the date.

- Review it for accuracy. Look at every item.

Make a copy of any applications you fill out at home or on the Internet. These will serve as a record of your job search, as well as supply a convenient source of information for filling out future applications.

SAMPLE EMPLOYMENT APPLICATION

DATE _____

PERSONAL INFORMATION

Name _____
      Last   First   Middle   Maiden

Current Address _____
      Number   Street   City   State   Zip

Mailing Address _____
      Number   Street   City   State   Zip

Telephone   Home ( ) _____   Cell ( ) _____   Other ( ) _____

E-mail Address _____

Are you 18 years or older? _____ Yes _____ No

Social Security Number _____

Position Applying For _____

Availability _____ Full-time _____ Part-time _____ On Call
_____ Any shift, if applicable _____ Overtime

Who referred you to our facility or how did you hear about this position? _____

Can you provide documentation that you are authorized to work in the U.S.? _____ Yes _____ No

Have you previously applied for a position at this facility? _____ Yes _____ No

Have you previously been employed by this facility? _____ Yes _____ No

EMPLOYMENT HISTORY

1. Current/Most Recent Employer

Company Name _____

Department and Supervisor's Name _____

Can We Contact as Reference? _____ Yes _____ No

Telephone Number _____

Address _____

Dates Employed   From _____ To _____

Job Title _____

(continued)

Major Duties _____

_____

_____

Reason for Leaving _____

2. Next Most Recent Employer

Company Name _____

Department and Supervisor's Name _____

Can We Contact as Reference? _____ Yes _____ No

Telephone Number _____

Address _____

Dates Employed   From _____ To _____

Job Title _____

Major Duties _____

_____

_____

Reason for Leaving _____

EDUCATION

High School
        Name _____
        City, State _____
        Graduated? _____ Yes _____ No

College/University
        Name _____
        City, State _____
        Degree Earned _____

College/University
        Name _____
        City, State _____
        Degree Earned _____

Technical School
        Name _____
        City, State _____
        Degree/Certificate Earned _____

Other
        Name _____
        City, State _____
        Degree/Certificate Earned _____

(continued)

SPECIAL SKILLS

Licenses, certificates, and/or registrations. Include the number and expiration date.
_____
_____

Working knowledge of computer software.
_____
_____

Other
_____
_____

OTHER INFORMATION

Have you ever been convicted of a misdemeanor or felony crime? _____Yes _____ No
If yes, please provide an explanation.
_____
_____
_____
_____

Have you served in the United States Armed Forces? _____ Yes _____ No
If yes, which branch of service? _____

INVITATION TO SELF-IDENTIFY

The following information is voluntary and will be kept confidential. It is used to help the facility comply with government reporting requirements and to evaluate its hiring practices.

Please check the appropriate spaces.
_____ Male _____ Female

Ethnic Background
_____ Hispanic or Latino
_____ American Indian or Alaskan Native
_____ Black or African American
_____ Asian
_____ White
_____ Two or more races

APPLICATION AGREEMENT

- I affirm that all information contained in this agreement is true and complete.
- I authorize the facility to investigate all statements made in this application, including Information from previous employers and references.
- I understand that if selected, my employment will be on an "at-will" basis which means that the employer and employee may terminate the employment at any time with or without notice or cause.

_____ I agree _____ I disagree (if you disagree, your application will not be considered.)

FIGURE 25–6 Example of a typical application for a health care position.

SUGGESTED LEARNING ACTIVITIES

1. Practice applying the listening skills described in Chapter 16 to everyday situations. It will pay off when you attend interviews and need to listen carefully to understand the needs and requirements of the employer.

2. Start writing down ideas for answering common interview questions.

3. Make a list of people who might serve as your references.

4. Review your wardrobe for clothes that are suitable for an interview.

5. Observe your own behavior. Do you make it a habit to be courteous? Do you speak clearly and in a pleasant tone?

6. Enlist the help of two friends, family members, or classmates and set up a practice interview. Choose a specific job to apply for. Give the "employer" questions from all the categories discussed in this chapter. Start the "interview" with a greeting and a handshake, and complete it with an appropriate closing. Have the second person observe and critique your performance.

7. Look on the websites of several health care facilities to review their application forms and procedures.

WEB ACTIVITIES

Very Well Health

https://www.verywellhealth.com/before-you-interview-for-a-medical-job-1736041

Before You Interview for a Medical Job

    List any new ideas presented in the articles you believe would be helpful in preparing for a job interview.

Monster

https://www.monster.com/career-advice/job-interview

Interviews

    This website contains many helpful articles about interviewing.

1. Using the links, choose five articles to read.

2. Based on what you learn, prepare a list of suggestions for applicants seeking jobs in health care.

FOX Rehabilitation

Interview video: https://www.foxrehab.org/video/prepare-for-healthcare-ot-pt-job-interview/

Rights and Not Quites (Interviewing for a Job in Health Care)

1. Watch the video, in addition to reading the transcript.

2. List the "do's and don't's" that Ms. Mendenhall explains and demonstrates with "interviewees."

3. What was the advice shared by her mother? How can that help you when you prepare for and attend interviews?

Glassdoor

https://www.glassdoor.com/blog/12-things-to-never-do-during-a-phone-interview/

12 Things to Never Do During a Phone Interview

1. List the suggestions about what not to do during a phone interview.

2. Based on these, how can you best prepare for this type of interview?

The Balance Careers

Thank You Email: https://www.thebalancecareers.com/thank-you-email-after-job-interview-2063958

Thank You Email After an Interview Examples

1. What are the advantages of sending a thank-you letter by email?
2. What should be included?
3. What suggestions are given to make your email effective and increase your chances for getting hired?

https://www.thebalancecareers.com/how-to-ask-why-you-didn-t-get-the-job-2062998

How to Ask Why You Didn't Get the Job

1. Why is it better to ask for feedback rather than asking directly why you didn't get the job?
2. What are examples of questions when asking for feedback?

REVIEW QUESTIONS

1. Why is it important to learn about the employer before a job interview?
2. How can job candidates prepare to present their technical and non-technical qualifications at job interviews?
3. What are five appropriate questions to ask a potential employer at a job interview?
4. What are three questions you should not ask at a job interview?
5. What are two examples of each of the following types of interview questions: general employment, behavioral (situational), and health-care specific?
6. What is the best way to answer difficult questions about sensitive issues?
7. What are five examples of questions that are illegal for employers to ask at a job interview?
8. What are three ways to respond to illegal interview questions?
9. Describe the ideal appearance of a man and a woman who is attending a health care job interview.
10. What is a reference? Give three examples of people who would be appropriate references.
11. What are letters of recommendation and what is their purpose?
12. What is the purpose of a professional portfolio?
13. What are eight documents that would be appropriate to include in the health care applicant's professional portfolio?
14. What are five items you should take to interviews?
15. How can you practice your interviewing skills?
16. What are examples of positive actions to take before an interview starts?
17. What are ten key points to help you do well during an interview?
18. What are four recent interview trends?
19. What are six actions to take after an interview to increase your chances of being hired?
20. What are five things an employer can require of a potential hire?
21. What are the proper ways to accept and decline job offers?
22. How should an applicant deal with being rejected for a job?
23. What are seven guidelines to follow when filling out a job application?

APPLICATION EXERCISES

1. Refer to the Case of the Modest Applicant at the beginning of the chapter. Describe how Sam could more effectively sell himself to an employer.

2. Carol-Ann LaRoche has completed her dental hygiene program. She is the first child in two generations to go to college, and her family is extremely proud of her. Carol-Ann did well in her courses. The most difficult part of her training was carrying on conversations with patients. She is very shy and feels unsure of herself socially. Although she is looking forward to working as a hygienist, she is terrified at having to attend job interviews. She just knows she'll get tongue-tied and be unable to make a good impression. Recommend a step-by-step plan that Carol-Ann can use to prepare for an interview successfully.

PROBLEM-SOLVING PRACTICE

Shawna is in the lucky position of having two good job offers to choose from. How can she use the five-step problem-solving process to help her make the best decision?

CHAPTER 26

Successful Employment Strategies

KEY TERMS

chain of command
employee handbook
grievance
integrity
job descriptions
minimum wage
performance evaluation
policies
probationary period
procedures
reasonable accommodations
risk management
sexual harassment
teams

OBJECTIVES

Studying and applying the material in this chapter will help you to:

1. List five important things that new employees should learn about the facility in which they work.
2. Explain the difference between policies and procedures.
3. List examples of typical contents of an employee handbook.
4. Explain the purpose of a probationary period.
5. Explain what is meant by "chain of command."
6. List the actions an employee should take in order to "give a full day's work."
7. Explain why being a good team member is important in health care work.
8. Explain how good teams contribute to the effectiveness of an organization.
9. List ten characteristics of a valued team member.
10. List six ways you can "go beyond the minimum" at work.
11. List and explain the purpose of the ten major employment laws presented in this chapter.
12. Explain the meaning of a grievance and how it should be handled.
13. Explain the meaning of sexual harassment, including examples, and the actions to take if it occurs.
14. Describe the contents of a typical performance evaluation.
15. Identify the steps to take when leaving a job voluntarily.
16. Describe what you can do to increase your changes of receiving a promotion.
17. Describe the actions employees should take when they are fired from a job.

The Case of the Irritating New Hire

Katie Cormack began her first job as a laboratory technician at Excelsior Medical Lab five weeks ago. She finds the work interesting and especially likes working with patients who come in to have blood drawn for various tests. Katie is surprised when the lab director, Gwen Hendricks, meets with her privately to let her know that other staff members have complained about the time they have to spend answering Katie's questions. Although they appreciate her

(continues)

enthusiasm and desire to do a good job, they are frustrated at having their work frequently interrupted to answer questions regarding common lab policies and procedures and the location of supplies and equipment. Ms. Hendricks explains to Katie that almost all the information she needs appears in the laboratory manuals or was presented in the new-employee orientation that she received when she started her job. This chapter explains the importance of accepting responsibility for learning a new job and explains the major methods and resources that new employees can use.

GETTING OFF TO A GOOD START

Obtaining the first job after graduation is exciting for the new health care professional. Beginning a new job represents a very important time in the health care professional's career. Your professional reputation starts to be established during your first few months of employment. The habits and relationships developed at this time contribute to future success.

Learning about the Job

Succeeding at a new job requires understanding the basics of the workplace. When Aileen McConnor reported for her first day of work as a health information technician at South Bay Hospital, her supervisor, Stan Bergman, conducted an orientation that included the following components:

- Tour of the facility
  - The medical records department
  - Location of files
  - Aileen's desk and work area
  - Lunch room and rest rooms
  - Storage of supplies
  - Personal storage area
- Explanation of safety rules and security precautions
- Demonstration of how to use equipment
- Introduction to coworkers
- Review of her job description

Aileen was glad for the opportunity to ask detailed questions about some of the job duties that were discussed during her employment interview. She also wanted to make sure that she clearly understood the work schedule that was discussed at the time of the job offer. Misunderstandings about these important issues can lead to employment nightmares. Aileen knew that Mr. Bergman would use her job description as a basis for judging her work performance. **Job descriptions** include important information about a specific job. They serve as guides for the actions and performance of the employee. See Table 26–1 for a description of the contents of a typical health care job description.

Policies and Procedures

Policies are the rules established and followed by an organization. **Procedures** are the specific steps taken to perform a task. Every facility develops and records its policies and procedures in order to ensure the quality and consistency of operations. Many health care policies and procedures are required by legal and regulatory agencies. Most facilities assemble manuals that contain all policies and procedures. Employees are expected to know and follow them. (See Figure 26–1.)

The **employee handbook** is a source of employment policies. It contains information specific to employment conditions, such as the following:

- Vacation policies
- Rules regarding overtime
- Paid holidays
- How to request a leave of absence

FIGURE 26–1 One of the first tasks of a new employee is to review the organization's policies and procedures.

Table 26–1 **Components of the Job Description**

Section Title	What It Contains	Examples
Job title	Exact name of the position	• Medical transcriptionist • Patient care assistant II • Ultrasound technician
Minimum requirements	Required knowledge, education, license or certification, and/or experience that must be demonstrated to qualify for the position	• Knowledge of medical terminology, anatomy and physiology (A&P), and English grammar • State nursing assistant certification • Registration with American Registry of Diagnostic Medical Sonographers (ARDMS)
Working conditions/physical requirements	Type of working environment. Physical abilities needed to perform the job	• Primarily sedentary work with use of earphones • Able to lift up to 30 pounds • Requires standing during 80% of workday
Reports to	Title of the supervisor who directly oversees the position	• Director of medical records • Director of health services • Imaging center director
Responsibilities, duties, and tasks	Specific work to be performed	• Transcribe daily dictation for outpatient surgical center • Transport patients to and from dining room • Perform diagnostic ultrasound procedures for abdominal and obstetrical/gynecological (OB/GYN) patients

• Benefits such as medical insurance

• Rules of conduct

If you are not shown these materials when you are hired, be sure to ask for them. Take time to study the sections that relate to your job. Ask questions about anything you do not understand. Manuals and handbooks serve as valuable references for both new and experienced staff members.

New employees sometimes do not understand the purpose of certain policies. Never refuse to follow policies with which you disagree. (The only exception is if they involve illegal or unsafe activities.) Courteously ask to have the purpose of the policy explained. The reason for it may not be obvious. For example, some facilities prohibit the wearing of colored nail polish. This may seem like a silly rule, but it is founded on principles of good hygiene. As pointed out in Chapter 13, colored polish can hide dirt beneath the nails and around the cuticles. The edges of chipped polish trap germs. Once understood, policies are easier to follow. New employees who have ideas for policy changes should wait until gaining some experience before suggesting "improvements."

Risk management refers to all the policies and procedures designed to ensure patient safety. Their purpose also includes protecting health care professionals and the public from various risks and they must be followed carefully. Many safety practices are mandated by law, and violating them can be a cause for immediate dismissal.

Probationary Period

Some employers have new hires begin with a **probationary period** that typically lasts between 60 and 90 days. This time allows the employer and employee to determine if they have a "match." The employer can evaluate the new hire's performance and decide if continued employment is advisable. This may be accomplished through a formal review process, which evaluates how the new employee has performed in areas such as the following:

• Cooperation with supervisor and coworkers

• Adequate skills to perform job tasks

FIGURE 26-2 Cooperation among coworkers is necessary to maintain a smooth-running health care facility.

- Ability to follow directions
- Willingness to learn
- Good attendance
- Appearance

(See Figure 26-2.)

GUIDELINES FOR WORKPLACE SUCCESS

There are certain basic guidelines that apply to all types of facilities and positions. Whether the health care professional works directly with patients, such as a physical therapist assistant, or provides a support service, such as a health information technician, the following recommendations will help ensure long-term career success.

Act with Integrity

Having integrity means conducting oneself honestly and morally. It means doing the "right thing" even under difficult conditions. For example, admitting an error and facing the consequences or spending extra time to redo a report until it is perfect, without being asked to do so, are two examples of acting with integrity.

Demonstrate Loyalty

Loyalty to the employer and to one's immediate supervisor is expected in all occupations. It is unacceptable to spend paid work time complaining about the supervisor or conditions of employment. This is especially true in a health care facility. It can cause serious problems. Patients who sense employee discontent or overhear negative comments may experience doubts about the quality of the facility, leading to a loss of confidence about their care. At best, patients feel uncomfortable. At worst, they sue for malpractice. All employees must realize that they represent the organization and therefore dedicate their work efforts to contributing to its success. Expand your view from simply achieving personal success to working for the success of the entire organization.

Being loyal, however, does not mean ignoring difficulties at work. On the contrary, these should be discussed directly and courteously with the supervisor. Problems that are not addressed do not disappear. They tend to become worse. Misunderstandings that could be cleared up in minutes can cause resentment and ruin working relationships. Give your supervisor the opportunity to work with you to create a positive working environment.

Employers appreciate employees who have thought through a problem and have ideas for solutions. This is a much more effective approach than simply presenting complaints.

When the health care professional finds it impossible to feel positive about and loyal to the place of employment, it is best to seek another job. There is too much at risk to do otherwise.

Follow the Chain of Command

Health care facilities organize their personnel so that there is a clear chain of command. This means that each person reports to a supervisor who, in turn, reports to another supervisor at the next higher level. This arrangement provides coverage of all necessary tasks along with quality control of employee performance. See Figure 26-3 for a sample organizational chart showing the various levels in a small medical office.

It is important for the health care professional to observe the chain of command. As discussed in the previous section, problems should be discussed with one's supervisor. Workplace problems should not be discussed with coworkers. Nor is it appropriate to go to the next higher level of management without first approaching the person directly involved. It is unfair to "report" your supervisor without giving him or her the opportunity to resolve the situation. It is also inefficient because it brings in another person who is not directly involved in the problem. (Exceptions to this are cases of serious improper behavior on the part of the supervisor, such as sexual harassment or intimidation. These should be reported immediately to the next level of management.)

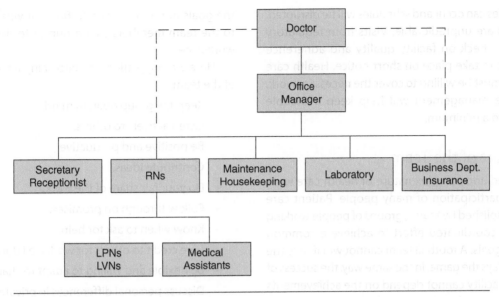

FIGURE 26–3 Sample organizational chart of a medical office.

Give a Full Day's Work

Consistent attendance and punctuality are essential when working in health care. Patients depend on services being provided as promised or required. In turn, employers depend on their employees to be available as scheduled to provide these services. Set perfect attendance as a goal. Plan backup childcare and transportation. Maintain good health habits, as discussed in Chapter 12. If an illness or emergency does require an absence, notify your supervisor with as much notice as possible so that the work can be covered.

While at work, focus fully on the job. Avoid making personal telephone calls and excessive socializing with coworkers. Do not use work time to discuss personal problems. Patients are annoyed when they are required to wait while health care professionals complete their personal business. It may be tempting to text your friends or send personal email messages when you are at work, but these activities should not be done at the workplace. You should also be aware that an increasing number of employers are monitoring their employees' emails, and inappropriate use and messages can result in dismissal.

Respect the time limits for breaks and meals. If your own tasks are completed and there is extra time, find something productive to do: volunteer to help a busy coworker, reorganize the supply cabinet, or practice a new skill. Devote all efforts to your employer during work hours.

Effective time management increases productivity and efficiency, which are important in today's cost-conscious environment. It also helps prevent frayed nerves and

Thinking It Through

Lack of information and failure to communicate are common causes of workplace conflict. Hank Stuart is experiencing a situation that really has him upset. He is a physical therapist assistant at a busy sports medicine clinic. He also has an interest in computers and worked in a large computer retail store while he went to school. It did not surprise Hank when one of the owners of the clinic, Kathy Chin, asked him to gather information about computer systems and software that could be used for patient management. Hank spent several hours of both work and personal time and gave his recommendation last week. It was then that he discovered that a system had already been purchased. The clinic's other owner had assigned the computer research task to another employee. Upset that his time and ideas were wasted, Hank has let everyone know just how disorganized and unfair his employers are. His coworkers are tired of hearing about it and wish Hank would just forget it.

1. Do you believe that Hank's reaction to the situation is appropriate? Why or why not?
2. How can he better deal with the situation?
3. What action would you recommend that he take?

the panic brought on when tasks are not completed on schedule. See Chapter 12 for a list of time-management techniques.

Emergencies can occur and schedules will be disrupted. Patient needs are unpredictable. Visits from regulatory agencies that check on facility quality and adherence to standards can take place on short notice. Health care professionals must be willing to cover the necessary work. Effective time management will help keep avoidable emergencies to a minimum.

Become Part of the Team

The specialized and complex nature of health care work requires the participation of many people. Patient care today is accomplished by **teams**, groups of people working together in a coordinated effort to achieve a common goal or set of goals. A football team cannot win if only the quarterback plays the game. In the same way, the success of a health care facility cannot depend on the achievements of just one person. A team may consist of all members of a department, or it may be a small group assigned to work on a specific project. Team goals may be ongoing, such as consistently providing high-quality patient care, or they may be short-term and project-oriented, such as computerizing the office record-keeping system.

Teams that work well can often accomplish more than individuals working separately. There are many ways that teams increase the effectiveness of a facility:

- They provide opportunities for mutual support and encouragement.
- Many viewpoints and ideas are available for solving problems.
- The members contribute a variety of skills.
- Creativity is generated through discussion.
- Work can be coordinated to take advantage of the interests and abilities of the members.
- Duplication of work and wasted effort can be avoided.

The variety of viewpoints and work styles that make teams successful can also be the source of frustration. For example, members who are very creative can contribute good ideas during brainstorming sessions, but become bored during discussions about the details and schedules necessary for the implementation of these ideas. It is necessary to be patient and take advantage of the strengths that each person brings to the group. If the entire group consisted of idea generators, there might be lots of discussion and little action.

New employees may be expected to become contributing members of one or more teams. Making a commitment to the organization and to coworkers is the first step toward becoming an effective team member. The needs of the group must be considered when making work-related decisions. Therefore, it is important to identify the goals of the team and to find out what is important to the team members as a group or to the goals of the workplace.

Here are suggestions for becoming a valued member of the team:

- Keep the group goals in mind.
- Listen actively to others.
- Be positive and productive.
- Contribute ideas.
- Do your fair share of the work.
- Follow through on promises.
- Know when to ask for help.
- Give credit to others for work well done.
- Be flexible and willing to adapt to changes.
- Discuss personal differences in private.

(See Figure 26–4.)

Staff meetings are a common way for team members to share ideas and information, plan work schedules, and keep up on issues of common interest. Workplace etiquette requires that employees arrive on time and be ready to participate. Respect others by paying attention. Avoid side conversations, looking at your phone, and other behaviors that indicate a lack of interest.

Meetings are not a place to discuss personal problems or grievances. Conduct these conversations in private with the appropriate person. Concentrate on issues important to the group. See Box 26–1 for an illustration of the consequences when there is a lack of teamwork.

Go Beyond the Minimum

Achieving professional success requires more than meeting minimum job requirements. It means setting high personal standards and striving to meet them every day. Developing the following habits will help lead to both professional success and personal satisfaction:

- Be enthusiastic: Develop an interest in your job. Be passionate about what you do.
- Project a positive attitude: Focus on the positive aspects of your work. Motivate yourself and others

FIGURE 26–4 Components of successful teamwork.

with a can-do attitude. Keep in mind that what you do each day contributes to the welfare of others. (See Figure 26–5.)

- Become a problem solver: Use your energy to think of solutions instead of voicing complaints. Enjoying the challenge of solving daily problems is an essential ingredient for a successful work life.

- Do more than is expected: Be willing to work extra time, if requested, to finish a task. If you finish your own work, offer to help others. Pitch in and help with major projects.

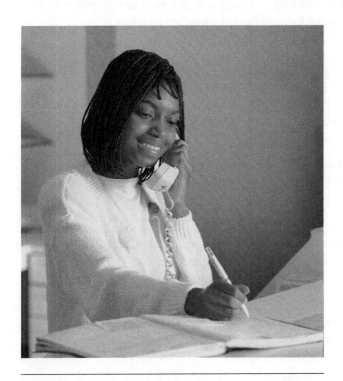

FIGURE 26–5 A positive attitude helps promote patient satisfaction.

- Practice quality control: Take the time to proofread your work. Memorize the abbreviations needed for charting. Practice procedures until you are proficient—on your own time, if necessary.

- Continue to learn: Add to your skills and knowledge. Participate in continuing education activities. (See Chapter 14.)

See Box 26–2 for a summary of the characteristics of great employees.

EMPLOYMENT LAWS

Job applicants and employees are protected by a number of laws. Some of these laws guarantee access to job opportunities. This means that it is illegal for employers to refuse to consider an applicant because of characteristics such as race, religion, and gender. The laws do not guarantee that a person will be hired; that depends on the applicant's qualifications.

Other laws protect the health and safety of employees. These are especially important in health care work because employees may be exposed to a number of potential risks. Table 26–2 contains a list of the most common laws that address the employer–employee relationship. The information provided here is a brief overview.

Not all the laws listed apply to all employers. For example, the Family Medical Leave Act applies only to organizations of a certain size. Laws prohibiting sexual harassment, however, apply to all employers, regardless of the number of employees.

In addition to the laws listed in the table, all states have laws that address **minimum wage** (the lowest hourly amount that an employee can be paid), overtime pay, and other issues regarding work conditions. These differ, so health care professionals should become familiar with the laws in their area.

Grievances

A **grievance** is a complaint about a circumstance considered to be unfair or potentially harmful. Employees have the right to present grievances to their employer.

Table 26-2 Major Employment Laws

Law	Purpose	Example
Age Discrimination in Employment (www.eeoc.gov/laws/types/age.cfm)	Prevents discrimination in hiring and the workplace against persons who are age 40 or older because of their age.	John Underwood, age 58, is proven to be the best qualified for a promotion at work. He cannot be denied the promotion because of his age.
Americans with Disabilities Act (www.eeoc.gov/laws/types/disability.cfm	Prevents employment discrimination against disabled applicants who are qualified to perform the job if **reasonable accommodations** are made (changes in equipment, special ramps for wheelchairs, etc.)	An applicant who is the most qualified for a medical transcription position cannot be denied the job because the arms of his or her wheelchair do not fit under the desks in the medical transcription area. A reasonable accommodation would be for the employer to furnish a higher desk or table.
Civil Rights Act of 1964 (www.eeoc.gov)	Prevents hiring discrimination on the basis of race, color, religion, sex, age, or national origin	A recently graduated nurse cannot be denied employment because she is 52 years old and the employer believes she will not follow directions as willingly as a younger person.
Title VII of 1964 Civil Rights Act (https://www.eeoc.gov/laws/types/sexual_harassment.cfm)	Prohibits sexual harassment, a form of sex discrimination	It is illegal for a medical laboratory director to continue to ask a lab technician under his supervision for dates when she has clearly stated that she is not interested in dating him.
Equal Pay Act of 1963 (www.eeoc.gov/laws/types/sex.cfm.)	Prevents wage discrimination for jobs that require equal skills, effort, and responsibility	A female medical assistant in an urgent care center must be paid the same hourly wage as a male medical assistant who does the same level of work and has comparable experience.
Fair Labor Standards Act (https://www.dol.gov/whd/regs/compliance/hrg.htm)	Sets the federal minimum wage. (States may have higher minimums.) Also requires 1½ overtime pay for hourly employees who work more than 40 hours in a workweek.	When Emily is hired as an occupational therapy aide, she must be paid no less than the federal minimum wage. A hospital orderly who works 46 hours one week, must be paid 1½ overtime pay for 6 hours.
Family and Medical Leave Act of 1993 (www.dol.gov/whd/fmla)	Allows employees up to 12 weeks of unpaid leave to meet family needs. Same or equivalent job must be given upon return	The father of a newborn infant cannot be dismissed for requesting 3 months to assist his wife in caring for their child.
Immigration Reform Act (https://www.eeoc.gov/eeoc/history/35th/thelaw/irca.html)	Prevents employment of persons who do not have the right to work in the United States	A home health agency that hires young women who do not have the legal right to work in the United States is subject to penalties under this law.
Occupational Safety and Health Act (https://www.osha.gov/law-regs.html)	Prevents unsafe working conditions	It is illegal for an employer to refuse to pay for a hepatitis B vaccination for a newly hired nurse who provides direct patient care and is exposed to blood and other bodily fluids.
Pregnancy Discrimination Act (www.eeoc.gov/laws/types/pregnancy.cfm)	A woman cannot be denied a job or promotion because of pregnancy or abortion. A pregnant employee cannot be fired or forced to go on leave.	Alison wants to continue working as long as possible during her pregnancy as a medical biller.

Many organizations have formal grievance policies that outline the steps required to file a grievance. Look in the employee handbook or ask your supervisor for a copy of the policy.

It is always best to try to resolve workplace issues at the lowest level possible. This means first presenting a problem to your supervisor for discussion and resolution. If the issue is not resolved satisfactorily, then it is appropriate to contact the next level of management. Grievances should be filed only after working up the chain of command, described in an earlier section.

Sexual Harassment

Sexual harassment refers to unwelcome actions that are sexual in nature. It is a form of sex discrimination that is prohibited by Title VII of the Civil Rights Act of 1964. Sexual harassment can occur in a variety of circumstances:

- The victim and the harasser may be a woman or a man. The victim does not have to be of the opposite sex.

- The harasser can be the victim's supervisor, a supervisor in another area, a coworker, or a nonemployee.

- The victim does not have to be the person directly harassed, but rather can be anyone affected by the offensive conduct.

  (*Source:* Adapted from Equal Employment Opportunity Commission. "Facts About Sexual Harassment," www.eeoc.gov/eeoc/publications/fs-sex.cfm.)

The following are examples of sexual harassment:

- A supervisor repeatedly asks an employee for a date after being turned down.

- A high-level manager promises promotional opportunities in exchange for sex.

- A coworker makes crude remarks about the body of a female coworker.

- An employee tells dirty jokes in the presence of coworkers who have stated their objections to such stories.

- A salesman visiting the facility touches a female employee inappropriately.

Mutual friendships and dating are not considered sexual harassment. Workplace romances, however, are not advised. If relationships end, working at the same facility can be uncomfortable and affect the quality of work performed by the people involved. For this reason, some facilities have policies that prohibit dating among employees who work in the same department.

The Equal Employment Opportunity Commission, a government agency that handles sexual harassment complaints that cannot be settled at the workplace, suggests that victims first speak directly to the harasser. Clearly identify the unwelcome behavior and state that it must stop. If the harassment continues, follow the facility's sexual harassment policy or grievance procedure to file a complaint. (*Source:* Equal Employment Opportunity Commission. "Facts About Sexual Harassment," www.eeoc.gov/eeoc/publications/fs-sex.cfm.)

Health care professionals can protect themselves against being accused of sexual harassment by avoiding the following behaviors:

- Discussing sexual matters that are not related to the job

- Telling "dirty" jokes

- Describing intimate details of their personal lives

- Joking around about sexual matters

- Touching coworkers and patients in suggestive ways

New employees should carefully observe and learn the level of formality that is customary in their workplace. Some workplaces are more casual than others. Behaviors that are acceptable in one may be considered unacceptable in others.

Employees who work together sometimes become friends and engage in playful conversation. The best way to prevent problems is to be aware of the reactions of others to your actions or conversation. If in doubt, ask them if they are uncomfortable, and immediately discontinue any conduct that they indicate is inappropriate.

TRACKING YOUR PROGRESS

Employees need to know how they are performing in order to grow professionally and improve their skills. If they are not meeting their employer's standards, evaluations provide an opportunity to learn about deficiencies and create plans to make improvements. Performance evaluations can be valuable learning experiences if approached with a positive attitude.

If the employer has a probationary period, it is common that an employee evaluation be conducted at the end of that period. When the mutual decision is to continue the employment, the evaluation meeting provides an excellent opportunity for the employee to ask questions that have come up during the probationary period. It is appropriate to ask for an honest appraisal of your performance and suggestions for improvement. If there have been any misunderstandings about the employer's expectations and priorities, this is the time to clarify them. Employees have the right to know the employer's expectations and the standards used for judging their performance.

The annual **performance evaluation** (review) usually takes place about one year after the hire date. If it is not scheduled within a few weeks after the first anniversary of hire, it is a good idea to check with your supervisor. These can be overlooked, and your interest in receiving a progress report is usually appreciated.

The evaluation typically consists of numerical ratings of the employee's performance of the duties outlined in the job description. It also includes ratings of important employee characteristics, such as cooperation. Performance evaluations may include a description of the employee's strengths, behaviors that require improvement, and goals to be met by the next evaluation. Box 26–3 contains a list of items that commonly appear on performance evaluations. Not every item will appear on every form.

Do not react defensively or show anger if you receive any low ratings. Ask for clarification and examples of how your work or behavior is below standard and suggestions for how to make improvements. Demonstrate a willingness to accept responsibility for your work and an interest in achieving higher standards.

This evaluation may or may not include a salary review. Some employers prefer to conduct the performance evaluation and salary review separately. They believe that this encourages a more honest appraisal of, and open discussion about, performance.

After discussing the contents with the employee, the supervisor places the evaluation in the employee's personnel file. Most states allow employees to see the contents of their files and request copies of documents placed there. This includes examining completed performance evaluations and any written warnings or disciplinary notices. It is a good idea to check your file periodically to remain aware of the contents.

You can better benefit from the evaluation if you conduct a self-appraisal in advance. In fact, some employers require this and ask you to bring your self-ratings to the meeting. Be honest about both your strengths and weaknesses. And be prepared to give examples that justify your "ratings."

MOVING UP

There are two ways to move up: within your organization and within your career. (They may overlap.) If you work in a one-physician office, there may be no opportunities for advancements. However, you may be able to learn and help with more procedures and you may get periodic salary raises, but the promotional opportunities will be limited.

In a larger organization, you may have chances to be promoted and/or given more responsibilities, possibly even a new job title in which you manage others. The following are ways to encourage promotions of this type:

- Share your professional goals for advancement with your supervisor
- Consistently practice the characteristics of the professional discussed in this chapter and in Chapter 13
- Demonstrate the leadership qualities listed in Chapter 13
- Network with your co-workers
- Take advantage of opportunities to volunteer at work for extra assignments, group projects, planning the company picnic, etc.

Box 26-3

Common Components of Performance Evaluations

- Accuracy: Performs work without errors
- Appearance: Maintains appropriate, professional appearance for position held
- Attendance and punctuality: Consistently on time and on duty during assigned hours
- Communication: Clear and effective oral and written communication; reports to supervisor as required
- Cooperation: Works well with others; contributes to team effort
- Dependability: Performs work without reminders
- Effectiveness under stress: Remains calm under demanding conditions and during emergencies

- Flexibility: Responds well to changing conditions as well as changing patient and facility needs
- Initiative: Willing and able to problem solve and make decisions
- Operation and care of equipment: Uses equipment safely and correctly; performs or requests maintenance as needed
- Quality of work: Performs tasks correctly; follows facility procedures
- Quantity of work: Completes tasks, meets deadlines, maintains work schedules
- Safety practices: Follows facility policies and standard precautions

- Attend any appropriate training workshops offered by your employer, your professional organization, local adult education, etc.

The second type of "moving up," is advancing your career by preparing for another position. For example, you may be working as a CNA (certified nursing assistant), but have an ultimate goal of becoming a registered nurse. This is known as "climbing the career ladder," discussed in Chapter 14. In this case, you will need additional education. (See Chapter 1 for more information about various occupations and the education and training needed for each, You can also contact the professional organizations listed in Appendix 1 for more information.) Some employers will help by giving you a schedule that enables you to attend classes; some have tuition reimbursement programs that will help you with school expenses.

MOVING ON

There are many reasons for leaving a job. It is important to do so for the right ones. No job is perfect, and you want to be sure that leaving is the right decision. Before deciding to resign, conduct an honest self-assessment. Sometimes we are part of the problem without realizing it. If this is the case, leaving a job is not necessarily an effective solution. Seeking ways to improve the situation may be a better plan.

If the dissatisfaction is limited to one department, a transfer to another part of the facility might be a workable solution. Requesting a promotion, if earned, can add needed challenges and interest to work that has become routine.

When considering whether to leave a job, it helps to review the working conditions that are most important to you. Rank them in order of importance and use your list to compare present and potential opportunities. The following list contains common reasons for changing jobs; you may want to add others.

- More opportunities to learn and apply new skills
- Higher level of job security
- Wider variety of duties
- Distribution of duties better suited to the employee's personality
- More education or training benefits available
- Better work schedule
- Opportunity to work with experts in the field of interest
- Better salary and benefits

It is usually advisable to obtain a new job before leaving the old one. Take care, however, that time at the current job is not spent conducting job search activities.

It is also unacceptable to use the current employer's supplies and equipment, such as paper and the copier, for preparing resumes or the fax machine to send them out. If you must attend interviews during the workday, schedule them during mealtimes or use personal time. Prospective employers will respect your efforts to be considerate of your current employer. It is also possible that you will ask the current employer to serve as a future reference. "Don't burn any bridges" is excellent employment advice.

Plan to have adequate savings or financial support if the decision is made to leave the present job before finding a new position. This prevents having to accept the first position that is offered, whether it is satisfactory or not.

Resigning the "right way" helps maintain a positive reputation in the health care community. The following professional courtesies are recommended:

- Give adequate notice. Two to four weeks is considered to be the usual minimum.
- Submit a letter of resignation. See Figure 26–6 for a sample letter.
- Do not list complaints or grievances in the letter.
- Tell your supervisor before telling anyone else at work.
- Complete all tasks and assignments.
- Do not slack off during the last few days.
- Leave everything in order.
- Offer to help train your replacement.

Thank your employer for the opportunity to work and learn. Ask for a reference letter, even if you have been hired elsewhere. You may need it in the future.

Employment situations occasionally present legal and ethical problems. If you are reasonably certain that any of the conditions listed here exist, report them to your supervisor immediately:

- You are required to perform duties that are clearly outside your scope of practice or for which you are not trained.
- Safe practices are not followed.
- Dishonest practices, such as improper insurance billing, are being done.
- Other illegal or unethical activities are allowed or encouraged.

If no corrective actions are taken, then it is appropriate to go up the chain of command and report to the next levels. If your concerns are still not addressed, then resignation may be the wisest alternative. Fortunately, these instances are rare. Most resignations serve as transitions to the next step in a successful career path.

2610 Flanders Court
Tampa, FL 33629
October 5, 20___

Grace Stonefield, Manager
Orthopedic Specialty Group
8884 Orange Parkway
Tampa, FL 33629

Dear Ms. Stonefield:

The purpose of this letter is to advise you of my decision to resign from my position as a Radiologic Technician at OSP. I will be relocating to Nashville in November. My last day of work will be October 25, 20___.

I have enjoyed my work at OSP and especially appreciate being given many opportunities to learn and expand my skills. The dedication to patient care and high level of team cooperation made this an excellent choice for starting my professional career.

Your guidance was especially helpful. Having a supervisor who was willing to give me so many opportunities to learn and take on additional responsibilities was an exceptional benefit. I hope I have a chance in the future to help a new technician in the same way.

I wish you and the staff continued success serving the needs of patients.

Respectfully,

Tyler Adams

Tyler Adams

FIGURE 26-6 Sample letter of resignation.

IF YOU ARE FIRED

Being fired from a job is never a pleasant experience. It can be emotionally upsetting and create doubts about personal worth. Try to remain calm and avoid lashing out verbally in anger or arguing. If this action is unexpected, ask for reasons why you are being fired. If you feel that this is the result of a misunderstanding or misinformation, request an opportunity to explain your side.

Your employer may dread having to dismiss an employee and try to conduct the firing as quickly as possible. They may state that the decision is final and that they are not allowed or willing to discuss it in detail. In this situation it may be best to leave as graciously as possible.

Do not be offended if you are accompanied to your work area, observed as you pack your belongings, and escorted to the door. This is standard procedure that employers are advised to follow. It does not necessarily mean that you are suspected of being dishonest.

Being dismissed can be a learning experience that contributes to future job success. This requires taking a hard look at yourself. The following are common reasons for dismissal:

- Lack of skills needed to perform required tasks
- Refusal to cooperate with supervisor or coworkers
- Theft
- Repeated failure to practice safe techniques
- Breach of patient confidentiality
- Continual attendance problems
- Dishonesty
- Poor interpersonal skills

Be honest with yourself. Blaming others will not help. Only by accepting responsibility can you develop a plan for positive change. Taking charge and making needed

Thinking It Through

Fran Nichols is angry. She can't believe what happened at work today and how unfairly she was treated by her supervisor, Dan Watson, RN. Dan has been on her case from the beginning, always criticizing her work. But she never thought he would actually fire her. Working an 8-hour shift as a nursing assistant is hard work, and it only makes sense to take some shortcuts to complete all the duties. The safety precautions that Dan insisted on were very time consuming and really didn't seem necessary. After all, the patients she worked with didn't have acquired immunodeficiency syndrome (AIDS) or anything, so it didn't really make sense to go to so much trouble with gloves and special waste disposal and so on.

1. Based on the information given, do you believe that Fran's dismissal was fair? Explain your answer.

2. What would you advise Fran if she wants to continue to pursue a career in health care?

changes is an empowering and positive experience. For example, if skills need improvement, contact your school to see if refresher training is available.

At the same time, if you truly believe you were fired because of your age, race, sexual orientation, or other illegal criterion, you may want to seek legal advice.

Feeling depressed after being fired is natural. Seek the support of friends and family. Talk over your feelings with someone you trust. Ask for their help as you conduct your self-assessment and make plans for the future.

SUGGESTED LEARNING ACTIVITIES

1. Learn about a professional organization in your occupational area(s) of interest. Using the list in Appendix 1, visit its website, call, or request information. Are the characteristics needed for successful employment identified? What are they?

2. Conduct an Internet search to investigate a variety of health care occupations. Which ones have the most growth? Which are expected to have increasing staffing needs in the future? In which geographical areas is the fastest growth taking place? What are the current salary ranges?

3. Identify friends, family, and acquaintances who are successful at their jobs. These can be in careers other than health care. Ask them what they believe makes them successful.

4. Prepare a list of questions you would want to know when starting a new job.

5. Look for opportunities to work with others on teams. For example, volunteer for a committee with an organization you are interested in. Help with a project at your child's school. Participate fully on group assignments given in your classes.

WEB ACTIVITIES

Way up

https://www.wayup.com/guide/alphasights-34660-sponsored-1-entry-level-job-advice/

How to Make a Great First Impression at an Entry-Level Job

1. List the suggestions given in the article.
2. Which do you think are the most helpful or important? Explain why.
3. Which can you start preparing for now?
4. Create a plan to implement the suggestions.

https://www.wayup.com/guide/6-things-to-do-in-your-first-week-at-a-new-job/

6 Things to Do in Your First Week at a New Job
   Some great suggestions to consider before starting the new job.

HR Daily Advisor

https://hrdailyadvisor.blr.com/2015/01/07/can-an-employer-prohibit-employees-from-dating-one-another/

Can an Employer Prohibit Employees from Dating One Another?

1. List the reasons given why employee dating is prohibited or discouraged by some employers.
2. Do you agree with these reasons? All? Some? If not, explain why not.

The Balance Career

https://www.thebalancecareers.com/what-you-should-ask-an-employer-when-you-re-fired-2063949

What You Should Ask an Employer When You Are Fired

1. List the questions you should ask.
2. Why is it important that you ask these questions?
3. Would you feel comfortable asking them? Why or why not?

REVIEW QUESTIONS

1. What are five important things a new employee should learn about the facility when starting a job?
2. What is the difference between a policy and a procedure?
3. What are typical contents of an employee handbook?
4. What is the purpose of a probationary period?
5. What is meant by the "chain of command"?
6. What actions should an employee take in order to "give a full day's work"?
7. Why is being a good team member important in health care work?
8. How do good teams contribute to the effectiveness of an organization?
9. What are the ten characteristics of a valued team member?
10. What are six ways you can "go beyond the minimum" at work?

11. What are the ten major employment laws presented in the chapter and what is the purpose of each?

12. What is a grievance and how should an employee handle it if he or she has one?

13. What is the meaning of sexual harassment, including examples, and what steps should a victim take?

14. What is included in a typical employee performance evaluation?

15. What steps should an employee take when leaving a job voluntarily?

16. What can you do to increase your chances of receiving a promotion?

17. What should an employee do when fired from a job?

APPLICATION EXERCISES

1. Refer back to the Case of the Irritating New Hire. Describe all the ways that Katie could have learned about her job to avoid burdening her coworkers with too many questions.

2. Ronnie Martinez, a medical assistant at a busy urgent care center, has an appointment in two weeks with his supervisor, Dr. Barnes, for his first annual performance review. His first review took place about three months after he was hired. At that time, Dr. Barnes indicated that Ronnie's overall performance was satisfactory. He did recommend that Ronnie spend some time working on his venipuncture skills and that he strive to always arrive at work on time, not a couple of minutes after 8 a.m. as sometimes happened. Ronnie feels that he has made progress in these areas. Describe how Ronnie should prepare for his performance evaluation meeting.

PROBLEM-SOLVING PRACTICE

Cameron has been working in the health information management department in a large facility for just over a year. He believes he is doing a good job but does not receive much feedback from his supervisor. He hopes to advance his career and "move up the ladder." How can he apply the five-step problem-solving process to identify ways to achieve career success?

Appendix 1
Health Care Professional Organizations

THERAPEUTIC AND TREATING OCCUPATIONS

Dental Occupations

American Dental Assistants Association
140 N. Bloomingdale Road
Bloomingdale, IL 60108
www.adaausa.org

American Dental Association
211 E. Chicago Avenue
Chicago, IL 60611-2678
www.ada.org

American Dental Hygienists' Association
444 N. Michigan Avenue, Suite # 400
Chicago, IL 60611
www.adha.org

Dental Assisting National Board, Inc.
444 N. Michigan Avenue, Suite 900
Chicago, IL 60611
https://www.danb.org

National Association of Dental Laboratories
325 John Knox Road, # L103
Tallahassee, FL 32303
www.nadl.org

Emergency Medical Occupations

National Association of Emergency Medical Technicians
132-A East Northside Drive
Clinton, MS 39056
www.naemt.org

National Registry of Emergency Medical Technicians
6610 Busch Blvd.
Columbus, OH 43229
www.nremt.org

Society of Emergency Medicine Physician Assistants
4950 W. Royal Lane
Irving, Texas 75063
www.sempa.org

Home-Care and Long-Term Care Occupations

American Health Care Association
1201 L. Street NW
Washington, DC 20005
www.ahcancal.org

National Association for Home Care & Hospice
228 Seventh Street SE
Washington, DC 20003
www.nahc.org

Massage Therapy Occupations

American Massage Therapy Association
500 Davis Street, Suite 900
Evanston, IL 60201
www.amtamassage.org

Associated Body & Massage Professionals
25188 Genesee Trail Road, Suite 200
Golden, CO 80401
www.abmp.com

Medical Office Occupations

American Academy of Physician Assistants
2318 Mill Street, Suite 1300
Alexandria, VA 22314
www.aapa.org

American Association of Medical Assistants
20 N. Wacker Drive, Suite 1575
Chicago, IL 60606
www.aama-ntl.org

American Medical Association
AMA Plaza
330 N. Wabash Avenue
Chicago, IL 60611-5885
www.ama-assn.org

American Medical Technologists Association
10700 W. Higgins, Suite 150
Rosemont, IL 60018
www.americanmedtech.org

American Osteopathic Association
142 East Ontario Street
Chicago, IL 60611
www.osteopathic.org

American Podiatric Medical Association
9312 Old Georgetown Road
Bethesda, MD 20814-1621
www.apma.org

American Society of Podiatric Medical Assistants
109 1st Street
Itasca, IL 60143
www.aspma.org

National Commission on Certification of Physician
   Assistants
12000 Findley Road, Suite 100
Johns Creek, GA 30097-1409
www.nccpa.net

Mental Health Occupations

American Association of Psychiatric Technicians
1220 S. Street, Suite 100
Sacramento, CA 95811-7138
www.psychtechs.org

American Psychiatric Association
800 Maine Ave.
Washington, DC 20024
www.psychiatry.org

American Psychological Association
750 First Street NE
Washington, DC 20002-4242
www.apa.org

Nursing Occupations

American Association of Colleges of Nursing
655 K. Street, NW, Suite 750
Washington, DC 20036
www.aacnnursing.org

American Nurses Association
8515 Georgia Avenue, Suite 400
Silver Spring, MD 20910
www.nursingworld.org

National Association for Practical Nurse Education
   and Service, Inc.
2071 N. Bechtle Avenue PMB 307
Springfield, OH 45504-1583
www.napnes.org

National League for Nursing
The Watergate
2600 Virginia Avenue NW, 8th Floor
Washington, DC 20037
www.nln.org

National Student Nurses' Association
45 Main Street, Suite 606
Brooklyn, NY 11201
www.nsna.org

Occupational Therapy Occupations

American Occupational Therapy Association
4720 Montgomery Lane, Suite 200
Bethesda, MD 20814-3449
www.aota.org

Pharmacy Occupations

American Association of Colleges of Pharmacy
1400 Crystal Drive, Suite 300
Arlington, VA 22202
www.aacp.org

American Pharmacists Association
2215 Constitution Avenue NW
Washington, DC 20037
www.pharmacist.com

Pharmacy Technician Certification Board
2215 Constitution Avenue NW, Suite 101
Washington, DC 20037
www.ptcb.org

Physical Therapy Occupations

American Physical Therapy Association
1111 North Fairfax Street
Alexandria, VA 22314-1488
www.apta.org

Respiratory Therapy Occupations

American Association for Respiratory Care
9425 N. MacArthur Boulevard, Suite 100
Irving, TX 75063-4706
www.aarc.org

Commission on Accreditation for Respiratory Care
P.O. Box 54876
Hurst, TX 76054-4876
www.coarc.com

National Board for Respiratory Care
10801 Mastin Street, Suite 300
Overland Park, KS 66210
www.nbrc.org

Surgical Occupations

Association of Surgical Technologists
6 West Dry Creek Circle, Suite 200
Littleton, CO 80120
www.ast.org

Veterinary Occupations

American Veterinary Medical Association
1931 N. Meacham Road, Suite 100
Schaumburg, IL 60173-4360
www.avma.org

National Association of Veterinary Technicians in America
1931 N. Meacham Road
Schaumburg, IL 60173
www.navta.net

Vision Care Occupations

American Optometric Association
243 N. Lindbergh Boulevard, Flr 1
St. Louis, MO 63141-7881
www.aoa.org

Association of Schools and Colleges of Optometry
6110 Executive Boulevard, Suite 420
Rockville, MD 20852
https://optometriceducation.org

Joint Commission on Allied Health Personnel in
    Ophthalmology
2025 Woodlane Drive
St. Paul, MN 55125-2998
www.jcahpo.org

Opticians Association of America
3740 Canada Road
Lakeland, TN 38002
www.oaa.org

DIAGNOSTIC OCCUPATIONS

Diagnostic Imaging Occupations

Alliance of Cardiovascular Professionals
P.O. Box 2007
Midlothian, VA 23113
www.acp-online.org

American College of Cardiology
Heart House
2400 N Street NW
Washington, DC 20037
https://www.acc.org

American College of Radiology
1891 Preston White Drive
Reston, VA 20191
www.acr.org

American Registry of Diagnostic Medical Sonographers
1401 Rockville Pike, Suite 600
Rockville, MD 20852-1402
www.ardms.org

American Registry of Radiologic Technologists
1255 Northland Drive
St. Paul, MN 55120
www.arrt.org

American Society of Echocardiography
2530 Meridian Parkway, Suite 450
Durham, NC 27713
www.asecho.org

American Society of Radiologic Technologists
15000 Central Avenue SE
Albuquerque, NM 87123-3909
www.asrt.org

Cardiovascular Credentialing International
1500 Sunday Drive, Suite 102
Raleigh, NC 27607
www.cci-online.org

International Society for Magnetic Resonance in Medicine
2300 Clayton Road, #620
Concord, CA 94520
www.ismrm.org

Joint Review Committee on Education in Diagnostic
   Medical Sonography
6021 University Boulevard, Suite 500
Ellicott City, MD 21043
www.jrcdms.org

Society of Diagnostic Medical Sonography
2745 Dallas Parkway, Suite 350
Plano, TX 75093-8730
www.sdms.org

Society of Vascular Ultrasound
4601 Presidents Drive, Suite 260
Lanham, MD 20706-4831
www.svunet.org

Medical Laboratory Occupations

American Medical Technologists Association
10700 W. Higgins Road, Suite 150
Rosemont, IL 60018
www.americanmedtech.org

American Society for Clinical Laboratory Science
1861 International Drive, Suite 200
McLean, VA 22102
www.ascls.org

American Society for Clinical Pathology
33 W. Monroe Street, Suite 1600
Chicago, IL 60603
www.ascp.org

HEALTH INFORMATION MANAGEMENT OCCUPATIONS

American Academy of Procedural Coders
2480 South 3850 West, Suite B
Salt Lake City, UT 84120
www.aapc.com

American Health Information Management Association
233 N. Michigan Avenue, 21st Floor
Chicago, IL 60601-5809
www.ahima.org

American Medical Billing Association
2465 E. Main
Davis, OK 73030
www.ambanet.net/AMBA.htm

Association for Healthcare Documentation Integrity
4120 Dale Road, Suite J8-233
Modesto, CA 95356
www.ahdionline.org

ENVIRONMENTAL OCCUPATIONS
Biomedical Engineering Occupations

Association for the Advancement of Medical
   Instrumentation
4301 N. Fairfax Drive, Suite 301
Arlington, VA 22203-1633
www.aami.org

Biomedical Engineering Society
8201 Corporate Drive, Suite 1125
Landover, MD 20785-2224
www.bmes.org

Dietary Services Occupations

American Dietetic Association
120 South Riverside Plaza, Suite 2000
Chicago, IL 60606-6995
2nd location—Washington office:
1120 Connecticut Avenue NW, Suite 480
Washington, DC 20036
www.eatright.org

Appendix 2
Useful Spanish Expressions for Health Care Professionals

Hello, hi.	Hola. (OH-lah)
Good morning.	Buenos días. (bway-nohs DEE-ahs)
Good afternoon.	Buenas tardes. (bway-nahs TAR-days)
Good evening, good night.	Buenas noches. (bway-nahs NO-chase)
Please.	Por favor. (por fah-VOR)
Thank you.	Gracias. (GRAH-see-us)
You're welcome.	De nada. (day NAH-dah)
Yes/No.	Sí/No (see/no)
My name is _____	Me llamo (may YAH-mo) _____ or
	Mi nombre es (me NOM-bray es) _____
What is your name?	¿Cómo se llama usted? (CO-mo say YA-mah oo-STED)
Nice to meet you.	Mucho gusto. (MOO-choh GOO-stoh)
Do you speak English?	¿Habla usted inglés? (AH-blah oo-STED eeng-GLACE)
Do you understand English?	¿Comprende usted inglés? (comb-PREN-day oo-STED eeng-GLACE)
Do you understand me?	¿Me comprende usted? (may comb-PREN-day oo-STED)
Repeat, please.	Repita usted, por favor. (ray-PEE-tah oo-STED por fah-VOR)
I don't understand Spanish very well.	No comprendo el español muy bien. (no comb-PREN-doh el es-pahn-NYOL moo-ee bee-EN)
How do you feel?	¿Cómo se siente? (CO-mo say see-EN-tay)
Good.	Bien. (bee-EN)
Fair.	Así, así or Regular. (ah-SEE, ah-SEE or ray-goo-LAHR)
Bad.	Mal. (mahl)
Do you have pain?	¿Tiene usted dolor? (tee-EN-ay oo-STED do-LOR)
Where?	¿Dónde? (DOHN-day)
Show me.	Enséñeme. (en-SEN-yeh-may)

Are you comfortable?	¿Está usted cómodo? (es-TAH oo-STED CO-mo-do)
What's the matter?	¿Qué pasa? (kay PAH-sah)
Do you want something?	¿Desea usted algo? (deh-SAY-ah oo-STED AHL-go)
It is important.	Es importante. (es eem-por-TAHN-tay)
Be calm, please.	Cálmese usted, por favor. (CALL-meh-say oo-STED, por fah-VOR)
Don't be frightened.	No tenga usted miedo. (no TANG-gah oo-STED mee-EH-doh)
We are here to help you.	Estamos aquí para ayudarle. (eh-STAH-mos ah-KEY pah-rah ah-you-DAR-lay)

Glossary

Abdominal cavity Located in the abdomen; contains the stomach, intestines, liver, gallbladder, pancreas, and spleen.

Account payable Amount owed to another business for services, supplies, or equipment.

Account receivable Amount due from a customer for services, supplies, or equipment.

Acronyms Abbreviations in which groups of letters are formed by taking the first letter of each word of a phrase.

Active listening Listening characterized by focusing fully on what a speaker is saying.

Acupuncture Chinese medicine treatment in which tiny needles are inserted into specific points in the body to alleviate pain and relieve various physical, mental, and emotional conditions.

Adult Someone who is 18 years of age or older.

Adult foster home A setting such as a family-style home that provides 24-hour personal care, meals, and supervision for a small number of residents.

Advance directives Written documents that detail the patient's wishes regarding health care decisions; consist of the living will and the durable power of attorney.

Adverse drug events Harm experienced by patients as a result of exposure to medications.

Advocate One who supports or promotes the interests of others.

Aerobic Requires oxygen to live.

Aerobic exercise A type of exercise that elevates the heart rate beyond normal resting rate.

Afebrile A temperature that is within the normal range.

Agency for Healthcare Research and Quality (AHRQ) Federal agency with the goals of enhancing the quality, appropriateness, and effectiveness of health care services.

Agenda A list of what is to take place at a meeting.

Agent Someone who has the authority to represent another person.

AIDS A disease that occurs when an HIV-positive person develops signs and symptoms of a weakened immune system.

Alternative medicine Health care systems, practices, and products that have not traditionally been performed by practitioners of Western medicine; practices used *instead of* conventional medicine.

Alzheimer's disease Progressive, degenerative disorder that attacks the brain's nerve cells resulting in memory loss, impaired thinking and language skills, and changes in behavior.

Ambulatory services Also known as **outpatient services**, they provide diagnostic, treatment, and rehabilitation services for patients who do not require hospitalization.

Amino acids Molecules that are the building blocks of protein.

Anaerobic Does not require oxygen to live.

Anaphylactic shock A life-threatening, severe allergic reaction resulting in swelling of the respiratory system that restricts breathing.

Anatomical position The body as viewed in a full upright position (standing), with the arms relaxed at the sides of the body, palms facing forward, feet pointed forward, and the eyes directed straight ahead.

Anatomy The study of the form and structure of an organism.

Angles The amounts of variance from a reference plane expressed in degrees.

Anorexia nervosa A disease based on the distorted belief that one is overweight, even when severely underweight, and the cutting of calories below the number necessary to maintain health.

Anterior (ventral) Toward the front of the body.

Anterior body cavity Consists of the thoracic, abdominal, and pelvic cavities; protects the internal organs; also called ventral body cavity.

Antibiotic Classification of medications capable of inhibiting the growth of, or destroying, microorganisms.

Antibodies Protective proteins that combat pathogens.

Antioxidants Substances that reduce damage in the body due to oxygen.

Antiseptics Chemical agents that prevent or inhibit growth of microorganisms.

Apex At the top (highest point).

Apnea Absence of respirations.

Apothecary system A measurement system that is used infrequently except for a measurement of weight (grain).

Artificial intelligence Sophisticated technology that enables machines and/or computers to make decisions traditionally believed to require human intelligence.

Asepsis (aseptic technique) Methods used to make the patient, the professional, and the environment as pathogen-free as possible.

Asking questions A communication technique used to request clarification and additional information.

Assault Any threatened or implied act, whether carried out or not.

Assertiveness The ability to express oneself freely in a non-threatening manner.

Assessment Gathering information; a step in charting the health care professional's impression of what is wrong with the patient, based on the signs and symptoms.

Assisted living residence Facility that provides housing, meals, and personal care to individuals who need help with daily living activities, but do not need daily nursing care; may also be referred to as supportive housing, residential long-term care facilities, adult residential care facilities, board-and-care, and rest homes.

Attitude How one mentally views a situation.

Autonomy Self-determination.

Bacteria One-celled microorganisms that can be either pathogenic or nonpathogenic.

Bacteriocidal A method or chemical that kills bacteria; also called germicidal.

Bacteriostatic A method or chemical that inhibits the growth of bacteria.

Barriers Blocks to communication.

Base At the bottom (lowest point).

Baseline Information obtained during a patient's history and physical exam.

Basic formula A method for converting and calculating drug dosages.

Battery Unauthorized touching of another person.

Behavioral questions Job-interview questions in which the applicant is given a situation and asked how he or she would handle it; or the applicant is asked to describe how he or she handled a real-life situation in the past.

Biases Having certain beliefs and feelings, usually negative, about a person because he or she belongs to a specific group or has certain characteristics. (Also known as prejudice.)

Binge eating The compulsive consumption of large quantities of food, beyond that needed to satisfy physical hunger.

Bioinformatics The organization of biological data into databases.

Bioterrorism Microbes or toxins used as weapons.

Block letter A written format in which all lines are flush with the left margin.

Body mass index (BMI) Measurement of the relationship of weight to height using a mathematical formula.

Body mechanics The correct positioning of the body for a given task, such as lifting a heavy object or typing; when the correct muscles are used and the body is in alignment, good body mechanics are being demonstrated.

Body systems Combinations of two or more organs to provide major body functions.

Bradycardia A heart rate that is below the normal range.

Bradypnea A respiratory rate that is below the normal range.

Breach of contract When one of the parties in a contract fails to fulfill its part of the agreement.

Bulimia Condition characterized by compulsive eating of huge quantities of food, followed by self-induced vomiting and/or the use of large amounts of laxatives.

Burnout A form of physical and emotional exhaustion that is caused by a variety of personal and environmental stressors experienced over an extended period of time.

Calories Units of heat energy; energy content of foods.

Capitation Payment of a fixed fee by an insurance company to a health care provider for each patient enrolled in a health care plan, regardless of services given to the patient.

Carbohydrates Food substances that are composed of units of sugar and provide the body with immediate energy.

Cardiopulmonary resuscitation (CPR) Manually providing respiratory and cardiac support for a patient who is not breathing and whose heart has stopped beating.

Carpal tunnel syndrome Compression of the median nerve as it travels through the wrist at the carpal tunnel.

Career ladders The various levels within an occupational area that require different amounts of education and training.

Caudal Closer to the coccyx (lower back).

Cell Smallest living structure of the body.

Celsius (C) Measurement of temperature based on a freezing point of 0° and a boiling point of 100°; also known as centigrade.

Centers for Disease Control and Prevention (CDC) A government agency that formulates safety guidelines to help prevent and control the spread of infectious diseases.

Cephalic (cranial) Closer to the head.

Certification The process of determining whether a person has met predetermined standards.

Chain of command The organization of employees in which each person reports to a supervisor who, in turn, reports to another supervisor at the next higher level.

Chain of infection Defines the six criteria that must be present for an infection to develop.

Charting Recording observations and information about patients.

Cheyne-Stokes A breathing pattern that has a period of apnea followed by a gradually increasing depth and frequency of respirations.

Chief complaint The patient's statement of the main reason he or she is seeking medical care.

Chiropractic Health care practice based on the belief that pressure on the nerves leaving the spinal column causes pain and dysfunction of the body part served by that nerve.

Cholesterol Waxy substance necessary to build cells but which in excess can clog arteries.

ChooseMyPlate Icon developed by the U.S. Department of Agriculture in 2011 to illustrate healthy food choices.

Chronic illness Health problem of long duration in which the disease condition shows little change or slowly gets progressively worse.

Chronological resume Employment resume that emphasizes work experience; the employment history section describes previous jobs in some detail.

Clinical depression Severe, persistent depression marked by specific symptoms, such as insomnia, feelings of worthlessness, and inability to experience pleasure in activities previously enjoyed.

Closed fracture When a bone is broken but does not protrude through the skin.

Closed-ended questions Inquiries that can be answered with a single word or a response of "yes" or "no."

Cloud storage Storage of digital data on multiple servers and sometimes at multiple locations.

Codes of ethics Principles created by professional organizations to serve as guides for the conduct of health care professionals in those occupations.

Cognitive development The growth of intellectual processes of thought, awareness, and the ability to rationally comprehend the world and determine meaning.

Coinsurance A cost-sharing provision in a health insurance contract that stipulates that the insured person is to assume a percentage of the costs of covered services.

Cold calling Calling or visiting employers to make the first contact.

Combining forms Root words plus vowels, in medical terms.

Combining vowel The letters *a, e, i, o,* or *u* when used to link the root word to the next element in a medical term.

Communicable disease A disease that can be transmitted either directly or indirectly from one individual to another.

Communication Process in which messages are exchanged and meanings interpreted between a sender and a receiver.

Compassion The sincere concern for others, especially those who are anxious, fearful, and in pain.

Compatibility The ability to be combined without unfavorable results.

Complementary medicine Health care practices, products, and approaches to health care that have not traditionally been performed in conventional medical offices; practices used *together* with conventional medicine.

Computer literate Having the knowledge and skills to efficiently perform the computer tasks required in one's work, as well as a basic understanding of how computers work and what types of health care applications are currently available.

Confidentiality Preserving the legal right of a patient to privacy concerning his or her medical affairs.

Consent To give permission; permission that is given.

Consonant Any letter except *a, e, i, o,* and *u.*

Constructive criticism Appropriate feedback on the performance of others, based on the belief that it can be improved.

Contaminated Infectious material is present.

Continuing care community Provides a variety of living arrangements that support lifestyles as they change from independent living to the need for regular medical and nursing care.

Continuing education Learning experiences beyond those needed to earn the initial certificate or degree to work in an occupation.

Continuing education unit (CEU) A credit granted for certain types of learning that take place after the completion of formal education; same as continuing professional education (CPE).

Continuing medical education (CME) Education and/or training to stay up-to-date in one's profession and/or to earn continuing education credits.

Continuing professional education (CPE) Education and/or training to stay up-to-date in one's profession and/or to earn continuing education credits.

Contraction The combined form of two words; for example, it is = it's.

Contracts Promises that are enforceable by law.

Controlled substance Prescription drug that has the potential for addiction.

Converting the fractions Changing all the denominators to the same number in order to add or subtract the fractions.

Copay The set amount that the patient pays when medical services are received.

Cost of money The amount that is lost when money is not invested; often used to refer to money that is owed to a business, but not collected in a timely way.

Cover letters Written documents sent with resumes as a way to introduce oneself and inform the employer why the resume is being sent.

Cranial cavity Located in the skull; contains the brain.

Cross-training Training that health care employees are given to perform tasks in addition to those traditionally assigned to their job titles.

Culture The values, shared beliefs and attitudes, social organizations, family and personal relationships, language, everyday activities, religious practices, and concepts of time and space of a given group of people.

Current Procedural Terminology (CPT) codes Numerical codes assigned to diseases and conditions, also known as diagnoses.

Damages Money to compensate for an injury or loss.

Database The organization of computerized information in a structured way that makes it easy to sort and access.

Decimals A linear arrangement of numbers based on units of 10, containing a point (decimal point) to separate the whole number from the fractional part of a number (e.g., 2.5).

Deductible An amount required to be paid under a health insurance contract by the insured before benefits become payable.

Deductive reasoning Drawing a logical conclusion from one or more statements.

Deep Farther from the body surface.

Defamation of character A legal charge for disclosing unauthorized information that could harm the reputation of another.

Defense mechanisms Behaviors that are usually performed unconsciously in response to perceived threats to self-esteem; often provide temporary relief from mental discomfort and anxiety.

Degrees Units of measurement used in angles, temperature readings, and depth of burns.

Dementia Decline in memory and/or other thinking skills.

Development The mental, emotional, and social growth of individuals as they progress through life stages.

Diagnosis Determination of a disease or syndrome.

Diagnostic Pertaining to identifying and determining the cause and extent of diseases and injuries.

Diagnostic procedures Tests performed to determine the diagnosis.

Diagnostic-related groups (DRGs) A classification system of patients based on their diagnoses to predetermine Medicare payments.

Diet The foods people habitually eat.

Discreet Being careful about what you say, preserving confidences, and respecting privacy.

Diseases Abnormal conditions created when the normal anatomy and physiology of the body are altered.

Disinfectants Agents or methods that destroy most bacteria and viruses.

Distal Farther from the reference base point.

Dominant culture Beliefs and behavior that are generally considered to be foundational for a society or country.

Durable power of attorney for health care Document, sometimes called a "health care power of attorney," in which an individual designates specific people to act on their behalf if they become unable to make health care decisions.

Dyspnea Labored breathing or difficulty with breathing.

Electronic health records (EHRs) Digital versions of patient records, such as history and physical, physician's orders, and test results. (Also called electronic medical records.)

Electronic mail A means of creating and sending messages from one computer to another, using the Internet system of networks. Commonly called e-mail.

Electronic medical records (EMRs) Digital versions of patient records, such as history and physical, physician's orders, and test results. (Also called electronic health records.)

Electronic spreadsheet Software that permits the user to apply the computer's ability to perform high-speed calculations of numerical data.

Emancipated minors Individuals younger than age 18 who are financially independent, married, or in the military.

Emergency preparedness plan Policy and procedures to be followed when an event occurs that has the potential to kill or injure a group of people.

Empathy Striving to understand another person's attitudes, feelings, and behavior.

Employee handbook A source of employment policies.

Environmental safety The identification and correction of potential hazards that can cause accidents and injuries.

Epidemics Widespread occurrences of infectious diseases.

Eponyms Terms identifying diseases, body structures, and procedures that are named for the person who identified or discovered them.

Ergonomics The science of designing and arranging things in the working and living environments to ensure maximum efficiency, health, and safety; a good ergonomic environment maximizes the comfort level and efficiency of the person while limiting possible exposure to discomfort or potential injury.

Erikson's stages of psychosocial development A theory based on the psychosocial challenges that are presented to individuals as they progress through life stages.

Estimating Expressing the approximate answer.

Ethical dilemma When the underlying principles of an ethical system appear to contradict each other and no clear answer emerges.

Ethics A system of principles (fundamental truths) a society develops to guide decision making about what is right and wrong; it helps people deal with difficult and complex problems that lack easy answers.

Etiology Study of the causes of diseases.

Etiquette Manners; acceptable conduct.

Eupnea Breathing that is within the normal range, is unlabored, and has an even rhythm.

Euthanasia Performing a deliberate action that results in a painless, easy death for individuals with an incurable disease; same as mercy killing.

Exclusive provider organization (EPO) A hybrid of an HMO and PPO in which services are covered only if providers and hospitals are in the plan's network, except in emergencies.

Exertion injuries Injuries caused by lifting, pulling, and pushing.

Exhalation The part of the respiratory cycle in which air is removed from the lungs.

Expanding consciousness A theory developed by Margaret Newman, RN, to assist patients in making their lives as meaningful as possible by focusing on their possibilities rather than their limitations.

Expenditures The money that must be spent in the process of doing business (e.g., the cost of resources required to maintain a health care delivery system).

Express consent Permission that is given orally or in writing to receive treatment; more formal than implied consent.

Express contract Result of the parties in a contract discussing and agreeing on specific terms and conditions.

External bleeding When blood drains to the outside of the body through a break in the skin.

External customers People who come to the health care provider for services; they may be referred to as customers, patients, or clients.

Fahrenheit (F) Measurement of temperature based on a freezing point of 32° and a boiling point of 212°.

False imprisonment A legal claim patients can charge if they are held against their will, unless they are mentally incompetent or a danger to themselves or others.

Fats Food substances that contain fatty acids and provide the most concentrated form of energy for the body.

Febrile A temperature that is elevated above the normal range.

Feedback A method by which participants in a communication encounter can check their understanding of the messages exchanged.

Fee-for-service Method of payment in which the patient pays the health care provider an amount from an established schedule of fees.

Fiber A substance in food that cannot be fully digested.

Fiber optics Technology that uses hair-thin cables to transmit data.

Fields Basic data categories in a database.

File A group of related computer records or documents.

Financing The source of money used to run a business.

First aid Emergency care provided to an accident victim or to someone who has become suddenly ill.

Flammable Easily set on fire; same as inflammable.

Fractional equation A method for solving proportion math problems.

Fractions A method used to express numbers that are not whole numbers; a fraction is read as parts (numerator) to a whole (denominator).

Fraud A form of dishonesty that involves cheating or trickery.

Free radicals Molecules that have unpaired, highly reactive electrons. In the body, they can damage normal cells.

Frontal plane Divides the body vertically into front and back portions.

Frostbite Condition in which the skin begins to freeze.

Functional resume Employment resume that emphasizes professional and general qualifications rather than one's work history.

Fungi (pl. of fungus) Microorganisms that represent a large group of organisms that are neither plant nor animal. They have unique characteristics that are not shared by other organisms and are thus placed in a kingdom of their own.

Gatekeepers Health care providers, often physicians, who serve as the patient's first contact when entering the health care system; also known as primary care providers.

Gene therapy The insertion of normal DNA into cells to correct a genetic defect or to treat certain diseases.

Genetics Determines one's inherited characteristics.

Germ theory A theory that states that specific microorganisms called bacteria are the cause of specific diseases in both humans and animals.

Gilligan's stages of the ethics of care A theory identifying the stages of development in women based on their caring effects on human relationships.

Golden rule A primary principle when assisting others, meaning to "do no further harm."

Good Samaritan Act A law to protect individuals from liability when they stop to assist someone who has been hurt or is ill.

Gram The basic metric unit for measuring weight.

Grammar A set of rules that determines proper word order, sentence construction, punctuation, and capitalization.

Grievance A formal complaint about a circumstance considered to be unfair or potentially harmful.

Growth Refers to the physical changes that normally take place as the body matures.

Health disparities Differences in the health status of different groups of people.

Health literacy The ability to obtain, process, and understand basic health information and services needed to make appropriate health decisions.

Hemorrhage Severe, heavy bleeding.

Hepatitis B A virus that causes a blood-borne infection. An occupational hazard for health care professionals.

HIPAA (Health Insurance Portability and Accountability Act of 1996) Government law mandating significant changes in the legal and regulatory environment governing the provision of health benefits, the delivery and payment of health care services, and the privacy and security of individually identifiable, protected health information in written, electronic, and oral formats.

Hippocrates Physician in ancient Greece, often referred to as the Father of Medicine.

HIV Abbreviation for human immunodeficiency virus that causes acquired immune deficiency syndrome (AIDS).

HIV positive The condition of being infected by the human immunodeficiency virus.

Holistic medicine Health care practices based on the belief that all aspects of the individual—physical, mental, emotional, spiritual, and environmental—contribute to states of health and disease.

Homeopathy A health care practice that is based on the idea that "like cures like." Disorders are treated with very small amounts of the natural substances that cause symptoms of the same disorder in healthy people.

Homeostasis Tendency of a cell or the whole organism to maintain a state of balance.

Hospice A facility or service that offers palliative (relieves but does not cure) care and support to dying patients and their families.

Hosts Living plants or animals from which microorganisms derive nourishment.

Household system A measurement system based on common household items used to measure length, volume, and weight.

Hypertension Condition in which the blood pressure is above the normal range.

Hyperthermia Condition in which the body temperature is above the normal range.

Hypotension Condition in which the blood pressure is below the normal range.

Hypothermia Condition in which the body temperature is below the normal range.

Illegal questions Job-interview questions that request information that cannot legally be used to make a hiring decision.

Illness A state experienced by the body when one or more of the control systems loses the ability to maintain homeostasis.

Immune response Defense used by the body to fight infection and disease by producing antibodies.

Implicit bias Bias that is unconscious and outside our immediate intentional control.

Implicit racism Racism outside one's consciousness or awareness.

Implied consent Permission for procedures indicated by the patient's actions; for example, showing up for a medical appointment. Or in an emergency situation when the patient is unable to give consent.

Implied contracts When the actions of the parties create contracts without them being detailed in a written format.

Improper fractions A fraction in which the numerator is larger than the denominator.

Incident report Written document that is filled out when any unexpected situation occurs that can cause harm to a patient, an employee, or any other person.

Independent clauses Parts of sentences that can stand on their own as complete sentences.

Infection control Procedures to be followed to prevent the spread of infectious diseases.

Infectious disease Disease caused by growth of pathogens.

Inferior Below.

Inflammable Easily set on fire; same as flammable.

Informed consent Permission given for a procedure to be performed after it and any possible consequences have been explained.

Inhalation The part of the respiratory cycle in which air enters the lungs.

Inpatient Admitted to, and treated within, a hospital.

Inservice training Training offered by an employer specific to the needs of employees.

Integrative medicine Combines treatments from conventional medicine with complementary and/or alternative medicine for which there is high-quality scientific evidence of safety and effectiveness; also called integrated medicine.

Integrity A personal characteristic reflected as honesty; choosing the right rather than the easy way; conducting oneself honestly and morally.

Integumentary The skin.

Intermediate nursing care facility (INCF) A type of nursing home that provides personal care, social services, and regular nursing care for individuals who do not require 24-hour nursing, but are unable to care for themselves.

Internal bleeding Blood loss that occurs inside the body.

Internal customers People who work within the health care industry—in other words, other health care professionals.

Internet A vast global system of computer networks linked with other networks that allows instant communication and the sharing of information.

International Classification of Diseases (ICD-10) codes List of numbers assigned to diseases and conditions.

Invasive procedures Punctures or incisions of the skin or insertion of instruments or foreign material into the body.

Job descriptions Lists of duties, responsibilities, and other important information about a specific job title.

Job interview A conversation between an applicant and a potential employer to determine if there is a match between the needs of the employer and the qualifications of the applicant.

Joint dislocation When a joint becomes disconnected from its socket.

Justice Fairness.

Kohlberg's moral stages A theory identifying the stages of moral development in humans.

Lasers Focused light rays that can cut and remove tissue.

Lateral Away from the center of body (toward the sides).

Leadership An approach to working with others that encourages people to work together and do their best to achieve common goals.

Leading questions Inquiries in which all or part of the answer is included in the wording of the question.

Learning objectives Educational goals; what students are to accomplish as the result of a lesson.

Legislation Laws.

Legumes Plants with seed pods that split along the sides when ripe. Foods that are legumes include peas, beans, peanuts, lentils, and soybeans.

Letters of recommendation Statements written on a job applicant's behalf by former employers and other professionals.

Libel A legal charge for defamation of character (damaging someone's reputation) committed in a written form.

Licensure A designation that means a person has been granted permission to legally perform certain acts.

Life review Telling the events of one's life as a form of self-evaluation and closure as the end of life approaches.

Lifelong learning All purposeful learning activities, both formal and informal, that take place throughout our lives.

Liter The basic metric unit for measuring volume.

Living will The part of an advance directive that outlines the individual's wishes regarding the type and extent of medical care to be given.

Malpractice Professional negligence.

Managed care Promotion of cost-effective health care through the management and control of its delivery.

Manual dexterity Skill in working with one's hands.

Massage therapy Manipulation of soft tissues by rubbing or kneading to achieve health benefits.

Math anxiety A strong negative reaction to math that interferes with the ability to concentrate, learn, and perform math calculations.

Medial Toward the midline or center of the body.

Medic Alert An organization that provides bracelets or pendants for patients to wear that contain information or warnings about specific medical problems.

Medicaid Federally funded but state-administered insurance plan for individuals who qualify due to low income.

Medical asepsis (clean technique) Procedures to decrease the numbers and spread of pathogens in the environment.

Medical documentation Notes and documents that health care professionals add to a patient's medical record.

Medical history Data collected on a patient that includes personal, familial, and social information.

Medical malls Facilities that offer a variety of outpatient services, some of which were previously provided by hospitals.

Medical record The collection of all documents that are filed together and form a complete chronological health history of a particular patient.

Medical terminology A language used by health care professionals that includes specialized terms and abbreviations.

Medicare A federally funded insurance program that is part of the Social Security Administration and provides health insurance for people aged 65 and older and others, such as the severely disabled, who qualify for social security.

Medication adherence Taking prescribed medications correctly as per timing, dosage, and frequency.

Meditation A process for quieting the mind by clearing it of thoughts.

Mentor A combination of coach and advisor who can provide information and encouragement.

Mercy killing Performing a deliberate action that results in a painless, easy death for individuals with an incurable disease; same as euthanasia.

Metabolism Processing and combining of nutrients to form tissue and/or produce energy for the body.

Meter Basic metric unit for measuring length.

Metric system A measurement system based on tens; basic units are length (meter), volume (liter), and weight (gram).

Microbes Microorganisms that are pathogenic.

Microorganisms Small, usually one-celled living plants or animals.

Microscope Instrument fitted with a powerful magnifying lens.

Midsagittal plane Passes through the midline and divides the body vertically into equal right and left portions.

Military time A method of telling time that is based on a 24-hour clock.

Minerals Substances derived from nonliving matter that the body needs in small quantities to grow and function properly.

Minimum wage The lowest hourly amount that an employee can legally be paid.

Mixed number A whole number and a fraction, such as 1½.

Modified block letter A written format in which all lines are flush with the left margin except the date, closing, and signature.

Muscle relaxation Releasing tension in the muscles.

Mutate When referring to bacteria, means they change in ways that reduce or eliminate the effectiveness of antibiotics to destroy them.

Negligence Failure to meet the standard of care that can be reasonably expected from a person with certain training and experiences.

Negotiated fees Amount negotiated between insurance companies and health care groups for the cost of services; depending on the plan, the patient either pays the difference in actual cost of service or the health care group accepts the negotiated amount as payment in full.

Networking Developing relationships with individuals who might help you meet your professional goals or secure job leads.

Networks Systems of computers that are linked so they can communicate and share data.

Neutropenic precautions Isolation procedures to protect an immunocompromised patient from infections.

Nomenclature Method of naming.

Nonverbal communication Meaning conveyed by tone of voice, body language, gestures, facial expressions, touch, and physical appearance.

Normal flora Microorganisms that commonly reside in a particular environment on or in the body.

Nosocomial infection Infection that occurs while the patient is receiving health care.

Nursing homes Facilities for the care of individuals who do not require hospitalization, but who do need general nursing care and assistance performing daily living activities.

Nutrients Substances needed by the body to grow and function properly.

Nutrition The process of obtaining food necessary for health and growth.

Obese A BMI of 30.0 or higher, which indicates the presence of considerably more body fat than is considered to be healthy.

Objective As an adjective, approaching situations from a factual rather than an emotional perspective; as a noun, a statement of your job goal.

Objective data Direct observations made by the health care professional to evaluate a patient's condition.

Occupational Safety and Health Administration (OSHA) A government agency that establishes minimum health and safety standards for the workplace and has the authority to enforce those standards.

Open fracture When a broken bone protrudes through the skin.

Open-ended questions Inquiries that require more than a one-word response; used to encourage patients to provide more detailed information or explanations.

Opinions Beliefs that are not based on certainty or are made without researching the facts.

Opioids pain medication Medications that relieve pain by reducing the intensity of pain signals reaching the brain.

Opportunistic infection Infection that occurs due to the weakened physiological state of the body.

Organic Relating to, or derived from, living matter.

Organic foods The results of certain methods of growing food and raising livestock, including the use of natural rather than chemical fertilizers and pesticides.

Organism The body as a whole.

Orthopnea When a patient has difficulty breathing unless in a sitting or standing position.

Orthostatic (postural) hypotension Rapid lowering of the blood pressure as a result of changing positions.

Osteopathy Health care practices based on the belief that the body can protect itself against disease if the musculoskeletal system, especially the spine, is in good order.

Osteoporosis Condition in which the bones lose their density and become fragile and more likely to fracture.

Outpatient services Health care services that do not require hospitalization; also referred to as ambulatory services.

Overweight A BMI of 25.0 to 29.9, which indicates the presence of more body fat than is considered healthy.

Palliative Reducing pain or severity of a disease or condition rather than curing it.

Pandemics Rapidly spreading diseases that attack many people at the same time.

Pantomime Using body movement and gestures to convey ideas or actions.

Paraphrasing Rewording the sender's message in the listener's own words and asking the sender for confirmation.

Parasite Organism that nourishes itself at the expense of other living things and causes them damage.

PASS Acronym for proper use of a portable fire extinguisher. (**P**ull the pin. **A**im the nozzle at the base of the fire. **S**queeze the handle. **S**weep back and forth along the base of the fire.)

Pathogens Disease-causing microorganisms.

Pathophysiology The study of why diseases occur and how the body reacts to them (changes in function caused by disease).

Patient Care Partnership New name for the American Hospital Association's Patient's Bill of Rights which contains 12 rights of hospitalized patients.

Pelvic cavity Located in the lower abdomen; contains the urinary bladder, rectum, and reproductive organs.

Percentages A method used to express a whole or part of a whole. The whole is written as 100%.

Performance evaluation An evaluation and rating of an employee's performance; also referred to as a performance review.

Peripheral Anatomical term meaning away from the center.

Personal health records (PHRs) Documents created and maintained by an individual patient to assist him or her in communicating with various health care providers to ensure greater continuity of care.

Personal space The distance at which people feel comfortable when carrying on a conversation.

Personalized medicine The prevention, diagnosis, and treatment of disease based on each patient's own biochemical makeup. (Also called precision medicine.)

Philosophy of individual worth A view based on the belief that every human being, regardless of personal circumstances or personal qualities, has worth.

Physical development The growth of the body, including motor sensory adaptation.

Physiological needs Level 1 in Maslow's hierarchy of needs that must be satisfied in order to maintain life; these needs include oxygen, water, and food.

Physiology The study of the functions (how and why something works) of an organism.

Piaget's cognitive stages A theory identifying the cognitive (intellectual) stages of development in children.

Plagiarism Copying the work of someone else and presenting it as one's own work.

Plan A step in SOAP charting that documents the procedures, treatments, and patient instructions that make up the patient's care.

Point-of-care charting Entering information about patients into the computer when at the patient's home or health care facility bedside.

Point of service (POS) An HMO and PPO hybrid in which members can see an in-network provider for a reduced rate or out-of-network provider for a higher rate.

Policies Rules established and followed by an organization.

Portfolio An organized collection of written documents to show to employers to support claims about a job applicant's qualifications.

Posterior (dorsal) Toward the back of the body.

Posterior body cavity Consists of the cranial and spinal cavity; protects the structures of the nervous system; also called dorsal body cavity.

Preauthorization Approval from an insurance company prior to receiving certain health care services, for the purposes of determining medical necessity and cost effectiveness.

Preferred provider organization (PPO) Health plan in which providers contract on a fee-for-service basis with employers, insurance plans, or other third-party administrators.

Prefixes Word elements that are attached to the beginning of roots and combining forms to add to or change their meaning.

Prejudice Negative feelings about a person because he or she belongs to a specific cultural or racial group.

Premium An agreed-upon amount paid to an insurance company for the benefit of having the company pay for a specified amount of future health care costs.

Prepaid plans A contracted type of insurance plan in which health care providers are paid a specific amount to provide certain health benefits.

Prevention (of disease) Behaviors that promote health and prevent disease.

Primary care providers (PCPs) Health care providers, often physicians, who serve as the patient's first contact when entering the health care system; also known as a gatekeeper.

Principles Fundamental truths.

Prioritize Ranking items that need to be done in order of importance.

Probationary period Typically the first 60–90 days of employment, which provide an opportunity for the employer and employee to determine if they have a "match."

Probing questions Inquiries that request additional information or clarification.

Problem-solving process A sequence of organized steps to follow when making decisions.

Procedures Specific steps taken to perform a task.

Processed foods Foods that are packaged in boxes, cans, or bags.

Professional development Continually striving to improve and be the best possible at your profession.

Professional distance A healthy balance in the health professional–patient relationship that involves demonstrating a caring attitude toward patients without the goal of becoming their friend.

Professionalism A set of characteristics and behaviors that enables one to do the best job possible to provide and maintain high-quality service to patients and employers.

Profit Amount of money remaining after all costs of operating a business have been paid.

Prognosis Prediction of the possible outcome of a disease and the potential for recovery.

Progress notes Written chronological statements about a patient's care.

Proportion A mathematical statement of equality between two ratios.

Proteins Food substances that contain amino acids, substances which are necessary for both building and maintaining the structural components of the body.

Protocols Standard methods of performing tasks.

Protozoa Microorganisms that are classified as animals.

Proximal Closer to the reference point.

Psychiatric hospitals Facilities that offer treatment to individuals with mental, emotional, and behavioral disorders.

Psychosocial development The maturation of emotions, attitudes, and other aspects of the mind, in addition to the individual's interactions and relationships with other members of society.

Psychosomatic Disorders, including physical illness, caused by mental or emotional factors.

Pulse deficit The rate of difference between a pulse point and an apical rate when they are taken simultaneously.

Pulse points Specific sites on the body where arterial pulsations can be felt.

Quality improvement Processes used to find ways to preserve or improve quality of care while decreasing costs.

Quotation Words written exactly as spoken.

RACE Acronym for responding to fires. (**R**emove patients. Sound the **A**larm. **C**ontain the fire. **E**xtinguish the fire or **E**vacuate the area.)

RAM An internal computer workspace that stores data only while the computer is on.

Ratios A method used to express the strength of a solution; it represents how many parts of one element are added in relationship to the parts of another element.

Reasonable accommodations Legal requirement to supply or make changes in equipment or other aspects of the environment if necessary to accommodate a disabled employee who is qualified to perform the job.

Receiver In communication, the person to whom the sender directs a message; also called the listener.

Reciprocal A fraction that has been "turned upside-down" during the process of dividing fractions.

Record A collection of related computerized data.

Reducing the fraction Finding a number that can be divided evenly into both the numerator and denominator.

Reference list A written list given to prospective employers upon request that includes contact information for people who will vouch for your job qualifications and character.

Reference plane A real or imaginary flat surface from which an angle is measured.

References People who will vouch for your qualifications and character.

Refined grains Grains modified so most nutrients are removed.

Reflecting A communication technique that involves prompting the sender to either complete or add more detail to the original message.

Registration Being placed on an official list after meeting the educational and testing requirements for a specific profession.

Reimbursed Paid back or paid for.

Reliable Trustworthy.

Repetitive motion injuries (RMIs) Injuries resulting from repeated movements that cause damage to a nerve, ligament, tendon, or muscle.

Requesting examples A communication technique to get additional, clarifying information.

Rescue breathing A technique in which the rescuer breathes for the victim.

Rescuer Person giving care during an emergency.

Respiration The process of taking air into and removing air from the lungs; one respiration includes one full cycle of inhalation and exhalation.

Respondeat superior Legal doctrine that makes an employer responsible for the behavior and actions of his or her employees.

Résumé Written summary of personal and professional qualifications.

Rickettsia A microorganism that is smaller than bacteria and has rod or spherical shapes.

Risk management All the policies and procedures designed to ensure patient safety.

Role model A person who serves as a positive example.

Roman numerals A numbering system based on I (1), V (5), X (10), L (50), C (100), D (500), and M (1000).

Rounding numbers Rules that determine whether a number is changed to zero, increased, or remains the same when digits are dropped from the right side.

Salutation Greeting.

Sample A group that represents a larger group when all members cannot be observed.

School career service Department that assists students and graduates with job-search skills such as résumé writing, interviewing, and dressing for success.

Scope of practice A description or list of skills that a specific occupational title is legally allowed to perform.

Search engine Computer software program capable of searching through and retrieving millions of documents on the Internet by using specific key words as identifiers.

Self-actualization Level 5 of Maslow's hierarchy of needs, defined as the achievement of one's greatest potential.

Self-directed learning All activities that an individual plans and participates in to increase knowledge and skills.

Self-esteem An individual's opinion of himself or herself.

Semi-block letter A written format similar to the block letter except that the first sentences of paragraphs are indented five spaces.

Sender In communication, the person who creates and delivers a message; also called the speaker.

Sexual harassment Unwelcome actions that are sexual in nature.

Signs Objective evidence gathered by health care professionals about a patient's condition.

Signs and symptoms The objective evidence (signs) observed by the health care professional and the subjective data (symptoms) reported by patients about their condition.

Simplifying the fraction Another term for reducing a fraction.

Site licenses Permission granting the installation of software on more than one computer.

Situational questions Job-interview questions in which the applicant is asked to describe how he or she would respond to a given situation.

Skilled nursing facility (SNF) A type of nursing home that provides nursing and rehabilitation services on a 24-hour basis; includes regular medical care for patients with long-term illnesses and those recovering from illness, injury, or surgery.

Slander A legal charge for defamation of character (damaging someone's reputation) committed in a spoken form.

SOAP A format for charting that uses a problem-oriented approach.

Sphygmomanometer An instrument that records the blood pressure.

Spinal cavity Located within the spinal column; contains the spinal cord.

Spore A thick capsule that a bacterium creates for self-protection.

Sprains Torn ligament fibers that result in a loosening of the joint.

Stages of dying Stages that dying people may experience as they face the fact of their own death. The five stages are denial, anger, bargaining, depression, and acceptance.

Standard precautions Practices designed to reduce the risk of transmission of microorganisms from both recognized and unrecognized sources of infection in health care settings.

Statistics The collection and analysis of large amounts of numerical data.

Sterile fields Areas designated to be free of microorganisms.

Sterilization Agents or methods that totally destroy all microorganisms, including viruses and spores.

Stethoscope An instrument that amplifies sounds so they can be heard coming from within the body.

Strains (muscle) Results of sudden tearing of muscle fibers during exertion; also referred to as pulled muscles.

Stress Physiological changes that occur in the body as it responds to danger, either real or imagined.

Stressors Any causes of stress to the individual.

Subjective As an adjective, referring to something that is dependent on or takes place in a person's mind and thus cannot be directly observed.

Subjective data Information the patient tells the health care professional about his or her condition, which cannot be directly observed.

Sucking wound A puncture into the respiratory system resulting in loss of air as the patient breathes.

Suffixes Word elements that are attached to the end of roots and combining forms to add to or change their meaning; any word ending.

Superficial Near or close to the body surface.

Superior Above.

Surgical asepsis (sterile technique) Procedures to completely eliminate the presence of pathogens from objects and areas.

Syllable Part of a word that has a single spoken sound.

Symptoms Subjective data reported to the health care provider by the patient.

Syndromes Not a precise disease but groups of related signs and symptoms.

Tachycardia A heart rate that is above the normal range.

Tachypnea A respiratory rate that is above the normal range.

Targeted drug therapy Use of drugs to block the growth and spread of cancer cells by preventing them from dividing or by destroying them.

Teach back Asking receivers (listeners) to explain what you have said in their own words.

Teams Groups of people working together in a coordinated effort to achieve a common goal or set of goals.

Telemedicine The practice of medicine, such as diagnosing and recommending treatment, via electronic communication.

Tendonitis Swelling, tenderness, or weakness in the tendons.

Terminal illness An illness from which the patient is expected to die because there is no known cure.

The Joint Commission An independent, not-for-profit organization that accredits and certifies health care organizations in the United States.

Therapeutic Relating to healing and assisting patients to regain or attain maximum wellness.

Therapeutic communication Communication that employs certain techniques specifically aimed at meeting the needs of patients.

Thoracic cavity Located in the chest; contains the heart, lungs, and major blood vessels.

Thoracic outlet syndrome Compression of the nerves, arteries, or veins in the passageway from the lower neck to the armpit.

Tissues Groups of cells that have a similar function.

Toxic Poisonous.

Traits Personal characteristics.

Trans fat Vegetable oil to which hydrogen has been added; has a harmful impact on cholesterol levels.

Transmission-based precautions Includes three types of isolation procedures (airborne, droplet, and contact precautions) required for preventing the spread of specific infections.

Transverse plane Divides the body horizontally into top and bottom portions.

Treatment Medications or procedures used to control or cure a disease or injury.

Triage system Guidelines to determine which patients to send where and what treatment will be given during an emergency.

Tuberculosis (TB) A disease caused by the contagious airborne pathogen *Mycobacterium tuberculosis*.

Type 2 diabetes Chronic disease characterized by high levels of sugar in the blood, a condition that can damage many parts of the body.

Utilization review (UR) Evaluation of the necessity, appropriateness, and efficiency of the use of health care services, procedures, and facilities.

Values Beliefs, ideals, and standards that provide the foundation for making decisions and guiding behavior.

Veterans Health Administration The largest integrated health care system in the United States serving nine million veterans in 1,250 health care facilities, including 172 medical centers and 1,069 outpatient sites.

Victim Person requiring care during an emergency.

Virtual communities Groups of individuals who use the Internet to communicate and share information with each other.

Virus smallest of the microbes. Not whole cells and therefore depend on living cells to provide food, nutrients, and a means of reproduction.

Vital signs Measuring the blood pressure, temperature, pulse, and respiration to give some indication of how the body is functioning.

Vital statistics The number of occurrences related to a specific event (e.g., births and deaths) for purposes of reporting.

Vitamins Substances derived from living matter that the body needs in small quantities to grow and function properly.

Vowel Any of the letters *a, e, i, o,* or *u.*

Wellness Promotion of health through preventive measures and the practice of good health habits; when the body is in a state of homeostasis.

Western medicine Based on a scientific approach, it treats symptoms and diseases using drugs, radiation, or surgery.

Whole grains Grains that contain all their original parts.

Whole numbers The traditional numbers we use to count (1, 2, 3, …).

Word parts The components of medical terms; each word part has its own meaning and location in the term and, like building blocks, they can be combined to create thousands of different words.

Word processing Using a software program for creating written documents on a computer.

Word root The part of the medical term that gives the main meaning to the word; often refers to the structure and function of the body.

Wound Damage to the soft tissue of the body as a result of violence or trauma.

References

Academy of Nutrition and Dietetics. (2019, February 11). *Processed foods: What's ok and what to avoid.* Retrieved from https://www.eatright.org/food/nutrition/nutrition-facts-and-food-labels/processed-foods-whats-ok-and-what-to-avoid

Acello. B. (2009). *Patient care: Basic skills for the health care provider.* Clifton Park, NY: Delmar Cengage Learning.

Acello, B., & Hegner, B. (2016). *Nursing assistant: A nursing process approach* (11th ed.). Boston: Delmar Cengage Learning.

A.D.A.M. Education. (2017). http://adameducation.com/aiaonline

Agarwal, S. (2017, December 28). *Physicians who refuse to accept Medicaid patients breach their contract with society.* Retrieved from https://www.statnews.com/2017/12/28/medicaid-physicians-social-contract/

Agency for Healthcare Research and Quality. (2018, October). *Understanding quality measurement.* Retrieved from https://www.ahrq.gov/professionals/quality-patient-safety/quality-resources/tools/chtoolbx/understand/index.html#useda

Agency for Healthcare Research and Quality. Patient Safety Network. (2018, April). *HealthGrades quality study: Fifth annual patient safety in American hospitals study.* Retrieved from https://psnet.ahrq.gov/resources/resource/7126/healthgrades-quality-study-fifth-annual-patient-safety-in-american-hospitals-study

Agency for Healthcare Research and Quality. Patient Safety Network. (2019, January). *Medication errors and adverse drug events.* Retrieved from https://psnet.ahrq.gov/primers/primer/23/Medication-Errors-and-Adverse-Drug-Events

Alexander Graham Bell Association. (1996). *Communicating with people who have a hearing loss.* [Brochure]. Washington, DC: Author.

Alonso-Zaldivar, R. (2012, September 7). The Associated Press. Report says U.S. health care system wasting $750 billion every year. *The Bulletin (Bend, OR),* pp. A1, A4.

Altman, D. (2015). The Wall Street Journal. *Health care deductibles: Climbing out of reach.* Retrieved from http://blogs.wsj.com/washwire/2015/03/11/health-care-deductibles-climbing-out-of-reach/

American Association of Naturopathic Physicians. (n.d.). *What is a naturopathic physician?* Retrieved from http://www.naturopathic.org/content.asp?contentID=60

American Cancer Society. (2015, June 8). *Depression.* Retrieved from https://www.cancer.org/treatment/treatments-and-side-effects/physical-side-effects/changes-in-mood-or-thinking/depression.html

American Heart Association. (2019). *HDL (good) LDL (bad) cholesterol and triglycerides.* Retrieved from https://www.heart.org/en/health-topics/cholesterol/hdl-good-ldl-bad-cholesterol-and-triglycerides

American Medical Association. (n.d.). *AMA Principles of medical ethics.* Retrieved from https://www.ama-assn.org/about/publications-newsletters/ama-principles-medical-ethics

American Sexual Health Association. (n.d.). *Healthcare providers.* Retrieved from http://www.ashasexualhealth.org/healthcare-providers

American Telemedicine Association. *What is telemedicine?* http://www.americantelemed.org/about-telemedicine/what-is-telemedicine#.VjHBBrdrLIU

American Transplant Foundation. (n.d.). *Facts: did you know?* Retrieved from https://www.americantransplantfoundation.org/about-transplant/facts-and-myths/

Anderson, R., Barbara, A., & Feldman, S. (2007). What patients want: A content analysis of key qualities that influence patient satisfaction. *Journal of Medical Practice Management, 22(5),* 255–261. Retrieved from www.drscore.com/press/papers/whatpatientswant.pdf

Baylor College of Medicine, (n.d.). *Introduction to infectious diseases.* Retrieved from https://www.bcm.edu/departments/molecular-virology-and-microbiology/emerging-infections-and-biodefense/introduction-to-infectious-diseases; https://www.beckershospitalreview.com/quality/where-does-the-us-rank-internationally-in-patient-satisfaction.html

Bend (OR) Bulletin, Health Response, June 1, 2018. From *The New York Times News Service.*

Berkeley Wellness. University of California. (2015, July 21). *Why you shrink as you age.* Retrieved from http://www.berkeleywellness.com/self-care/preventive-care/article/why-you-shrink-you-age

Bidwell, A. (2013, October 28). *Early childhood poverty damages brain development, study finds.* Retrieved from https://www.usnews.com/news/articles/2013/10/28/early-childhood-poverty-damages-brain-development-study-finds

Blumberg, Y. CNBD. Makeit. (2018, March 22). *Here's the real reason health care costs so much more in the US.* Retrieved from https://www.cnbc.com/2018/03/22/the-real-reason-medical-care-costs-so-much-more-in-the-us.html

Brown, P. L. (2018, May 14). California tests food as medicine for chronically ill patients. *Bend (OR) Bulletin.* Page A4.

Bureau of Labor Statistics. Occupational Outlook Handbook. (2019, April 12). Retrieved from https://www.bls.gov/ooh/healthcare/home.htm

Career Builder. (2011, April 14). *More than one-in-five hiring managers say they are less likely to hire a candidate who didn't send a thank-you note, finds new careerbuilder survey.* Retrieved from www.careerbuilder.com/share/aboutus/pressreleasesdetail.aspx?id=pr631&sd=4/14/2011&ed=04/14/2011

CDC Online. www.cdc.gov (Ch 10, msp 81)

Centers for Disease Control and Prevention. (2013). *Medication adherence.* Retrieved from http://www.cdc.gov/primarycare/materials/medication/docs/medicaton-adherence-01ccd.pdf

Centers for Disease Control and Prevention. (2016, May 16). *Occupational HIV transmission and prevention among health care workers.* Retrieved from https://www.cdc.gov/hiv/workplace/healthcareworkers.html

Centers for Disease Control and Prevention. (2017, May 26). *Deaths from Alzheimer's disease.* Retrieved from https://www.cdc.gov/features/alzheimers-disease-deaths/index.html

Centers for Disease Control and Prevention. (2018, August 13). *Adult obesity facts.* Retrieved from https://www.cdc.gov/obesity/data/adult.html

Centers for Disease Control and Prevention. (2018, November 6). *Frequently asked questions about estimated flu burden.* Retrieved from https://www.cdc.gov/flu/about/disease/us_flu-related_deaths.htm

Centers for Disease Control and Prevention. (n.d.). *Defining health literacy.* Retrieved from https://www.cdc.gov/healthliteracy/training/page572.html

Centers for Disease Control and Prevention. (n.d.). *Handwashing and hand sanitizer use.* Retrieved from https://www.cdc.gov/handwashing/pdf/hand-sanitizer-factsheet.pdf

Centers for Disease Control and Prevention. (n.d.). *Travelers' health. Vaccines. Medicines. Advice.* Retrieved from https://wwwnc.cdc.gov/travel

Centers for Disease Control and Health. Alcohol and Public Health. *Facts sheets – alcohol use and your health.* Retrieved from https://www.cdc.gov/alcohol/fact-sheets/alcohol-use.htm

Centers for Disease Control and Prevention. Antibiotic/Antimicrobial Resistance. (2018, September 10). *Combating antibiotic resistance, a global threat.* Retrieved from https://www.cdc.gov/drugresistance/index.html

Centers for Disease Control and Prevention. (2018, September 10). *Antibiotic/Antimicorbial resistance. Biggest threats and data.* Retrieved from (https://www.cdc.gov/drugresistance/biggest_threats.html)

Centers for Disease Control and Prevention. (2018, December 10). *West Nile Virus.* Retrieved from https://www.cdc.gov/westnile/index.html

Centers for Disease Control and Prevention. Healthcare-Associated Infections. (2019, January 9). *Clostridium difficile infection.* Retrieved from https://www.cdc.gov/HAI/organisms/cdiff/Cdiff_infect.html

Centers for Disease Control and Prevention. HIV/AIDS. (2016, November 7). *Occupational HIV transmission and prevention among health care workers.* Retrieved from https://www.cdc.gov/hiv/workplace/healthcareworkers.html

Centers for Disease Control and Prevention. Influenza. (2017, April 19). *Past seasons burden averted estimates.* Retrieved from https://www.cdc.gov/flu/about/burden-averted/2015-16.htm

Centers for Disease Control and Prevention. Influenza. (2017, November 1). *Flu Vaccination Coverage, United States, 2015-16 Influenza Season.* Retrieved from https://www.cdc.gov/flu/fluvaxview/coverage-1516estimates.htm

Centers for Disease Control and Prevention. Influenza. (2019, February 19). *Disease burden of Influenza.* Retrieved from https://www.cdc.gov/flu/about/disease/burden.htm

Centers for Disease Control and Prevention. Influenza. (2019, March). *Remembering the 1918 influenza pandemic.* Retrieved from https://www.cdc.gov/features/1918-flu-pandemic/index.html

Centers for Disease Control and Prevention. (2019, December 31). *Tuberculosis. Data and statistics.* Retrieved from https://www.hiv.gov/hiv-basics/overview/data-and-trends/statistics)

Centers for Disease Control and Prevention. National Center for Health Statistics. (2016, June 13). *Obesity and overweight.* Retrieved from https://www.cdc.gov/nchs/fastats/obesity-overweight.htm

Centers for Disease Control and Prevention. Opioid Overdose. (2018, December 19). *Drug overdose deaths.* Retrieved from https://www.cdc.gov/drugoverdose/data/statedeaths.html

Centers for Disease Control and Prevention. Smoking & Tobacco. (n.d.). *Fast facts.* Retrieved from https://www.cdc.gov/tobacco/data_statistics/fact_sheets/fast_facts/index.htm

Centers for Disease Control and Prevention. The National Institute for Occupational Safety and Health. (2010). *NIOSH: Occupational Hazards in Home Healthcare.* Retrieved from https://www.cdc.gov/niosh/docs/2010-125/default.html

Centers for Disease Control and Prevention. The National Institute for Occupational Safety and Health. (2014). *Back belts – do they prevent injury?* Retrieved from www.cdc.gov/niosh/docs/94-127/default.html

Centers for Disease Control and Prevention. The National Institute for Occupational Safety and Health. (2017, January 13). *Healthcare workers.* Retrieved from https://www.cdc.gov/niosh/topics/healthcare/default.html

Centers for Disease Control and Prevention. The National Institute for Occupational Safety and Health. (2018). *Healthcare workers.* Retrieved from https://www.cdc.gov/niosh/topics/healthcare/default.html

Centers for Disease Control and Prevention. Tuberculosis. (2018, December 31). *Data and statistics*. Retrieved from https://www.cdc.gov/tb/statistics/default.htm

Cimon, K., Featherstone, R. (2017, March). U.S. National Library of Medicine. Canadian Agency for Drugs and Technology. *Jewellery and nail polish worn by health care workers and the risk of infection transmission: A review of clinical evidence and guidelines*. Retrieved from https://www.ncbi.nlm.nih.gov/pubmed/29533568

Cleveland Clinic. Consult QD. (2016, November 22). https://consultqd.clevelandclinic.org/code-lavender-offering-emotional-support-holistic-rapid-response/

Davis, N. (2018, April 5). The Guardian. *Humans produce new brain cells throughout their lives, say researchers*. Retrieved from https://www.theguardian.com/science/2018/apr/05/humans-produce-new-brain-cells-throughout-their-lives-say-researchers

De Bord, J. (2014). *Informed consent*. University of Washington School of Medicine. Retrieved from https://depts.washington.edu/bioethx/topics/consent.html

Devine, P. G., Forscher, P. S., Austin, A. J., & Cox, W. T. L. (2012, November). *Long-term reduction in implicit race bias: A prejudice habit-breaking intervention*. Retrieved from https://www.ncbi.nlm.nih.gov/pmc/articles/PMC3603687/

Diabetes Association. (2019, January 30). *The cost of diabetes*. Retrieved from http://www.diabetes.org/advocacy/news-events/cost-of-diabetes.html

Dressner, M. (2017, June). U.S. Bureau of Labor Statistics. Monthly Labor Review. *Hospital workers: An assessment of occupational injuries and illnesses*. Retrieved from https://doi.org/10.21916/mlr.2017.17

Epstein, L. (2019, February 4). Investopedia. *6 reasons healthcare is so expensive in the U.S.* Retrieved from https://www.investopedia.com/articles/personal-finance/080615/6-reasons-healthcare-so-expensive-us.asp

Equal Employment Opportunity Commission. "Facts About Sexual Harassment," www.eeoc.gov/eeoc/publications/fs-sex.cfm.)

Estes, M. E. Z. (2011). *Health assessment and physical examination* (5th ed.). Clifton Park, NY: Cengage Learning.

Flight, M. (1998). *Law, liability, and ethics for medical office professionals* (3rd ed.). Clifton Park, NY: Delmar Cengage Learning.

Flight, M. (2004). *Law, liability, and ethics for medical office professionals* (4th ed.). Clifton Park, NY: Delmar Cengage Learning.

Flight, M. (2011). *Law, liability, and ethics for medical office professionals* (5th ed.). Clifton Park, NY: Delmar Cengage Learning.

Fox, M. (2018). *Texas Children's Hospital nurse fired after post about measles patient*. Retrieved from https://www.nbcnews.com/storyline/measles-outbreak/texas-children-s-hospital-nurse-fired-after-post-about-measles-n905146

Gordon, J. E., Deland, E., & Kelly, R. E. (2015, June 22). Columbia Medical Review. *Let's talk about improving communication in healthcare*. Retrieved from https://medicalreview.columbia.edu/article/communication-healthcare/

Harrington, C., Wiener, J., Rose, L., & Musumeci, M. (2017, October 27). *Key issues in long-term services and supports quality*. Henry J. Kaiser Family Foundation. Medicaid. Retrieved from https://www.kff.org/medicaid/issue-brief/key-issues-in-long-term-services-and-supports-quality/

Harvard Health Publishing. Harvard Medical School. (2018, April). *Reading the new blood pressure guidelines*. Retrieved from https://www.health.harvard.edu/heart-health/reading-the-new-blood-pressure-guidelines

Harvard Medical School. Division of Sleep Medicine. *Sleep, learning, and memory*. Retrieved from http://healthysleep.med.harvard.edu/healthy/matters/benefits-of-sleep/learning-memory

Harvard T. H. Chan School of Public Health. (n.d.). *Salt and sodium*. Retrieved from https://www.hsph.harvard.edu/nutritionsource/salt-and-sodium/

HCPro. (2010, June 7). Stressed Out Nurses Weekly. *In the know: Don't forget the three checks in medication administration*. Retrieved from http://www.hcpro.com/NRS-251960-4931/In-the-know-Dont-forget-the-three-checks-in-medication-administration.html

Health Cost and Utilization Project. (n.d.). *HCUP Fast Stats: Most common diagnoses for inpatient stays*. Retrieved from https://www.hcup-us.ahrq.gov/faststats/NationalDiagnosesServlet

HealthIT.gov. (2019, April 9). *What are the differences between electronic medical records, electronic health records, and personal health records?* Retrieved from https://www.healthit.gov/faq/what-are-differences-between-electronic-medical-records-electronic-health-records-and-personal

Healthline. (2013, July 27). *99,000 Americans die of healthcare acquired infections every year*. Retrieved from www.cdc.gov/washington/~cdcatWork/pdf/infections.pdf

Henry J. Kaiser Family Foundation. HIV/AIDS. (2019, March 25). *The HIV epidemic in the United States: The basics*. Retrieved from https://www.kff.org/hivaids/fact-sheet/the-hivaids-epidemic-in-the-united-states-the-basics/

HIPAA Journal. Cybersecurity Articles. Retrieved from https://www.hipaajournal.com/category/healthcare-cybersecurity/

Hogan, M., & Grument, J. (2016, June). *Suicide prevention: An emerging priority for health care*. Retrieved from https://www.healthaffairs.org/doi/full/10.1377/hlthaff.2015.1672

HIV.gov. (2019, March 13). *U.S. Statistics. Data & trends. Fast facts*. Retrieved from https://www.hiv.gov/hiv-basics/overview/data-and-trends/statistics

Home Care Institute. (2009). *Therapeutic communication in special situations*. Retrieved from www.hciclient.com/pdfs/Therapeutic_Communication_Special.pdf

Institute for Healthcare Communication. (2011, July). *Impact of communication in healthcare*. Retrieved from https://healthcarecomm.org/about-us/impact-of-communication-in-healthcare/

Institute for Healthcare Improvement. (2017, September 28). *How to reduce implicit bias*. Retrieved from http://www.ihi.org/communities/blogs/how-to-reduce-implicit-bias

Institute for Safe Medication Practices. (2017, October 2). *List of error-prone abbreviations*. Retrieved from https://www.ismp.org/recommendations/error-prone-abbreviations-list)

Krogstad, J. M., & Gonzalez-Barrera, A. (2017, August 29). University of California. Latino News Briefs. *A majority of English-speaking Hispanics in the U.S. are bilingual*. Retrieved from https://ucanr.edu/blogs/blogcore/postdetail.cfm?postnum=25033

Lindh, W., Pooler, M., Tamparo, C., & Dahl, B. (2010). *Delmar's comprehensive medical assisting: Administrative and clinical competencies* (4th ed.). Clifton Park, NY: Delmar Cengage Learning.

Lindh, W., Tamparo, C., Dahl, B., Morris, J., & Correa, C. (2018). *Clinical medical assisting* (6th ed.) Boston: Cengage Learning.

Maichou, L., Xiong, P., Park, L., Schwei, R. J., & Jacobs, E. A. (2017, March). *Western or traditional healers? Understanding decision making in the Hmong population*. Retrieved from https://www.ncbi.nlm.nih.gov/pmc/articles/PMC5010786/

Marino, K. (2000). *Resumes for the health care professional*. New York: John Wiley & Sons.

Martini, F. H., & Bartholomew, E. F. (2008). *Essentials of anatomy and physiology* (4th ed.). San Francisco, CA: Benjamin Cummings Publishing.

Mayo Clinic. (2017, February 7). Nutrition and healthy eating. *Carbohydrates aren't bad, but some may be healthier than others*. Retrieved from https://www.mayoclinic.org/healthy-lifestyle/nutrition-and-healthy-eating/in-depth/carbohydrates/art-20045705?p=1

Mayo Clinic. Nutrition and Healthy Eating. *Added sugars: Don't get sabotaged by sweeteners*. Retrieved from https://www.mayoclinic.org/healthy-lifestyle/nutrition-and-healthy-eating/in-depth/added-sugar/art-20045328

Mayo Clinic. Nutrition and Healthy Eating. *Mediterranean diet: A heart-healthy eating plan*. Retrieved from https://www.mayoclinic.org/healthy-lifestyle/nutrition-and-healthy-eating/in-depth/mediterranean-diet/art-20047801

McMains, V. Johns Hopkins University. (2016, May 3). *Johns Hopkins study suggests medical errors are third-leading cause of death in U.S.: Physicians advocate for changes in how deaths are reported*. Retrieved from https://hub.jhu.edu/2016/05/03/medical-errors-third-leading-cause-of-death/

MedlinePlus. (2019, January 29). MRSA. https://medlineplus.gov/mrsa.html and the CDC.

Milliken, M. E., & Honeycutt, A. (2004). *Understanding human behavior* (7th ed.). Clifton Park, NY: Delmar Cengage Learning.

Milliken, M. E., & Honeycutt, A. (2018). *Understanding human behavior: A guide for health care providers* (9th ed.). Clifton Park, NY: Cengage Learning.

National Council on Aging. (n.d.). *Elder abuse facts*. Retrieved from https://www.ncoa.org/public-policy-action/elder-justice/elder-abuse-facts/

National Institute on Deafness and Other Communication Disorders. (2016, December 15). *Quick statistics on hearing*. Retrieved from https://www.nidcd.nih.gov/health/statistics/quick-statistics-hearing

National Institute for Occupational Safety and Health (NIOSH). (2017, January 13). *Healthcare workers*. Retrieved from https://www.cdc.gov/niosh/topics/healthcare/default.html

National Institutes of Health. MedlinePlus. (2018). *The end of antibiotics? Drug-resistant bacteria: On the edge of a crisis*. Retrieved from https://medlineplus.gov/magazine/issues/winter18/articles/winter18pg8-11.html

National Center for Complementary and Integrative Health, Complementary, Alternative, and Integrative Health: What's In a Name? (2018, July).

National Center for Biotechnology Information, National Library of Medicine. *Patient experience in adult NHS services: Improving the experience of care for people using adult NHS services: Patient experience in generic terms. Knowing the patient as an individual*. Retrieved from https://www.ncbi.nlm.nih.gov/books/NBK115223/

Occupational Safety and Health Administration. (n.d.). *Laws and regulations*. Retrieved from https://www.osha.gov/law-regs.html

Pinder, G. MEDAPTUS. (2018, January 4). *13 principles to reduce medical errors in hospitals*. Retrieved from https://www.medaptus.com/13-systems-principles-reduce-medical-errors-hospitals/

Poverty USA. (2019). *The population of poverty USA*. Retrieved from https://povertyusa.org/facts

Preidt, R. (2016, April 25). *Many Americans turn to prayer for healing*. Retrieved from https://www.cbsnews.com/news/many-americans-turn-to-prayer-for-healing/

Reinberg, S. (n.d.). *Most doctors oppose physician-assisted suicide*. Medicine Net. Retrieved from https://www.medicinenet.com/script/main/art.asp?articlekey=173522

Rudowitz, R., Garfield, R., & Hinton, E. (2019, May 6). *10 Things to know about medicaid: Setting the facts straight*. Kaiser Family Foundation. https://www.kff.org/medicaid/issue-brief/10-things-to-know-about-medicaid-setting-the-facts-straight/

Science Daily. (2013, September 16). *TV drug ads: The whole truth?* Retrieved from https://www.sciencedaily.com/releases/2013/09/130916140455.htm

Science Daily, Boston University School of Medicine. (2017, September 18). *New lung cell type discovered*. Retrieved from https://www.sciencedaily.com/releases/2017/09/170918163424.htm

Sipherd, Ray, CNBC (2018, February 22). *The third-leading cause of death in US most doctors don't want you to know about*.

Retrieved from https:www.cnbc.com/2018/02/22/medical-errors-third-leading-cause-of-death-in-america.html

Smith, F. (2019, January). National Geographic Special Issue: The Future of Medicine. *Every body is unique.*

Sormunen, C., & Moisio, M. (2009). *Terminology for allied health professionals* (6th ed.). Clifton Park, NY: Cengage Learning.

Szalavitz, M. (2010, March 1). Psychology Today. *Touching empathy: Lack of physical affection can actually kill babies.* Retrieved from https://www.psychologytoday.com/us/blog/born-love/201003/touching-empathy

Tamparo, C. D., & Lindh, W. Q. (2008). *Therapeutic communications for health care* (3rd ed.). Clifton Park, NY: Cengage Learning.

Tamparo, C. D., & Lindh, W. (2017). *Therapeutic communication for health care professionals* (4th ed.). Boston: Cengage Learning.

Taylor, C., Lillis, C., & LeMone, P. (2006). *Fundamentals of nursing: The art and science of nursing care* (6th ed.). Philadelphia, PA: Lippincott-Raven Publishers.

TechLectures.com

TED. https://www.ted.com/talks

Tello, M. (2017, January 16). *Racism and discrimination in health care: Providers and patients.* Harvard Health Publishing. Harvard Medical School. Retrieved from https://www.health.harvard.edu/blog/racism-discrimination-health-care-providers-patients-2017011611015

Thomas, W. (2007). *What are old people for? How elders will save the world.* Acton, MA: VanderWyk & Burnham.

The Joint Commission. (2018, September 14). *Facts about the official "do not use" list of abbreviations.* Retrieved from http://www.jointcommission.oorg/facts_about_do_not_use_list

The Guardian. (n.d.). *Humans produce new brain cells throughout their lives, say researchers.* Retrieved from https://www.theguardian.com/science/2018/apr/05/humans-produce-new-brain-cells-throughout-their-lives-say-researchers

U.S. Census Bureau. (2018, September 13). *Hispanic heritage month 2018.* https://www.census.gov/newsroom/facts-for-features/2018/hispanic-heritage-month.html

U.S. Department of Health and Human Services. AIDSinfo. (2018). *The basics of HIV prevention.* Retrieved from https://aidsinfo.nih.gov/understanding-hiv-aids/fact-sheets/20/48/the-basics-of-hiv-prevention

U.S. Department of Health and Human Services. HIV.gov. (2018, June14). *Who should get tested?* Retrieved from https://www.hiv.gov/hiv-basics/hiv-testing/learn-about-hiv-testing/who-should-get-tested

U.S. Department of Health and Human Services. Organ Procurement and Transplant Network. *How organ allocation works.* Retrieved from https://optn.transplant.hrsa.gov/learn/about-transplantation/how-organ-allocation-works/

U.S. Department of Justice. Drug Enforcement Administration. Diversion Control Division. (n.d.). *Controlled substances schedules.* Retrieved from https://www.deadiversion.usdoj.gov/schedules

U.S. Department of Labor. (2016, September). *Handy reference guide to the fair labor standards act.* Retrieved from https://www.dol.gov/whd/regs/compliance/hrg.htm

U.S. Department of Labor. Wage and Hour Division. (n.d.). *Family and medical leave.* Retrieved from www.dol.gov/whd/fmla

U.S. Equal Employment Opportunity Commission. (n.d.). *Age discrimination.* Retrieved from www.eeoc.gov/laws/types/age.cfm

U.S. Equal Employment Opportunity Commission. (n.d.). *Disability discrimination.* Retrieved from www.eeoc.gov/laws/types/disability.cfm

U.S. Equal Employment Opportunity Commission. (n.d.). *Facts about sexual harassment.* Retrieved from https://www.eeoc.gov/eeoc/publications/fs-sex.cfm

U.S. Equal Employment Opportunity Commission. (n.d.). *Immigration reform act.* Retrieved from https://www.eeoc.gov/eeoc/history/35th/thelaw/irca.html

U.S. Equal Employment Opportunity Commission. (n.d.). *Pregnancy discrimination.* Retrieved from www.eeoc.gov/laws/types/pregnancy.cfm

U.S. Equal Employment Opportunity Commission. (n.d.). *Sex-based discrimination.* Retrieved from www.eeoc.gov/laws/types/sex.cfm

U.S. Equal Employment Opportunity Commission. (n.d.). *Sexual harassment.* Retrieved from https://www.eeoc.gov/laws/types/sexual_harassment.cfm

University of California San Francisco. HIV InSite. (2011, August 3). *Is HIV always fatal?* Retrieved from http://hivinsite.ucsf.edu/hiv?page=basics-00-14

University of Illinois at Chicago. (n.d.). *Cybersecurity: How can it be improved in health care?* Retrieved from https://healthinformatics.uic.edu/resources/articles/cybersecurity-how-can-it-be-improved-in-health-care/

University of San Francisco Health. (n.d.). *Communicating with people with hearing loss.* https://www.ucsfhealth.org/education/communicating_with_people_with_hearing_loss/

Vestal, V., and Kautz, D. D. (2009). International perspectives: Responding to the similarities and differences between Filipino and American nurses. *Journal of Nursing Administration,* 39, 8-10. DOI: 10.1097/NNA.0b013e31818fe726.

Veterans Health Administration. https://www.va.gov/health/

Wick, J. Y. (2016, August 29). *How to communicate effectively with dementia patients.* Retrieved from http://contemporaryclinic.pharmacytimes.com/chronic-care/how-to-communicate-effectively-with-dementia-patients

Williams, S. (2005). *Essentials of health services* (3rd ed.). Clifton Park, NY: Delmar Cengage Learning.

Zimmerman, B. (2016, May 3). Beckers Healthcare. *Where does the U.S. rank internationally in patient satisfaction?* Retrieved from https://www.beckershospitalreview.com/quality/where-does-the-us-rank-internationally-in-patient-satisfaction.html

Index

Note: Following page numbers, b refers to boxed material; f to figures; p to procedures; and t to tables.

A

Abbreviations, for medical terms, 99, 99t–100t
Abdominal cavity, 135, 135f
Abuse
  of children, 76, 77t
  of elders, 76–77, 77t
  spousal, 50t, 76
Acceptance stage, of dying, 200–201, 204–205
Accidents
  physical and mental changes increasing risk of, 261t
  reporting, 262
Account payable, 489
Account receivable, 489
Acetabulum, 147
Acquired immunodeficiency syndrome (AIDS), 161, 249t
Acromegaly, 177
Acting out, 331t
Active listening, 345
Activities of daily living (ADLs), assessment of, 419
Acupuncture, 48, 213
A.D.A.M., 389
Addison's disease, 177
Adolescence, 189t, 193, 193f, 197t
Adrenal glands, 177
Adrenaline, 179t
Adrenals, 179t
Adrenocorticotropic hormone (ACTH), 178t
Adult, definition of, 73
Adult day care, 56t
Adult foster homes, 55
Advance directives, 75–76
Adverse drug events (ADEs), 502
Adverse drug incidents, 387
Advocates, 505
Aerobic exercise, 285
Aerobic microorganisms, 220
Afebrile patients, 420
Affection needs, 327, 329

Affordable Care Act (ACA), 72, 83, 488–489
Age, creativity and, 195b
Age Discrimination in Employment, 556t
Agency for Healthcare Research and Quality (AHRQ), 500
Agendas, 372
Agent, 81
Aging population, 43
AIDS (Acquired immunodeficiency syndrome), 161, 249t
Airborne pathogens, 250
Airborne precautions, 242
Aldosterone, 179t
Alexander technique, 213
Allergic reactions, emergency procedures for, 445, 445p–447p
Alternative medicine, 45–48, 46t
Alveoli, 162f, 163
Alzheimer's disease, 51, 176, 349
Ambulatory services, 55, 56t
Amenorrhea, 181
American Hospital Association, 500
American Sign Language (ASL), 350, 350f
Americans with Disabilities Act, 556t
Amino acids, 277
Amputations, 452p
Amyotrophic lateral sclerosis (ALS), 175
Anaerobic microorganisms, 220
Anaphylactic shock, 445
Anatomy, 141
Androgens, 179t
Anemia, 160
Aneurysms, 160
Anger, communication and, 352
Anger stage of dying, 200, 204
Angina pectoris, 160, 467p
Angles, 118–119, 119f
Anorexia nervosa, 284
Anterior body cavity, 135, 135f
Anterior, definition of, 135t
Anthrax, 270t
Antibiotics, 219, 221t
  resistance to, 52–53, 251, 252t

Anticonvulsant drugs, 176
Antidiuretic hormone (ADH), 179t
Antioxidants, 281
Antiseptics, 232, 235–236
Anvil (incus), 170
Anxiety, communication and, 350
Aorta, 155, 156f
Apex, definition of, 135t
Aphasia, 175, 351
Apical pulse, 420t, 426, 426p–427p
Apnea, 428
Apostrophes, 366
Apothecary system, 122, 122t
Appearance
  of patient, assessment of, 416
  professional, 301–302, 535–536
Appendages, 152, 153
Appendicitis, 165
Appendicular skeleton, 145, 145f
Aqueous humor, 169
Arm, 147
Aromatherapy, 46t
Arteries, 154, 155, 156f, 157, 157f
Arteriosclerosis, 160
Arthritis, 148
Artificial intelligence, 386–387
Ascites, 165
Asepsis (aseptic technique), 224–239
  medical (clean technique), 224–225
  surgical (sterile technique), 225
Assault, 74
Assertiveness, 293
Assessment, 7
  observation and data collection *vs.*, 415
  physical. *See* Physical assessment
Assisted living residences, 55–56
Astigmatism, 171
Atelectasis, 163
Atherosclerosis, 160
Athlete's foot, 153
Atria, 155
Atrioventricular (AV) node, 155
Atrophy, 151

Attitude
professional, 299–300
Auditory nerve, 170
Aural (tympanic) temperature, 423p
Auricle, 170
Auscultation, 416
Autoimmune diseases, 161
Autonomic nervous system, 174
Autonomy, 70t, 73–76
Autonomy *vs.* shame and doubt stage, 189t, 191
Axial skeleton, 145, 145f, 146–147, 146f, 147f
Axillary temperature, 422p
Axons, 174
Ayurveda, 46t

B

Baby boomers, 195
Bacilli, 221t
Back belts, 214, 217f
Back pain, 149
Bacteria, 220–222
Bacteriocidal action, 232
Bacteriostatic action, 232
Bandaging, 466, 475p–478p
Bargaining stage of dying, 200, 204
Barrier devices, for resuscitation, 443, 444f
Bartholin's glands, 181
Base, definition of, 135t
Baseline, 415
Basic formula method, 115
Battery, 73
Bed scales, 435
Behavioral questions, 534
Beliefs, about health care, culture and, 324–326
Benign prostatic hypertrophy (BPH), 183
Bernhardt, Sarah, 195b
Biases, 6
Binge eating, 284
Bioelectromagnetic-based therapies, 46t
Biofield therapies, 46t
Bioinformatics, 388
Biomedical engineer, 31t
Biomedical equipment technician, 31, 31t
Biomedical equipment technologist, 31, 31t
Bioterrorism, 270t
Bird flu (H5N1), 251
Bites, first aid for, 462, 464p
Bleeding
emergency procedures for, 447, 448p–452p
external, 447, 448p–449p
internal, 447, 450p

Block letters, 368, 369f
Blood-borne pathogens, 239–241
Blood pressure, 420t, 429–430, 431p–432p, 432–433
diastolic, 429, 429t
systolic, 429, 429t
taking manually, 431p–432p, 432f
Blood vessels, 154, 155, 157, 157f, 158f
changes in, increasing risk of injuries and accidents, 261t
Body language, 344–345
Body mass index (BMI), 283
calculation, 283b
chart, 436f
Body mechanics, 205–216
back belts and, 214
lifting and, 211b, 211f, 212f
prevention and, 206
repetitive motion injuries and, 206–210, 207t
sitting and, 209b
standing and walking and, 209b
Body systems, 130, 131f, 142–184, 142t–143t
for movement and protection, 142, 142t, 144–154
for providing energy and removing waste, 143t, 154–168
reproductive, 180–184
for sensing, coordinating, and controlling, 168–180
Body temperature, 420, 421p–423p, 421t
Body weight, measuring, 433–436, 434f–436f, 436b
Boils, 153
Bone injuries, emergency procedures for, 447, 452, 453p–455p
Bone marrow, 144, 145
Botulism, 270, 270t
Bowman's capsule, 166
Brachial pulse, 424, 424f
Bradypnea, 428
Brain, 172, 172f, 173f
Brain stem, 173
Breach of contract, 81
Breasts, 181
Breathing difficulty, emergency procedures for, 466p
Bronchioles, 163
Bubonic plague, 270t
"Buffalo hump," 177
Bulbourethral gland, 183
Bulimia, 284
Bundle of His, 155, 156f
Burnout, 292–293

Burns, George, 195b
Burns, 452, 458f, 459, 459p–461p
chemical, 452, 460p
electrical, 452, 460p–461p
emergency procedures for, 452, 458f, 459, 459p–461p
radiation, 452, 460p
thermal, 452, 458f, 459p
Business letters, 367–368
effective, writing, 368
form, 368
formats for, 368, 369f–371f
preparing for mailing, 372, 372f
reminder letters as, 360
salutation in, 366
with test results, 360
Bystanders, enlisting help of, in emergency situations, 444

C

Calcitonin, 179t
Calcium, 278t
Calmness, in emergency situations, 444
Calories, 279
Cancer
of lung, 163
of skin, 153
of the skin, 153
Capillaries, 154
Capitalization rules, 363
Capitation, 487
Carbohydrates, 277, 279
Cardiac care units (CCUs), 54
Cardiac muscle, 133, 150
Cardiac sphincter, 164
Cardiologist, 15b
Cardiopulmonary resuscitation (CPR), 442, 444
Cardiopulmonary system, 162
Cardiovascular system, 154–159, 156f–159f
Cardiovascular technologist, 27, 27t
Career fairs, 519
Career ladders, 9, 314
Career orientations, 519
Careers. *See* Health care careers
Carotid pulse, 424, 424f
Carpal tunnel syndrome, 149, 207, 207t
Carpals, 147
Carriers, 224
Cartilage, 145
Cataract, 171
Catholicism, health care beliefs and, 324
Caudal, definition of, 135t
Cell body, 174
Cells, 130, 130b, 131f, 132f
Cellulitis, 153

Celsius (C) scale, 124
Centers for Disease Control and
    Prevention (CDC), 58, 58t, 225
Centers for Medicare and Medicaid
    Services (CMS), 485, 499
Central nervous system (CNS), 172–174,
    172f, 173f
Cephalic, definition of, 135t
Cerebellum, 173
Cerebral cortex, 173, 173f
Cerebral palsy, 175
Cerebrospinal fluid (CSF), 174
Cerebrovascular accident (CVA), 175
    emergency procedures for, 472p
Cerebrum, 172–173, 172f
Certification, 10
    in resume, 520
Certified coding specialist (CCS), 30, 30t
Certified medical assistant (CMA), 16t
Certified nursing assistant (CNA), 18–19,
    18t
Certified registered nurse anesthetist
    (CRNA), 18t
Certified registered nurse practitioner
    (CRNP), 18t
Certified Surgical Technician (CST), 22,
    23t
Cervix, uterine, 180
Chain of command, in workplace, 552,
    553f
Chain of infection, 224–226
    breaking, 225–226
Chair scales, 434, 435f
Charting, 399. See also Medical records
    by exception, 405, 405f
    narrative, 405, 405f
    problem-oriented, 404–405, 405f
Charting by exception (CBE), 405, 405f
Chemical burns, 452, 460p
Chemical-dot thermometers, 420, 421f
Chemical disinfectant agents, 235
Chemical hazards, 268
Chest pain, 467p
Cheyne-Stokes respirations, 428
Chief complaints, 404
Child abuse, 50t
Chinese medicine, 46t, 325
Chiropractic, 47, 47f, 47t
Cholecystitis, 165
Cholelithiasis, 165
Cholesterol, 279–280
ChooseMyPlate, 281, 282f
Choroid, 168–169
Chronic illness, 194
Chronic obstructive pulmonary disease
    (COPD), 163
Chronological resumes, 521, 522f

Cilia, 163
Ciliary muscles, 168–169
Circulatory system, 143t, 154–161
    assessment of, 417
Cirrhosis, 165
Civil Rights Act of 1964, 556t
Clavicles, 147
Clean technique. See Medical asepsis
Clinical decision-support systems
    (CDSS), 387
Clinical depression, 349
Clinical experiences, finding job leads
    through, 518
Clinical Psychologist (PhD, PsyD), 17t
Clinical social worker, 17t
Clitoris, 181
Closed-ended questions, 342, 343t
Closed fractures, 447
Cloud storage, 393
Cocci, 220t
Coccobacilli, 221t
Cochlea, 171
Code of Hammurabi, 67b
Codes of ethics, 68, 68b
Coding, 490
Cognitive development, 188, 198, 198t
Coinsurance, 485
Cold calling, 518
Colon cancer, 165
Colonies, bacterial, 220
Colons (punctuation), 366
Combining forms, 90–91, 91t
Commas, 366
Communicable diseases, 245
Communication, 337–358
    barriers to, 348–352
    computers and, 389–391
    creating the message and, 342–343
    delivering the message and, 343–345
    evaluating the encounter and, 347
    feedback and, 346–347
    goals of, 340–342
    gossip and patient privacy and,
        354–355
    importance of, 338–340
    listening to the response and,
        345–346, 346b
    nonverbal, 344
    patient education and, 353–354, 353t
    presentations to groups and, 354
    by telephone, 353
    therapeutic, 340
    through life span, 347–348
    written. See Business letters;
        Computers; Letters; Written
        communication
Community career centers, 515

Compassion, in health care
    professionals, 3f
Compatibility, of chemicals, 268
Compensation, 331t
Complementary and alternative
    medicine (CAM), 45–48, 46t
Computed tomography (CT), 384t
Computed tomography technologist,
    26t
Computer literacy, 380f
Computer networks, 379, 389
Computer viruses, 393–394
Computerized inventory system, 379
Computerized physician order entry
    (CPOE) system, 387
Computers, 378–397
    communication using, 389–391
    diagnostics and, 384–385
    documents and, 382, 382b
    in education, 389
    effective use of, 392–393
    electronic health records and,
        405–408
    information management and, 380,
        382
    learning about, 394
    maintaining the human touch with,
        394
    patient monitoring using, 388
    in research, 388–389
    security and, 393–394
    spreadsheets and, 382–384, 383f
    telemedicine and, 391–392
    telepharmacies and, 387
    in treatment, 386–387
    virtual communities, 391
    visual problems with, 208–209, 210b
Concrete operational stage, 198t
Conductive hearing loss, 171
Cones (retinal), 169
Confidentiality, 78–80, 354
    of written materials, 374
Confused patients, communication
    with, 349
Congestive heart failure, 160
Conjunctiva, 169
Conjunctivitis, 171
Connective tissue, 133
Consciousness
    lack of, emergency procedures for,
        473p
    level of, assessment of, 416
Consent, 73–75
    to treat, in emergency situations, 443
Consonants, 90, 364t
Constipation, 165
Constructive criticism, 505, 506f, 507b

Contact dermatitis, 154
Contact precautions, 244f
Contamination, 246
Continuing care communities, 56
Continuing education units (CEUs), 310–312
Continuing medical education (CME), 310
Continuing professional education (CPE), 308, 310
Contractions, 366
Contracts, 80–81
Contractures, 151
Control, 331t
Controlled substances, 77, 78b, 291
Controlled Substances Act, 77, 78b
Conventional moral stage, 198t, 199t
Convolutions, of brain, 172, 172f
Convulsions, emergency procedures for, 470p–471p
Copays, 487
Cornea, 168
Cornell note-taking system, 4, 5f
Coronary arteries, 155, 156f
Corpus callosum, 173
Corpus, uterine, 180
Corrections on medical documentation, 401–402, 402f
Cortisone, 179t
Cost of money, 489
Costs of health care. See Health care costs
Coughing, 417
Cover letters, 524–528, 525f–527f
Cowper's gland, 183
Cranial, definition of, 135t
Cranial cavity, 134, 135f
Cranial nerves, 174
Cranium, 146, 146f
Creativity, age and, 195b
Criticism
  constructive, 505, 506f, 507b
  destructive, 505–506, 507b
  professional acceptance of, 303
Crohn's disease, 165
Cross-training, 367, 491
Culture, 320–323, 320f
  cultural differences, 322–323
  dominant, 321
  individuals and, 321–322
Cumulative Index to Nursing and Allied Health Literature (CINAHL), 388
Current Procedural Terminology (CPT) codes, 490
Cushing's syndrome, 177

Customer service, 502–508
  customer satisfaction and, 505, 505f, 506t
  internal customers and, 505–508
  taking responsibility for quality and, 504–505
Cyanosis, 417
Cystitis, 167
Cybersecurity, electronic health records, 409

D

Damages, 81
Databases, 380, 380b
Data collection, assessment vs., 415
Deafness. See Hearing loss
Death and dying, 200–205, 348
  euthanasia and, 71–72
Decimals, 109–110, 110f, 111t, 112, 113t
Deductibles, 485
Deep, definition of, 135t
Defamation of character, 80
Defense mechanisms, 330, 331t
  against infections, 224
Definitive observation units, 54
Degenerative joint disease, 148
Degrees, 118, 119f
Dementia, 51, 176, 349
Demographic changes, 309
Dendrites, 174
Denial, 331t
Denial stage, of dying, 200
Dental assistant (CDA or RDA), 12t, 13
Dental hygienist (RDH), 12, 12t
Dental laboratory technician, 12t, 13
Dentist (DDS or DMD), 12t
Depression
  communication and, 349
  stage of dying, 200, 204
Dermatitis, 154
Dermis, 152
Destructive criticism, 505–506, 507b
Detached retina, 171
Development. See Growth and development
Diabetes, 176
Diabetes insipidus, 180
Diabetes mellitus, 177
  emergency procedures for, 467p–468p
  type 2, 282
Diagnoses, 141
Diagnostic imaging, 384, 384t, 385f
Diagnostic medical sonographer, 26–27, 27t
Diagnostic procedures, 141

Diagnostic-related groups (DRGs), 485
Diagnostics
  computerized, 384–385
  remote, 384–385
Diagnostic vascular technologist, 27, 27t
Dial (aneroid) sphygmomanometer, 430f
Dialysis, 167
Diaphragm, 163
Diaphysis, 144
Diarrhea, 165
Diastolic pressure, 429, 429t
Diencephalon, 173
Dietetic aide, 31t
Dietetic assistant, 31t
Dietetic technician (DTR), 30–31, 31t
Dietitian (RD), 31t
Diets, 277. See also Nutrition
  vegetarian, 283–284
  weight-loss, 283
Digestive system, 143t, 164f
  assessment of, 418
Digital sphygmomanometers, 430f
Diplobacilli, 221t
Diplococci, 220t
Discretion, 70t, 78–80
Diseases, 141
Disinfectants, 235
Disoriented patients, communication with, 349
Displacement, 331t
Distal, definition of, 135t
Diverticulitis, 165
Diverticulosis, 165
Documentation. See Medical documentation; Medical records
Domestic violence, 77
Dominant culture, 321
Dorsal, definition of, 135t
Double-bagging, 243
Downloading, 394
Dressing, for safety, 259
Droplet precautions, 243f
Drowning, emergency procedures for, 470p
Drug abuse, 77, 291, 461, 462p
Drug names, 97
Drugs, prescription. See Prescription drugs
Dwarfism, 180
Dysentery, 223
Dysmenorrhea, 181
Dyspnea, 417

E

Eardrum, 170
  ruptured, 171

Ears, 143t, 170–171, 170f, 171, 172
assessment of, 418
injuries to, 457p
Eating, healthy, 281
Eating disorders, 284
Ebola virus, 251
Ectopic pregnancy, 181
Eczema, 154
Edema, 167
Education. *See also* Learning; Lifelong
learning
computers in, 389
continuing, 308, 310–312
of patients, 353–354, 353t, 373–374
in resume, 520
Educational Resources Information
Center (ERIC), 388
Efficiency, health care costs and,
491–492
Elder abuse, 76–77, 77t
Eldercare, 76b
Electrical burns, 452, 460p–461p
Electrical impedance tomography (EIT),
384t
Electrocardiography (ECG) technician,
27–28, 27t
Electroencephalographic technologist,
27t, 28
Electroneurodiagnostic technologist,
27t, 28
Electronic health records (EHRs), 379,
405–406
advantages of, 407
challenges of, 407–408
example of, 406–407
provider's concerns, 408
safeguarding, 408–410
Electronic mail (email), ethics and, 68b
Electronic medical records (EMRs),
405–408
Electronic sphygmomanometers,
430, 430f
Electronic thermometers, 420, 421f
Emancipated minors, 73
Embolus, 161
Embryo stage, 189
Emergency code system, 270, 271f
Emergency departments, 54
Emergency medical responder, 14t
Emergency medical technicians (EMTs),
13, 14t
Emergency physician, 15b
Emergency preparedness plan, 270–271
Emergency procedures, 441–480
for allergic reactions, 445, 445p–447p
bandaging and, 466, 475p–478p

for bleeding and wounds, 447,
448p–452p
for bone, joint, and muscle injuries,
447, 452, 453p–455p
for breathing difficulty, 466p
for burns, 452, 458f, 459, 459p–461p
cardiopulmonary resuscitation as,
442, 444
for chest pain, 467p
for diabetes, 467p–468p
for drowning, 470p
for facial injuries, 452, 456p–457p
for fainting (syncope), 469p
for fever (hyperthermia), 469p
figure-eight wraps and, 476p–477p
for hyperventilation, 467p
for poisoning, 461–462, 463p
for seizures (convulsions), 470p–471p
for shock, 471p
situations and, 442–444
slings and, 474p–475p
spiral wraps and, 475p–476p
for stroke or cerebrovascular accident,
472p
for temperature-related illness, 462,
464p–465p
for unconsciousness, 473p
Emotional status, assessment of, 416
Empathy, 300
Employee handbook, 550–551
Employees, great, 555, 555b
Employment. *See also* Health care
accepting, 540, 542
declining, 542
dismissal/firing from, 561
general questions, 533–534
guidelines for success in, 552–555
laws governing, 555, 556t, 557
leaving/resigning, 559, 560f
performance evaluations and,
557–558, 558b
promotional opportunities, 558–559
starting out in, 550–552
Encephalitis, 176
Endocarditis, 161
Endocardium, 155
Endocrine system, 143t, 177–180, 178f,
178t–179t
assessment of, 418
Endocrinologist, 15b
Endometriosis, 181
Endosteum, 144
Energy therapies/theories, 46t, 48
Enrollees, 487
Entamoeba coli, 224f
Envelopes, addressing, 372, 372f

Environment
assessing, in emergency situations,
443
physical, communication and, 345
Environmental control, standard
precautions for, 239
Environmental hazards, 260t
Environmental safety, 258–271
bioterrorism and, 269–270, 270t
chemical hazards and, 260t
emergency code system and, 270,
271f
emergency preparedness plan for,
270–271
fire and electrical hazards and, 263–
268, 264f–266f, 266t–267t
general guidelines for, 259–262
importance of, 259
infectious waste and, 268–269
oxygen hazards and, 269
radiation hazards and, 268
workplace violence and, 260t
Epidemiology, 219
Epidermis, 152
Epididymitis, 183
Epigastric region, 136
Epiglottis, 162
Epilepsy, 176
Epinephrine, 179t
Epiphyses, 144
Epithelial tissue, 133
Eponyms, 97
Equal Employment Opportunity
Commission, 557
Equal Pay Act of 1963, 556t
Ergonomic hazards, 260t
Ergonomics, 206
Erikson, Erik, 188
Erikson's stages of psychosocial
development, 188, 189t, 191–195
Escherichia coli, 219
Esophagus, 164
Esteem needs, 327, 329
Estimating, 116
Estrogen, 180
Ethics, 64–87
of care, Gilligan's stages of, 199, 199t,
202, 202t
codes of, 68, 68b
dilemmas in, 65, 66t, 84
guiding principles of, 69, 70t, 71–82
health care and, 66–82
law and, 65–66
patient rights, 82–84
purpose of, 65
Etiology, 141

Etiquette, 368
Eupnea, 428
Eustachian tubes, 170–171
Euthanasia, 71–72
Evil eye, 324
Examples, for obtaining feedback, 346–347
Exclusive provider organization (EPO), 486
Exercise, aerobic, 285
Exercises, for computer users, 210t
Exertion injuries, 210–211. *See also* Repetitive motion injuries (RMIs)
   lift team/specialized equipment usage, 212
   preventing, 212–213, 212f
   safe lifting techniques, 211b, 213
Exhalation, 428
Exocrine glands, 177
Expanding consciousness, 44
Expenditures, 489
Express consent, 73
Express contract, 81
External auditory canal, 170
External bleeding, 447, 448p–449p
External customers, 503. *See also* Patients
Eyebrows, 169
Eyelashes, 169
Eyelids, 169
Eyes, 143t, 168–169, 168f, 169f, 171
   assessment of, 418
   injuries to, 456p
   protection for, 232
Eyestrain, preventing, 208, 210b

F

Face shields, 232
Facial expressions, 345
Facial injuries, emergency procedures for, 452, 456p–457p
Fahrenheit (F) scale, 124, 125, 125f, 125t
Fainting, emergency procedures for, 469p
Fair Labor Standards Act, 556t
Faith healing, 324
Fallopian tubes, 180
False imprisonment, 75
Family and Medical Leave Act of 1993, 556t
Family breakdown, 50t
Family practice physician, 16b
Fascia, 150
Fats, 277
   cholesterol, 279–280
   trans, 280

FDA Adverse Event Reporting System (FAERS), 387
Febrile patients, 420
Federal Child Abuse Prevention and Treatment Act, 76
Feedback, 346–347
Feedback mechanism, 177
Fee-for-service, 484
Female reproductive system, 143t, 180–182, 181f, 419
Femoral pulse, 424, 424f
Femur, 147
Fetus, 189
Fever, 420
   emergency procedures for, 469p
Fiber optics, 386
Fibers, 279
Fibroid tumors, 182
Fibromyalgia, 151
Fibula, 147
Fields, in databases, 380
Figure-eight wraps, 476p–477p
Files, 360, 380
Fimbriae, 180
Financing, 489
Fingernails, 301
Fingers, bandaging, 478p
Fires
   responding to, 263–268, 264f–266f, 266t–267t
   types of, 266t
Firing, 561
First aid, 442
First-degree burns, 452, 458f
First responder, 14t
Flagella, 220
Flammable liquids, 266t
Flexitarian (semi-vegetarian), 284
Folate, 278t
Follicle-stimulating hormone (FSH), 178t
Food. *See* Diets; Nutrition
Food and Drug Administration (FDA), 58t
Form letters, 368
Formal operational stage, 198t
Fox, Michael J., 330
Fractional equation method, 114
Fractions, 110–112, 112f, 112t, 113t
Fractures, 149, 149f
   closed, 447
   first aid for, 453p–455p
   open, 447
Fraud, 78
Free radicals, 278t
Frontal plane, 134, 134f
Frostbite, 462, 464p

Full-thickness burns, 452, 458f
Functional resumes, 521, 523f
Fundus, uterine, 180
Fungi, 223
Furuncles, 153

G

Gallbladder, 165
Gandhi, Mahatma, 195b
Gangrene, 151
Gastric ulcers, 166
Gastritis, 165
Gastroenteritis, 165
Gastroesophageal reflux disease (GERD), 166
Gastrointestinal system, 164
Gatekeepers, 487
Gene therapy, 42
General survey, 415–416
Generalized infections, 218
Generativity *vs.* stagnation stage, 189t, 194
Genetics, 141–142
Genitalia, female, 181
Germ theory, 220
Germicidal action, 232
Gerontologist, 16b
Giardia lamblia, 223f
GIDEON (Global Infectious Diseases and Epidemiology Network), 387
Gigantism, 180
Gilligan's stages of the ethics of care, 199, 199t, 202, 202t
Glaucoma, 171
Glomerulonephritis, 167
Glomerulus, 166
Gloves
   nonsterile, applying and removing, 229, 229f, 230p–231p
   sterile, applying and removing, 237p–239p
Glucagon, 179t
Glucocorticoids, 179t
Golden rule, 442
Gonadocorticoids, 179t
Good Samaritan Act, 442, 442b
Good Samaritan laws, 82
Gossip, 354–355
Gouty arthritis, 148
Government health programs, 484–486
Government health services, 58
Government institutions, 483
Gowns, 232
Graafian follicles, 180
Gram (g), 121
Gram staining, 222

Grammar, 363
Grandma Moses, 195b
Grave's disease, 180
Grievances, 555, 557
Group presentations, 354
Growth and development, 187–204
    care considerations and, 196,
        196t–197t, 198
    death and dying and, 200–202
    future trends and, 199–200
    Kohlberg's theory of, 198–199, 198t
    life stages and, 188–196, 189t
    Piaget's theory of, 198, 198t
Growth hormone (GH), 178t
Guided imagery, 46t, 47t
Guidelines for weighing patients, 435,
    436b

H

Habits, changing, 277
Hair, 153
Hammer (malleus), 170
Handwashing
    for infection control, 226–228
    procedure for, 227p–228p
    when to do, 226f
Hard drive, 393
Harmony, health and, 324–325, 325b
Hashimoto's disease, 161
Health care, 36–63
    affordability and, 48–49
    aging population and, 43
    approaches to, 44–48
    beliefs, culture and, 324–325, 325b,
        326b
    career ladders, 314
    challenges, 48–53
    changes in, keeping up with, 309–310,
        309t–310t
    consolidation of services, 57
    cost of, 43–44
    eliminating racism, 50
    facilities and services, 53–58, 54f
    facilities, types of, 57–58, 58b
    future of, 48
    government services in, 58, 58t
    of long-term care services, 49, 49t
    quality of care, 50–51
    specialization in, 42
Health care careers, 1–35
    in biomedical engineering
        occupations, 31, 31t
    in diagnostic imaging occupations,
        26–28, 26t–27t
    in diagnostic occupations, 11, 24,
        26–31, 567–568

educational programs for, 3
in emergency medical occupations,
    13, 14t
in environmental occupations, 30, 568
growing health care jobs, 2, 2t
in health information management
    occupations, 29–30, 29t–30t, 568
in massage therapy occupations, 13,
    15t
in medical laboratory occupations,
    28–29, 28t
in medical office occupations, 13,
    16, 16t
in mental health occupations, 16–17,
    17t
in nursing occupations, 17–19, 18t
in nutrition and dietary service
    occupations, 30–31
in occupational therapy occupations,
    19–20, 20t
in pharmacy occupations, 20, 21t
in physical therapy occupations,
    20–21, 21t, 22f
in respiratory therapy occupations,
    21–22, 22t
in therapeutic and treatment
    occupations, 12–24, 565–567
thinking skills for, 6–9
in veterinary occupations, 23, 24f, 24t
in vision care occupations, 23–24, 25t
Health care costs, 43–44, 481–496
    controlling organizational costs and,
        489–490, 489f
    government programs, 484–486
    health care institutions and, 483
    health care professionals' impact on,
        490–492
    history of reimbursement for, 484
    impact on individuals, 483
    managed care and, 486–487
    payment methods for, 484, 484f
    providing affordable health care,
        488–489
    quality of care and, 498
    rising, 482–483
Health care industry
    ethics and, 66–82
    facilities and services provided by, 483
    rationing of care and resources and,
        72
Health care institutions, 483
Health care instructions, 75
Health care professionals
    costs and, 490–492
    employment and. See Employment;
        Health care careers

essential core qualities of, 3–4
ethics and. See Ethics
infection risk for, 218, 245–251
job search and. See Job interviews;
    Job search; Resumes
reporting of accidental exposure by,
    253
standards for, 10–11
Health Care Reform Act of 2010, 83
Health care specific questions, 534–535
Health care surrogate/representative,
    75
Health insurance Portability and
    Accountability Act of 1996 (HIPAA),
    409
Health maintenance organization
    (HMO), 486
Healthy lifestyle. See Diets; Lifestyle
    management; Nutrition; Stress
Healthy weight maintenance, 282–284
Hearing loss, 171
    assessment of, 418
    communication and, 350–351
    increasing risk of injuries and
        accidents, 261, 261t
Heart, inflammation of, 161
Heartburn, 166
Heart-healthy foods 162
Heat cramps, 465p
Heat stroke, 465p
Height, measuring, 433
Hemiplegia, 175
Hemodialysis, 167
Hemophilia, 161
Hemorrhage, 447
Hemorrhoids, 166
Hepatitis, 166
Hepatitis A, 247t
Hepatitis B, 246, 247t
Hepatitis C, 248t
Hepatitis D, 248t
Hepatitis E, 248t
Herbal remedies, 325
Herpes zoster, 176
High-density lipoprotein (HDL), 280
HIPAA (Health insurance Portability and
    Accountability Act of 1996), 409
Hippocrates, 66
Hippocratic Oath, 66, 67b
Hirsutism, 177
Hitchcock, Alfred, 195b
HIV positive, definition of, 246
Hodgkin's disease, 161
Holistic medicine, 44–45
Home health aide, 18t, 19
Home health care providers, 56–57

Homelessness, 50t
Homeopathic medicine, 46t
Homeopathy, 47–48, 47t
Homeostasis, 130
Honesty, 70t, 77–78
Hormone, 177
Hospice, 57
Hospice Patient Rights, 84
Hospitals, 53–55
Hosts, 220
    reservoir, 224
Household system, 119–120, 120f, 120t
Human body
    abdominal descriptions of, 136,
        136f, 137f
    anatomy and physiology of, 141
    basis of life and, 130–133, 131f
    cavities of, 134–135, 135f
    describing, 136–137
    directional terms for, 134, 134f, 135t
    planes of, 134, 134f
    structural organization of, 130, 131f
    systems of. See Body systems
Human Genome Project, 388
Human immunodeficiency virus (HIV),
        246, 249, 249t
Humerus, 147
Humor, in communication, 343
Humors, 325
Hydrotherapy, 213
Hyperglycemia, 177, 467p–468p
Hyperopia, 171
Hyperparathyroidism, 177
Hypertension, 141, 161, 429, 433
Hyperthermia, 462
    emergency procedures for, 469p
Hyperthyroidism, 180
Hyperventilation, emergency
        procedures for, 467p
Hypochondriac regions, 136
Hypogastric region, 136
Hypoglycemia, 468p
Hypoparathyroidism, 177
Hypotension, 429
    orthostatic (postural), 432
Hypothalamus, 173
Hypothermia, 462, 464p–465p
Hypothyroidism, 180

I
ICD-10 codes, 490, 491b
Ileocecal valve, 165
Iliac regions, 136
Ilium, 147
Illegal questions, 535
Illness, 141
    chronic, 194

Image-guided surgery, 386
Immigration Reform Act, 556t
Immune response, 160, 161, 219
Implicit bias, 319
Implicit racism, 50
Implied consent, 73
Implied contract, 81
Improper fractions, 111
Incus, 170
Independent clauses, 366
Individual worth, philosophy of, 319
Industry vs. inferiority stage, 189t,
        193
Infancy, 189t, 191, 196t
Infant, 191
Infection control, 217–257
    asepsis for. See Asepsis (aseptic
        technique)
    importance of, 218–219
    microorganisms and, 219–224
    reporting accidental exposure and,
        253
    risks to health care professionals and,
        218, 245–251
Infections
    chain of infection and, 224–226
    cutaneous, fungal, 223
    drug-resistant, 252t
    generalized (systemic) and localized,
        218
    nosocomial, 219
Infectious diseases, 37, 218
Infectious hazards, 260t
Infectious waste, 268–269
Inferior, definition of, 135t
Inflammable liquids, 266t
Inflammation, of heart, 161
Information, collecting in
        communication process, 341–342
Information management, 380, 382
Informed consent, 73
Ingestion injuries, 462, 463p
Inhalation, 428
Inhalation injuries, 462, 463p
Injuries, physical and mental changes
        increasing risk of, 261, 261t
Inner ear, 170, 171
Inorganic substances, 278
Inpatients, 54
Insect bites and stings, first aid for,
        446p–447p
Insertion, of muscles, 150
Inspection, 416
Insulin, 179t
Insurance companies, 484
    government, 485
    premium for, 484, 487

prepaid plans for, 487
    private, 488
Integrative medicine, 45
Integrity, 3, 552
Integrity vs. despair stage, 189t, 194
Integumentary system, 142t, 152–154,
        152f, 153f
    assessment of, 417
Intensive care units (ICUs), 54
Intermediate nursing care facilities
        (INCFs), 55
Intermittent fever, 420
Internal bleeding, 447, 450p
Internal customers, 503, 505–508. See
        also Health care professionals
International Classification of Diseases
        ICD-10 codes, 490, 491b
Internet, 389–391
    electronic mail and, 390–391
    evaluating sources on, 390, 390t
    finding job leads on, 516–518, 517b,
        518f
    for research, 389–390
    social and professional networking
        sites on, 391
Internist, 15b
Interstitial cell-stimulating hormone
        (ICSH), 179t
Intervertebral disks, 146, 147f
Intimacy vs. isolation stage, 189t, 193
Invasive procedures, 73
Inventory systems, computerized, 379
Involuntary nerves, 174
Iris, 168
Iron, 278t
Iron-deficiency anemia, 160
Ischium, 147
Islam, health care beliefs and, 324

J
Job applications, 542, 543f–545f
Job descriptions, 550, 551t
Job fairs, 518–519
Job interviews, 531–540
    checklists, 537–538
    follow-up activities for, 539–540
    making a good impression in,
        538–539, 538f, 539f
    preparing for, 532–540
    recent trends in, 539
Job search, 513–519. See also Job
        interviews; Resumes
    accepting a job and, 540, 542
    declining a job and, 542
    expectations and, 513–514
    finding job leads and, 515–519
    organizing time and space for, 514

professional image and, 514–515
self-evaluation for, 513
The Joint Commission, 499–500
Joint Commission on Accreditation of
    Healthcare Organizations (JCAHO),
    399
Joint dislocations, 447, 453p–455p
Joint injuries, emergency procedures for,
    447, 452, 453p–455p
Justice, 70t, 76–77
Justified text, 368

K

Kevorkian, Jack, 71
Key words, 388
Kidney calculi, 167
Kidney failure, 167
Kidney infections, 167
Kidneys, 166–167
Kohlberg's moral stages, 198–199, 198t
Kübler-Ross, Elisabeth, 200–205
Kyphosis, 149, 149f

L

Labia majora, 181
Labia minora, 181
Labyrinthitis, 171
Lacrimal glands, 169
Lactation, 181
Lactogenic hormone (LTH), 179t
Lacto-ovo vegetarian, 284
Lacto-vegetarian, 284
Language barriers, 352
Large intestine, 165
Laryngitis, 163
Larynx, 162
Lasers, 386
Later adulthood, 189t, 194–196,
    194f, 197t
Lateral, definition of, 135t
Laws. *See* Legislation
Leadership, 303–304
Leading questions, 342, 343t
Learning. *See also* Education
    about computers, 394
    continuing education and, 308
    lifelong. *See* Lifelong learning
    for mastery, 4
    self-directed, 312–314
Learning objectives, 353
Left lower quadrant (LLQ), 136, 136f, 137
Left upper quadrant (LUQ), 136, 136f,
    137
Legislation
    on abuse, 76
    on advance directives, 75
    Affordable Care Act (ACA), 488–489

employment, 555, 556t, 557
ethics and, 65–66
Good Samaritan laws, 82, 442, 442b
Health Care Reform Act of 2010, 83
Patient Protection and Affordable
    Care Act, 79, 488–489
protective, 77, 78b
Legumes, 277
Lens (of eye), 168
Letters
    cover, 524–528, 525f–527f
    form, 368
    of recommendation, 536
    reminder, 360
    of resignation, 559, 560f
    thank-you, following job interviews,
        539–540, 541f
Leukemia, 161
Libel, 80
Licensed practical/vocational nurse
    (LPN/LVN), 18, 18t
Licenses, in resume, 520
Licensure, 10
Life, preservation of, 69, 70t, 71–72
Life review, 201, 204
Life stages, 188–196, 189t
Lifelong learning
    continuing education units and,
        310–311
    importance of, 309–310
    self-directed, 312–314
Lifestyle management, 275–297
    changing habits for, 277
    diet and nutrition and. *See* Diets;
        Nutrition
    eating disorders and, 284
    helping patients with, 293
    importance of, 277
    minimizing health risks, 290–293
    physical activity and, 284–285
    preventive measures, 285–286, 286f
    sleep and, 285
    stress and. *See* Stress
Lifting
    back belts for, 214
    body mechanics and, 211b, 211f, 212f
Ligaments, 150
Lightning injuries, 460p–461p
Limited X-ray machine operator, 27, 27t
Linen, standard precautions for, 239
Lister, Joseph, 40t
Listening, 345–346, 346b
Liter (l or L), 121
Liver, 165
Living will, 75
Localized infections, 218
Long-term care facilities/services, 49, 49t

Lordosis, 149, 149f
Losses, dealing with, 330–331
Lou Gehrig's disease, 175
Love needs, 327, 329
Low-density lipoprotein (LDL), 280
Loyalty, to employer, 552
Lumbar regions, 136
Lung cancer, 163
Lungs, 163
Luteinizing hormone (LH), 178t
Lymph nodes, 159f, 160
Lymphatic ducts, 159
Lymphatic system, 159–160, 159f–160f

M

Macular degeneration, 171
Mad cow disease, 251
Magnesium, 278t
Magnetic resonance imaging (MRI),
    384t, 385f
Magnetic resonance technologist, 26t
Malaria, 224
Male reproductive system, 143t,
    182–184, 183f, 419
Malingering, 331t
Malleus, 170
Malnutrition, 50t
Malpractice, 82
Mammary glands, 181
Managed care
    goals of, 486
    negotiated fees, 487
    prepaid plans, 486–487
    primary care providers, 487
    review of services, 487
    types of, 486
Mandela, Nelson, 195b
Manual dexterity, 12
Masks, 232
Maslow's hierarchy of needs, 327–330
Massage therapists, 13
Massage therapy, 46t, 47, 47t, 213
Master gland, 177
Math, 106–128
    angles and, 118–119, 119f
    basic calculations in, 107, 109–116
    importance in health care, 107
    math anxiety and, 107, 108t–109t
    measurement systems and, 119–124
    medication safety and, 124
    military time and, 116–117, 117f, 117t
    Roman numerals and, 118, 118t
    temperature conversion and,
        124–125, 125f, 125t
Measurement systems, 119–124
    converting between, 122–124, 123t
Mechanical lift scales, 434–435, 435f

Medial, definition of, 135t
Medic Alert, 443
Medicaid, 79, 484–485
Medicaid recipients, 485b
Medical asepsis, 224–243
   antiseptics and disinfectants for, 232,
      235–236
   breaking chain of infection using,
      225–226
   standard precautions and, 236, 240f
Medical aspects
   neutropenic precautions and,
      244–245
   transmission precautions and,
      241–243, 241f, 242f
Medical assistant (MA), 13, 16
Medical documentation, 399. *See also*
      Medical records
   good, characteristics of, 400–401, 401f
   HIPAA and, 409
   making corrections on, 401–402, 402f
   purposes of, 399–400
Medical equipment repairer, 31
Medical errors, 83, 110, 124
Medical floor, 54
Medical history, 402, 403f
Medical laboratory assistant, 28t, 29
Medical laboratory technician, 28t, 29
Medical laboratory technologist (MT),
      28t, 29
Medical malls, 57–58, 58b
Medical practice management system,
      flow of information in, 380, 381f
Medical records, 360, 399
   contents of, 402–405
   HIPAA and, 409
Medical records clerk, 30t
Medical specialists, 15b–16b
Medical terminology, 89–105, 92f
   abbreviations and symbols in, 99,
      99t–100t
   building blocks of, 90–96
   deciphering, 96–97
   dictionary of, 101
   drug names, 97
   eponyms, 97
   importance of, 90
   learning and using, resources for,
      102b–103b
   mastering, 101–102, 102t
   spelling of, 97–98, 97f, 98t, 99f
   words with special meanings, 97
Medical transcriptionist (MT), 29t, 30
Medicare, 485
Medication(s). *See also* Prescription
      drugs
   adherence, 52

communication and, 349
converting, 115–116
errors, 502
errors, reducing/minimizing, 110, 124
Medications. *See* Prescription drugs
Medigap policies, 485
Meditation, 46t, 47t, 288f, 289–290, 290b
Mediterranean diet, 282
MEDLINE/PubMed, 388
Medulla, of kidney, 167
Medullary cavity, 144
Meeting agendas, 372
Meeting minutes, 372–373
Meetings, professional, 519
Melanin, 152
Melanocyte-stimulating hormone
      (MSH), 178t
Melatonin, 179t
Memos, 372, 373f
Meniere's disease, 171
Meninges, 174
Meningitis, 176
Menorrhagia, 181
Menstrual disorders, 181
Mental function, changes in, increasing
      risk of injuries and accidents, 261t
Mental health technician, 16, 17t
Mental status, assessment of, 416
Mentors, 313–314
Mercury thermometers, 420
Mercy killing, 71
Message. *See* Communication
Metabolism, 278t
Metacarpals, 147
Metatarsals, 147
Meter (m), 121
Methicillin-resistant *Staphylococcus
      aureus* (MRSA), 252, 252t
Metric system, 120–121, 121t, 122f
Microbes, 220–222
Micrococci, 220t
Microorganisms, 219–224
Microscope, 219
Middle adulthood, 189t, 194, 194f, 197t
Middle ear, 170–171
Middle-old, 189t, 197t
Midsagittal plane, 134, 134f
Mind maps, 362, 362f
Mind–body connection, 325
Mind–body medicine, 46t
Mineralocorticoids, 179t
Minerals, 278, 278t
Minimum wage, 555
Ministrokes, 175
Minors, 73
Minutes of meetings, 372–373
Mixed number, 111

Modified block letters, 368, 370f
"Moon face," 177
Moral development, 198–199, 198t
Motor fibers, 174, 174f
Mouth, 163
Movement
   safe, 260
   of victims in emergency situations,
      danger of, 444
Mucous membranes, 163
Mucus, 162
Multiple sclerosis, 176
Muscle injuries, emergency procedures
      for, 447, 452, 453p–455p
Muscle relaxation techniques, 288–289,
      288f, 289b
Muscle spasms, 151
Muscle sprain, 151, 455p
Muscle strain, 152, 455p
Muscular dystrophy, 152
Muscular system, 142t, 150–152, 151f
Muscular tissue, 133
Musculoskeletal and nerve injuries,
      treatment of, 213–214
Musculoskeletal hazards, 260t
Musculoskeletal system, assessment of,
      417
Mutate, 53
Myasthenia gravis, 152
MYCIN, 386–387
Myelin, 174
Myocardial infarction (MI), 160
Myocarditis, 161
Myocardium, 155
Myopia, 171

N

Nails, 153
Narrative charting, 405, 405f
National Council Licensure Exam
      (NCLEX), 389
National Institute for Occupational
      Safety and Health (NIOSH), 214
National Institutes of Health (NIH), 58t
Naturopathic medicine, 46t, 47
Needs, Maslow's hierarchy of,
      327–330
Negligence, 82
Negotiated fees, 487
Neonate, 191
Nephritis, 167
Nephrons, 166
Nerve and musculoskeletal injuries,
      treatment of, 213–214
Nervous system, 143t, 172–180
   assessment of, 418
   central, 172–174, 172f, 173f

divisions of, 175, 176f
    peripheral, 174, 174f
Nervous tissue, 133
Networking
    to find job leads, 515–516, 517f
    for professional development, 308
Networks (computers), 379, 389
Neuralgia, 176
Neuritis, 176
Neurodiagnostic technologist, 27t, 28
Neurological changes, increasing risk of
    injuries and accidents, 261t
Neurons, 174–175, 175f
Neurotransmitters, 175
Neutralism, 220
Neutropenic precautions, 244–245
Newman, Margaret, 44
Niacin, 278t
Nomenclature, 119
Nonprofit institutions, 483
Nonverbal communication, 344
Norepinephrine, 179t
Normal flora, 219, 226
Nose, 162
    injuries to, 457p
Nosocomial infections, 219
Numbers, writing correctly, 367
Nursing career ladders, 314f
Nursing homes, 55
Nutrients, 277–279
Nutrition, 277
    diets and, 277–281
    eating disorders and, 284
    food labels and, 280
    healthy eating, 281
    healthy weight maintenance, 282–284
    organic foods and, 280–281

O

"Obamacare," 488–489
Obesity, 282–284
Objective data, 7, 141
    in resume, 519
Obligate intracellular parasites, 223
Observation, assessment *vs.*, 415
Obstetrician, 16b
Occupational hazards, 291–292
Occupational Outlook Handbook, 32
Occupational Safety and Health Act,
    556t
Occupational Safety and Health
    Administration (OSHA), 58t, 65,
    77, 219
Occupational therapist (OTR), 20t
Occupational therapy aide, 20, 20t
Occupational therapy assistant (COTA),
    19, 20t

Oil glands, 153
Old-old, 189t, 197t
O*Net, 32
On-the-job training, 10
Open-ended questions, 342, 343t
Open fractures, 447
Operating room technician (ORT),
    22, 23t
Ophthalmic assistant, 25t
Ophthalmic laboratory technician,
    24, 25t
Ophthalmic medical technician,
    24, 25t
Ophthalmic medical technologist, 25t
Ophthalmic technician, 25t
Ophthalmologist (MD), 25t
Opinions, 7
Opioid pain medications, 52
Opioids, 52
Opportunistic infections, 219
Optic nerve, 168
Optician, 25t
Optometric assistant/technician, 25t
Optometrist (OD), 25t
Oral temperature, 421p–422p
Orbit (eye), 169
Orchitis, 183
Organ systems, 130, 131f
Organ transplantation, 72
Organic, definition of, 278
Organic and conventional farming
    methods, 280, 281t
Organic foods, 280–281
Organs, 130, 131f
Orientation, assessment of, 416
Origin, of muscles, 150
Orthopedist, 15b
Orthopnea, 417
Orthostatic hypotension, 432
Ossicles, 170
Osteoarthritis, 148
Osteomyelitis, 149
Osteopathy, 47, 47t
Osteoporosis, 149, 285
Otitis externa, 171
Otitis media, 171
Otolaryngologist, 15b
Otorhinolaryngologist, 15b
Outer ear, 170
Outlines, 362, 362f
Outpatient services, 55, 56t
Oval window, 170
Ovaries, 180
Overweight, 282–284
Ovum, 180
Oxygen hazards, 269
Oxytocin, 179t

P

Pain
    in chest, 467p
    communication and, 349
    evaluation of, 419, 419f
Palliative care, 57
Palpation, 416
Pancreas, 165, 177, 179t
Pancreatic cancer, 166
Pancreatitis, 166
Pandemics, 37
Pantomime, 345
Paramedic, 14t
Paraphrasing, 346
Paraplegia, 176
Parasites, 220
    intracellular, obligate, 223
Parasitic conditions, 220
Parasympathetic nervous system, 174,
    175t
Parathormone (PTH), 179t
Parathyroid, 179t
Parathyroid glands, 177
Parkinson's disease, 176
Partial-thickness burns, 452, 458f
Partnership for Patients, 499
PASS, 264, 265t, 266t
Patella, 147
Pathogens, 218
Pathologist, 16b
Pathologist (MD), 28t
Pathophysiology, 141
Patient care assistant, 18t
Patient-care equipment, standard
    precautions for, 232
Patient Care Partnership, 82–83, 500
Patient care technician, 18t, 19
Patient education, 353–354, 353t
    written materials for, 373–374
Patient monitoring, computerized, 388
Patient outcomes, 498, 499
Patient Protection and Affordable Care
    Act, 79, 488–489
Patient record systems, computerized,
    379
Patients, 317–336
    angry, 352
    communication barriers and, 348–352
    culture and, 320–323, 320f
    dealing with loss and, 330–331
    defense mechanisms used by, 330, 331t
    health care beliefs of, 324–325, 325b,
        326b
    helping with lifestyle management, 293
    as individuals, 318–320, 331–332,
        332b

Patients (Continued)
maintaining the human touch with, 394
Maslow's hierarchy of needs, 327–330
non-English speaking, 352
placement of, standard precautions for, 239
safety of, 260–261, 261t
satisfaction, 300, 498, 505, 505f, 506t
services sought by, 503, 503b
terminally ill, 348
Pediatrician, 16b
Pelvic cavity, 135, 135f
Pelvic inflammatory disease (PID), 182
Penis, 182
Peptic ulcers, 166
Percentages, 111, 112f
Percussion, 416
Performance evaluations, 557–558, 558b
Pericardium, 155
Periods (punctuation), 364
Periosteum, 144
Peripheral, definition of, 135t
Peripheral nervous system, 174, 174f
Peristalsis, 164
Peritonitis, 166
Pernicious anemia, 160
Personal care aide, 19
Personal efficiency, health care costs and, 491–492
Personal health records (PHRs), 408
Personal protective equipment (PPE), 229, 229f, 232p–235p
Personal space, 322
Personalized medicine, 48
Phagocytosis, 158
Phalanges, 147
Pharmaceutical software programs, 379
Pharmaceuticals, 387
Pharmacist (PharmD), 21t
Pharmacy Aide/Helper/Clerk, 21t
Pharmacy technician, 20, 21t
Pharyngitis, 163
Pharynx, 162
Philosophy of individual worth, 319
Phimosis, 183
Phlebitis, 161
Phlebotomist, 28t, 29
Phosphorus, 278t
Physiatrist, 15b
Physical activity, 284–285, 285f
Physical assessment, 413–440
general, 414–419
of height and weight, 433–436, 434f–436f, 436b
of vital signs, 416, 419–433, 420t, 421p–423p

Physical development, 188
Physical disinfectant methods, 235
Physical hazards, 260t
Physical observations, 416–419
Physical therapist (PT), 21t
Physical therapist aide, 20–21, 21t
Physical therapist assistant (PTA), 20, 21t
Physiological needs, 327, 328
Physiology, 141
Piaget's cognitive stages, 198, 198t
Pineal gland, 179t
Pitocin, 179t
Pituitary glands, 177–178, 178t–179t, 180
Plagiarism, 390
Plague, 270t
Plans, 405
Plant-based diets, 283
Plant medicines, 325
Plasma, 158, 159
Plastic surgeon, 15b
Platelets, 158, 159
Pneumocystis pneumonia, 224
Pneumonia, 163
Pneumonic plague, 270t
Pneumothorax, 163
Point-of-care charting, 388
Point of service (POS), 486
Poisoning, emergency procedures for, 461–462, 463p
Policies, 550–551
Polydipsia, 177
Polyuria, 177
Popliteal pulse, 424, 424f
Portfolios, 537
Positron emission tomography (PET), 384t
Positron emission tomography technologist, 26t
Postconventional moral stage, 198t, 199t
Posterior, definition of, 135t
Posterior body cavity, 134, 135f
Postural hypotension, 432
Potassium, 278t
Poverty, 50t
Practicing, for job interviews, 538
Prayer, 46t
Preauthorization, 50, 487
Precision medicine, 48
Preconventional moral stage, 198t, 199t
Preferred provider organization (PPO), 486
Prefixes, 95, 95t–96t
Pregnancy Discrimination Act, 556t
Prejudice, 319–320
Premenstrual syndrome (PMS), 182
Premiums, 484, 487

Prenatal development, 189–190, 189t, 190t, 196t
Preoperational stage, 198t, 201t
Prepaid plans, 486–487
Presbyopia, 171
Preschoolers, 189t, 192, 192f, 197t
Prescription drugs
computer applications and, 387
increased risk of injuries and accidents and, 261t
medication adherence, 52
reducing medication errors and, 110, 124
television ads for, 53
Presentations to groups, 354
Pressure sores, 153
Prevention, 141
Preventive measures, against health problems, 285–286, 286f
Primary care providers (PCPs), 486, 487
Primary prevention, 141
Prioritizing, 287
Privacy, 354–355
Probationary period, 551–552
Probing questions, 342, 343t
Problem-oriented charting, 404–405, 405f
Problem-solving process, 6–9
Procedures, 550–551
Processed foods, 280
Professional development, 308
Professional distance, 302, 302f
Professional image, projecting, 514–515
Professional licensing exams, 389
Professional meetings, 519
Professional networking sites, 391
Professional organizations, 32, 308, 565–568
Professionalism, 298–306
acceptance of criticism and, 303
appearance and, 301–302, 535–536
attitude and, 299–300
behaviors, 300–301
continuing education and, 308, 310–312
definition of, 299
handling difficult situations, 302–303
leadership and, 303–304
outside workplace, 303
professional distance and, 302, 302f
professional organizations and, 32, 565–568
technical skills and, 301
Professionals. See Health care professionals; specific types of professionals
Profit, 486

Progesterone, 180
Prognosis, 141
Progress notes, 402, 404–405
Progressive relaxation, 47t
Projection, 331t
Prolactin, 179t
Proofreading, 374, 374b
Proportions, 114–115
Proprietary (for-profit) institutions, 483
Prostate gland, 182
Prostatic hypertrophy, 183
Protected health information (PHI),
    409–410
Proteins, 277
Protozoa, 223–224
Proximal, definition of, 135t
Psoriasis, 154
Psychiatric aide, 17, 17t
Psychiatric clinical nurse specialist, 17t
Psychiatric hospitals, 54
Psychiatrist (MD), 17t
PsychINFO, 388
Psychosocial development, 188,
    189, 189t
Psychosocial hazards, 260t
Psychosocial observations, 416
Psychosomatic disorders, 45
Pubis, 147
Public health, 52
Pulmonary arteries, 155, 156f
Pulse, 424–428
    apical, 420t, 426, 426p–427p
    deficit, 427
    points, 424
    radial, 420t, 424p–425p
    rhythm of, 424–425
Punctuation rules, 364, 366–367, 367b
Pupil (of eye), 168
Purkinje fibers, 155, 156f
Pyelonephritis, 167

Q

Qi Gong, 46t, 47t
Quadriplegia, 176
Quality control
    quality improvement, 499–501, 500b
    quality of care, 498–499
    reducing medical errors, 501–502
Quality improvement, 499–501, 500b
Quality of care, 50–51, 498–499
Questions
    asked by interviewers, 533–535
    behavioral, 534
    difficult, 535
    general employment questions,
        533–534
    health care specific, 534–535

illegal, in job interviews, 535
for job interviews, 533
maximizing effectiveness of, 343
to request clarification, 346
situational, 534
types of, 342, 343t
Quotation marks, 366
Quotations, 363

R

RACE, 265, 266t
Radial pulse, 420t, 424, 424f, 424p–425p
Radiation burns, 452, 460p
Radiation hazards, 268
Radiographer, 26, 26t
Radiologic technologist (RT), 26, 26t
Radiologist, 15b
Radius, 147
RAM, 393
Rationalization, 331t
Rationing, of care and resources, 72
Ratios, 112
Reasonable accommodations, 556t
Receiver, 338
Reciprocals, 111
Records, in databases, 380
Rectal temperature, 422p
Red blood cells, 144, 158
Red marrow, 144–145
Reeve, Christopher, 330
Reference lists, 536
Reference plane, 118, 119f
References (for job), 536
Refined grains, 279
Reflecting, 346
Reflexes, slowed, increased risk of
    injuries and accidents and, 261t
Reflexology, 46t
Registered health information
    administrator (RHIA), 29t
Registered health information
    technician (RHIT), 29t, 30
Registered medical assistant (RMA), 16t
Registered nurse (RN), 17, 18t
Registered radiologic assistant, 26t
Registration, 10
Regression, 331t
Regulatory agencies, 219
Rehabilitation, 387
Reiki, 46t
Reimbursement, 484–486
Rejection, 542
Relaxation techniques, 288–289, 288f,
    289b
Release of information, 79, 79b
Reliability, of facts, 8
Religious beliefs, health and, 324

Reminder letters, 360
Remote diagnostics, 384–385
Renal calculi, 167
Renal failure, 167
Repetitive motion injuries (RMIs),
    206–210, 207t
    computer use and, 207, 209b
    preventing, 207–208, 208f, 209b
    visual problems, 208–209, 210b
Reporting, of unsafe conditions and
    accidents, 262
Reports, 360
Repression, 331t
Reproductive system, 143t, 180–184,
    419
Request forms, 360
Rescue breathing, 444
Rescuer, 443
Research
    computers in, 388–389
    Internet for, 389–390
Reservoir host, 224
Resident flora, 226
Resigning from a job, 559, 560f
Respirations, 420t, 428–429, 428p, 429t
    counting, 428p
    rates at, 428, 429t
Respiratory system, 143t, 161–163, 162f,
    417
Respiratory therapist, 21–22, 22f, 22t
Respondeat superior, 81
Resumes, 519–524
    contents of, 519–521
    cover letters for, 524–528, 525f–527f
    formats for, 521, 522f, 523f, 524
    guidelines for, 524
    recent trends for, 524
Resuscitation, barrier devices for, 443,
    444f
Retina, 169
Retina (of eye), 168
Reverse isolation, 244
Rheumatoid arthritis, 148
Rhinitis, 163
Riboflavin, 278t
Ribs, 146–147
Rickettsia, 223
Right lower quadrant (RLQ), 136,
    136f, 137
Right upper quadrant (RUQ), 136,
    136f, 137
Risk management, 551
Robertson, Anna Mary, 195b
Robotic surgery, 386
Rods (retinal), 169
Role models, 313
Roman numerals, 118, 118t

S

Roosevelt, Eleanor, 195b
Rounding numbers, 112–113, 114t
Ruptured eardrum, 171

Safe sex, 292
Safety. See Environmental safety
Safety needs, 327–329
Salt (sodium), 280
Salutation (in business letter), 366
Sample, 116
Scapulae, 147
Scheduling programs, computerized, 379
School-age children, 189t, 192–193, 192f, 197t
School career service, 515, 515f
Sciatica, 176
Sclera, 168
Scoliosis, 149, 149f
Scope of practice, 6
Search engine, 390
Sebaceous glands, 153
Secondary prevention, 141
Second-degree burns, 452, 458f
Security, computer, 393–394
Security needs, 327–329
Seizures, 176
    emergency procedures for, 470p–471p
Self-actualization needs, 327, 329–330
Self-directed learning, 312–314
Self-esteem needs, 327, 329
Semi-block letters, 368, 371f
Semicircular canals, 171
Semicolons, 366
Seminal vesicles, 182
Sender, 338
Senile dementia, 176
Sensorimotor stage, 198t, 201t
Sensory fibers, 174, 174f
Sensory hearing loss, 171
Septicemia, 161
Sexual harassment, 557
Sexual practices, safe, 292
Sexually transmitted diseases (STDs), 182, 183, 292
Sharp instruments, blood-borne pathogens and, 239
Shiatsu, 213
Shingles, 176
Shock
    anaphylactic, 445
    emergency procedures for, 471p
Shoulder girdle, 147
Sickle cell anemia, 160
Sign language, 350, 350f

Signs, 7, 141
Single mothers, 50t
Sinoatrial (SA) node, 155, 156f
Sinuses, 162
Sinusitis, 163
Site licenses, 393
Sitting, body mechanics and, 209b
Situational questions, 534
Skeletal muscle, 133, 150
Skeletal system, 142, 142t, 144, 144f
    age-related changes in, 152
    bone structure and, 144–146, 144f, 145f
    diseases and disorders of, 148–149, 149f
    preventive measures for, 152
Skilled nursing facilities (SNFs), 55
Skin cancer, 153
Slander, 80
Sleep, 285
Slings, 474p–475p
Small intestine, 165
Smallpox, 270t
Smoking, 290–291
Smooth muscle, 133, 150
SOAP charting, 404–405, 405f
SOAPIE charting, 405
Social conditions, health care delivery and, 49–50, 50t
Social networking sites, 391
Spanish expressions, 569–570
Spasticity, 151
Specialization, 42
Speech impairment, communication and, 351, 351f
Spelling
    of medical terms, 97–98, 97f, 98t, 99f
    in written communication, 362–363, 364t, 365t
Sphincters, 150
Sphygmomanometers, 430, 430f
Spinal cavity, 134, 135f
Spinal cord, 173–174
Spinal cord injury, 176
Spinal nerves, 174
Spiral wraps, 475p–476p
Spirilla, 221t
Spirochetes, 221t
Spleen, 160
Sports medicine physician, 15b
Spousal abuse, 50t, 76
Sprains, 151, 455p
Spreadsheets, 382–384, 383f
Stages of dying, 200, 203
Standard precautions, 236, 240f
    in emergency situations, 443–444
    environmental control and, 239

handwashing as, 227p–228p
    linen and, 239
    patient-care equipment and, 232
    patient placement and, 239
    personal protective equipment for, 229, 229f, 232p–235p
Standards, for health care professionals, 10–11
Standing balance scale, 434, 434f
Standing, body mechanics and, 209b
Stapes, 170
Staphylococci, 220t
Statements (documents), 360
Statistics, 116
Step-down units, 54
Sterile field, 225
Sterile technique, 225, 236, 237p–239p
Sterilization, 235–236
Stethoscope, taking apical pulse using, 426, 426f, 426p–427p
Stings, first aid for, 446p–447p
Stirrup (stapes), 170
Stomach, 164–165
Streptobacilli, 221t
Streptococci, 220t
Stress, 286–290
    external and internal stressors, 286–287
    meditation and, 288f, 289–290, 290b
    muscle relaxation techniques, 288–289, 288f, 289b
    prioritizing for dealing with, 287
    time management and, 287–288
Stressors, 286–287
Stroke, 175
    emergency procedures for, 472p
Study techniques, for medical terminology, 101, 102t
Subcutaneous tissue, 152
Subjective data, 8, 141
Substance abuse, 50t, 291
Sucking wounds, 451p
Sudoriferous glands, 153
Suffixes, 93, 93t–94t, 364t
Sugars, 279
Suicides, prevention, 53
Superficial, definition of, 135t
Superficial burns, 452, 458f
Superior, definition of, 135t
Superior vena cava, 155
Surgeon, 15b
Surgery
    image-guided, 386
    robotic, 386
Surgical asepsis, 225, 236, 237p–239p
Surgical floor, 54
Surgical physician assistant, 23t

Surgical technologist, 22, 23t
Sweat glands, 153
Swine flu (H1N1), 251
Syllables, 364t
Symbiosis, 220
Symbols, 99, 100t
Sympathetic nervous system, 174, 175t
Symptoms, 8, 141
Synapses, 175
Syncope, emergency procedures for, 469p
Syndromes, 141
Systemic infections, 218
Systemic lupus erythematosus, 161
Systolic pressure, 429, 429t

T

Tachypnea, 428
Tai chi, 47t, 213, 325
Targeted drug therapy, 42
Tarsals, 147
Teams, in workplace, 554, 555b
Telemedicine, 391–392
Telepharmacies, 387
Telephone communication, 353
Temperature, 420, 421f, 421p–423p, 421t
Temperature-related illness, emergency procedures for, 462, 464p–465p
Temperature scales, 124, 125t
Temporal artery temperature, 423p
Temporal pulse, 424, 424f
Tendonitis, 207, 207t
Tendons, 150
Terminal illness, 200, 203
Tertiary prevention, 141
Testes (testicles), 182
Testicular cancer, 183
Tetany, 177
Thalamus, 173
Thank-you letters, following job interviews, 539–540, 541f
Therapeutic communication, 340
Therapeutic (healing) touch, 46t
TherapyEdge–HIV, 387
Thermometers, 420, 421f
Thiamin, 278t
Third-degree burns, 452, 458f
Thomas, William H., 199–200, 202–203
Thoracic cavity, 135, 135f
Thoracic outlet syndrome, 207, 207t
Thoracic surgeon, 15b
Thrombosis, 161
Thymosin, 179t
Thymus, 179t
Thyroid glands, 179t, 180
Thyroid-stimulating hormone (TSH), 178t

Thyroxine (T_4), 179t
Tibia, 147
Time
    management, 287–288
    military, 116–117, 117f, 117t
    organizing for job search, 514
Tinnitus, 171
Tissues, 130, 131f, 133, 133f
Title VII of 1964 Civil Rights Act, 556t
Titles, writing correctly, 367
Toddlers, 189t, 191–192, 191f, 196t
Tonsillitis, 161, 163
Touch
    in communication, 345
    culture and, 322
Toxic chemicals, 268
Toxins, bacterial, 220
Toxoplasmosis, 224
Traditional Chinese medicine, 46t
Transcutaneous electrical nerve stimulation (TENS), 213
Trans fats, 280
Transient flora, 226
Transient ischemic attacks (TIAs), 175
Transitional care units (TCUs), 54
Transmission-based precautions, 241–243, 241f, 242f
Transverse plane, 134, 134f
Trauma centers, 54
Treatment, 141
    computers in, 386–387
Triage system, 271
Triangular slings, 474p–475p
Trichomoniasis, 223
Triiodothyronine (T_3), 179t
Trust vs. mistrust stage, 189t, 191
Tuberculosis, 163, 250–251, 251t
    latent and active, 250, 251t
Tympanic membrane, 170
Tympanic thermometers, 420, 421f

U

Ulcerative colitis, 166
Ulcers, 166
Ultrasonography, 384t, 385f
Umbilical region, 136
Unconsciousness, emergency procedures for, 473p
Unsafe conditions, reporting, 262
Upper respiratory infection, 163
Uremia, 167
Ureters, 167
Urethra, 167, 182–183
Urethritis, 167
Urinary bladder, 167
Urinary incontinence, 167
Urinary retention, 167

Urinary system, 143t, 166–168, 167f, 418
Urinary tract infection (UTI), 167
Urologist, 15b
U.S. Department of Agriculture (USDA), dietary guidelines of, 281, 282f
Uterus, 180–181
Utilization management (UM), 500, 501b
Utilization review (UR), 500, 501b

V

Vagina, 181
Vaginitis, 182
Values, 69
Vancomycin-resistant Enterococcus (VRE), 252, 252t
van Leeuwenhoek, Anton, 39
Varicose veins, 161
Vasopressin, 179t
Vegans, 283
Vegetarian diets, 283–284
Veins, 154, 155, 157, 158f
Venereal disease, 182
Ventral, definition of, 135t
Ventricles, of heart, 155
Venules, 157
Vertebrae, 146, 147f
Vertigo, 171
Veterans Health Administration, 485
Veterinarian (DVM or VMD), 24t
Veterinary assistant, 24t
Veterinary technician, 23, 24t
Veterinary technologist, 23, 24t
Vibrios, 221t
Victim, 443
Villi, 165
Violence, 50t
    in workplace, 259, 260t
Virtual communities, 391
Viruses
    computer, 393–394
    pathogenic, 222, 222f
Visual changes, increasing risk of injuries and accidents, 261t
Visual impairment, 171
    communication and, 351
Visual problems, with computers, 208–209, 210b
Vital signs, assessment of, 416
Vitamins, 278, 278t
Vitreous humor, 169
Vowels, 364t

W

Wage, minimum, 555
Walking, body mechanics and, 209b
Water, 278

Weakness, increased risk of injuries and accidents and, 261t
Weight. *See* Body weight
Weight-loss diets, 283
Wellness, 44
West Nile virus, 251
Western health care, history of, 37, 38t–42t
Western medicine, 45
Wheelchair scales, 434, 435f
White blood cells, 144, 158
White coat syndrome, 432
Whole grains, 279, 279f
Whole numbers, 109
Williams, Stephen, 44
Withdrawal
  from addictive drugs, 462p
  as defense mechanism, 331t
Womb, 180-181

Word parts, 90–96
Word processing software, 363
Word roots, 90–91, 91t, 92t
Work experience, in resume, 520–521
Workplace habits, 3–4
Workplace violence, 206t, 262–263
Wounds
  emergency procedures for, 447, 450p
  sucking, 451p
Wright, Frank Lloyd, 195b
Written communication, 359–377.
    See also Letters; Medical
    documentation; Medical records
  computers and. *See* Computers
  confidentiality and, 374
  grammar and, 363
  meeting agendas and, 372
  meeting minutes and, 372–373

memos and, 372, 373f
organizing content for, 361, 362, 362f
for patient education, 373–374
proofreading, 374, 374b
spelling and, 362–363, 364t, 365t

X
Xiphoid process, 147

Y
Yellow marrow, 144
Yin and yang, 325
Yoga, 46t, 47t, 213
Young adulthood, 189t, 193, 193f, 197t
Young-old, 189t, 197t

Z
Zinc, 278t